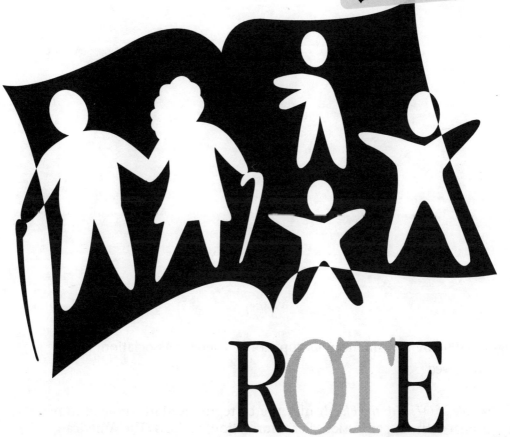

ROTE

the Role of OT with the Elderly

Edited by

K. Oscar Larson, MA, OTR

Regena G. Stevens-Ratchford, PhD, OTR/L, FAOTA

Lorraine Pedretti, MS, OTR

Jeffrey L. Crabtree, MS, OTR/L, FAOTA

The American Occupational Therapy Association, Inc.

Table of Contents

Chapter 16
Health Education in Occupational Therapy 805
Elizabeth Walker Peterson, MPH, OTR/L

Chapter 17
Client- and Family-Practitioner Relationships: Collaboration as an Effective Approach to Treatment 833
Deborah Walens, MHPE, OTR/L, FAOTA, and Laurie Rockwell-Dylla, MS, OTR/L

Chapter 18
Keeping Current with Laws and Public Policy Issues That Influence Practice 861
Jeffrey L. Crabtree, MS, OTR/L, FAOTA

Editorial Review Board

Preface

Why are 1976, 1986, and 1996 important years for gerontic occupational therapists? As coincidental as it may appear, each of these 10-year dates has been a milestone: in 1976 the Representative Assembly approved the formation of the initial Special Interest Sections, one of which was the Gerontology SIS; in 1986 the original *Role of Occupational Therapy with the Elderly, ROTE,* was produced as a seminar workshop and accompanying study guide; and now, in 1996, AOTA and the GSIS are presenting the second edition of ROTE in a textbook format.

The original ROTE divided the text into four modules, each with several chapters. Module I addressed physical and psychosocial aging. Module II discussed gerontic occupational therapy. Module III presented treatment approaches. And, Module IV focused on service management issues. In the revised edition, we have followed a similar four-module format, but have organized some of the topics differently, added current information about aging and interventions, and reflected on the changes in service delivery in the contexts of community treatment, home care, and wellness models of practice.

Module I, which I edited, asks the question, "What is gerontic occupational therapy?" Parallel questions that each take a chapter (or more) to answer are "Who provides services to older adults?" and "What are the lives of aging people like?" This module presents an overview of gerontology, service delivery systems (in and outside of the health care system), the organization of gerontic occupational therapy, and the normal and pathological changes that people experience as they age.

The Uniform Terminology for Occupational Therapy (AOTA, 1994) has given an important framework for this module, especially in regard to defining the domain of concern for occupational therapy practitioners. Based on the Uniform Terminology, the concepts of *performance areas, performance components,* and *performance contexts* help to determine what aspects of living occupational therapy practitioners may be able to affect. The authors describe these aspects both in terms of how an older person may live and how an occupational therapy practitioner may provide services. Also, the authors explore the potential relationships between one aspect of performance and another.

Module II, edited by Regena Stevens-Ratchford, reviews service delivery within healthcare and community systems. The context of therapy becomes the focus of this module: primary care, rehabilitation and subacute rehabilitation, home health care, home and environmental design, and adult day treatment programs. While each chapter has its defining boundaries, the authors describe the continuum of care. They not only address the emphasis of intervention in a particular setting, but also consider the process for the older adult working within that system. To this end, issues about initiating, planning, providing, and terminating services are discussed.

Module III, edited by Lorraine Pedretti, delves more deeply into the specific interventions offered by occupational therapy practitioners. As you would expect, the core ideas explored in this module are evaluation, treatment planning, and service provision. However, to explain these steps in occupational therapy terminology, the authors have organized their discussions around occupational performance. Several authors collaborate to review interventions for performance components, such as sensorimotor, cognitive, and psychosocial components. And several authors review interventions in performance areas, such as self-maintenance, work and productivity, and leisure activities. Additional topics that this module addresses include the transition from the hospital or rehabilitation facility to home, and servicing people with terminal illnesses.

Module IV, edited by Jeffrey Crabtree, closes the text with discussions about service management issues. The first three chapters of this module are about education: how to use groups to provide therapy to older adults, how to inform consumers of your services, and how to educate the older adult and his or her family about treatment and follow-up care. One chapter reviews the legislation and public agendas that affect our practice, as well as how we can become involved in the process of setting the agenda. Another chapter explores the processes of assuring quality care and being accountable for the services that we provide to our clients.

The knowledge base in occupational therapy and gerontology has grown much in the past 10 years, and will continue to grow in the years to come. This text attempts to synthesize that knowledge that we currently have available. We hope that students who read this text will be able to develop a foundation for their clinical practice with aging adults and will generate ideas for future research. Those clinical experiences and research explorations will provide greater insights that can influence future revisions of this text!

K. Oscar Larson, MA, OTR

Reference

American Occupational Therapy Association. (1994). Uniform terminology for occupational therapy (3rd ed.). *American Journal of Occupational Therapy, 48,* 1047–1054.

Module I

K. Oscar Larson, MA, OTR
Editor

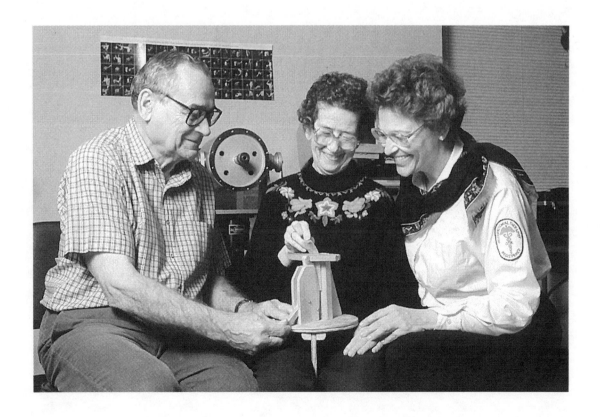

Author Biographies

Marlene J. Aitken, PhD, OTR/L, is an associate professor in the School of Pharmacy and Allied Health Professions, Department of Occupational Therapy, at Creighton University in Omaha, Nebraska. She is a graduate in occupational therapy from the University of Iowa. Ms. Aitken received her doctorate in public health and gerontology from the University of Illinois at Chicago. Her primary areas of teaching are research and instructional methods. She has published chapters and articles in the areas of theories of aging, breast cancer, older adult sexuality, and home care for children on ventilators. She is the current editor of the Gerontology Special Interest Section Newsletter.

Joseph Cipriani, MA, OTR/L, is an assistant professor in the Department of Occupational Therapy at College Misericordia in Dallas, Pennsylvania. He earned his bachelor of arts degree in psychology from Wilkes College, Wilkes-Barre, Pennsylvania, his bachelor of science degree in occupational therapy from College Misericordia, and his master of arts degree in psychology from Wichita State University, Wichita, Kansas. He is a doctoral candidate in higher education at Nova Southeastern University, Ft. Lauderdale, Florida. He engages in clinical practice in acute care and rehabilitation settings. His research interests are in occupational therapy education, human development, and geriatrics.

Debra David, PhD, is a professor and the director of the Gerontology Program at San Jose State University. She received her doctorate in sociology from the University of California, Berkeley, and completed a National Institute on Aging postdoctoral traineeship in the Counseling Psychology Department at Northwestern University. She is currently the president of the California Council on Gerontology and Geratrics. Her publications focus on reminiscence, ethnogerontology, and ethical issues in long-term care.

Diane Foti, MS, OTR, received her master's and bachelor's degrees in occupational therapy from San Jose State University. Her clinical practice has been in a variety of settings, with emphasis on the treatment of physical disabilities and gerontic occupational therapy. She is a part-time lecturer in the Department of Occupational Therapy at San Jose State University and a contributing author to Occupational Therapy Practice Skills for Physical Dysfunction, by Lorraine Pedretti.

Beverly P. Horowitz, DSW, OTR/L, is Associate Professor and Co-Chair of the Occupational Therapy Department at Touro College, Barry Z. Levine School of Health Sciences, in Dix Hills, New York. She received her bachelor of arts from the State University of New York at Stony Brook and her master of science in occupational therapy from Columbia University. Fordham University awarded her a Doctor of Social Work degree with a concentration in gerontology. In addition to her work at Touro College, Dr. Horowitz is in private practice, specializing in home care and adult/geriatric rehabilitation. Dr. Horowitz is an active speaker and is a reviewer for the *American Journal of Occupational Therapy*. Soon-to-be released publications include a chapter in *A Therapist's Guide to the Evaluation and Treatment of Vision Dysfunction and Low Vision*.

K. Oscar Larson, MA, OTR, is proprietor of On Task in Alexandria, Virginia. He received his bachelor of arts degree in occupational therapy from San Jose State University and a master of arts degree from New York University, focusing on role adaptation in bereavement. He has worked at Payne Whitney Clinic–New York Hospital in New York City and at the Mental Health and Behavioral Center at Alexandria Hospital. He was on the standing committee of the Gerontology Special Interest Section for AOTA, editing the Gerontology Special Interest Section Newsletter for 3 years. He has been pre-

senter at the annual conference of AOTA and the 1994 congress of the World Federation of Occupational Therapists. Other recent publications include vignettes in the *Mental Health Service Delivery Guidelines* and work sheets in *Life Management Skills, IV*.

Linda L. Levy, MA, OTR/L, FAOTA, is an associate professor of occupational therapy at Temple University and a faculty associate of the Geriatric Education Center of Pennsylvania. She has a master's degree in social gerontology and health planning and a bachelor's degree in occupational therapy from the University of Pennsylvania. She has extensive clinical experience in psychiatric and geriatric issues, having directed occupational therapy programs at the Hospital of the University of Pennsylvania and the Philadelphia Psychiatric Center. She has published widely and presented numerous seminars on geriatric rehabilitation and the impact of dementia on individual behaviors, rehabilitation, and the family. Ms. Levy served as a health systems agency planner in mental health, developmental disabilities, and long-term care services.

Lela A. Llorens, PhD, OTR, FAOTA, is professor emeritus of San Jose State University and a recognized leader in the field of occupational therapy. She earned her bachelor of science degree in occupational therapy from Western Michigan University, her master of arts degree in vocational rehabilitation from Wayne State University, her doctorate from Walden University, and her certificate in gerontology from San Jose State University. Dr. Llorens served as chair and graduate coordinator in the Departments of Occupational Therapy at San Jose State University and the University of Florida. She is currently a member of the CORE faculty of the Stanford Geriatric Education Center, which focuses on ethnogeriatrics.

Helene Lohman, MA, OTR/L, has a master's certificate in gerontology. She has taught occupational therapy courses at Creighton University, Omaha, Nebraska, and has written numerous articles. She is the author of a book on the geriatric code of practice (in press) and of *Introduction to Splinting: A Critical Thinking and Problem Solving Approach.*

Joan C. Rogers, PhD, OTR, FAOTA, is a professor of occupational therapy and an assistant professor of psychiatry, Division of Geriatrics and Neuropsychiatry, at the University of Pittsburgh Medical Center. A charter member of the Academy of Research, she is also a recipient of the Eleanor Clarke Slagle Lectureship. Her degrees include a bachelor of science degree in biology from Canisius College in Buffalo, a master of arts degree in occupational therapy from the University of Southern California, and a doctorate in educational psychology (life-span human development) from the University of Illinois at Urbana-Champaign.

Learning Outline

SECTION 5.

SECTION 6.

Chapter 4
Older Adults: Living Lives

SECTION 1.

SECTION 2.

Cognition and the Aging Adult. 199
Linda L. Levy, MA, OTR/L, FAOTA

SECTION 3.

Adaptation and the Aging Adult. 211
Linda L. Levy, MA, OTR/L, FAOTA

SECTION 4.

Mental Disorders in Aging Adults. 221
Linda L. Levy, MA, OTR/L, FAOTA

SECTION 5.

Ability and Disability: The Performance Areas 230
Joan C. Rogers, PhD, OTR, FAOTA

Introduction to Module I

To begin this exploration of the role of the occupational therapist in serving elderly people, I asked three questions.

- Who are the professionals involved in assisting people as they age and what is the discipline of gerontology?
- Who are the occupational therapists who consider themselves gerontic specialists, and how do they define their professional role?
- Most important, who are aging adults, and how do they live their lives? This first module will set out to answer these questions.

David opens the first chapter with a discussion of gerontology and its history. Foti continues with a more detailed review of occupational therapy's involvement with aging adults. Cipriani describes the process of maturation for people in their senior years.

Each of the following three chapters clarifies these themes to prepare the reader for organizing the material presented in the remaining modules of this text. Aitken and Lohman enumerate the variety of professionals working to assist older adults through the existing medical and social systems. Larson and Horowitz discuss the organization of the specialty of gerontic occupational therapy. Levy, Rogers, Llorens, and Larson describe the lives of older adults, focusing on the interrelationship of occupational performance components, areas, and contexts.

As I began to discuss this project with the authors and gather their input, I realized what an extensive number of ideas we were attempting to synthesize into four chapters. We put as much effort into deciding what would not fit into the text as what would. We grant to the reader that your professional experiences may bring you into contact with other professionals whom we have not credited, may direct you to practice areas that we have not identified, and may offer you additional insights into the lives of all of us who age. We have attempted here to define the most relevant aspects of the role of occupational therapy with the elderly.

K. Oscar Larson, MA, OTR
Co-Editor, ROTE, revision 1996

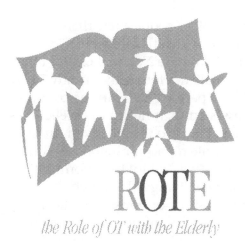

ROTE

the Role of OT with the Elderly

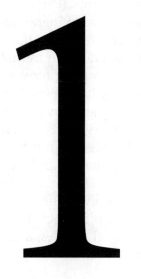

Introduction to ROTE

Section 1. Gerontology: The Study of Aging and Older Adults

Debra David, PhD

Abstract

The author provides an overview of the demographic and social trends that led to the development of gerontology, as well as a discussion of future directions for the field.

Demographics of the Aging Population

During the 20th century, Americans have witnessed a dramatic rise in the number and proportion of persons age 65 and over. The 3.1 million older Americans in 1900 made up about 4% of the population. By 1994, there were 33.2 million older Americans, making up almost 13% of the population (U.S. Bureau of the Census, 1995). The relative growth of the "oldest old" segment of the population—those age 85+—has been even sharper; it increased from 123,000 in 1900 (about .2% of the population) to an estimated 3,620,000 in 1995 (about 1.3% of the population; U.S. Bureau of the Census, 1994).

The main reasons for this "demographic revolution" have been a sharp rise in average life expectancy and an overall drop in birth rates (despite relatively high birth rates during the "baby boom" years of 1946 to 1964). Life expectancy at birth was about 47 years in 1900 (46 for men and 48 for women). By 1991, it had jumped to 76 years (72 for men and 79 for women). Because women now live about 7 years longer than men, on the average, the ratio of older women to older men becomes greater with age. Among those age

65+, there are about 3 women for every 2 men; among those age 85+, there are about 5 women for every 2 men. As a consequence, older men are almost twice as likely as older women to be married (75% vs. 41%), and older women are about three times more likely than men to be widowed (48% vs. 14%; U.S. Bureau of the Census, 1995).

In the first half of the 21st century, the older population will continue to grow substantially, especially beginning in 2011, when the oldest members of the "baby boom" generation reach age 65. By 2050, it is projected that the number of persons age 65+ will more than double to 68 million (almost 23% of Americans). Those age 85+ will exceed 15,000,000 (about 5% of the population; U.S. Senate Special Committee on Aging, 1991). These projections, which represent the "middle" estimates of the Bureau of the Census, may be modified by changes in mortality (death rates), fertility (birth rates), and migration. However, they are likely to be reasonably accurate: everyone who will be 65 or older by 2050 has already been born!

About 4 out of 5 men age 65+ live in a family setting with their spouses or other family members, compared with 57% of women in that age group. Therefore, men are more likely to have a family caregiver to assist them if they become ill or disabled. The likelihood of living in a family setting declines with age for both sexes. More than 95% of older adults live in community, rather than institutional, settings (U.S. Bureau of the Census, 1990). Even among those who need assistance with activities of daily living, at least two persons live in the community for every one who resides in a nursing home (U.S. Senate Special Committee on Aging, 1991).

Most older people view their health positively. A Health Interview Survey conducted by the National Center for Health Statistics found that nearly 71% of elderly persons living in the community assessed their health as excellent, very good, or good. Similarly, most older people report no significant limitations in their ability to perform activities of daily living (ADL), such as bathing, eating, or transferring from bed to chair, or in home management tasks (often called instrumental activities of daily living, IADL) such as laundry, cleaning, shopping, or managing finances. However, almost 20% of adults age 65+ who live in the community report at least one ADL or IADL difficulty; more than half of those age 85+ have at least one difficulty. Women and Blacks are significantly more likely than men and Whites to report difficulties (U.S. Senate Special Committee on Aging, 1991).

The older population in the United States is becoming more diverse in its racial and ethnic composition. The U.S. Bureau of the Census (1995) estimates that 1 in 10 elderly persons were a race other than White in 1990; that proportion is projected to double by 2050. Similarly, the proportion of older adults who are Hispanic is expected to grow from 4% to 16% (Hispanics may be of any race). Due to high rates of immigration among Asian and Hispanic groups and high mortality and fertility rates among most minority populations, they have a smaller proportion of older members than Whites (Angel & Hogan, 1994). For example, about 8% of Blacks, 7% of other races (Asian, Native American, Eskimo, and Aleut), and 6% of Hispanics were age 65+ in 1990. However, these proportions are projected to reach 13% for Blacks, 16% for other races, and 13% for Hispanics by 2030.

The economic status of older adults is more varied than that of any other age group; relying on age group averages in income can be very misleading. Older adults are about as likely as other adult age groups to have incomes below the poverty line. In 1989, 11.4% of persons age 65+ were below the poverty line, compared with 10.2% of those age 18 to 64. Another 15% of older adults had incomes just slightly above the poverty line (between 100% and 150% of poverty). However, many older people are financially comfortable. If assets such as homes, savings, and investments are included, people over age 65 are likely to have higher net worth than younger adults. There are many subgroups of elders who are at high risk of poverty, including women, minority group members, the very old, and those who live alone (U.S. Senate Special Committee on Aging, 1991). The cost of extended long-term nursing home or home health care can also impoverish persons with considerable assets, because most older people have no insurance coverage for chronic health care.

Developing Interest in Older Adults

The study of older adults and the processes of aging has emerged with the sharp increase in the older population outlined earlier. According to Robert Kastenbaum (1987), the term *gerontology* was coined in 1903 by French biologist M. Elie Metchnikoff to describe the scientific study of old age. Kastenbaum noted that contemporary gerontology also includes scientific studies of processes associated with aging, studies from the perspective of the humanities, and applications of knowledge for the benefit of mature and aged adults.

The earliest scientific studies of aging focused on its biological aspects. Late in the 19th century, Russian biologist S. P. Botkin conducted physiological analyses of nearly 3,000 older residents of St. Petersburg and made distinctions between normal and pathological aging (i.e., diseases that may speed aging processes). One of the first major studies of psychological aging was *Senescence, the Last Half of Life*, published in 1922 by the American developmental psychologist G. Stanley Hall. Social scientists began to study aging in the 1930s. E. V. Cowdry's *Problems of Ageing* (1939) is an early example of this work (Birren & Clayton, 1975).

In the public arena, the growth of the older population and a drop in the status held by many older adults in pre-industrial society made the problems of aging increasingly visible. Biological models of aging as inevitable decline justified ageism (prejudice against older people) and age discrimination in employment. Most industrializing nations began to establish retirement policies and public pension systems. According to retirement expert Robert Atchley (1994), the main purpose of retirement "was and is to keep down the number of persons holding or looking for jobs" (p. 287). Supporting people too old or disabled to work or rewarding people for service were secondary goals.

In the United States, the first national policy for older adults was the Social Security Act, passed in 1935. This program set a precedent that dominated policies for older adults for more than 50 years: old people (defined as those age 65 or older) became "entitled" to government assistance to address the special problems of aging (Achenbaum, 1983; Torres-Gil, 1992).

A focus on the special problems of older adults also dominated much early scientific research. Age-associated deficits in physical and cognitive performance were often assumed to be caused by aging. Many studies compared age groups, attributing differences to age per se (Rowe & Kahn, 1987).

The formal development of gerontology accelerated with the founding of the Gerontological Society of America (GSA) in 1945 and the publication of the first major periodical, the *Journal of Gerontology*, beginning in 1946. From its inception, GSA has been multidisciplinary. Most early members represented the biological, medical, and behavioral sciences, but the membership has now expanded to include social scientists, humanists, policy analysts, and practitioners (Havighurst, 1987).

Scientific interest in normal aging grew in the 1940s and 1950s with the establishment of several major research centers by the National Institutes of Health (NIH), Duke University, and the University of Chicago, which all began longitudinal studies to follow changes in normal individuals over a period of time (Hooyman & Kiyak, 1991). The NIH center, founded in 1946, launched the Baltimore Longitudinal Studies to examine physiological and psychological functions; headed by the physician, Nathan Shock, these studies continue today under the direction of the National Institute on Aging. The Duke Longitudinal Study examined medical, psychological, and social data for a group of volunteers age 60 to 90 from mid-1955 until 1976. The University of Chicago, under the leadership of Robert Havighurst, conducted the Kansas City Studies of Adult Life from 1952 to 1962. These studies examined social psychological adaptation to aging through cross-sectional interviews with 750 individuals aged 40 to 70 in the mid-1950s and a six-year longitudinal study of 280 persons aged 50 to 90.

Through these pioneering studies and later longitudinal research, many assumptions about the problems of older adults have been challenged, along with notions that age-related declines in physical, cognitive, and social performance are an inevitable part of normal aging. For example, the possibility of stability and even improvement in some areas of performance is recognized. It is now known that many age-related losses are due to factors such as lifestyle, habits, and psychosocial conditions; some may be prevented or modified. Heterogeneity within age groups now receives considerable research attention and multiple causes of differences between age groups are examined (Ferraro, 1990; Rowe & Kahn, 1987). It is interesting to note that all three social theories of aging described later in this chapter (disengagement, activity, and identity continuity) were supported by data from the Kansas City Studies, leading one of its principal researchers, Bernice Neugarten (1968, 1987), to conclude that there are diverse patterns of adaptation to aging and no single optimum model of development.

The federal government has responded to the growing numbers of older Americans through the passage of major legislation to protect their health, income, and social welfare. Among the most important laws have been the following:

1. Medicare (1965), a universal health insurance program for elderly and disabled persons

2. Older Americans Act (OAA; 1965), establishing the Administration on Aging (AoA) and an "aging network" of services

3. Age Discrimination in Employment Act (ADEA; 1967, with major amendments in 1978 and 1986), to outlaw age discrimination and, in 1986, abolish mandatory retirement

4. Supplemental Security Income (SSI; 1974), a welfare program to assure a minimum income floor to aged, blind, and disabled persons

5. Employees Retirement Income Security Act (ERISA; 1974), protecting private pension programs.

In addition, the National Institute on Aging (NIA) was established in 1975. Major changes in the Social Security Act in 1983 increased taxes and raised the age of retirement with full benefits from 65 to 67 by the year 2027.

Public attention to older adults has increased significantly in recent decades. For example, the American Association of Retired Persons (AARP, founded in 1958) now claims over 32 million members age 50+, and its magazine, *Modern Maturity*, has the largest circulation in the world. And, according to Ken Dychtwald (1990), major corporations have discovered the "mature market."

The growth of academic interest in aging and older adults from the 1960s to the present has been phenomenal. An attempt to compile a bibliography of research from 1954 to 1974 located 50,000 titles (Woodruff, 1975). Today, there are dozens of multidisciplinary and specialized journals on gerontology and life span development. From small academic programs offering gerontology education at the University of Chicago, Duke University, and the University of Michigan in the mid-1960s, it is estimated that over 1,600 colleges and universities offered at least one formal course related to aging in 1992 (Peterson, Wendt, & Douglass, 1994).

Social Trends

Increasing longevity and the growth in the size of the older population have led to major changes in individual lives, family relationships, and the structure of our society. For the first time in history, most people can expect to survive to old age.

One consequence of longer life spans and age-based pension policies has been an extended period of retirement for most individuals. It is estimated that 2/3 of men over age 65 in 1900 were in the labor force; unemployment or health problems kept most of the remainder from working. In 1989, about 17% of men and 8% of women aged 65+ were employed (U.S. Senate Special Committee on Aging, 1991). Retirement is an invention of the 20th century, and many people now choose to retire as soon as they can afford to do so. The average age of retirement is now 62, and most people look forward to a variety of leisure and volunteer roles.

A less positive consequence of longevity has been an increased likelihood of becoming dependent on others due to poor health or disability (Verbrugge, 1984). Advances in medicine and improvements in sanitation and health practices have enabled more people to prevent, delay, or minimize the risks of life-threatening illnesses. Although these changes mean that more people enjoy good health for longer periods, they are also more likely to survive long enough to develop chronic, disabling conditions that may require rehabilitation or long-term care.

Family and other social relationships have also been affected by aging and related demographic changes. One major trend has been toward long-lasting bonds. Despite high divorce rates, the number of marriages that reach their 50th, 60th, or even 75th anniversary is growing. Sibling ties of eight or nine decades are common. Approximately 10% of adults over age 65 still have a living parent. Four-generation families are becoming the norm. For the first time in history, most parents survive for an extended "postparental" period when their children are adults. In fact, women are likely to spend, on average, more years with parents over 65 than with children under 18 (Cantor, 1991; Hagestad, 1988).

Changing family patterns are likely to significantly affect the future availability of caregivers. Despite popular images that families "abandon" their elderly members, current studies demonstrate that family members provide about 80% of services to older adults with disabilities. The primary caregivers are likely to be daughters (29%), wives (23%), other female relatives such as daughters-in-law and sisters (20%), and husbands (13%) (Stone, Cafferata, & Sangl, 1987).

However, smaller families with fewer children, the increasing number of women in the labor force, and increasing incidence of divorce, stepfamilies, and single-parent families may reduce the ability of families to provide care for impaired members (Cantor, 1991).

Social ideas about age-appropriate behavior (age norms) and the timing of events in the life cycle have been changing in major ways. Although we now recognize more life stages than in agricultural societies, differences between life stages are blurring and age norms are becoming more flexible (Neugarten & Neugarten, 1986). Ironically, our laws and social policies have become more age-based during a period when the utility of age distinc-

tions may be decreasing. Sociologists Matilda and John Riley (1994) have attributed this phenomenon to "structural lag," which means that social roles and institutions have not changed quickly enough to keep up with new social realities. They argued that more age integration and a more flexible life course that allows for cyclical periods of education, work, and leisure make greater sense than linear stages, given increasing numbers of robust long-lived people who need meaningful, productive roles.

The age-based public policies established in the United States between the 1930s and the 1980s are becoming highly controversial in the 1990s as their costs increase with the growing older population. Social welfare expert Fernando Torres-Gil (1992), Assistant Secretary on Aging in the Clinton Administration, has proposed that those policies need to be revised in response to changing longevity, diversity, and generational interests before the "baby boom" generation reaches retirement age. Like the Rileys, he suggested more age-integration, with most benefits contingent on need. He proposed postponing eligibility for age-based programs until age 70. Whether or not politicians agree with Torres-Gil's views, there is broad consensus that meeting the needs of an older population will be a major challenge in the 21st century.

Future Directions

The field of gerontology and the lives of older adults are likely to change dramatically in the decades ahead. Geriatrician Robert Butler (1987) predicted that biomedical research will lead to major advances in many areas, including identifying genetic markers of disease; finding lower-risk and less expensive treatments; using micro-processors plus prostheses to compensate for physical disabilities; preventing, diagnosing, and treating Alzheimer's disease and other dementias; and stimulating the immune, endocrine, and neurotransmission systems. Exercise and other health maintenance practices may also improve wellness throughout the lifespan (Buskirk, 1985).

Many experts expect that a "cyclic" life course will become common, with most people experiencing multiple careers, lifelong learning, serial marriages, and more opportunities for leisure activities throughout the life span (Atchley, 1994; Dychtwald, 1990; Riley & Riley, 1994).

A likely rise in the number of very old people with disabilities, coupled with smaller families, may mean that caring for older parents may become more typical (Brody, 1985). New strategies for dealing with long-term care needs, such as assisted living and home sharing, may also increase. The "independent living" movement, which helped lead to the passage of the Americans with Disabilities Act in 1991, may increase opportunities available to disabled elders.

Changes in the broader society will affect the status of older adults in the future. For example, future cohorts of computer-literate older adults will be able to use the "information superhighway" from their homes to bank, shop, and communicate with health providers and others. Technological improvements may make homes and highways more accommodating to persons with physical disabilities. However, a growing split between workers in complex, sophisticated industries that rely on information systems and participate in the global economy, and unskilled workers in low-paying service jobs could result in a growing divide between fortunate retirees with high assets and income and less fortunate older adults who must continue to work or depend on support from families or the government. Changes in public policies for elderly individuals will also shape the opportunities and problems that they face.

Forecasts of the future are highly uncertain. However, given the demographic patterns that are well-established, it is clear that issues of aging and older adults will become increasingly important.

Activities

1. According to Bernice and Dail Neugarten, age norms have become more flexible than they were in previous generations. Compare the actual and anticipated timing of major events in your life course (such as completing school, beginning one's first full-time job, marriage, childbearing, retirement, etc.) to that experienced by your parents. Then discuss whether the Neugartens' observation fits your own family's case.

2. Imagine your "ideal" situation when you are 75 years old. Consider your work or retirement status, physical condition, level and sources of income, living arrangements, activities, social relationships, and any other issues that you consider relevant. Based on the social trends covered in this module, discuss how likely it is that this "ideal" situation will be possible.

3. Describe a new product or service for older adults that you think will become "marketable" by the year 2030. Outline a marketing plan to support its development.

Review Questions

1. How has the size and proportion of the older population in the United States changed since the year 1900? And what changes are projected by the year 2050?

2. What early ideas about aging were modified as a result of longitudinal studies of normal aging individuals?

3. About what proportion of older adults age 65+ need assistance with activities of daily living? About what proportion of older adults age 85+ need such assistance?

4. What assumptions underlie current public policies for older adults in the United States? Why are those assumptions being challenged in the 1990s?

5. Give at least two examples of how the "typical" life course of Americans has changed during the past century.

6. How are changes in family patterns likely to affect the availability of caregivers in the future?

References

Achenbaum, W. A. (1983). *Shades of gray: Old age, American values, and federal policies since 1920*. Boston: Little, Brown.

Angel, J. L., & Hogan, D. P. (1994). The demography of minority aging populations. In *Minority elders: Five goals toward building a public policy* (2nd ed., pp. 9–21). Washington, DC: Gerontological Society of America.

Atchley, R. C. (1994). *Social forces and aging: An introduction to social gerontology* (7th ed.). Belmont, CA: Wadsworth.

Birren, J. E., & Clayton, V. (1975). History of gerontology. In D. S. Woodruff & J. E. Birren (Eds.), *Aging: Scientific perspectives and social issues* (pp. 15–27). New York: Van Nostrand.

Brody, E. (1985). Parent care as a normative family stress. *Gerontologist, 25,* 19–30.

Buskirk, E. R. (1985). Health maintenance and longevity: Exercise. In C. E. Finch & E. L. Schneider (Eds.), *Handbook of the biology of aging* (2nd ed., pp. 894–931). New York: Van Nostrand.

Butler, R. N. (1987). Future trends. In G. L. Maddox (Ed.), *The encyclopedia of aging* (pp. 265–267). New York: Springer.

Cantor, M. H. (1991). Family and community: Changing roles in an aging society. *Gerontologist, 31,* 337–346.

Cowdry, E. V. (Ed.). (1939). *Problems of ageing*. Baltimore: Walhams & Wilkins.

Dychtwald, K. (with Flower, J.). (1990). *Age wave: The challenges and opportunities of an aging America*. New York: Bantam Books.

Ferraro, K. F. (1990). The gerontological imagination. In K. F. Ferraro (Ed.), *Gerontology: Perspectives and issues* (pp. 3–18). New York: Springer.

Hagestad, G. O. (1988). Demographic change and the life course: Some emerging trends in family realm. *Family Relations, 37,* 405–410.

Hall, G. S. (1922). *Senescence, the last half of life*. 1972. Reprint of the 1923 ed. New Hampshire: Ayer.

Havighurst, R. J. (1987). Gerontological Society of America. In G. L. Maddox (Ed.), *The encyclopedia of aging* (pp. 287–288). New York: Springer.

Hooyman, N. R., & Kiyak, H. A. (1991). *Social gerontology: A multidisciplinary perspective* (2nd ed.). Boston: Allyn and Bacon.

Kastenbaum, R. (1987). Gerontology. In G. L. Maddox (Ed.), *The encyclopedia of aging* (pp. 289–290). New York: Springer.

Neugarten, B. L. (Ed.). (1968). *Middle age and aging: A reader in social psychology*. Chicago: University of Chicago Press.

Neugarten, B. L. (1987). The Kansas City Studies of Adult Life. In G. L. Maddox (Ed.), *The encyclopedia of aging* (pp. 372–373). New York: Springer.

Neugarten, B. L., & Neugarten, D. A. (1986). Changing meanings of age in the aging society. In A. Pifer & L. Bronte (Eds.), *Our aging society: Paradox and promise* (pp. 33–51). New York: W. W. Norton.

Peterson, D. A., Wendt, P. F., & Douglass, E. B. (1994). *Development of gerontology, geriatrics and aging studies programs in institutions of higher education*. Washington, DC: Association for Gerontology in Higher Education.

Riley, M. W., & Riley, J. W., Jr. (1994). Age integration and the lives of older people. *Gerontologist, 34*, 110–115.

Rowe, J. W., & Kahn, R. L. (1987). Human aging: Usual and successful. *Science, 237*, 143–149.

Stone, R., Cafferata, G. L., & Sangl, J. (1987). Caregivers of the frail elderly: A national profile. *Gerontologist, 27*, 616–626.

Torres-Gil, F. M. (1992). *The new aging: Politics and change in America*. New York: Auburn House.

U.S. Bureau of the Census. (1990). Marital status and living arrangements: March 1989. *Current Population Reports* (Series P-20, No. 445). Washington, DC: U.S. Government Printing Office.

U.S. Bureau of the Census. (1994). *United States population estimates, by age, sex, race, and Hispanic origin, 1990 to 1994* (release PPL-21). Washington, DC: U.S. Bureau of the Census, Population Division.

U.S. Bureau of the Census. (1995). *Sixty-five plus in the United States* (Statistical Brief SB/95-8). Washington, DC: Author.

U.S. Senate Special Committee on Aging. (1991). *Aging America: Trends and projections* (DHHS Publication No. FCoA 91-28001). Washington, DC: U.S. Department of Health and Human Services.

Verbrugge, L. M. (1984). Longer life but worsening health? Trends in health and mortality of middle-aged and older persons. *Milbank Memorial Fund Quarterly, 62*, 475–519.

Woodruff, D. S. (1975). Introduction: Multidisciplinary perspectives of aging. In D. S. Woodruff & J. E. Birren (Eds.), *Aging: Scientific perspectives and social issues* (pp. 3–14), New York: Van Nostrand.

Section 2. Gerontic Occupational Therapy: Specialized Intervention for the Older Adult

Diane Foti, MA, OTR

Abstract

In this section, the author provides a historical perspective of the field of gerontic occupational therapy, summarizes current treatment approaches, and discusses future trends in the field.

Introduction

The population in the United States is graying, while the demand for health care services is expanding. Accordingly, occupational therapy practitioners are needed at all levels of health care, including preventative, acute, subacute, extended, skilled nursing, rehabilitation, home health, and community care programs. In order to work with the aging individual, professionals must have a comprehensive knowledge base of physical, psychiatric, and psychosocial dysfunction. The elderly individual is not only changing as a result of aging, but may also have multiple medical problems that impair function. Therefore, physical and mental health problems may concurrently cause limitations for the aging individual. Social concerns, such as whether a partner, son, or daughter will be able to assist the patient, can also compound the situation.

The elderly population includes the well-elderly, the acutely disabled, (such as those individuals with a cerebral vascular accident [CVA] or depression) and those with long-term physical or psychiatric disability. For example, a person with a spinal cord injury that occurred in his twenties, but who is now 65 years old, and a person with bipolar disorder who is now aging, both fall into the scope of practice for the gerontic occupational therapist.

The combination of disability, disease, aging, and the individual's personality and social situation creates a challenging area of practice. Because the aging population is so diverse, occupational therapy practitioners need to have a knowledge base that includes an understanding of specific diseases and disabilities, and of the aging process. Further knowledge of developmental theories, models of adaptation and learning, culture, and family dynamics are also essential in order to appropriately treat the aging individual. Kiernat (1991b, p. 7) described the gerontic occupational therapist as the "master generalist." She said, "The occupational therapist serving older adults must have advanced knowledge of physical rehabilitation and behavioral health and be a specialist in independent living and the repertoire of community agencies and social support services."

Before discussing occupational therapy and the elderly any further, the terminology used in this discussion needs to be clarified. The terms needing clarification are *geriatrics, gerontology,* and *gerontic*. These terms are frequently used interchangeably, and although related, each is distinct. *Geriatrics* refers to the medical practice that deals with diseases that are associated with older people and aging. *Gerontology* is the study of aging. *Gerontic* means pertaining to old age (Lewis, 1989a). The term *gerontic* is more appropriate in reference to the clinical practice of working with elderly individuals because the practice is not always related to diseases of aging nor is it always a scientific study of the aging process. However, it always pertains to the aging person (Rogers, 1981). As occupational therapy practitioners working with aging persons we often borrow from the knowledge base in the field of geriatrics and gerontology (disease and the aging process). But it would be limiting to purely define our practice with elderly individuals as focusing only on the disease process or on the aging process. Our scope of practice encompasses a more holistic approach to working with the aging person. Therefore, the term *gerontic occupational therapist* is more aptly applied to the specialist in this field of practice.

Over the last five decades the field of gerontic occupational therapy has developed. This discussion will take a historical perspective so that the reader can appreciate the evolution of this field of practice.

Initial recognition of the special area of practice with the elderly began in the 1940s, but the preponderance of growth has occurred since the mid-1970s. Occupational therapy literature reflects that practitioners saw the need for a special focus with the elderly as far back as the 1940s (Hildenbrand, 1949a, 1949b). The demographics of the time reflected the significant lengthening of the human life span from 42 years in 1900, to 65 years in 1940, and it was clear this trend of greater life expectancy would continue.

In 1940, occupational therapists had already been treating individuals who had diseases or disabilities of old age, such as CVA or arthritis. Occupational therapists were concerned about the institutionalized elderly individual's ability to maintain a sense of self-worth. For well-elderly persons, the concern was how to adapt to the new trend of forced retirement.

In 1947 Hildenbrand described the goals of geriatric medicine and occupational therapy to prolong life span and help aging persons to enjoy better health and vitality, adjust to senescent changes, and prove useful to society. Occupational therapy was seen as providing activities to promote change and adjustment, while supporting the client's sense of self-worth and contributions to society (Hildenbrand, 1947).

Early Activity Intervention with the Elderly

During this period, the trend of forced retirement at age 65 was evolving. Health professionals from this period were concerned that inactivity and role loss with forced retirement was neither good for the economy nor for the individual. (Hildenbrand, 1949b; King, 1951; Lang & Waterman,1959). There was concern about the lack of planning for retirement and the economic impact on the unemployed aging individual without a pension plan. Foresight was expressed by Hildenbrand (1949b) when she described concerns about the impact of forced retirement on the aging individual. She suggested a need for job analysis of the physical and mental abilities required for each job (now required by the American Disabilities Act in 1990) and for an assessment of these same abilities in the individual to determine a match. The job analysis would eliminate age as the criteria for acquiring a job; instead, the individual would be judged based on qualifications. Society was seen as needing to change to accommodate aging individuals, or else they would become a burden due to limited income and cost of medical care.

Activities related to vocation or hobbies were used to assist with psychological adjustment, provide preventive or diversional therapy, or provide functional therapy. Preventive therapy addressed the emotional and social needs of the individual, and functional occupational therapy addressed improvement or maintenance of physical deficits (Hildenbrand, 1949a; Murphy, 1949).

The 1940s and 1950s began a period of expanding occupational therapy services to include constructive activities and to teach activities of daily living, work simplification, and rehabilitation techniques for the "handicapped homemaker" (Spackman, 1968). These changes reflected the emergence of the rehabilitation movement, which continued into the 1950s, 1960s, and 1970s.

THE REHABILITATION MOVEMENT

The decades of the 1950s and 1960s brought greater information about the special needs of the aging population based on physiological and psychological aspects of aging. The role of occupational therapy practitioners was expanding. Willard and Spackman's (1963) third edition of *Occupational Therapy* includes for the first time a chapter on occupational therapy in geriatrics. It is significant that the authors of a primary occupational therapy text considered the physical, emotional, social, cognitive, and psychological needs of the aging individual to be vital knowledge for the entry level occupational therapist.

Other professionals were also contributing to the knowledge of gerontol-ogy. Gregg and Sherrill (1957) described eye problems of the aging individual, the relationship to activities, and ways that activities could be modified. Pincus (1968) described factors that may inhibit learning for the aging individual and methods to adapt the environment to promote optimum learning.

During this period, occupational therapy practitioners and other health professionals involved in activity programming continued to explore the meaning of activities and the psychological impact of the activities. Hildenbrand (1953) and Lakin and Dray (1958) both acknowledged the psychological needs of the aging individual who suffers role loss due to retirement or limitation of activities and social disruption due to institutionalization. They identified the need for occupational therapy practitioners to facilitate adjustment, develop new roles and consider psychological needs when designing activity programs. The Lakin and Dray study (1958) is the first research on the aging individual in the occupational therapy literature. It is a qualitative study with very loose guidelines and observations of findings but, nonetheless, the beginnings of research. A quantitative study by Pearman and Newman (1968) demonstrated that despite age, the study group showed a need to be involved in meaningful activities, especially in regard to a work-oriented program. Models of practice identifying the special needs of the aging individual continue to be sorted out. Tendo (1961) reported on the need for the aging population in a psychiatric setting to be treated separately from the younger population because its needs are different.

ENVIRONMENTAL AND SOCIOLEGAL CHANGES

During the 1950s and 1960s the majority of occupational therapy practitioners worked in institutions, although at this time several new models of practice were emerging. Roles for occupational therapists as consultants and in public health were developing. Occupational therapy practitioners in long-term care facilities provided activities which had personal and social implications for the individual (Kaplan, 1957; Lakin & Dray, 1958). But not all long-term care facilities, mental health centers, or community agencies had occupational therapy practitioners on staff. Consequently, the role of consultant emerged for the occupational therapist. The consultant role allowed the occupational therapist to provide services to a larger number of people (Mazer, 1969; Schroepfer, 1961). The occupational therapy consultant helped the organization define its needs regarding activity for the aging resident and identify resources and methods to implement change.

Legislative acts have significantly affected the practice of gerontic occupational therapy. As social needs for the aging person have become recognized, and with the public supporting the need for government intervention, laws have been established to address the needs of the aging population. Several different laws have been enacted that affect care of elderly persons and the practice of gerontic occupational therapy. (A few of these are discussed as they affected the growth of gerontic occupational therapy, but for more information about legislation affecting practice with older adults refer to chapter 18). The Medicare program, the Older Americans Act, and the Americans with Disabilities Act (ADA) of 1992 have influenced practice by providing a source for reimbursement, a climate for acceptance of program development for elderly individuals, and opportunities for occupational therapy practitioners to explore new roles.

The Medicare program has affected occupational therapy practitioners the most by providing opportunities for development of occupational therapy roles and providing for reimbursement of services. Medicare is the largest single payer for occupational therapy services. In 1985, approximately 20% of occupational therapy practitioners served Medicare beneficiaries (American Occupational Therapy Association [AOTA], 1987).

The federal Medicare program was implemented in 1965. Individuals over age 65 were eligible for Medicare, which covered a percentage of the cost for inpatient hospital services, extended care, home health, and outpatient medical services. Occupational therapy services were identified as covered services for extended care, Part A only, home health, and outpatient medical treatment. Occupational therapy assistant services were also covered when provided under the supervision of an occupational therapist. Medicare Part A coverage in extended care required that the client need skilled services and that coverage not exceed 100 days. Occupational therapy service for Part B coverage in extended care was initiated in the 1980s and allowed for reimbursement of services as long as the client was making weekly progress.

The Older Americans Act of 1965 addressed many areas of concern for aging individuals. Some of the needs included the establishment of the administration on aging, senior centers, nutrition programs, library services for the homebound, and job opportunities and training for older adults. The implementation of the

Older Americans Act has provided the opportunity for occupational therapists to offer services and develop some of the programs that were identified for the older adult.

The Americans with Disabilities Act of 1992 addressed needs of the disabled individual in three areas:

1. Employment opportunity
2. Community accessibility
3. Public transportation accessibility.

It is still relatively new legislation, and the effect on older adults has not yet been determined. This legislative act could potentially improve employment for those individuals who do not wish to retire at age 65 but need to be matched to a job suited to their abilities. The ADA will also create a more negotiable community for those with physical limitations. The ADA guarantees older adults with disabilities equality in the workplace and the community (Bachelder, 1994). For the occupational therapy practitioner, the ADA has opened up numerous opportunities as consultants and private practitioners.

Roles in public health began emerging in satellite clinics and in home care in the 1960s and 1970s (Wiemer & West, 1970). The movement toward home care indicated a need to assist the individual with the transition to resuming previous roles or adapting to new roles in the home environment. The need to become a therapist not just to the patient but also to the family was stressed (Mendoza, 1969). The methods used by occupational therapy practitioners in home care included adapting the environment, providing family education, transitioning leisure and self-care activities taught in the hospital to home, and facilitating community support (Meeske & Jacoby, 1952; Moss & Stewart, 1959).

Expansion of the knowledge of gerontic occupational therapy. Immense growth in the areas of gerontology and geriatrics began in the 1970s and continues into the 1990s. Occupational therapy practitioners have borrowed theories, models of treatment, and research methods from the social sciences and the biological sciences. In conjunction with other gerontologists, gerontic occupational therapists have contributed to the knowledge of the aging process, models of practice and their applications to the elderly, the evaluation process, program development, specific occupational therapy skill development, and research about treatment outcomes, program effectiveness, and education.

The Model of Human Occupation (Kielhofner, 1985) and the Occupational Performance Model (Pedretti, 1996b) have both been applied to working with the elderly. Rogers (1986) applied the occupational performance model to working with the client with depression. Olin (1984) applied the Model of Human Occupation to working with the client with dementia. Models of treatment approaches have also been borrowed from the field of psychology. Miller (1986) used psychodynamic and cognitive models to consider a variety of treatment approaches when working with the depressed client. Bonder (1986) considered how family systems theory applied to intervention for the family and client with Alzheimer's disease. These examples demonstrate how the gerontic occupational therapist has taken models of treatment from our own practice and the practices of other professionals to support and rationalize various assessment and treatment approaches.

Gerontic occupational therapy has also been wrestling with various practice models. There has been debate in the field regarding how independent living, rehabilitation, and the medical models influence treatment. The medical model is externally driven by physicians; therapists receive prescriptive treatments, and the patient is treated. The focus is typically on the disease process and preventing sickness.

The rehabilitation model and independent living model share the focus of function in the areas of self-care, work, and leisure. The rehabilitation model continues to be driven by health professionals, but with a team-oriented approach, and the client continues to be treated, but also provides some input as to the goals to be achieved. The independent living model is client driven, with the overall goal of modifying the environment to create independence. The occupational therapist becomes a resource person. The gerontic occupational therapist should be aware of the various models and consider the implications of the way treatment is approached. Frequently, we are practicing with a mixture of these models. The referral may come from the physician, but the practitioner may be practicing in the community with clients with an independent living approach, in which the client sets goals and establishes the treatment plan.

INCREASING KNOWLEDGE OF AGING CHANGES

Physical changes that occur with aging have been summarized by several occupational therapy practitioners regarding specific physiological systems. Vision has been covered by Cristella (1977) and McGrath (1983); the nervous system by Hasselkus (1974); and hearing by Falconer (1985–1986). Maloney (1987) has contributed to the understanding of all

sensory modalities, typical changes with aging, and methods of assessment. In addition to identifying the physical changes that occur with aging, these authors have described the effects on treatment and how treatment with elderly persons can be modified.

Our understanding of cognition in normal aging has been researched and expanded by several occupational therapists. Dorfman and Ager (1989) studied memory, and their results indicated that although memory skills tend to decrease with age, recent and continued mental stimulation are predictive of higher levels of memory retention. Ager (1986) reviewed the literature about age-related changes in learning and tied it to an information processing model. She then recommended teaching strategies for use with elderly individuals. Working memory has been explored to determine its impact on treatment and teaching the older adult (Andiel & Liu, 1995). Allen (1992) expanded her model of cognitive levels to go beyond assessment and be applied to treatment. She provided a model of treatment intervention for each level of cognition and identified suitable teaching style and methods, along with environmental considerations.

FAMILY INTERVENTION

Psychosocial aspects of aging have also been examined by the geriatric occupational therapy literature. Kirchman and Schulte (1989) studied the morale of elderly persons living in a sheltered environment and those in the traditional community setting. Their studies indicated that those in the sheltered environment had a higher level of morale. Teitelman (1982) and Foy and Mitchell (1990) provided a review of current literature to consider motivation and learned helplessness by elderly individuals. Teitelman presented recommendations for increasing the aging person's sense of control by providing choices, structuring a predictable environment, helping to establish realistic outcomes, and considering the impact of staff attitudes.

Aspects of caregiving and family dynamics have become critical information for the occupational therapist working with elderly individuals. Treatment is rarely provided without inclusion of caregivers, who may be family members or friends. Involving the family in treatment requires an understanding of family dynamics and the potential for caregiver stress, as well as cultural sensitivity (Baum, 1991). In terms of considering culture, Raphael (1988) and McCormack, Llorens, & Glogoski (1991) discussed the impact of culture. Raphael studied Hispanic families and the role of the grandparents. Selected ethnic minority groups were presented and treatment implications for developing rapport and nonverbal communication were discussed in the literature (Barney, 1991; McCormack et al. 1991). Hasselkus (1989) studied the meaning of caregiving activities to the caregiver and explored the implications for occupational therapy practice. Taking another viewpoint, Clark, Corcoran, and Gitlin (1995) explored how occupational therapists develop relationships with caregivers and the effect on the therapeutic relationship. All these studies are examples of how gerontic occupational therapy has developed in terms of the family dynamics.

ASSESSMENTS

The typical nonstandardized assessments have come under scrutiny as to the objectivity and accuracy of the information and measurements. New evaluation techniques have been developed by occupational therapy practitioners or have been taken from other areas of practice and applied to the aging population. An example of a recently developed assessment tool is the Assessment of Motor and Process Skills (AMPS; Fisher, 1993). The AMPS is designed to evaluate instrumental ADL skills and the effects of performance component deficits. The Barthel Self-Care Index is an example of an assessment used in other areas of practice but now used to evaluate the elderly. Hasselkus (1982) found that the Barthel Self-Care Index is sensitive to the levels of performance in activities of daily living and may help define service needs of the elderly community.

Other evaluations were designed to assess performance components such as cognition. Allen (in Kehrberg, Kuskowski, Mortimer, & Shoberg, 1992) expanded on her model of cognitive levels and redesigned her assessment to suit the older client with sensory impairments. The assessment now includes not only identification of the cognitive level but appropriate activities to use environmental requirements, and the most appropriate teaching method.

Occupational therapy practitioners continue to borrow assessments from other professions to provide a more comprehensive evaluation. Barrett (1986) debated whether the practice needs more objective cognitive assessments for the person with dementia. She recommended use of the Luria-Nebraska Neuropsychological Battery to provide a functional profile of a client and to assist in treatment planning.

Practitioners are continually judging the type of assessments used to determine the most suitable type for generating the information needed. In order to get a more comprehensive overview of the type of assessments used in practice, refer to chapter 11.

Program Development

Entire programs have been developed to address specific performance areas, disabilities, and diseases occurring with aging. A complete issue of the journal, *Physical and Occupational Therapy in Geriatrics*, was devoted to the identification and description of innovative programs for impaired elderly individuals (Killeffer, Bennett, & Gruen, 1984). Some examples of how the gerontic occupational therapy practitioner role has expanded with program development to address performance area deficits are driver evaluation (Kerr, 1995), work therapy (Griffin & Mouheb, 1987; Ward, 1971), gardening programs, ADL skill maintenance programs, and social adjustment programs.

Roles for occupational therapy practitioners related to specific diseases, disabilities and conditions are extensive. Some examples are day treatment and respite programs for persons with dementia (Rabinowitz,1986), stroke education classes (Evans, Held, Kleinman, & Halar, 1985), hospice for the terminally ill (Oelrich, 1974; Pizzi, 1983), and programs to prevent and treat depression (Taira,1986).

TREATMENT MODALITIES

Treatment modalities have expanded for the gerontic occupational therapist. As described earlier, initially craft and work activities were the primary treatment modalities. With the rehabilitation era came the use of homemaker activities and activities of daily living. Biomechanical and neurodevelopmental treatment approaches were also used with aging individuals with diagnoses such as stroke and rheumatoid arthritis. These included such approaches as splinting, exercise (Riccio, Nelson, & Bush, 1990), and use of Brunnstrom (Pedretti, 1996a) or Bobath (Davis, 1996) techniques.

The modern era brought in the use of treatment modalities such as use of poetry (Curley, 1982), computers (O' Leary, Mann, & Perkash, 1991; Zemke,1986), use of reminiscences to promote social skills (Buechel, 1986), pet therapy, and reality orientation to promote satisfactory life adjustment. Treatment was not only provided to address psychosocial and cognitive deficits, but also to address the physical impairments due to aging and many different disease processes. Some of these treatment modalities included wheelchair sitting posture (Herzberg, 1993; Shafer & Washburn, 1986), adaptive equipment (Bennett, 1989; Breuer, 1982; Mann, Hurren, & Tomita, 1993), energy conservation and work simplification, and dysphagia assessment and treatment (Lewis, 1989b).

The perspective of the independent living movement is now applied to elderly individuals. The environment is seen as the aspect that needs to change to promote the independence of the elderly person. Models of practice have been written from a perspective of the environment being the primary focus. Kiernat (1982) suggested that the environment be viewed as another modality to be shaped to promote the client's independence. The environment has particularly been emphasized as a compensation method for the person with Alzheimer's or a dementia (Skolaski-Pellitteri, 1983). Some examples are using labeling and signs to cue the client and conducting evaluations for safety for the clients with dementia or a physical deficit.

Gerontic occupational therapy knowledge has expanded as practitioners have shared their clinical experience through research, and in part, in collaboration with other health professionals working with older adults. Models of practice and frames of reference have been explored to determine how they apply to work with the aging person. The development of the knowledge has included understanding physiological and psychosocial changes occurring with aging, with a developmental perspective. A wide array of activities and functionally based skills and treatment interventions have evolved. Programs have developed to encompass well elderly persons and those with specific skill deficits or specific disease processes. To share concerns and expertise, occupational therapy practitioners have joined together in the Gerontology Special Interest Section, and to further pass on our knowledge to future generations of practitioners, experts in the field have developed the *Role of Occupational Therapy with the Elderly* (ROTE).

GERONTOLOGY SPECIAL INTEREST SECTION AND THE ROLE OF OCCUPATIONAL THERAPY WITH THE ELDERLY (ROTE)

Special interest sections were initially established in 1976 and 1977 by the American Occupational Therapy Association. The purpose of the special interest sections, as stated by a new bylaw established in 1976, is to:

1. Develop knowledge and skills in specific areas of occupational therapy practice

2. Promote continuing education, publications, and research within each Special Interest Section

3. Function as a resource or collaborate with any member of the association

4. Respond to emerging issues, both internal and external to the association, as they relate to specialty areas of occupational therapy (Loar, 1979).

The first chairperson of the Gerontology Special Interest Section was appointed in 1977. By 1978, the membership numbered 1,860 (Chermak, 1978). The structure is designed to support the practitioner. There is a standing committee that coordinates efforts made by the entire special interest section. There is a list of practitioners in the field who have volunteered to share their expertise in specific areas of gerontic occupational therapy. On a statewide level, there is a designated state liaison, available to discuss issues and represent practitioners at a national level. The Gerontology Special Interest Section also meets annually at the American Occupational Therapy Association Conference to discuss pertinent issues in practice.

Several articles in the occupational therapy literature seem to suggest that within the profession there was some question regarding the actual need for a geriatric specialty. In support of the Gerontology Special Interest Section, Joan Rogers (1981) described the occupational therapist who works in the area of geriatrics as the master specialist, a practitioner who requires skills from many areas of practice and requires knowledge of gerontology and geriatric medicine. Hasselkus and Kiernat (1989) described the aging individual as experiencing a complex developmental stage within the context of age-related physical and psychosocial changes, such as sensory losses and family transitions. There is also a changing balance of time spent in work, play and self-care. As with other specialty areas, the gerontic occupational therapist requires a knowledge of the developmental stage of the individual being treated, applied in unison with skills practiced by many of the other specialty areas.

The Gerontology Special Interest Section supports a range of information about specific skills and program development, integrating frames of reference with gerontic occupational therapy practice, the normal aging process, quality of care issues, reimbursement and legislative issues, and current research. The special interest section serves as a resource on literature, research, and practice issues. Members are encouraged to get involved in other organizations that also work with the elderly, so that the practitioner has new resources from which to learn and other health practitioners can be enlightened about the contribution occupational therapy practitioners can make to the care of the aging person. The newsletter has provided a forum for occupational therapy practitioners to share ideas and knowledge and to recognize that working with the aging individual requires a unique blend of skills and knowledge.

In order to ensure an ongoing contribution to the knowledge of geriatrics and gerontology and to ensure quality of care for the client, educating the occupational therapy practitioner is a concern. Several models of teaching have been presented in the literature. Models of teaching have been both didactic and experiential, such as development of interdisciplinary teamwork (Miller, 1988), teaching clinical reasoning through self-talk (Rogers, 1982), and combining coursework, research and clinical practice (Breines, 1992; Maynard, 1986). Gerontological content needs to be integrated into the occupational therapy course curricu-

lum in order to prepare entry-level occupational therapy practitioners to serve the older client (Stone & Mertens, 1991).

Teaching materials were developed in the late 1970s (Lewis, 1979) and continue to be developed in the field of practice (Kiernat, 1991a; Lewis, 1989). In response to a need for a more comprehensive approach to teaching about work with the aging person the *Role of Occupational Therapy With the Elderly* (Davis & Kirkland, 1986) was compiled and written by experts in the field. The curriculum was produced under a grant from the U.S. Department of Health and Human Services, Office of Human Development Services, Administration on Aging. It was soon followed by a guide to be used by faculty to assist with application of the information in undergraduate and graduate level courses (Brooks, Davis, Kirkland, & Nystrom, 1987).

The first edition involved a multi-step process to determine the content of the curriculum. First, a literature review was completed covering a multitude of topics, including education standards, terminology, role delineations, and multidisciplinary books and journals.

Next, a survey was conducted of occupational therapists and occupational therapy assistants to identify work roles and functions and to identify basic compentencies needed to work with the aging individual. One of the aspects that makes this publication unique is the development of gerontic practice competencies. The competencies could potentially be used by fieldwork practices to evaluate student training and as a model for curriculum design for gerontic occupational therapy practitioners.

The occupational therapy department at the State University of New

York at Buffalo surveyed entry-level occupational therapy students. The survey results were used to determine the extent of gerontological training among faculty and the content of entry-level education about aging.

The final phase in preparation for writing the ROTE was having a national panel of experts review the data collected to determine roles and functions of the gerontic occupational therapy practitioner.

Future Trends

The U.S. Bureau of Labor Statistics, which tracks the nation's labor force, projected occupational therapy to be among the 20 fastest growing professions from 1992 to 2005. An estimated growth of between 53 and 62% was predicted from 1992 to 2005. The estimated growth for the same period for Certified Occupational Therapy Assistants and Occupational Therapy Aides was about 78% (Silvergleit, 1994a).

The data are not available to identify the exclusive need for occupational therapists in the field of geriatrics. The demographics of the population demonstrate that the number of older adults is increasing significantly. If occupational therapists stay true to historical trends of filling a need once it is identified, the tendency will be for an increasing number of occupational therapy practitioners to provide services to elderly persons.

The future path for the field of gerontic occupational therapy provides an array of choices and possibilities for how practice may evolve. Therapists' response to the outside forces of managed health care and potential legislative changes, modifying current Medicare and Medicaid guidelines, will alter practice. Practice will evolve based

on occupational therapy practitioners' ability to identify the effects of occupational therapy intervention especially in terms of function and to support the significance of their activity. Occupational therapists' ability to market themselves and provide a vision for future occupational therapists will also affect how practice will evolve. Occupational therapists' response to the aging individual as the center of practice may also alter practice. There is a need to stress quality of life and consider its impact on the individual.

Managed Health Care

Our future role as practitioners with the aging person is being molded from outside the practice by the managed health care movement. Managed health care is reforming how care is typically provided. Services are being streamlined, there is an increased demand to validate outcomes of services provided, and costs and services are being cut.

Managed health care creates a difficult balancing act. The heaviest users of health care services typically are older individuals. Thus, as the aging population increases, the demands on the health care system are greater. On one hand, there is a demand for services, and on the other, a demand to cut costs. Managed health care is attempting to reduce costs through health maintenance and rehabilitation, therefore avoiding more costly acute care. There is a demand that health care practitioners understand and support the rationale for treatment and services. There is a shift in emphasis from reimbursement based on physician prescribed services to management of the health of the patient.

Services such as occupational therapy now become a critical component in the continuum of health maintenance and illness or disability prevention. Multidisciplinary standards of care and critical pathways are being developed to determine the most effective treatment intervention for specific diagnoses. There is a demand to demonstrate effectiveness of treatment through outcome criteria that are functionally based and prove cost effectiveness (Foto, 1995). Managed health care can appear to be a formidable monster, overcoming practice, or it can be viewed as an opportunity to support the roots and basis for occupational therapy practice.

Function and Activity

The focus in the gerontology community is on the function of the aging person. Occupational therapists have assumed that all other health professionals understand that occupational therapy's primary concern is function. This has been a naive viewpoint. Because occupational therapists have not made their role obvious, other professionals have attempted to fill the role. It is imperative at this point that each professional considers how he or she presents the scope of occupational therapy practice. This is an opportune moment, as the fields of gerontology and geriatrics are growing and health care is reformed, to provide a solid picture of what occupational therapy has to offer to the aging person.

In order to support the importance of function there is a need to research "normal" function in the areas of self-care, work, and leisure. In the specialty area of pediatrics there are parameters for what is considered normal development, and parameters of "normal" activity for the older adult are needed in the areas of self-care, work, and leisure. Results of the research could only be applied as guidelines, as there are many other factors that could influence function. In the realm of function, occupational therapists must consider the importance of using standardized testing to document progress and the impact of treatment. As the aging client passes through the continuum of care, from therapist to therapist, and ADL evaluation to ADL evaluation, there is inconsistency in the data collection methods. If there was continuity in the assessment tools used, data could be collected about the effectiveness of occupational therapy.

In the same vein as researching function, the significance of activity needs further research. Occupational therapists consider theirs to be an activity based practice but need further proof about the effect activity has on the individual. This is particularly true of the significance of activity in maintaining mental health and quality of life. The physical aspects of activity are continually being researched. For example, cardiovascular exercise has been researched sufficiently to show how a given amount of physical activity increases longevity. But there is little research on the effect of activity on aging individuals' perception of themselves and their outlook on life, and therefore its impact on quality of life.

Quality of life issues will come to the forefront of practice as the aging population increases. Because chronic disability increases with age, occupational therapy practitioners must consider how their practice can impact prevention of chronic disability. Can occupational therapists evaluate the well elderly person's activity in terms of risk factors that may lead to chronic disability? After gathering an occupational history and identifying problem activities, the occupational therapy practitioner could teach and advise the client on methods to change behavior that could potentially prevent chronic disability.

Many occupational therapy referrals are generated from acute medical problems, when the aging individual actually could have benefitted from services much earlier. In the mode of preventing chronic disability or inability to participate in selected activities, isn't there a need for the occupational therapist to provide treatment and interventions prior to severe limitations? For example, an older person with limitations in activity due to degenerative joint disease may become depressed due to inactivity. This person may not be referred to occupational therapy until he or she has a hip arthroplasty, when in actuality the person could have used intervention much earlier. Early intervention could have ensured that the individual maintained activity with self-care, leisure, and work activities. Activities could be prioritized according to those most significant to the individual and according to those that cause the greatest or least joint stress. The occupational therapist could then recommend modification to activities. Occupational therapy will not prevent a potential hip arthroplasty, but may prevent depression and unnecessary inactivity. This in turn could result in a patient who has a more positive affect before entering surgery because he or she has not been totally inactive, and therefore this person may recover more easily from surgery. Early intervention conforms with the Model of Human Occupation's premise that individuals need to maintain a sense of competency and control over their lives in order to continue to live with purpose and dignity (Kielhofner & Burke, 1983). This example also supports the premise that managed health care is attempting to promote with early intervention and a more cost-effective treatment approach.

PATIENT AND FAMILY EDUCATION

As our society becomes more and more culturally diverse, the future requires that occupational therapists consider the influence of culture on the entire process of working with a client. Attention to the client's cultural background is not entirely new, but bears repeating as it is still not integrated totally into the evaluation process. There is a need for sensitivity regarding the client's needs and goals. For example, some cultures may not highly value independence as a goal as a person ages. In fact, time to spend sharing life experience and wisdom may be the priority. This client may need assistance with self-care. The occupational therapist must then reevaluate his or her role. In this situation, the emphasis may be on teaching the family or caregivers how to care for the aging individual. Respecting cultural differences is an important aspect in supporting the individual's sense of control over his or her environment, thus supporting maintenance of quality of life.

Care for the elderly individual has brought to the forefront the integral need to include the family in treatment. Approximately 95% of elderly persons live in the community; therefore, it is imperative to include education of the family or caregiver as a primary treatment goal. Shortened lengths of stay and transitions to a number of health settings prior to discharge home have made the issue of patient and family education more complex. There is frequently little time to teach in the acute care setting, and in long-term care facilities, family instruction is often put off until just before discharge. At the time of discharge families are frequently overwhelmed with information and the degree of comprehension and retention is questionable.

Families need to be involved from the beginning of care. Goals need to be set by the family and the patient. This poses a difficult problem because families often do not have the background to see the elderly person's potential for independence. Therefore, their goals may be short-sighted or the family may lack the knowledge to understand the client's deficits and so may have unrealistic expectations. The therapist must have skill in presenting the client's potential to the family and allow the family to participate in therapy early on so they can appreciate the progress of the aging individual and develop realistic expectations of the patient's personal care needs.

ADVOCATING OCCUPATIONAL THERAPY

As the need for services increases, there is an increasing shortage of occupational therapy personnel. The American Occupational Therapy Association projects the shortage of occupational therapists to be around 35 to 40% (Silvergleit, 1994b). In order to fill the need for services while there is a shortage of personnel, a reformation of the occupational therapist's role is required. There is a need for occupational therapists to take the lead as case managers. Occupational therapists have the variety of skills needed to manage patients whose primary needs are functionally based. To implement this role, the issue of occupational therapists as primary referral sources (Foto, 1995) and as primary care providers must be addressed. Currently, in the home health setting, according to Medicare guidelines, an occupational therapist is not permitted to be a case manager or open a case without a physical therapist or nurse on the case. Filtering occupational therapy referrals through other health professionals leaves it up to others to determine the need for occupational therapy. Several recommendations are posed, including the need to change the current Medicare guideline and the need for each occupational therapist to educate the staff who may be determining the need for occupational therapy. Occupational therapists have the potential to be excellent case managers for individuals with functional deficits and perhaps are better suited because they straddle medical, psycho-social, and environmental boundaries.

As the concept of managed health care has evolved, the image of a multi-skilled caregiver has developed. To prevent duplication of services and improve continuity of care, the concept of combining the roles of health professionals has been considered. This brings up an enormous amount of uncertainty among health professionals. It is unclear whether the implementation of a multiskilled caregiver means entirely eliminating one profession or combining two professions.

Certainly, there is something to be said for simplifying the number of providers working with one elderly individual. Patients are frequently unsure as to what each professional's role involves and instruction from many different professionals can be inconsistent and confusing. On the other hand, does one profession—nursing, physical therapy, or occupational therapy—have the breadth of knowledge and skill to be the primary provider to a client who has not only medical and physical needs but functional and emotional deficits? To clarify this question, occupational therapy practitioners need to clearly define their scope of practice, areas of expertise, and level of services (skilled versus nonskilled) that they are able to provide (Foto, 1995).

In some cases, as with the need to screen for services, the occupational therapist could be considered the multiskilled caregiver. As hospital stays shorten, patients are being screened for functional deficits in the emergency rooms. The occupational therapist has the skill to evaluate the client from an emotional, cognitive, perceptual, and physical perspective to determine if a client could return home safely or if further inpatient rehabilitation services are needed.

For example, an elderly individual may be admitted to the hospital or emergency room for a medical condition that has actually evolved because the patient was depressed and failed to take medication. The occupational therapist has skills in assessing both the cognitive and physical changes associated with the medical condition and in determining the type of interventions needed. An occupational therapist could also apply these same skills in other scenarios, such as for the client in a residential facility who has had a change in function. The client may have a change in sleep patterns, reduced interest in activities, increased tearfulness, and somatic complaints. The occupational therapist could screen the client for cognitive and emotional deficits that may be contributing to the change in function. Recommendations for more specific evaluation by a psychiatrist or psychologist may be made to determine if the client actually has an evolving case of dementia or is depressed. These case examples demonstrate how an occupational therapist could function in the role of screening a client for physical, perceptual, cognitive, and emotional deficits, thus making recommendations for a client to receive further rehabilitation services and potentially services from other medical personnel.

Education

Educating future occupational therapists about gerontic occupational therapy is imperative. Many new graduates are entering the field and immediately working with the elderly as there are many job openings in the field. The new practitioner must be equipped with the knowledge, skills, and sensitivity to provide satisfactory treatment. Knowledge of geriatrics and gerontology can be integrated into the current curriculum. For example, human development courses can be designed to give the same weight to the development of the aging adult as is given to other developmental stages. Skill courses can integrate case studies involving older persons into skill practice and discuss special considerations regarding sensory and cognitive changes with treatment for the aging person. Medical conditions courses can discuss the complexity of medical conditions of the older adult, not as if these conditions occur individually, but with the focus that they often occur simultaneously. Courses about psychiatric and psychosocial disorders can integrate changes that occur with aging with cognitive and potential emotional changes, as well as the complex social dynamics of the aging person and the family. Practicum and fieldwork sites can be created that offer experience with the aging adult. More specifically, specialty fieldwork sites in gerontic occupational therapy for the certified occupational therapy assistant and occupational therapist can be offered. Colleges and universities can support fieldwork supervisors by providing continuing education about student supervision and gerontic occupational therapy. Instructors and experienced gerontic occupational therapists need to pass on the vision that occupational therapists are facilitators of adaptation and that the elderly client has potential for change. Occupational therapists have the knowledge and skills to promote adaptation to physical, emotional, sensory-perceptual, and cognitive changes by working with the client and the family.

Summary

The historical perspective demonstrates that occupational therapy's roots are based in activity and that occupational therapy practitioners anticipated early on the greater need for more services for elderly persons. Many practitioners and educators have contributed to the growth of the knowledge base of gerontic occupational therapy. Contributions have been made regarding knowledge of normal aging, models of practice and application to the elderly, the evaluation process, program and role development, treatment methods, and educational models. Our national organization, AOTA, acknowledges the special skills and knowledge needed by the gerontic occupational therapist by supporting the Gerontology Special Interest Section. *Role of the Occupational Therapist with the Elderly* was developed when a need for educational material to teach entry level therapists about gerontic occupational therapy was identified. ROTE was developed with contributions from many occupational therapy practitioners in the community, with the support of the American Occupational Therapy Association, and with support of a federal grant.

The future of the practice of gerontic occupational therapy appears quite challenging. Occupational therapists need to work with others in the health care community to promote a managed health care system that meets the needs of aging clients. Clinicians and educators need to research the founda-tions of occupational therapy practice—both the function and the benefits of activity. Occupational therapists must learn to document the outcome of occupational therapy intervention. Families and cultural differences need to be considered when providing services to elderly persons. Occupational therapists must continue to educate team members about their roles and take on the challenge of creating new roles, such as that of case manager or possibly multiskilled caregiver. A proactive approach will help ensure the growth of, and ongoing contributions by, gerontic occupational therapy practitioners.

Activities

1. Find one article written prior to the 1970s about the physiological or psychological changes that occur with aging and one article on the same topic written in the 1980s and/or 1990s. Is there a difference in the understanding of how aging changes are portrayed? How is the information the same? How is the information different?
2. Review three to four issues of the *Gerontology Special Interest Newsletter*. What are the primary issues regarding practice? Is a trend reflected from newsletter to newsletter?

Review Questions

1. How have occupational therapists contributed to the knowledge base of gerontic occupational therapy?
2. What are some of the issues facing gerontic occupational therapy in the future?
3. What effect has the Gerontology Special Interest Section and the development of ROTE had on the practice of occupational therapy?
4. Describe some specific examples of how gerontic occupational therapy practice has changed since the 1970s.

References

Ager, C. (1986). Teaching strategies for the elderly. *Physical and Occupational Therapy in Geriatrics, 4,* 3–14.

Allen, C. K. (1992). Modes of performance within the cognitive levels. In: Allen, C. K., Earhart, C. A., & Blue, T. (1992). *Occupational Therapy Treatment Goals for the Physically and Cognitively Disabled.* Rockville, MD: The American Occupational Therapy Association, Inc., 85–102.

American Occupational Therapy Association. (1987). *Occupational therapy medicare handbook.* Rockville, MD: Author.

Americans with Disabilities Act of 1990. (Public Law 101–336), 42 U.S.C. 12101.

Andiel, C., & Liu, L. (1995) Working memory and older adults: Implications for occupational therapy. *American Journal of Occupational Therapy, 49,* 681–686.

Bachelder, J. (1994). Implications of the Americans with Disabilities Act of 1990 for elderly persons. *American Journal of Occupational Therapy, 48,* 73–81.

Barney, K. (1991). From Ellis Island to assisted living: Meeting the needs of older adults from diverse cultures. *American Journal of Occupational Therapy, 45,* 586–593.

Barrett, C. (1986). In search of brain-behavior relationships in dementia and the Luria-Nebraska neuropsychological battery. *Physical and Occupational Therapy in Geriatrics, 4,* 113–139.

Baum, C. (1991). Addressing the needs of the cognitively impaired elderly from a family policy perspective. *American Journal of Occupational Therapy, 45,* 594–606.

Bennett, S. (1989). Low vision aids for the elderly: An overview for occupational therapy personnel. *Physical and Occupational Therapy in Geriatrics, 12,* 4–5.

Bonder, B. (1986). Family systems and Alzheimer's Disease: An approach to treatment. *Physical and Occupational Therapy in Geriatrics, 5,* 13–24.

Breines, E. (1992). Preparing occupational therapy students for practice with the elderly. *Physical and Occupational Therapy in Geriatrics, 10,* 47–55.

Breuer, J. (1982). A handbook of assistive devices for the handicapped elderly: A new help for independent living. *Physical and Occupational Therapy in Geriatrics, 1.*

Brooks, B., Davis, L., Kirkland, M., & Nystrom, E. (Eds.). (1987). *ROTE II: The role of occupational therapy with the elderly: Faculty guide.* Rockville, MD: American Occupational Therapy Association.

Buechel, H. (1986). Reminiscence: A review and prospectus. *Physical and Occupational Therapy in Geriatrics, 5,* 25–37.

Chermak, J. (1978). Membership and organization of section. *Gerontology Specialty Section Newsletter, 1,* 1–2.

Clark, C., Corcoran, M., & Gitlin, L. (1995). An exploratory study of how occupational therapists develop relationships with family caregivers. *American Journal of Occupational Therapy, 49,* 587–594.

Cristella, M. (1977). Visual functions of the elderly. *American Journal of Occupational Therapy, 31,* 432–440.

Curley, J. (1982). Leading poetry writing groups in a nursing home activities program. *Physical and Occupational Therapy in Geriatrics, 1,* 23–34.

Davis, J. (1996). Neurodevelopmental treatment of adult hemiplegia: The Bobath approach. In L. Pedretti (Ed.), *Occupational therapy practice skills for physical dysfunction.* St. Louis, MO: Mosby.

Davis, L., & Kirkland, M. (Eds.). (1986). *The role of occupational therapy with the elderly (ROTE).* Bethesda, MD: American Occupational Therapy Association.

Dorfman, C., & Ager, C. (1989). Memory and memory training: Some treatment implications for use with the well elderly. *Physical and Occupational Therapy in Geriatrics 7,* 21–41.

Evans, R., Held, S., Kleinman, L., & Halar, E. (1985). Family stroke education: Increasing patient and family involvement in rehabilitation. *Physical and Occupational Therapy in Geriatrics, 2,* 63–72.

Falconer, J. (1985–1986). Aging and hearing. *Physical and Occupational Therapy in Geriatrics, 4,* 3–20.

Fisher, A. G. (1993). The assessment of IADL motor skills: An application of many-faceted Rasch analysis. *American Journal of Occupational Therapy, 47,* 319–338.

Foto, M. (1995). New president's address: The future—challenges, choices, and changes. *American Journal of Occupational Therapy, 49,* 955–959.

Foy, S., & Mitchell, M. (1990). Factors contributing to learned helplessness in the institutionalized aged: A literature review. *Physical and Occupational Therapy in Geriatrics, 9,* 1–23.

Gregg, J., & Sherrill, S. (1957). Eye problems of aging patients. *American Journal of Occupational Therapy, 11,* 313–319, 339.

Griffin, R., & Mouheb, F. (1987). Work therapy as a treatment modality for the elderly patient with dementia. *Physical and Occupational Therapy in Geriatrics, 5,* 67–72.

Hasselkus, B. (1974). Aging and the human nervous system. *American Journal of Occupational Therapy, 28,* 16–21.

Hasselkus, B. (1982). Barthel self-care index and geriatric home care patients. *Physical and Occupational Therapy in Geriatrics, 1,* 11–22.

Hasselkus, B. (1989). The meaning of daily activity in family caregiving for the elderly. *American Journal of Occupational Therapy, 43,* 649–656.

Hasselkus, B., & Kiernat, J. (1989). Not by age alone: Gerontology as a specialty in occupational therapy. *American Journal of Occupational Therapy, 43,* 77–79.

Herzberg, S. (1993). Positioning the nursing home resident: An issue of quality of life. *American Journal of Occupational Therapy, 47,* 75–77.

Hildenbrand, G. (1947). Geriatrics and occupational therapy. *American Journal of Occupational Therapy, 1,* 159–161.

Hildenbrand, G. (1949a). Found horizons for the aging. *American Journal of Occupational Therapy, 3,* 128–133.

Hildenbrand, G. (1949b). Geriatrics and economic plight of our aging. *American Journal of Occupational Therapy, 3,* 137–139.

Hildenbrand, G. (1953). Psychological problems with geriatric patients. *American Journal of Occupational Therapy, 7,* 68, 80–81.

Kaplan, J. (1957). The social care of older persons in nursing homes. *American Journal of Occupational Therapy, 11,* 240–243.

Kehrberg, K., Kuskowski, M., Mortimer, J., & Shoberg, T. (1992). Validating the use of an enlarged easier-to-see Allen Cognitive Levels Test in geriatrics. *Physical and Occupational Therapy in Geriatrics, 10,* 1–14.

Kerr, T. (1995). Driving home some points about road safety. *Advance for Occupational Therapists, 11*(35), 13, 16.

Kielhofner, G. (1985). *Model of human occupation: Theory and practice.* Baltimore: Williams & Wilkins.

Kielhofner, G., & Burke, J. (1983). The evolution of knowledge and practice in occupational therapy: Past, present and future. In G. Kielhofner (Ed.), *Health through occupation: Theory and practice in occupational therapy* (pp. 3–54). Philadelphia: Davis.

Kiernat, J. (1982). Environment: The hidden modality. *Physical and Occupational Therapy in Geriatrics 2,* 3–12.

Kiernat, J. (Ed.). (1991a). *Occupational therapy and the older adult.* Gaithersburg, MD: Aspen.

Kiernat, J. (1991b). The rewards and challenges of working with older adults. In Kiernat, J., *Occupational therapy and the older adult* (pp. 2–10). Gaithersburg, MD: Aspen.

Killeffer, E., Bennett, R., & Gruen, G. (1984). Handbook of innovative programs for the impaired elderly. *Physical and Occupational Therapy in Geriatrics, 3.*

King, W. (1951). Progressive steps in geriatrics. *American Journal of Occupational Therapy, 5,* 110–112.

Kirchman, M., & Schulte. (1989). A study of morale in the elderly. *Physical and Occupational Therapy in Geriatrics, 7,* 29–41.

Lakin, M., & Dray, M. (1958). Psychological aspects of activity for the aged. *American Journal of Occupational Therapy, 12,* 172–187.

Lang, V., & Waterman, T. (1959). Geriatrics as a community problem. *American Journal of Occupational Therapy, 13,* 121–124.

Lewis, S. (1979). *The mature years: A geriatric occupational therapy text.* Thorofare, NJ: SLACK.

Lewis, S. (Ed.). (1989a). *Elder care in occupational therapy.* Thorofare, NJ: SLACK.

Lewis, S. (1989b). Modalities and treatment in occupational therapy. In S. Lewis (Ed.), *Elder care in occupational therapy.* Thorofare, NJ: SLACK.

Loar, B. (1979). The gerontology specialty section: An historical view. *Gerontology Specialty Section Newsletter, 2,* 2.

Maloney, C. (1987). Identifying and treating the client with sensory loss. *Physical and Occupational Therapy in Geriatrics, 4,* 31–46.

Mann, W., Hurren, D., & Tomita, M. (1993). Comparison of assistive device use and needs of home-based older persons with different impairments. *American Journal of Occupational Therapy, 47,* 980–987.

Maynard, M. (1986). An experiential learning approach: Utilizing historical interview and an occupational inventory. *Physical and Occupational Therapy in Geriatrics 5,* 51–69.

Mazer, J. (1969). The occupational therapist as consultant. *American Journal of Occupational Therapy, 23,* 417–421.

McCormack, G., Llorens, L., & Glogoski, C. (1991). Culturally diverse elders. In J. Kiernat (Ed.), *Occupational therapy and the older adult.* Gaithersburg, MD: Aspen.

McGrath, L. (1983). Functional low vision assessment. *Physical and Occupational Therapy in Geriatrics, 3,* 55–59.

Meeske, R., & Jacoby, R. (1952). Occupational therapy in home care. *American Journal of Occupational Therapy, 6,* 9–12, 32.

Mendoza, N. (1969). The role of occupational therapy in a home setting. *American Journal of Occupational Therapy, 23,* 141–144.

Miller, P. (1986). Models for treatment of depression. *Physical and Occupational Therapy in Geriatrics 5,* 3–12.

Miller, P. (1988). Teaching process: Its importance in geriatric teamwork. *Physical and Occupational Therapy in Geriatrics, 6,* 121–131.

Moss, F., & Stewart, G. (1959). A program for geriatric patients from hospital to community. *American Journal of Occupational Therapy, 13,* 268–271.

Murphy, L. (1949). Problems in geriatrics and chronic illness. *American Journal of Occupational Therapy, 3,* 134–137.

Oelrich, M. (1974). The patient with a fatal illness. *American Journal of Occupational Therapy, 28,* 429–432.

O'Leary, S., Mann, C., & Perkash, I. (1991). Access to computers for older adults: Problems and solutions. *American Journal of Occupational Therapy, 45,* 636–642.

Olin, D. (1984). Assessing and assisting the persons with dementia: An occupational behavior perspective. *Physical and Occupational Therapy in Geriatrics, 3,* 25–32.

Pearman, H., & Newman, N. (1968). Work-oriented occupational therapy for the geriatric patient. *American Journal of Occupational Therapy, 22,* 300–303.

Pedretti, L. (1996a). Movement therapy: The Brunnstrom approach to treatment of hemiplegia. In L. Pedretti (Ed.), *Occupational therapy practice skills for physical dysfunction.* St. Louis, MO: Mosby.

Pedretti, L. (1996b). Occupational performance: A model for practice in physical dysfunction. In L. Pedretti (Ed.), *Occupational therapy practice skills for physical dysfunction.* St. Louis, MO: Mosby.

Pincus, A. (1968). New findings on learning in old age: Implications for occupational therapy. *American Journal of Occupational Therapy, 22,* 300–303.

Pizzi, M. (1983). Hospice and the terminally ill geriatric patient. *Physical and Occupational Therapy in Geriatrics, 3,* 45–54.

Rabinowitz, E. (1986). Day care and Alzheimer's disease: A weekend program in New York City. *Physical and Occupational Therapy in Geriatrics, 4,* 95–103.

Raphael, E. (1988). Grandparents: A study of their role in Hispanic families. *Physical and Occupational Therapy in Geriatrics, 6,* 31–62.

Riccio, C., Nelson, D., & Bush, M. (1990). Adding purpose to the repetitive exercise of elderly women through imagery. *American Journal of Occupational Therapy, 44,* 714–719.

Rogers, J. (1981). The issue: Gerontic occupational therapy. *American Journal of Occupational Therapy, 35,* 663–666.

Rogers, J. (1982). Teaching clinical reasoning for practice in geriatrics. *Physical and Occupational Therapy in Geriatrics, 1,* 29–37.

Rogers, J. (1986). Occupational therapy assessment for older adults with depression: Asking the right questions. *Physical and Occupational Therapy in Geriatrics, 5,* 13–33.

Schroepfer, M. (1961). A state occupational therapy program for the aged. *American Journal of Occupational Therapy, 15,* 145–148.

Shafer, A., & Washburn, B. (1986). Applications of materials technology in solving familiar problems in nursing homes. *Physical and Occupational Therapy in Geriatrics, 4,* 61–68.

Silvergleit, I. (1994a, September 8). The work force of the '90's. *Occupational Therapy Weekly,* 20–23.

Silvergleit, I. (1994b, September 15). The high demand for OTR's and OTA's. *Occupational Therapy Weekly*, 20–22.

Skolaski-Pellitteri, T. (1983). Environmental adaptations which compensate for dementia. *Physical and Occupational Therapy in Geriatrics, 3*, 31–44.

Spackman, C. (1968). A history of the practice of occupational therapy for restoration of physical dysfunction: 1917–1967. *American Journal of Occupational Therapy, 22*, 67–71.

Stone, R., & Mertens, K. (1991). Educating entry-level occupational therapy students in gerontology. *American Journal of Occupational Therapy, 45*, 643–650.

Taira, E. (Ed.). (1986). Community programs for the depressed elderly: A rehabilitation approach. *Physical and Occupational Therapy in Geriatrics, 5*.

Teitelman, J. (1982). Eliminating learned helplessness in older rehabilitation patients. *Physical and Occupational Therapy in Geriatrics 1*, 3–10.

Tendo, H. (1961). Occupational therapy for the aged psychiatric patient. *American Journal of Occupational Therapy, 15*, 153–156.

Walker, A. (1963). Occupational therapy in geriatrics. In H. Willard & C. Spackman (Eds.), *Occupational therapy* (3rd ed., 157–166). Philadelphia: Lippincott.

Ward, R. (1971). Review of research related to work activities for aged residents of long-term-care institutions. *American Journal of Occupational Therapy, 25*, 348–351.

Wiemer, R., & West, W. (1970). Occupational therapy in community health care. *American Journal of Occupational Therapy, 24*, 323–325.

Willard & Spackman, (Eds.). (1963). *Occupational therapy* (3rd ed.). Philadelphia: Lippincott.

Zemke, R. (1986). Taking a byte of the apple: Computer activities in a senior day care center. *Physical and Occupational Therapy in Geriatrics 4*, 39–48.

Section 3. Maturation: Development of the Older Adult

Joseph Cipriani, MA, OTR/L

Abstract

The author discusses various theories of development in older adults, including the biophysical, cognitive, affective, and social domains.

Introduction

Development can be defined as changes in the structure, thought, and behavior of a person as a function of both biological and environmental influences (Craig, 1989). The related concept of *maturation* refers to achieving full or optional development of a component or skill (Schuster, 1992). The number of influences that can affect the development of an organism as complex as the human being is extraordinary. Using a holistic approach, Schuster (1992c) defined five major domains in which human developmental change occurs: biophysical, cognitive, affective, social, and spiritual. Because developmental theories attempt to explain in what ways a person changes, and sometimes how the changes occur, theory and research in human development represent an important knowledge base for the profession of occupational therapy. For example, by understanding normal developmental processes, a therapist can recognize abnormal function and engage in an intervention process that can help "normalize" the developmental interruption (Simon & Daub, 1993).

Early theory and research in human development tended to focus on infancy through adolescence. Older adulthood, if conceptualized at all, was seen as a period of stagnation or adjustment to declining function. The advent of research in gerontology helped significantly to change perspectives on the older adult. Currently, human development can be viewed as a *lifelong process*, in which an organism is engaged in adaptation with the environment from the moment of conception to death. Breines (1989) noted that understanding how developmental change occurs is critical for occupational therapists, because change is the essence of adaptation, and adaptation is a core concept of the profession.

Because there is not yet an all-encompassing theory of human development that effectively integrates the process of change within and among the five domains of development, each existing theory provides information on one domain or part of a domain. These theories for the older adult can be described as primarily biophysical, personality, or social.

Biophysical Theories

For the older adult, one category of theories attempts to explain the process of aging. Aging is referred to as a universal, biologically based process that occurs with the passage of time alone (Davis, 1986). In essence, these theories attempt to explain the physical process of aging up to death. Biological theories of aging address questions such as how cells age, what triggers the process of aging, and what age-related processes occur independently of pathological or external influences (Miller, 1992). A sampling of these theories follows, as described by Ashburn (1992).

BIOLOGICAL PROGRAMMING THEORY

In this theory, an aging chronometer (biological clock) exists that controls the speed of metabolic processes, and ultimately aging. Locations of this aging control center have been hypothesized to be in the brain or individual cells.

FREE RADICAL THEORY

Here, free radicals are formed as by-products of normal cellular processes. These chemicals alter molecules of cell membranes, and also cause chromosomal mutations. Cumulative effects are gradual contributions to changes associated with aging.

CROSS-LINKAGE THEORY

This theory proposes that with age the molecular strands of selected cellular proteins (i.e., DNA, collagen, enzymes) connect crosswise. Over time, with the formation of new cross-links, these proteins are altered structurally and functionally. These alterations can cause failures in related cells, tissues, and organs.

GENE THEORY

In this view, one or more genes are programmed to initiate or stop functioning of specific processes throughout a person's life span. It is used to explain correlation data on longevity over generations within families.

AUTOIMMUNE THEORIES

These theories propose that as age advances, the immune system begins to form antibodies against its own proteins, incorrectly identifying them as antigens. In essence, the immune system of a person's body attacks and destroys its own body cells.

No biological theory of aging is universally accepted by researchers (Ashburn, 1992). Miller (1992) offers several conclusions on what is known of biological aging:

1. Biological aging occurs in all living organisms.
2. Biological aging is natural, inevitable, irreversible, and progressive with time.
3. The course of aging varies from individual to individual.
4. The rate of aging for different organs and tissues varies among individuals.
5. Biological aging is influenced by nonbiological factors.
6. Biological aging processes are different from pathological processes.
7. Biological aging increases one's vulnerability to disease.

It is important for the occupational therapist to take a holistic view when considering biological aging, as psychosocial factors are an important variable of influence (Ashburn, 1992; Davis, 1986). Stereotyping groups of older adults in terms of sensorimotor skills or other performance components perpetuates the myth of older adults as a "homogenous" group. One of the more consistent findings in recent gerontological research is that as people age, they become less and less like others of the same age, on virtually every measure (Miller, 1992).

Personality Theories

Historically, little attention was paid by theorists to personality development of older adults, as opposed to childhood. Myers (1993) defined personality as "an individual's characteristic pattern of thinking, feeling and acting" (p. 345). Most theories of personality describe developmental tasks that are to be mastered for successful development to occur. Some of the best known theories are the following.

ERIKSON

Erik Erikson is perhaps the most well-known, pioneering theorist in this area. He identified eight stages of development, using the psychodynamic perspective, that highlighted his observations on the contributions of the socialization process to development (Schuster, 1992b). Each stage revolves around a psychosocial conflict that the person must resolve to progress developmentally. The conflict for older adults is one of ego integrity versus despair. Ego integrity refers to a sense of coherence and wholeness to one's life. Persons accept life, see meaning in it, and believe that they did the best they could under the circumstances (Levy, 1993). The virtue developed is one of wisdom. An important result of successful resolution of this conflict is an acceptance of death as a natural outcome to life. If integrity does not predominate, despair occurs. Death is feared, and a person wishes for another chance (Levy, 1993). Erikson attributed despair to a lack of built-up inner resources from successful handling of previous psychosocial dilemmas (Cech & Martin, 1995).

HAVIGHURST

Robert Havighurst, an educator, described at each life phase a set of developmental tasks for a person to master. His view of development is one of a cognitive learning process. His tasks for older adults include:

1. Adjusting to retirement and reduced income
2. Adjusting to decreasing physical strength and health
3. Adjusting to death of spouse
4. Establishing satisfactory physical living arrangements (Schuster, 1992a; 1992b).

Many of Havighurst's tasks are consistent with intervention approaches used by occupational therapists (e.g., environmental adaptation, health maintenance). However, the lack of a more "positive" focus on developing new skills, roles, and means of achieving quality of life for older adults is a major limitation of Havighurst's approach. Also, Havighurst's theory has been criticized as reflecting a 1960s middle-class set of values (Schuster, 1992b).

PECK

Developmental tasks of the older adult are also a focus in the theory of Robert Peck. His tasks include:

1. Ego differentiation versus work role preoccupation
2. Body transcendence versus body preoccupation
3. Ego transcendence versus ego preoccupation.

For example, ego differentiated adults possess a sense of self-identity and worth that is defined along several dimensions, versus work role preoccupied individuals, whose sense of identity and worth is still totally based upon their career. The advent of retirement can produce a declining sense of well being in the work-preoccupied individual (Bornstein, 1992). In occupational therapy an intervention focus on multiple performance areas (i.e., self-care, work, and play and leisure), along with the acknowledgment of an individually referenced balance between them, complements Peck's focus on multiple dimensions of self-identity and worth.

MASLOW

Abraham Maslow, considered a founder of the humanistic view of development, created the well-known pyramid of needs. This pyramid is supported at the bottom by fulfillment of physiological needs and culminates at the top with the attainment of self-esteem and self-actualization (Hasselkus, 1993). For the older adult, this can be a time of striving for full maximization of potential, or a regression to focusing on meeting lower level motivational needs such as safety and belongingness when necessary. For example, an older adult with declining vision and hearing may focus on safety needs. The occupational therapist, by helping the older client increase safety and by improving functional performance in self-care, work, or leisure areas, can "free up" the individual to pursue higher order needs.

Limitations of Personality Theories

Many personality theories are "stage" theories. Stage theories conceptualize development as a series of relatively discrete, abrupt changes, rather than conceptualizing change as subtle, elemental, and continuous (Breines, 1989). Lost in a stage conceptualization is how an individual person builds unique adaptive skills cumulatively and continuously. The danger lies in the temptation for occupational therapists to apply "cookbook" intervention using group norms, such as Havighurst's "adjust to declining physical strength" for *every* older adult they engage with clinically.

Social Theories

These theories are of special interest to occupational therapists because the focus is on what happens to people's involvement in life activities as they age. Examples are disengagement theory, activity theory, and identity continuity theory.

DISENGAGEMENT THEORY

This highly controversial theory was based on three premises. One was that society benefits (due to minimizaton of disruption) by the disengagement of those members most likely to die (i.e., older adults). Second, older adults self-disengage through general reduction in energy levels, less societal involvement, and an increased preoccupation with their own needs and desires. Third, well-being in older adulthood is a function of the congruency between society's expectations and the needs of the older adult. Therefore, if reduced activities were wanted and expected by the individual and society, well-being would occur (Bornstein, 1992). The image of an older adult living with family, who only half-heartedly comes down from his or her room to dinner would be consistent with this theory. It is doubtful many occupational therapists would feel comfortable applying this theory to their practice, as active engagement is a basic concept in the profession.

ACTIVITY THEORY

Here the maintenance of high levels of activity for older adults is seen as positively affecting well-being. It is a commonly cited theoretical argument for creating activity programming for older adults (Bornstein, 1992). Activities in this theory are broadly defined as physical, psychological, and social. New activities can be substituted for old ones, and current activities can be adapted. The older adult who says "I just like to keep busy" is an unwitting proponent of this theory. Occupational therapists may feel a natural link to this theory; however, activity here is not strongly individually referenced as in the identity continuity theory.

IDENTITY CONTINUITY THEORY

This theory assumes that well-being is associated with the ability of the individual to maintain patterns of behavior that existed prior to older adulthood. Life satisfaction is related to a continuity over time in lifestyle performance, regardless of the level of activity represented in those patterns and styles. Of the three theories, empirical evidence is the strongest for the identity continuity theory (Bornstein, 1992). The Lifestyle Performance Model (Fidler, 1996), a model of occupational therapy practice, reflects an emphasis on continuity of lifestyle performance over time. The model is designed to be used across all levels of the life span, and across different cultures.

Issues of Gender and Culture

Much of the research generated historically on adult development has been with all male subjects, or was written from the perspective of male authors. In a review of conceptual and empirical adult development literature, Caffarella and Olson (1993) stated that maintaining relationships and a sense of connectedness to others was central to the overall developmental process throughout a woman's lifetime. Even within the literature on female development, a lack of diversity of age, race, and socioeconomic status of subjects makes generalization difficult (Caffarella & Olson, 1993).

Using this perspective, issues of gender and culture must continuously influence the thinking of the clinician working with older adults. One interesting study by O'Bryant (1991) logically hypothesized that because self-sufficiency is highly valued in America, the life satisfaction of widows would be related to their ability to perform tasks as independently as possible. Yet for widows in certain circumstances, it appears interdependence was more

highly valued, perhaps because such social interactions reduce feelings of loneliness and social isolation, and may also provide evidence there are people who care about them.

Conclusions

Because there is no all-encompassing theory of human development for older adults, existing knowledge limits the ability of an occupational therapist to integrate an understanding of changes in the biophysical, cognitive, affective, social and spiritual domains into an existing whole. Yet rapid advances in knowledge about older adults is occurring via gerontology research, and the future looks promising for improved practice in gerontologic occupational therapy. It is critical that members of the occupational therapy community contribute to this knowledge base directly, as they best understand the philosophical foundations of the profession and are motivated to improve the quality of life of older adults through engagement in occupation.

Activities ▬▬▬▬▬▬▬▬▬▬▬▬▬▬▬▬

1. Define "development" and "maturation." Why are these terms relevant to occupational therapy practitioners?

2. Review one of the case studies from later chapters of the text. Identify information concerning biophysical, personality, or social theories of aging that affect the person's life and the occupational therapy practitioner's intervention.

3. Review Miller's eight conclusions about biological aging. Identify some example of each of these conclusions based on your life and professional experiences.

4. How has neglect of gender and cultural influences affected the development of knowledge in gerontology? How might occupational therapy researchers guard against similar biases?

References

Ashburn, S. S. (1992). Biophysical development during middlescence. In C. S. Schuster & S. S. Ashburn (Eds.), *The process of human development: A holistic life span approach* (pp. 756–778). Philadelphia: Lippincott.

Bornstein, R. (1992). Psychosocial development of the older adult. In C. S. Schuster & S. S. Ashburn (Eds.), *The process of human development: A holistic life span approach* (pp. 831–850). Philadelphia: Lippincott.

Breines, E. B. (1989). Development, change and continuity theories: An analysis. *Canadian Journal of Occupational Therapy, 56*(3), 109–112.

Caffarella, R. S., & Olson, S. K. (1993). Psychosocial development of women: A critical review of the literature. *Adult Education Quarterly, 43*(3), 125–151.

Cech, D., & Martin, S. (1995). *Functional movement development across the life span.* Philadelphia: Saunders.

Craig, G. J. (1989). *Human development* (3rd ed.). Englewood Cliffs, NJ: Princeton Hall.

Davis, L. J. (1986). Gerontology in theory and practice. In L. J. Davis & M. Kirkland (Eds.), *The role of occupational therapy with the elderly* (pp. 29–39). Rockville, MD: American Occupational Therapy Association.

Fidler, G. (1996). Life-style performance: From profile to conceptual model. *American Journal of Occupational Therapy, 50,* 139–147.

Hasselkus, B. R. (1993). Functional disability and older adults. In H. L. Hopkins & H. D. Smith (Eds.), *Willard and Spackman's occupational therapy* (8th ed., pp. 742–753). Philadelphia: Lippincott.

Levy, L. L. (1993). Late adulthood. In H. L. Hopkins & H. D. Smith (Eds.), *Willard and Spackman's occupational therapy* (8th ed., pp. 130–137). Philadelphia: Lippincott.

Miller, C. A. (1992). Biophysical development during late adulthood. In C. S. Schuster & S. S. Ashburn (Eds.), *The process of human development: A holistic life span approach* (pp. 804–830). Philadelphia: Lippincott.

Myers, D. G. (1993). *Exploring psychology* (2nd ed.). New York: Worth.

O'Bryant, S. L. (1991). Older widows and independent lifestyles. *International Journal of Aging and Human Development, 32*(1), 41–51.

Schuster, C. S. (1992a). Development frameworks of selected stage theorists. In C. S. Schuster & S. S. Ashburn (Eds.), *The process of human development: A holistic life span approach* (pp. 893–896). Philadelphia: Lippincott.

Schuster, C. S. (1992b). Study of the human life span. In C. S. Schuster & S. S. Ashburn (Eds.), *The process of human development: A holistic life span approach* (pp. 4–23). Philadelphia: Lippincott.

Schuster, C. S. (1992c). The holistic approach. In C. S. Schuster & S. S. Ashburn (Eds.), *The process of human development: A holistic life span approach* (pp. 24–49). Philadelphia: Lippincott.

Simon, C. J., & Daub, M. M. (1993). Human development across the life span. In H. L. Hopkins & H. D. Smith (Eds.), *Willard and Spackman's occupational therapy* (8th ed., pp. 95–130). Philadelphia: Lippincott.

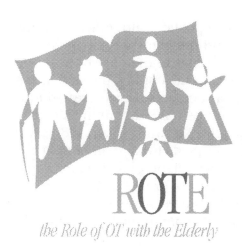

the Role of OT with the Elderly

Health Care Systems: Changing Perspectives

Marlene J. Aitken, PhD, OTR/L
Helene Lohman, MA, OTR/L

Abstract

The authors discuss belief systems about health and aging and provide an overview of the various professionals who work with elderly individuals and the settings in which such services are provided.

Belief Systems About Health and Aging

MEDICAL MODEL

Pathology and Reductionism

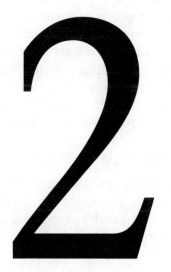

Medicine in the early part of the 20th century focused on becoming a more scientific discipline and began its long history of reductionism and determinism. Patients were viewed in terms of their pathology and reduced to what was wrong with their various parts or systems. The role of the physician was to "repair" these parts to return the patients to health. Kielhofner (1992) noted that this created a problem in the physicians' understanding of occupational therapy (OT) because this concept of looking only at parts of the patient did not correlate well with the OT tradition of looking at the total person and focusing on function and occupation. However, because occupational therapists were struggling with their professional image especially in the late 1950s and early 1960s, many therapists embraced medicine's philosophy and moved to become more scientific in their practice (Mosey, 1971). It has taken several years for the profession to shift away from this medical model and some believe occupational therapy has not completely accomplished the adoption of the new paradigm described by Kielhofner (1992) and others.

Although many health professionals are moving away from the reductionism of the 1960s and 1970s, some still approach treatment of older adults in terms of their pathology. Patients seem to be nameless entities and are called the "total hip," the "stroke in 315," or the "bad cardiac." In the author's experience, some physicians seem to be guilty of dehumanizing older patients by reducing them to their pathology. One plastic surgeon chastised an 80-year-old woman with arthritis for having an infection in "his skin graft" on her knee. She promptly reminded him that the knee was still connected to her body and was not his possession.

Disease Cure and Prevention

Some of the difficulties that some medical professionals, especially physicians, encounter when working with elderly individuals is that they have been trained to "cure." Because many of the medical problems of elderly individuals are chronic, the likelihood of ever seeing a complete cure is nil. Persons over 65 may have more than one chronic problem (American Association of Retired Persons [AARP], 1994). Effective management of chronic, disabling illness, as exemplified by rehabilitation, requires a major deviation, or paradigm shift, from the traditional medical model as noted previously (Hoenig et al., 1994).

In light of the increasing longevity of this group, we could see an increasingly disabled population. Should the health care system focus more on prevention? Because most deaths from infectious diseases have been eliminated, many public health officials strongly support programs that encourage people to change their lifestyles. In the Alameda County study, physical activity was associated with a decreased mortality risk, as was maintaining a moderate weight (Kaplan & Haan, 1988). Dietitians predict that maintaining a reasonable weight, exercising regularly, and selecting a proper diet may retard the aging process and delay certain debilitating conditions common in old age (i.e, osteoporosis, hypertension, dementia, and diabetes; Posner, Fanelli et al., 1987).

The two top causes of mortality, heart disease and cancer, are linked by extensive research to poor health habits and destructive lifestyles (Kaplan & Haan, 1988). Longitudinal studies such as the Alameda County and Framington studies have provided evidence that changes in diet and habits have been effective in reducing heart disease. Health promotion activities and increased screening for cancer and heart disease have been advocated for the older adult.

Science and Technology

There have been many advances in science and technology that provide an improvement in diagnosis and treatment. These have contributed to the increasing longevity of the older adult. Arthritis sufferers can reduce pain and in many instances increase their mobility through joint replacement. The most common replacement surgery is for the hip, but knee, shoulder, ankle, and finger joints can also be replaced.

GERONTOLOGY

Gerontology is a discipline devoted to the study of the nonphysical aspects of human aging and includes the psychological, social-psychological, and social aspects of aging (Atchley, 1991).

Social gerontology is a subfield that deals primarily with the nonphysical side of aging. Physical aging is of interest to gerontologists only as it influences the ways individuals and societies adapt to one another. However, because physical aging is the root of all aspects of aging, all gerontologists must understand it.

Aging affects everyone because nearly everyone has the potential to grow old and all the groups in which we live have older members. But although aging has always been a part of human life, the systematic study of aging, especially its social aspects, is relatively young. For example, the Gerontological Society of America—an organization of researchers, practitioners, and educators interested in aging—was not founded until 1945. The behavioral and social sciences section of this society was not established until 1956, and social gerontology as a concept was not developed until the late 1950s (Tibbits, 1960). However, since 1960, research on aging has expanded so rapidly that in 1990 research and education on social aspects of aging was conducted at more than 1,000 colleges and universities in the United States alone (Atchley, 1991).

The numerous processes of changes in physical functioning related to aging are studied as a part of biological aging. In psychological aging, certain dimensions diminish with age while others increase or remain constant. For example, abstract problem solving ability generally declines with age, vocabulary usually increases, and habits tend to remain fairly constant (Atchley, 1991). Variability is as great as that found in physical aging. Social aging is more of a process of establishing what is appropriate to, or expected of, people of various ages, not based on research about what people of various ages are capable of doing. Statements of "that's great for someone her age" are evidence of a culture's expectations of what *is* appropriate for "her age."

Gerontologists note that aging is not one process but many, and the possible outcomes can be positive and negative. Both kinds of outcomes exist and understanding these are important. However, it is also important to acknowledge that in the older population as a whole, positive outcomes outnumber the negative at least two to one (Atchley, 1991).

Defining aging or the aged by chronological age may misclassify some proportion of the population. At 65, persons are eligible for Medicare, and the Department of Labor classifies the older worker as over 40. At 60, people are eligible to participate in senior centers, and at 72, restrictions on earnings by Social Security recipients no longer are applied. The range of age in government programs and local agencies is phenomenal, resulting in a hodgepodge of definitions that reveal no consensus about when old age begins chronologically.

Defining age by function relies on observable individual attributes to assign people to age categories. Physical appearance, mobility, strength, activities of daily living, coordination, and mental capacity are examples of such functional attributes. Gray hair, wrinkles, stiff joints, confusion, and hearing problems are just some of these attributes. Anyone who has *all* of these is surely old regardless of his or her chronological age. Because only a few people have even one or more of these attributes, classifying people into age categories based on functional attributes is an uncertain process. However, in everyday life these definitions give us a general feeling of where to place people along a continuum of age categories. Often by using a combination of physical and social attributes, people can be categorized into broad life stages, such as adolescence, young adulthood, adulthood, middle age, later maturity, and old age. Some gerontologists further classify old age as young old, middle old, and the old old. The chronological boundaries of many life stages are fuzzy and may differ across cultures. Middle age is a stage marked by transitions at home, on the job, and in the family. During later maturity (usually considered to begin in the 60s), declines in physical functioning and energy availability become more common as do incidences of chronic illness and activity limitation. Old age is characterized by extreme physical frailty usually occurring in the late 70s; however, many people in their 80s, 90s, and even centenarians show no signs of this (Atchley, 1991; Kropf & Pugh, 1995).

Social gerontology research focuses on concepts and perspectives of individual aging as well as the societal responses to aging. Mental aging research includes studies on the senses, perception, motor capacity, mental ability, and personality. Social aging research on the individual may include social roles, self-concept, self-esteem, life course, age norms, age grading, social support, and exchange theory. Studies on individual adjustment to aging include compensation, conflict management, and coping with role loss. The research on aging and society covers a broad area of topics such as retirement, age discrimination disengagement, the elderly subculture, advocacy groups, and the care of the elders (Atchley, 1991).

WELLNESS AND PREVENTION

Until very recently, prevention efforts in the United States were focused on the young. Persons over age 60 were excluded from most prevention trials, such as the Multiple Risk Factor Intervention Trials (MrFIT) and the Lipid Research Centers Coronary Primary Prevention Trial (Omenn, 1990). Work to study whether older adults can also benefit from health promotion efforts began only recently. Early results are encouraging. Studies at the Center for Health Promotion in Older Adults at the University of Washington demonstrated the effectiveness of smoking cessation for both the old and the young. Specific objectives for older adults in the health promotion goals for the Year 2000 (U.S. Department of Health and Human Services [USDHHS] 1990) have encouraged more efforts to prevent disease and disability among older people. Although funding for the Health Promotion Year 2000 programs has not been approved, many health departments include the objectives in their community plans.

Life Style

The entire wellness movement is predicated on the notion that there are identifiable life-style factors that can prevent or delay the onset of serious illness or disability. Millions of people today are attempting to keep their levels of blood cholesterol low and engaging in regular exercise in an attempt to lower their chances of having a heart attack. As noted earlier, these efforts seem to be working because a decrease in heart disease has been demonstrated in the past decade.

People are controlling their weight to avoid high blood pressure; others are eating foods high in fiber to reduce their risk of colon cancer. Millions have quit smoking to reduce their chances of health problems such as heart disease and emphysema. Although only about 11% of the country's population is over 65, this group contains 30% of the adult, confirmed smokers (Riley, 1983). These older adults continue to smoke and do not accept the connection between smoking and lung cancer. Some even have mistaken beliefs such as that any and everything causes cancer, and they are not interested in smoking cessation programs. The Great American Smoke-outs held each fall seem to have been more positively associated with quitting for younger smokers, whereas individual counseling-type approaches were found to be more appealing to the older adults (Heinold, 1984). Older smokers have smoked for over 40 years and can't see what difference quitting would make on their health at such a late date. Few of their physicians encourage them to quit because they also question the value of older adults quitting at that time in their lives. Until recently, little was known regarding the reversibility of the effects of smoking following cessation by those who have had a long history of chronic cigarette smoking. Studies have demonstrated the reversibility of physiological alterations linked to cigarette smoking and lowering the risk of heart attack (Jajich, Ostfeld, & Freeman, 1984) or stroke (Rogers, Meyer, Judd, & Mortel, 1985). This information could be of value in motivating the elder person to stop smoking even after a lifetime as a smoker. Direct evidence from current research might decrease physicians' reluctance to encourage their older smokers to quit. The Alameda County Study examined changes in smoking status in older persons and the impact of changes in smoking status on mortality (Kaplan & Haan, 1988). Even when there is statistical adjustment for a number of factors, including the presence of chronic conditions and symptoms at baseline, those who have quit smoking have lower risk than continuing smokers. The evidence is consistent enough to stress the importance of the smoking and health association even in the sixth and seventh decades of life.

Ethnic minorities are disadvantaged on most indicators of health wellness, yet health services have not been adequately responsive to this group's needs. Part of the problem has been found to be related to availability, accessibility, and acceptability (Mokuau & Fong, 1994). A wellness program was conducted for elderly Black females aimed at increasing cardiorespiratory and muscular endurance, flexibility, balance, and muscular strength. The nurses that initiated this program felt that it was successful in helping these women develop new skills for health promotion and health maintenance and positively influenced their general self-image (Toliver & Banks-Scott, 1987).

By looking ahead and taking sensible precautions, millions of people will lead healthier, more vigorous lives as older people.

Growth, Change, and Adaptation

Adaptation is the process of adjusting to fit a situation or environment. We usually adapt to age changes in appearance gradually and routinely, but adapting to disability that may appear as we grow old usually requires all the coping skill and social support we can muster.

What is it about aging that requires adaptation? Many physical, psychological, and social changes may accompany aging and alter the individual's circumstances in ways that require some sort of adjustment. Continuity is an important adaptive strategy for people who are aging. Internal continuity refers to the persistence of a personal structure of ideas based on memory. External continuity refers to living in familiar environments and interacting with familiar people. Continuity does not mean that nothing changes; it means that new life experiences occur against a solid backdrop of familiar and relatively persistent attributes and processes for both the self and the environment. Continuity is an adaptive response to both internal and external pressures.

Anticipation is another important adaptive strategy for the older adult. Wellness programs, financial planning, and planning for long-term care needs help elders realize what might happen and allow them to take action to minimize or eliminate negative aspects of possible changes.

Compensation involves taking actions that could offset or make up for a loss of function. Hearing aids and eyeglasses are the most common examples of compensations for physical age changes. Environmental adaptations in living spaces can help older adults adapt to impaired mobility and lives in wheelchairs. Church membership, civic clubs, and garden clubs can provide compensation for social losses.

The outcome of these adaptations should be successful aging. Havighurst, Neugarten, and Tobin (1963) noted that, in general, if older persons are satisfied with their present and past lives, they have adapted to aging. The authors identified five components of life satisfaction:

1. Zest—being enthusiastic and demonstrating vitality in many life areas

2. Resolution and friends—accepting responsibility for one's own life

3. Completion—feeling accomplishment in life

4. Self-esteem—feeling worthwhile

5. Outlook—being optimistic and having hope (Havighurst et al., 1963).

This scale has been used in hundreds of studies, and the findings indicate that the majority of elders have high life satisfaction. Based on this criterion, a majority have successfully adapted to aging.

Service Systems for Older Adults

MEDICAL/SOCIAL MODELS OF DELIVERY

With the growth of the geriatric population, it is inevitable that occupational therapists will treat elder patients in many areas of the medical system. It is a myth that geriatric patients reside only in nursing home facilities. A sophisticated knowledge of the different areas for medical delivery will help the astute therapist best meet the needs of the elder patient. As these systems are reviewed, keep in mind the following general themes:

1. Elder patients usually enter the health care system through an admission to an acute care hospital. They reside there for a very short time period and many are discharged back to the community. (Some elders may now enter the health care system through an admission to a subacute unit.)

2. Sicker patients who are not "cured" leave the acute care system where, depending upon their needs, they may be admitted to one of many health care settings including home health care, rehabilitation hospitals, subacute units, skilled nursing homes, or outpatient rehabilitation. These systems are designed to deliver more cost-efficient treatment.

3. Both private and federal third-party payers are carefully monitoring care so that patients do not stay too long in any one system. Managed care is increasingly playing a strong role in the health care system. Third-party

payers are looking for cost-effective treatment with functional outcomes.

4. Patients may move around from system to system. For example, a patient may start in an acute hospital and then be discharged to a subacute unit for further rehabilitation. Then, he or she may be discharged home and receive therapy through home health care.

5. The majority of elder patients will eventually end up back in the community. Ninety-five percent of all elders at any given time reside in the community (AARP, 1994).

DEFINITION OF TERMS

The term *medical model* refers to a traditional approach to diagnosis and treatment of illness as practiced by physicians (Anderson, Anderson, & Glanz, 1994). Usually treatment is based on medical diagnosis and includes some type of medical regimen. Traditionally in the medical model, members of the health care team follow guidelines of the physician and are concerned about the physical well-being of the patient. Some of the benefits of a medical model are clear lines of communication and institutional efficiency in the system in which it is provided. An acute care hospital is an example of a system utilizing the medical model. Some adult day care programs may operate from a social model of delivery in which the patient is considered in terms of social and recreational needs.

The Acute Care System (Hospital)

The elder patient enters the acute care hospital directly from home or as a transfer from another setting such as from a nursing home. In either case, the elder will usually have an acute condition, whether from an accident or illness, that requires inpatient hospital-ization. Older people account for 36% of all hospital stays and 46% of all days of care in the hospital (AARP, 1994).

The primary goal of this system is to quickly discharge patients by stabilizing their medical conditions but not necessarily curing them. For those inpatient elders who have Medicare insurance, the hospital will receive a fixed payment based on diagnosis. This prospective payment system, which started in 1983, uses diagnostic-related groups (DRGs) as a means of determining payment. For example, if an elder patient sustains gall bladder surgery, the hospital receives a set amount of money as long as the patient stays within the prescribed days mandated by the DRGs. Since the advent of DRGs, the stay of the elderly individual in the acute care system has dramatically shortened. The average length of hospital stay for an older person is 8.2 days as compared to 14 days in 1968 (AARP, 1994). Shortened stays coupled with sicker patients have resulted in discharges to other more cost effective systems such as outpatient care, subacute units, and home health care programs.

The occupational therapist working in the acute care setting. Approximately 15.6% of occupational therapists (OTRs) and 9.4% of certified occupational therapy assistants (COTAs) consider the general hospital to be their primary site of employment (AOTA, 1991). Working in an acute care hospital is usually fast paced with a large variety of patient diagnoses. Therapists need to be flexible to adjust to a constantly changing caseload. With the quick patient discharges, it is not uncommon that a patient for whom OT was ordered be discharged before being seen.

The elder patient in the acute care setting. For the elder patient, being admitted to an acute care hospital can be a difficult experience.

According to Strumpf (1994) "the elder is at risk for a reduction in physical function and mobility, changes in cognition and behavior and adverse drug reactions. Additionally there is risk for the elder to develop incontinence, pressure sores, infections, and fall-related injuries" (p. 523; see also Creditor, 1993; Hirsch, Sommers, Olsen, Mullen, & Winograd, 1990; Keating, 1992).

The hospital experience itself can be quite traumatic for the elder because of the following reasons:

1. The environment is very hectic. During the day shift there is a constant stream of health care professionals and workers in the hospital halls and patient rooms. This can create a large amount of background noise, different from that which the elder is used to hearing, making it especially difficult for those with auditory problems. Additionally, the daily schedule is not always delineated for the patient. Health care professionals may come and go, doing their duties without taking into consideration a patient's need for rest and recovery. Sensory problems coupled with fatigue and constant change can contribute to an elder's sense of powerlessness, confusion, or depression in the hospital environment.

2. The environment is not adapted for the elder's chronic sensory deficits. Although the elder population constitutes a large proportion of hospital patients, the hospital room environment is usually very generic in order to suit a patient with any diagnoses or of any age. It is designed for the provision of services in the most cost-efficient manner. Typically, no accommodations have been made for sensory deficits. Elders can function with sensory deficits in a familiar environment, but can have difficulty functioning in an environment that is dramatically different (Cristenson, 1983). The room may have inadequate lighting or it may not be adapted for hearing deficits.

3. The elder patient may experience feelings of overwhelming loss and fears about the future. An acute hospitalization may result in numerous emotions for those elders who were previously independent. Depression is common in the hospital environment and often is not addressed. Blazer (as cited in Kurlowicz, 1994) found that 12% to 16% of elders hospitalized for medical illness suffer from major depression and 20% to 30% suffer from depressive symptoms. For some elders, loss of functional abilities can be very devastating. This may occur because of a disability or simply because the patient's caregivers perform self-care tasks for the patient. The elder's perceptions about hospitalization may affect his or her progress. For example, the patient may misperceive that sustaining a hip fracture leads to a spiral downhill course eventually resulting in loss of independence and institutionalization. Additionally, many elders are transferred to another setting, such as a subacute unit, for interim therapy prior to going home. If the transfer is not properly explained, it could reinforce the elder's misperception of becoming permanently institutionalized. For all these reasons, it is imperative that health care workers spend time addressing the psychosocial concerns of the patient as well as his or her physical needs.

Advantages and disadvantages of the acute care system. Advantages of an elder being in the acute care system include readily available access to physicians, technological treatment, strong in-house support services, and a comprehensive treatment team. In an effort to better meet the elder patient's needs, many acute care hospitals have developed integrated services of care including one or more of the following services: adult day care, emergency response system, geriatric acute care unit, geriatric clinics, comprehensive geriatric assessment, respite care, and senior member programs. Of these, the single most popular service is an emergency response system (Anderson, 1993). Although the elder may have numerous chronic conditions, the elder is treated for his or her primary admitting condition. In the acute care hospital, there may be minimal contact between the different departments with few organized health care team meetings. Therefore, it is paramount in the acute care system to make strong efforts to communicate with other health professionals.

Rehabilitation Settings

Quick discharges of elder patients from acute care hospitals have impacted all areas of the health care system, including rehabilitation settings. As an interim step to going home, many elder patients who have amendable functional disabilities are often transferred to a rehabilitation unit or hospital. The rehabilitation system is increasingly scrutinized for cost efficiency. This has influenced rehabilitation practice to be faster paced. Elder patients are admitted sooner, sicker, and for shorter stays. In a recent comprehensive study of rehabilitation facilities, the mean length of stay for patients decreased over a 3-year period from 28 days in 1990 to 23 days in 1993 (Granger, Ottenbacher, & Fiedler, 1995).

The objective of a rehabilitation setting is to maximize independence and enhance quality of life. In this setting, members of an interdiscipli-

nary team may include, but are not limited to, occupational, physical, speech, and recreational therapists; psychologists; social workers; chaplains; dietitians; and nurses. They work with patients and their families to obtain optimal functional outcomes. The team is often headed by a physiatrist, a physician who specializes in physical medicine and rehabilitation. Other ancillary team members may include an orthotist who specializes in braces and splinting, a prosthetist who specializes in artificial limbs, an audiologist who specializes in the diagnoses and treatment of hearing disorders, a pharmacist, and a supplier of durable medical equipment.

Rehabilitation hospitals are exempt from the prospective payment system mandated for acute care hospitals. Under Medicare guidelines, in a free-standing rehabilitation hospital or in a rehabilitation unit in an acute care hospital, patients are required to receive a minimum of 3 hours of daily structured therapy from the combined rehabilitation disciplines. Managed care is also an important third party payer in the rehabilitation system. It has become increasingly important to educate the third party payers on the benefits of rehabilitation. Outcome measures and studies showing the efficacy of treatment are helpful (Aavik, 1994; Granger et al., 1995; Joe, 1995; Polk, 1992).

The elder patient in the rehabilitation setting. Diagnoses of elder patients seen in rehabilitation settings include, but are not limited to, patients with neurological problems such as cerebral vascular accidents (CVAs), orthopedic problems such as hip fractures, cardiac conditions, respiratory conditions, cancer, and arthritis. Granger et al. (1995) found in their comprehensive study that the majority of the patients receiving rehabilitation in an inpatient hospital are White and female with the mean age being 69 years old. Sixty-six percent of rehabilitation patients were living with others prior to admission rather than alone in the community. This statistic indicates a strong need for caregiver or family support and education. Active participation in the rehabilitation process is a strong expectation for the patient and his or her family. The rehabilitation team works with the patient to help maximize independent functioning. Issues addressed in treatment are broad and based on the particular needs of the patient. Generally, the patient's day is very structured to fit in specific therapies and groups.

Members of the team provide a holistic approach by addressing psychosocial, physical, mental, and economic concerns. It is important to consider psychosocial issues as patients may be grieving loss of function or other losses. Some patients and their families may require the extra support of the psychologist on the health care team. Many patients benefit from informal and formal peer support provided in structured groups. Rehabilitation programs generally have a wide variety of patient groups that vary from setting to setting. Examples of possible groups are ROM groups, feeding groups, community skills groups, and wheelchair mobility groups (Elmore & Smith, 1993).

It is important that the members of the health care team display patience and support of patient progress. The functional effects from an elder patient's chronic conditions should never be ignored. Social service is available to consult about economic concerns. However, all members of the treatment team should be aware of the insurance and economic issues related to each patient's care in order to provide the best care.

The ultimate goal of the treatment team is for the patient to return home. For example, the occupational therapist on the health care team may have the elder patient engaged in simulated home activities of daily living such as cooking a meal. Some rehabilitation centers have special programs that can simulate living in the community or programs that help with community reintegration (Joe, 1994). Other centers encourage community reintegration through support groups for caregivers and members of the patient's family (Raffaele & Zackowski, 1993). Many rehabilitation centers have adaptive driving programs. These programs can be very beneficial for all elders and especially for those with visual problems. The home setting should also be evaluated to enable the elder to have a good transition home. The occupational therapist may recommend home modifications in order to help the transition.

The occupational therapist working in rehabilitation. Rehabilitation centers have traditionally been one of the largest employers of occupational therapists. Approximately 11.4% of practicing OTRs and 10.9% of practicing COTAs are employed by rehabilitation centers (AOTA, 1991). Working in a rehabilitation center requires the skills of being a good communicator with the patient, treatment team, and caregivers. In addition, one needs to be a patient advocate making sure the patient gets the services he or she needs during hospitalization and after discharge. There are numerous community services available such as home health, adult day care, Visiting Nurses Association, and Meals on Wheels that can enable the elder to remain at home. It is important to have a realistic attitude regarding patient outcomes. Not all patients return to maximal independence but most improve to some degree on the continuum from dependence to independence. This needs to be communicated to the patient and his or her family in a tactful and realistic manner.

Advantages and disadvantages of the inpatient rehabilitation system. The rehabilitation system provides many advantages for patient care including:

1. A strong and comprehensive interdisciplinary team involved in regular patient care conferences

2. Regular physician contact commonly under medical guidance by a physiatrist

3. Strong peer patient support both formally and informally

4. A positive environment.

Generally, there is a hopeful expectation in rehabilitation settings that most patients will eventually be discharged to the community.

Some of the disadvantages to working in a rehabilitation setting include the following:

1. Insurance and managed care providers have great expectations. As discussed earlier, patients are now staying for shorter time periods, and there is the expectation from third party payers that treatment will quickly result in functional outcomes or the patient will be discharged. This can be especially disconcerting if the elder patient, perhaps due to depression, is not motivated to work on rehabilitation goals. It can also be unsettling for those motivated patients who are not making measurable progress. However, on the other hand, many managed care providers are working in concert with rehabilitation services to optimize patient care. As their goal is to get patients to a functional level and back home as quickly and efficiently as possible, they are often able to facilitate patients

getting timely treatment and facilitate availability of resources. Managed care will continue to grow, and it is beneficial for health care providers in rehabilitation hospitals to establish a good working relationship with representatives from the managed care organization. The future of many rehabilitation facilities will depend upon this good working relationship (S. Luehring, personal communication, August 23, 1995).

2. The 3 hours of structured rehabilitation can be a difficult goal to accomplish with frail elders who may not be able to tolerate the expected amount of intensive therapy.

Outpatient Rehabilitation

Outpatient rehabilitation is beneficial for medically stable patients who need continued support from rehabilitation services. Often outpatient services are associated with a rehabilitation or acute care therapy department. With the advent of DRGs in the acute care setting, outpatient rehabilitation has dramatically increased. Currently, there is not a per diem system of reimbursement in an outpatient rehabilitation setting. However, there may be one in the future. Patients are reimbursed for therapy considered to be "reasonable and necessary." Under Medicare Part B, patients are expected to attend therapy three times weekly. Again the ultimate goal for therapy is to maximize the patient's ability to perform activities of daily living independently. In this setting, it is particularly important to establish home programs for the patient and caregivers. Compliance with home programs is necessary for the patient to improve.

Advantages and disadvantages of outpatient rehabilitation. There are numerous advantages to rehabilitation in an outpatient setting:

1. Outpatient rehabilitation is a very cost-efficient method of treatment. Treatment costs are dramatically reduced because there are fewer overhead costs compared to inpatient hospitalization.

2. The patient may be more comfortable and more accepting of treatment because he or she is living at home instead of in an unfamiliar hospital environment. In addition, therapy may seem more relevant because it can apply to activities in the home setting.

Outpatient rehabilitation has the following disadvantages:

1. In some outpatient settings the team is not as strong as in the inpatient setting. Multidisciplinary team members evaluate the patient separately and communicate recommendations via written note or phone communication. Scheduled team meetings can be a rare occurrence (Rodriguez & Goldberg, 1993). However, in an organization accredited by the Commission for Accreditation of Rehabilitation Facilities (CARF), a strong team approach in outpatient rehabilitation is a necessity (S. Luehring, personal communication, August 23, 1995).

2. Outpatient rehabilitation is not feasible unless the patient has adequate transportation to the setting.

Subacute Care

Subacute care is a new area for comprehensive patient treatment in the health care market. This service fills the treatment gap between acute and long-term care and operates from a medical model of care (Joint Commission on Accreditation of Healthcare Organizations [JCAHO], 1995). Presently subacute care is new, unregulated, and there are no specific reimbursement criteria for this type of care (Gill & Balsano, 1994).

Survey guidelines have been developed by the Joint Commission on Accreditation of Healthcare Organizations for units that choose to be accredited (JCAHO, 1995).

Patients are triaged to subacute units primarily from acute care and rehabilitation hospitals, although some patients can be admitted directly from home (Gill & Balsano, 1994). These inpatient programs can be found in diverse settings including acute care hospitals, rehabilitation hospitals, and nursing homes. Typically they are associated with, or attached to, a long-term care facility and are usually considered to be distinct entities (Walsh, 1994). However, in some rural settings a few patients can make up a subacute program because the program rather than the physical setting is important (M. Tellis-Nayak, personal communication, July 27, 1995).

Subacute programs can address the following types of patient needs: ventilator, wound management, cardiac care, orthopedic care, and neurological (JCAHO, 1995). In subacute units there is diversity in patient age range. Not all patients are of the elder population. Programs can be targeted to be specifically rehabilitative in orientation. Approximately 30% to 40% of services provided on a subacute unit are rehabilitation while the other 60% to 70% services have a medical orientation (Stahl, 1994). Subacute programs are expected to become the rehabilitation units of the future.

Managed care providers are major reimbursers for this system. Managed care providers estimate, track, and oversee the cost of delivery for all services including rehabilitation services (Hoffman & Heller, 1994). Critical pathways is an approach to care that efficiently delineates patient outcomes in a coordinated program within specified time frames. It is often used to guide patient stays (Anderson, Anderson, & Glanz, 1994).

Definition of subacute care.
Subacute care has been defined by the JCAHO (1995) as goal-oriented, comprehensive, inpatient care designed for someone who has had an acute illness, injury, or exacerbation of a disease process. It is rendered immediately after, or instead of, acute hospitalization to treat one or more specific, active, complex medical conditions, or to administer one or more technically complex treatments in the context of a person's underlying long-term conditions and overall situation. Generally, the condition of an individual receiving subacute care is such that the care does not depend heavily on high-technology monitoring or complex diagnostic procedures.

Subacute care requires the coordinated services of an interdisciplinary team, including physicians, nurses, and other relevant professionals who are knowledgeable and trained to assess and manage these specific conditions and perform the necessary procedures. It is given as part of a specifically defined program, regardless of the site.

Subacute care is generally more intensive than traditional nursing facility care and less intensive than acute inpatient care. It requires frequent (daily to weekly) patient assessment and review of the clinical course and treatment plan for a limited time period (several days to several months), until a condition is stabilized or a predetermined treatment course is completed (p. 3).

Table 2–1 includes four identified levels for subacute care provision.

Advantages and disadvantages of the subacute care system. Subacute care is considered to be cost effective for provision of patient care. Compared to an acute care hospital, costs per patient are reduced by 30% to 60% (Garfinkle, 1994). Other advantages of the subacute care unit are reduced lengths of patient stay, increased nursing hours, advanced technologies, and specialized staff (Singleton, 1994).

It is predicted that the demand for subacute care will continue to increase for the following reasons (Stahl, 1994; Timmreck, 1989):

1. The aging of the elder population

2. Hospital restructuring

3. Increasingly competitive health care environment

4. Need for integrated health care delivery

5. Government financing mechanisms

6. The growth of managed care.

A disadvantage of the subacute care system is that it is new and unregulated at this time. Additionally, as with other systems, there is pressure from third party payers to quickly discharge patients.

Nursing Home Facilities (Long-Term Care)

It is a myth that the majority of the elder population are in nursing homes. Presently only 5% of those 65 and older reside at any one time in nursing home facilities (AARP, 1994). This percentage increases with age. Between the ages of 65 and 74, 6% of elders reside in nursing homes, and in the over 85 age group, 24% of elders reside in nursing homes (AARP, 1994). In the future, residence in nursing homes is expected to increase as the frail elder population continues to grow.

Nursing homes offer a variety of services. In addition to therapy, additional services may include respite care, hospice beds, and a subacute unit. Although some nursing homes hire their own rehabilitation staff, others purchase therapy services through corporate services. Approximately 6.4% of OTRs and 20.1% of COTAs consider a

Table 2–1. Four Categories for Subacute Care Provision

Type	Location	Clientele	Length of Stay
Transitional Subacute Care	Often attached to a hospital, (substitutes for continued hospital stays) or HMO owned	Serves very sick patients (cardiac, stroke, pulmonary oncology, decubitus wound management, complex medical conditions).	Short stay transitional units 5–30 days
General Subacute Care	Often located in nursing facilities	Serves clients with general rehabilitation needs, intravenous therapy needs, and those without significant medical complications. (includes many Medicare patients)	10–40 days
Chronic Subacute Care	Long-term care hospital	Serves patients that are comatose, are permanently on a ventilator, or have a progressive neurological impairment. There is little hope for functional independence.	60–90 days (Stabilized patients are discharged after this time period either to home, or to a nursing facility.)
Long-Term Transitional Hospitals	Often licensed as a hospital, but exempt from the prospective payment system	Serves patients with complex medical needs or acute ventilator-dependent patients.	25+ days

Note: Adapted from Griffen, K.M. (1995) *Handbook of Subacute Health Care* pp. 6–7; and *Survey Protocol for Subacute Programs*, Joint Commission on Accreditation of Healthcare Organizations (1995).

skilled nursing home or intermediate care facility as their primary employment setting. Skilled nursing homes are the primary work setting for COTAs (AOTA, 1991).

Since the implementation of DRGs in the acute care system, nursing homes have gone through significant changes. Before DRGs, nursing homes were considered to be institutions for long-term placement for patients with chronic illnesses to receive custodial care for the remainder of their lives (Burton, 1994; Tresch, Duthie, & Gruchow, 1989). Chronic disease accompanied by impaired function and lack of an informal support system in the community were, and still are, reasons for permanent nursing home placement (Ellis, 1986).

Table 2–2 illustrates differences between an acute care system and a nursing home facility. These differences are becoming less distinct. In this table, the nursing home facility has two emphases: a rehabilitation focus and a custodial care focus.

Patients in a long-term care setting. Although nursing home facilities still have patients requiring custodial care, an increasing number are admitted for rehabilitation or medical treatments (Shaughnessy & Kramer, 1990). Some nursing homes can be thought of as an extension of an acute care hospital, where the therapy that was initiated in the acute care hospital is continued (Tresch et al., 1989).

Admission to a nursing home can be a stressful experience for patients as they make the adjustment to a new system. Some patients in the nursing home setting experience a sense of powerlessness when they perceive they have no control over their lives. These feelings may be manifested by depression or angry behavior. Nursing home staff can contribute to the perceived loss of control by doing for the patient rather than encouraging patient independence. The occupational therapist and other health professionals can help patients by providing choices, increasing the predictability of the environment, involving patients in goal setting, and maintaining a positive attitude when working with elders (Teitelman, 1982). Patient rights are now addressed by federal regulations.

Patients are increasingly admitted in a sicker condition to nursing home facilities. This admission of sicker and more frail elder patients has had repercussions on the nursing home system including a higher death rate. Approximately half of all nursing home residents come from the hospital (Burton, 1994; Shaughnessy & Kramer, 1990; Strumpf, 1994). Additionally, 15% of discharges from nursing homes are for hospitalizations (Burton, 1994; Strumpf, 1994; Shaughnessy & Kramer, 1990; Tresch, et al., 1989).

Under Medicare guidelines, patients in a skilled nursing home can be certified according to a level of care. With Medicare Part A, (Inpatient Medicare), patients who are residing in skilled qualified facilities can receive occupational therapy services for any reason with a physician order. However, treatment must be "reasonable and necessary" in order to sustain Medicare payment.

Advantages and disadvantages in a nursing home system. Like any health care system, a nursing home setting has disadvantages and advantages. Nursing homes serve the medical needs of most patients, especially those recovering from an illness who only require regular nursing supervision. Additional strengths of this system are strong team involvement and concern for the patient's rights and quality of life.

Table 2–2. Differences Between the Approach to the Elder in the Acute Care and a Nursing Facility

Characteristics	Acute Care	Nursing Facility
View of Problem	Biomedical base	a) Biomedical base b) Psychosocial base
Goal of System	Evaluate, treat, and discharge as quickly as possible	a) Rehabilitate patients to go home b) Provide psychosocial support and promote quality of life
Therapeutic Aim	Cure or stabilize the condition	a) Improve function so that the patient can go home b) Maintain quality of life in the nursing home setting
Entry to the System	Physician order	Patient or family choice (with physician order)
Diagnoses	Address primary physical complaint (chronic problems not usually addressed)	a) Address primary diagnosis in rehabilitation with multiple secondary diagnoses b) Address chronic physical and sensory problems
Client	Has passive, dependent role, minimal impact on system	Participates in care; has a large impact in the nursing home setting (Omnibus Budget Reconciliation Act of 1987 [OBRA] regulations)

Table 2–2. Differences Between the Approach to the Elder in an Acute Care and a Nursing Facility (Continued)

Characteristics	Acute Care	Nursing Facility
Decision Making	Physician directed	Team and patient directed
Physician Involvement	Daily	According to OBRA regulations upon admission, the physician follows the patient minimally once every 30 days for the first 90 days and once every 90 days thereafter.
Medical Teams	Minimal	Numerous team meetings

a = Rehabilitation services in an LTC facility
b = Traditional custodial LTC facility (Stryker, 1983)

The Omnibus Budget Reconciliation Act. Many positive changes occurred in the long-term care system with the enactment of the Omnibus Budget Reconciliation Act (OBRA) of 1987. This act, which revolutionized the nursing home system, focuses on the physical, mental, and psychosocial well-being of nursing home residents. It applies to all nursing homes that receive federal money for Medicare or Medicaid patients. OBRA centers on providing quality of patient care and attending to patient rights (Moon-Sperling & Pinson, 1991). Included in this act is a comprehensive screening tool, the Minimal Data Set (MDS), which is coordinated by a registered nurse. The occupational therapist can contribute information to the MDS. Strict guidelines have been established to complete the MDS and care plans within specific time frames. Restraint reduction, a small part of the MDS, has become a great concern. The nursing facility is required by OBRA to show evidence of consultation by an occupational therapist or physical therapist to consider the means of less restrictive intervention (K. Brown, personal communication, August 22, 1995). Areas included in the MDS are:

1. Cognitive patterns
2. Communication or hearing patterns
3. Vision patterns
4. Physical functioning and structural problems
5. Continence
6. Psychosocial well-being
7. Mood and behavioral patterns
8. Activity pursuit patterns
9. Disease diagnoses
10. Health conditions
11. Oral or nutritional status
12. Oral/dental status
13. Skin condition
14. Medication use
15. Special treatments and procedures.

A prime disadvantage of nursing homes is a lack of regular medical direction because, traditionally, physicians have not been active participants (Vladeck, 1989). Consequently, federal regulations have been established for minimal physician visits. Additionally, as compared to an acute care system, there tend to be fewer nurses and nursing assistant staff to provide care. Staff turnover can be high, resulting in poor continuity of care. In some settings, poor staffing can be frustrating for patients waiting to have simple needs met such as assistance with transferring from the bed to the chair.

Home Health Care

Home health care (HHC) is the fastest growing area of the health care system (Hing, 1994). Between 1986 and 1992 the number of home health care agencies increased 88% (as cited in Thiers, 1994). Since 1963 the number of home health agencies has grown from 1,100 to 15,000 (National Association for Home Care, 1994). HHC is expected to expand in the future unless there are substantial payment restrictions from third party payers. Practice in HHC primarily involves caring for the elder population, especially those 85 or older (Thiers, 1994).

Defining home health. There is a variety in the provision and types of home health care agencies. As Ozminkowski and Branch (1995) related, "This diversity may leave the elder and family unaware of the range of services available or eligibility for service use" (p. 225). Some HHC agencies are part of the services provided by a comprehensive hospital system. Others are associated with a pharmaceutical or medical supply company. Some agencies are freestanding. Certain agencies specialize in the care of particular diagnoses. For example, some HHC programs service mentally ill elders who have unique needs for care including mental and physical concerns (Lindbeck-Perkins, 1993; Menosky, 1995).

The Joint Commission on Accreditation of Healthcare Organizations (JCAHO, 1992) defines home health as:

> Services provided by health care professionals in an individual's place of residence on a per-visit or per-hour basis to clients who have or are at risk of an injury, an illness, or a disabling condition, or who are terminally ill and require short-term or long-term intervention by health professionals. These services may include dental, medical, nursing, occupational therapy, pediatric, physical therapy, speech language pathology, audiology, social work, and nutrition counselling services, and may be provided directly or through contract with another organization or individual (p. 29).

Care of the patient is provided by a treatment team guided by a physician. The team should be broad, including all people who have regular contact with the elder patient. In addition to the team members listed in the JCAHO definition, the home health aide and family members should also be included. Although occupational therapists are members of the treatment team, only approximately 3.6% of all practicing OTRs and 1.5% of all practicing COTAs consider home health care to be their primary employment setting (AOTA, 1991).

The key for successful team work in HHC is communication and collaboration of treatment. Generally, the treatment team is coordinated by a team member who acts as a case manager who considers all the patient's needs. This case manager serves as a patient advocate and as a liaison between the patient, family, and service providers (Young & Youngstrom, 1995).

The ultimate goal of therapeutic treatment is patient independence and safety in the home environment. Evaluation and treatment should not be confined to just the specific physical and mental needs of the patient but should include the home environment. Simple home modifications can dramatically improve a patient's functional abilities (Rodriguez & Goldberg, 1993). Informal evaluation is beneficial to identify the coping abilities of the family members in dealing with the patient's illness.

Many agencies are certified to provide care to Medicare patients (Hing, 1994). Home health care is the fastest growing Medicare benefit, increasing by 583% since 1980 and 26% since 1990 (Stone, 1995). To be eligible for Medicare reimbursement the patient is required to be homebound. This means that trips away from home are infrequent and usually for medical care visits. Under current Medicare guidelines, occupational therapy is not considered to be a skilled qualifying service. Either a RN, speech therapist, or physical therapist will need to see the patient prior to the occupational therapist. The government relations section of AOTA is working on changing this stipulation.

The patient in home health care. Hing (1994) found in a comprehensive study of 1,500 home health care agencies that home health patients are predominantly White (70%), female (66%), widowed (44%), or married (35%). The majority of home health patients received help with either an ADL or IADL, which indicates a high degree of functional dependence among the elder patients (Hing, 1994).

Characteristics of a therapist working in home health care. Working in a home health care system presents its unique requirements. The following are some suggestions.

1. It is very important to have good team communication because team members work alone with minimal face-to-face contact with the exception of scheduled meetings.

2. It is helpful to have prior work experience preferably in a rehabilitation setting (Thiers, 1994).

3. Flexibility is a necessity in order to adapt treatment to a home environment. Therapists learn to work with minimal equipment that they transport in their cars. Home health therapists often adapt treatment from readily available equipment found at home. For example, a therapist might use canned items in a strengthening program.

4. It is beneficial to have good organizational skills in order to coordinate a schedule considering other team member's visits.

5. The therapist should include family members in the patient's care. Consideration of the family involves the sensitivity of being a visitor in another person's home. The therapist may have excellent ideas to improve the home setting but these may not be agreeable to the family. For example, the therapist may want to put in bathroom hand rails, but the family may find them unaesthetic in their living environment.

6. The therapist should be sensitive to culture issues and consider cultural rituals that occur in the home.

Advantages and disadvantages of practice in home health care. Home health care is considered to be a preferred site of care for elderly persons for the following reasons:

1. The elder is treated in a familiar environment where he or she is most comfortable. This allows the treatment team to find interventions to obstacles encountered in real life situations (Rodriguez & Goldberg, 1993).

2. Treatment is realistic, employing activities that the patient does at home.

3. Treatment activities usually include the family and caregivers.

Home health care can be a challenging area of practice for an entry-level therapist because there is minimal team contact and the therapist is expected to work independently (Joe, 1993). Home health care requires an expansive amount of documentation with the demands especially high for Medicare documentation. Additionally, being out in the community can pose safety risks such as theft that can easily be dealt with by commonsense safety interventions (Williams, 1994).

Adult Day Care

Adult day care (ADC) is a community-based service for elders and adults with mental or physical limitations who need support. ADCs provide comprehensive group programs and health, social, and related support services. Some programs specialize in certain patient diagnoses such as Alzheimer's disease or mental illness (Plotkin & Wells, 1993; Wimo, Mattson, Adolfsson, Eriksson, & Nelvic, 1993).

The National Institute on Adult Day Care (1990) defines ADCs as:

> A community-based group program designed to meet the needs of adults with functional impairments through an individual plan of care. It is a structured comprehensive program that provides a variety of health, social, and related support services in a protective setting during any part of a day but less than 24-hour care.

Individuals who participate in adult day care attend on a planned basis during specified hours. Adult day care assists its participants to remain in the community, enabling families and other caregivers to continue caring at home for a family member with an impairment. (p. 1)

There are a variety of models for provision of ADC. Programs run the continuum from social and recreational to medically based (Conrad, Hanrahan, & Hughes, 1990). ADCs can be staffed by nurses, social workers, recreational therapists, and activity directors. Rehabilitation services such as occupational, physical, and speech therapy can be provided directly by staff or more commonly provided as contractual services. Less than 1% of all OTRs and 1.7% of all COTAs are primarily employed in an adult day care setting (AOTA, 1991).

The client in adult day care. Weissert et al. (1989) found in their study of adult day care settings that clients differed from nursing home patients. They were slightly younger and displayed more independence in activities of daily living. Additionally, a high percentage of ADC participants suffered from some type of mental disorder (Weissert et al., 1989).

Advantages and disadvantages. There are numerous advantages to an ADC program including:

1. The provision of much-needed respite for caregivers. This substantial benefit can make enough difference for some elders to remain in the community.

2. The presence of peer social interaction in a safe environment. This is especially helpful for those elders who are unmarried or widowed and living alone.

3. The provision of emotional and sensory stimulation, health promotion or disease prevention, and socialization through structured groups. A variety of groups can be provided in this setting including, but not limited to, activity groups, psychosocial

groups such as reminiscence groups, ADL groups, community education groups, exercise, and health educational groups.

4. The provision of case management services. These include, but are not limited to, provision of health assessment, nutritional education, therapeutic diets, transportation, and access to community support services such as Meals on Wheels and Life Line.

Although ADCs are considered to be a cost-efficient form of service because they help keep elders in the community, the primary disadvantage is the cost of program provision. It is often difficult to get adequate funding to support an ADC. Some ADC programs benefit by being associated with a hospital. Poor funding, however, can influence obtaining adequate staffing. At the present time, there is minimal insurance coverage for ADC programs. This can eliminate those clients who are not eligible for Medicaid and are in the middle income class. Operating on a limited budget can influence the ability of an ADC to market services to caregivers in the community. Finally, some believe that there are not enough ADC centers to meet the needs of elders in the community (P. MacGinn, personal communication, July 1995). Presently there are 3,000 adult day care programs in the United States, and the demand for ADC programs is expected to be 10,000 by the year 2000 (Cox & Reifler, 1994; National Institute on Adult Day Care, 1990).

Hospice

Hospice is a unique area of practice that provides service for terminally ill individuals. It differs from the medical model of care because its mission is to provide quality of life to the dying. As Pizzi (1992) remarked,

"quality of life is not simply about pain control and keeping people comfortable—it is about enhancing the ability to perform activity important to the person and family system, helping those we serve develop competence, mastery, and control when life-threatening illness takes control, creating opportunities to live fully and productively until death." (p. 1)

The philosophy of hospice states, Hospice is a special kind of care designed to provide sensitivity and support for people in the final phase of a terminal illness. Hospice care seeks to enable patients to carry on an alert, pain-free life and to manage other symptoms so that their last days may be spent with dignity and quality at home or in a home-like setting (NHO,1994).

Because hospice is a philosophy of care, it can take place in many settings including a hospital, long-term care facility, home health agency, or adult day care facility. Table 2–3 lists basic characteristics of a hospice program. The hospice program is an autonomous, centrally administered program of coordinated outpatient and inpatient services primarily concerned with home care, with back-up inpatient services when home care is not feasible.

The patient in a hospice setting. The majority of patients serviced by hospice are White (85%) and living with their spouse (55%), in their own personal residence (77%) (NHO, 1993). Most (78%) are diagnosed with cancer. The other diagnoses serviced are heart disease (10%), AIDS (4%), renal disease (1%), Alzheimer's disease (1%), and assorted diagnoses (6%) (NHO, 1993). The fact that people are living longer increases their chances of having a terminal illness (Woodard, 1995). Patients

Table 2–3. Characteristics of a Hospice Program

Characteristic	Description
Primary Unit of Care	Patient and family: total patient care includes dealing with family and other significant patient relationships.
Symptom Control	Physical: pain, nausea, vomiting, and other symptoms are controlled as effectively as medically possible. Emotional: behavioral sciences are important in helping patient and family cope with emotional distress accompanying impending death. Spiritual: attention to human spiritual concerns is as important as pain care and is integral to a hospice program.
Physician-Directed Interdisciplinary Care	All health care is provided under the direction of a qualified physician. The interdisciplinary areas include social work, physical, occupational and speech therapy, pastoral care, and a wide variety of consultant services (e.g., psychiatric, radiologic, pediatric, oncologic).
Trained Volunteers	Volunteers are specially selected and extensively trained; they augment staff services and are not engaged in lieu of staff. Volunteers provide vital services other than clinical (e.g., transportation, companionship, recreational and other services).
Services Available on Call	Hospice services are available on a 7-day week, 24-hour basis. Hospice nursing staff bear primary responsibility and call on other program resources as necessary.
Staff Support and Communication	Opportunities for staff to discuss their concerns—either one-to-one, or in a group, on a structured or unstructured basis—are imperative. Channels for staff discussion, support, and mutual evaluation are established.
Bereavement Follow-Up	Hospice services are extended to the family during the period of bereavement. Extent and length of bereavement care is based on factors prior to and following death of patient.
Hospice Services Based on Need	Hospice services are based on need rather than ability to pay.

Note: Information provided courtesy of the American Cancer Society.

in the hospice setting are in varying levels of functional decline. Some patients are referred to a hospice program at a time they can benefit from full services of an interdisciplinary team. Others are referred very late and die soon after starting the hospice service.

Prior to admission to a hospice program, the patient will face the issue of having a terminal illness. Patients who are in a Medicare-certified hospice are diagnosed by their physician as having six months or less to live. Some patients are at peace with dying whereas others may have unresolved fears. The fears a dying person may feel can be tremendous, based individually on each patient. Team members need to be sensitive to any patient fears and allow the patient to express them. Additionally, each patient has his or her own values, attitudes, and religious beliefs about death. It is important that the treatment team respect the patient's beliefs. The patient needs support and it can come from many sources. Many hospice teams access people from the patient's religious practice to provide spiritual support.

Treatment is provided by an interdisciplinary team that can include physicians, nurses, social workers, and rehabilitation personnel. A strong component of many hospice programs are lay volunteers who usually receive formal training. The team works collectively to maximize the patient's quality of life.

Patients in hospice settings receive help in controlling symptoms of pain, not only related to physical pain, but also to psychological, social, and spiritual pain. Controlling a patient's pain rather than attempting to cure the condition is referred to as palliative care (AOTA, 1987). Patients in hospice programs know and should have accepted the fact that their medical condition is terminal and they will no longer receive aggressive treatment. A large component of treatment is working with the patient and family on closure (Woodard, 1995). The occupational therapist works with patients to maintain independence and control in their dying days. Hospice programs strongly support the family as a unit of care and usually provide bereavement counseling.

Characteristics of a therapist working in a hospice setting. Every Medicare hospice is federally mandated to have a contractual agreement with an occupational therapist (Pizzi, 1992). The mandate does not delineate the frequency of therapy services. In the recent AOTA Member Data Survey, no OTRs or COTAs listed the hospice setting as their primary employment (AOTA, 1991). It is felt that occupational therapy is underutilized in a hospice setting partially because of physician team leaders who do not understand the contribution that occupational therapists can make (Thiers, 1993).

Working in a hospice setting can be quite emotionally demanding as well as rewarding. The following are helpful characteristics for the therapist who chooses to work in this setting:

1. The occupational therapist will need to have a good understanding of hospice philosophy in order to provide appropriate patient treatment as well as to articulate the hospice philosophy to physicians, other health care workers, patients, and their families.

2. The occupational therapist will need to have an acceptance of death as a part of life. This may be a difficult concept to accept, considering that we live in a death-denying society.

3. The occupational therapist will need to have an acceptance that a patient's function will decline. This may be particularly difficult for ther-

apists trained in hospital systems where the goal is to cure rather than to maintain function.

4. The occupational therapist will need good team communication skills, especially if the hospice is located in a home health setting.

5. The occupational therapist will need to be flexible and creative with treatment interventions. Hospice treatment truly involves a holistic approach to patient care.

6. The occupational therapist will need to have a strong background in both mental health and physical rehabilitation occupational therapy in order to provide holistic treatment.

Advantages and disadvantages of working in a hospice setting. Hospice can be a rewarding system to work in for those who find meaning in helping others enhance their quality of life. It is also rewarding to provide holistic treatment to patients. Another advantage is the strong team component.

Hospice can be a frustrating system to work in when family caregivers and healthcare workers do not understand its mission. For example, caregivers may panic and call emergency services if the patient loses consciousness rather than letting him or her die peacefully. Physicians who do not understand the philosophy of hospice care may unknowingly order aggressive treatment. Some primary physicians may demonstrate lack of involvement in the patient's care due to a perception that the patient who is dying is a personal failure. Occupational therapists trained in rehabilitation philosophy may be uncomfortable with the hospice philosophy of palliative care (Holland & Tigges, 1981).

THE GERIATRIC SPECIALIST

Geriatric MD (Geriatrician)

The geriatric specialty in medicine has only been certified since 1988. Through 1994 approximately 6,000 physicians have been certified. Over 90% of these certified geriatric physicians have received their certificate through a "grandfather" clause. If over 25% of their patients were over 65 and if they had been in practice over four years, they did not have to demonstrate any proof of additional education in geriatrics. After 1994, however, additional education was required prior to certification in geriatrics (Benson, 1994).

Internists certified in geriatric medicine are expected to have specific knowledge of the aging process and specific skills in the diagnostic, therapeutic, preventive, and rehabilitative aspects of illness in the elderly. These specialists care for the geriatric patients in the patients' homes, in the doctor's office, and in the long-term care facility. They are trained to recognize unusual presentations of illness and drug interactions, to utilize community social services, and to assist with the special ethical issues in the care of the elderly.

Most of the physicians caring for the older adults are primary care or internal medicine physicians. Because of the high rates of functional disability in this population, medical organizations have recommended that functional assessment be routinely performed by primary care physicians. Early identification and intervention by primary care physicians could reduce functional decline (Keller & Potter, 1994). However, these physicians continue to underrecognize functional disability (Hoenig, 1993; Williams & Lowenthal, 1995).

Physician education pertinent to geriatric functional disability is inadequate. Improving physicians' understanding of the initial management of functional disability and the role of rehabilitation is important if they are to be able to use the payment mechanisms available to support geriatric rehabilitation. Formal medical education in rehabilitation seems to be lacking and is reported to be poor at best. In 1975, only an average of four hours instruction on exercise was included in medical school curricula. In 1983, of 115 medical schools, 45 did not include physical medicine and rehabilitation in their education programs. Only 36% of residency programs in internal medicine during 1988 and 1989 had any requirements for geriatric education.

The primary purpose of geriatric training in medical school is to improve the care of elderly individuals by practitioners in every specialty by increasing their knowledge base and fostering interest in older patients. Of 126 fully accredited medical schools in the United States, only 13 require either a course or a rotation in geriatrics (U.S. House of Representatives, 1992). Elective experiences in geriatrics are not popular and only less than 5% of students participate in these. The second goal is to interest some students in geriatric medicine as a career. Although this geriatric training has been strongly recommended for over 10 years, there are still relatively few programs and only a very few schools require this training (Barry, 1994).

One more recent positive sign is the mandate from internal medicine accreditation requiring that all internal medicine residents become familiar with medical rehabilitation services (*Directory of Graduate Medical Education Programs* as cited in Hoenig, 1993).

The shortage of geriatrics teachers exists because most geriatricians are in practice outside of academic medical centers. Relatively few geriatricians have received the kind of formal training desirable for substantial academic careers that those in more classic subspecialties have received (Benson, 1994). In addition to the scarcity of qualified faculty, medical schools also have an already overcrowded curriculum, lack of appropriate training sites, negative faculty attitudes, and limited financial resources (Morley, 1993).

In a U.S. House of Representatives conference on health care professionals caring for elderly patients, it was reported that fellowships in geriatric medicine have not been very effective in providing additional service to elderly individuals. Over 50% of those physicians completing a geriatric fellowship return to academic placements (U.S. House of Representatives, 1992).

Geriatric Nurse Practitioner

The initial development of the geriatric nurse practitioner (GNP) was to meet the need for consistent, accessible, and quality care for residents of nursing homes (Radosevich et al., 1990). In the late 1980s, it was estimated that there were 750 GNPs compared to the projected need for 25,000 in the year 2020 to fill this role in nursing homes (USDHHS, 1987). However, today the GNP scope of practice includes skilled nursing facilities, retirement centers, day care centers, community clinics, physicians' offices, and in some cases, independent practice.

A GNP is educated in a graduate nursing program that offers a master's degree in nursing along with practitioner knowledge and skills. Following the academic program, the GNP must complete an eight-month internship under the guidance of a geriatrician, internist, or gerontologic nurse practitioner. Upon completion of this program, the GNP may be certified for expanded practice by several states and the American Nursing Association. The GNP is then certified to assume mid-level medical management of clients and can take histories, perform physical exams, evaluate laboratory tests, monitor and manage common acute, chronic health problems of the aged, and in some states, prescribe medications. In the nursing home, the GNP provides crucial input into evaluative assessments and the development of programs to meet the needs of the staff and residents. In the community the GNP may have many roles as a primary caregiver and case manager to aged individuals. In addition, the GNP can provide education for home health staff.

In Tucson, Arizona, the practitioner not only cares for elderly individuals in their homes and neighborhoods but teaches them to maintain their health. In the Carondelet Community Nursing center, they monitor the clients' blood pressure, cholesterol, and blood sugar levels and teach them about disease processes, symptom management, and medications (Hey, 1993).

In addition the GNP may provide weekly health clinics in housing units and monitoring and education in senior centers. In a clinic located in an apartment building housing primarily the elderly, nurses provided for the physical and emotional needs of their clients. Additional services requested by the participants included programs for coping with depression and stress, alcoholism, and arthritis (Pulliam, 1991).

In small communities and in rural areas, the GNP may operate community clinics to provide care when no physician is available. The extent to which the GNP can supply comprehensive clinic services depends on federal and state laws governing practice and reimbursement policies (Ebersole & Hess, 1994b).

The GNP is very involved in caring for the nation's elderly persons; 79% of family nurse practitioners, 78% of adult nurse practitioners, 99% of gerontologic, and 42% of women's health practitioners see patients over the age of 65 (U.S. House of Representatives, 1992).

Gerontologic Clinical Nurse Specialist

The gerontologic clinical nurse specialist (GCNS) is also prepared at the master's level and is seen as a caregiver, educator, and advocate of and for aged individuals. The GCNS also initiates wellness programs in care plans for elderly persons in institutional and community programs. Acting in a consultant role, the GCNS assists those who are involved in planning care such as social service, staff, and discharge planners. Although both the GNP and the specialist work as case managers, the specialist more often directs the discharge planning because of the GCNS' extensive knowledge of aging, the community resources, the family situation and the elderly person's choice and level of independence. The GCNS is found in hospitals, outreach programs and as an independent consultant (Ebersole & Hess, 1994b).

An example of a managed care model using the GCNS is a program in North Little Rock, Arkansas. There a GCNS acts as the team coordinator in a community seniors' health program, and a geriatrician from the University Medical Center acts as a consultant. This team sees clients in their homes or in one of three clinics. One clinic serves primarily Black clients with low socioeconomic status, and two clinics are in high-rise apartments with Black and racially mixed clients in the lower to middle socioeconomic range. An additional clinic serves a White middle socioeconomic clientele. The GCNS and the team help the older adults in maintaining or improving their health and in continuing to live in their own homes.

This managed care model, although it does provide direct service delivery, focuses on disease prevention and health promotion (Leath & Thatcher, 1991).

Geriatric Social Worker and Case Manager

The geriatric social worker has several roles in the care of the older adult. In acute care, this professional works with the family and the other members of the health care team in discharge planning. In long-term care settings, the social worker acts as an advocate for patients' rights, addresses caregiver concerns, and participates in care plans.

As the population ages, the social worker has had an increasing role in case management. Case management involves the coordination of an array of resources to make them more accessible, appropriate, and cost effective. It gives social workers an opportunity to use their clinical understanding and skills in providing services for clients who require ongoing care in the community (Soares & Rose, 1994).

Geriatric Occupational Therapist

As the numbers of OTRs increase to 40,000 and of COTAs to over 10,000, more of these therapists are reporting geriatrics as their primary practice focus. This, of course, may reflect the aging of our population, and these growing numbers represent a larger proportion of those needing rehabilitation services. Approximately 30% of OTRs and almost 40% of COTAs

reported that they work with geriatric patients (AOTA, 1991). The most frequent health problem of clients across the membership of both groups was CVA/hemiplegia, reported by almost 30% of the membership. The specific roles of the occupational therapist were presented in the service systems described earlier.

Geriatric Physical Therapist

There are a growing number of physical therapists who report that their primary area of practice is in geriatrics. In addition, many of those in general practice are treating an increasing number of elderly clients. In 1995, 4,747 members of the American Physical Therapy Association (APTA) were listed as members of the Geriatric Special Interest section of the association. In 1992, a certification exam was initiated in this specialty area and to date (1995), 115 physical therapists have passed this exam (M. Goldstein, APTA, personal communication, August 1995).

The purpose of geriatric physical therapy intervention is to improve or maintain the functional status of the individual. In the nursing home, the physical therapists can be part of the Minimum Data Set (MDS) assessment team. They are primarily involved with the section on physical function and structural problems. The seven areas in this section include bed mobility, transfers, locomotion, dressing, eating, toilet use, personal hygiene, bathing, body control problems (e.g., contractures, amputations, hemiplegia, balance), and mobility appliances and devices.

Prevention of impairments and disabilities in patients in and outside of nursing homes is one of the priorities of physical therapists, and new models of service delivery are being considered. Some even suggest looking into the benefits of group programs to reduce per patient costs and integrate therapeutic activities into the daily lives of the older adult. These activities could include maintenance of muscle function, joint mobility, proper posture, and balance (Rothstein, 1992).

Geriatric Researcher

Research on the older adult includes the same designs and methodology as that used with younger groups. Initially those interested in this group as the target population had to contend with testing instruments or measures that had not been standardized on persons over 65. Much of the earliest research was methodological, the collection of data on normal older adults to use as guidelines or baseline to compare to older adults with various dysfunctions.

Research methods in gerontology differ from those in other social sciences in the need to distinguish age differences from age changes and period or cohort effects. Age differences can come from comparing individuals at a given point in time and could result from a number of factors other than aging. Age changes are changes in a given individual over time. Period effects result from variations in social conditions over time. In addition, period and age effects can interact so that the consequences of being a particular age depend somewhat on when in history one experiences that age. For example, those older people who experienced the economic hardships of the Depression may have different perceptions of their current status in today's society. To some statisticians, some lower income elderly persons should be classified as poor, but these older people feel that compared to their earlier days, they are much better off.

WELLNESS AND PREVENTION

Community Services

Over the past few years, as the U.S. population ages, more people are demanding services in the community that meet their needs and interests in activity as well as health education and prevention. The location or setting for these events is generally related to the level of impairment of the older individual seeking these services.

Residential and assisted living facilities, physical and social environments. Only about 5% of those persons over 65 live in institutions such as nursing homes. The other 95% are living in their own homes, with their children, or in various types of retirement settings. One such category of setting is the continuing care retirement community (CCRC). It is estimated that there were approximately 800 of these centers in 1994, and their number was expected to double by the year 2000 (Petit, 1994). It was estimated that a quarter of a million people, with an average age of 82, live in the CCRCs. Many of these communities employ a "wellness" nurse whose goal is to maintain the health of the residents by understanding relocation trauma, by providing continuity of care, and by offering educational programs and wellness programs. In addition, advocacy, assessment, and coordination of services may be components of the wellness nurse position.

In addition to the CCRCs, programs have been developed in high-rise apartments for older residents. One such program was a nurse-managed stay well center in midtown Manhattan for older performing artists. A visiting nurse monitored the residents' health, provided health education, and encouraged fitness activities (Smith & Sorrell, 1989).

In their social environments, many older adults are involved in activities to promote healthier lifestyles. Many have joined health and fitness clubs and square dance groups and participate in nutrition seminars offered in the community. Health screening programs conducted in shopping malls are very popular with this age group.

Senior center programs. The earliest senior centers were initiated by social workers in New York in 1943 because of their concern for their older clients' need for escape from their loneliness and isolation. These first programs provided the space, some refreshments, and games but little else. During the following decades, the concept of the multiservice senior center was adopted by an ever-increasing number of communities across the country (Lowy, 1985).

Most multipurpose centers offer at least three basic services: education, recreation, and information and referral or counseling. More recently, centers have added volunteer opportunities and health and social services. Some centers have reported that their participants have become older with some decline in health. Others report that their participants seem healthier and are demanding more active programming (Krout, 1994). In responding to this more active group, many centers have instituted physical fitness programs, which may include ping-pong, golf, horseshoes, and other activities enjoyed by the older adult. In addition, there are activities that incorporate rhythmic action and stretching, and provide improvement in, or maintenance of, cardiopulmonary function, muscle tone, and mental stimulation. Weiss (1995) contended that the senior centers can be "universities for the second phase of life." He described wellness programs and programs for peer support and normalizing the aging process.

Adult Education

Persons are retiring earlier and are healthier than their counterparts a decade ago. Although many have retired from their jobs, many are interested in pursuing other careers or learning new subjects. There has been an increase in these "nontraditional" students in all levels of higher education. In some universities, courses are offered for individuals over 60 at a reduced fee. They may choose to complete coursework for a degree or just audit courses for enjoyment or enrichment.

In addition, many retired executives are participating in educating their peers in preparing tax returns or preparing for their own retirement. A group of retired executives work with persons starting business to provide them with organization and development advice (Personal communication with an executive from the local Service Corps of Retired Executives, August 18, 1995).

Community colleges. Community colleges have assumed much of the responsibility for providing low-cost, accessible educational programs for citizens within their areas. They have been a wonderful resource for older persons who want to develop a specific skill or knowledge base. Many of these local colleges offer preretirement programs, job reentry skills, and second career guidance counseling. In some cases, retired elderly individuals teach the community college courses. In response to the growing aging population, many community colleges have developed Older Adult Institutes or Centers to provide programs and activities of special interest to these groups. Health and wellness clinics are often a part of these institutes.

Public libraries. The public library system is targeting the geriatric population and instituting programs to meet informational and recreational needs. From retirement planning, visual aids, and screening, to making library material accessible to elderly individuals, the public library system attempts to meet the challenge of providing service to this population. Although not a formal group, the library has inherent therapeutic effects that benefit those who participate in their programs (Smyer & Hillman, 1991).

Some libraries have created innovative programs specifically targeting elderly persons. Some of these include large-print books and magazines, mail delivery to the homebound, low-vision reading aids, 24-hour audio reader service through a closed circuit radio station, kits designed to stimulate reminiscing, and one-to-one reading service in several languages.

Elder hostel. The elder hostel program is an international adult education program based on the youth hostel concept that was originated in 1974 at the University of New Hampshire. Today programs are offered on campuses throughout the world. There are now more than 90,000 participants (over 60) in this extremely successful educational program. Most of those who participate live in the dorm rooms and eat in the dining halls while taking three-week noncredit college courses taught by regular faculty or specialists in particular fields. Some of the reasons noted for participating in the hostel program were the opportunity to go somewhere or do something different, short time frame for learning, low fixed cost, suitable course content, no tests or homework, and opportunities to develop new interests and reexplore old ones. Older citizens wishing intellectual stimulation and personal enrichment should be encouraged to investigate these programs (Ebersole & Hess, 1994a).

Hospital/agency-based education. Hospitals are increasing their roles in health promotion and illness prevention as part of their vision and mission to serve their communities. One hospital established a senior care unit to help patients over the age of 62 maintain their current physical and mental abilities while recovering from an acute illness. The staff of the unit provided teaching materials on most disease entities, medications, home environmental needs, and normal age-related changes. Teaching that began at the hospital continued at home with take-home brochures and pamphlets (Parks, 1994).

Many hospital-sponsored wellness programs offer a variety of activities ranging from nutrition assessment to individual counseling and disease awareness programs. Especially popular with older adults have been nutrition programs conducted by a registered dietitian (Hickerson & Gregoire, 1992).

One hospital has a program called Age Well that it has developed for older adults. It was created as a community service that offers many programs that are either complimentary or available at reduced cost. Programs offered include health-related seminars, health screenings, a wellness center (health club), walking club, exercise group, and education on fitness. In addition, the hospital offers its Age Well members discounts on weight loss programs, eyeglasses, hearing aids, and prescriptions (personal communication with Age Well at Immanuel Hospital, Omaha, NE, August 17, 1995).

Self-Help/Support Groups

Self-help groups can provide support, guidance, and education to persons caring for elderly relatives, particularly those who are ill, handicapped, or mentally impaired. By sharing their common experiences, such persons learn from each other, adapt better to their disorganizing situations, and lessen the stress and despair under which they live.

When people come together in some formal way to find or exchange solutions to common problems, they form self-help or mutual support groups. These groups tend to focus on a single issue that their constituents have in common. There are a wide range of services offered by these organizations: outreach, small discussion groups, one-on-one helping, newsletters, public education, and advocacy, as well as social activities (Silverman, 1980). In many of these groups, problems are not defined as illness or as consequences of some deficit in the individual's ability. Instead, they are seen as appropriate reactions that anyone suffering from that condition or in that type of situation would experience. Participants' feelings are legitimated, and they are no longer alone with them. Most of the groups provide education and information that help the participants cope with their problems or situations. Some examples of these groups are mental health groups, drug or alcohol addiction, multiple sclerosis groups, Alzheimer's, or other disease-specific support groups. These groups vary across communities and states.

In most communities, the area Agency on Aging office has a listing of support or self-help groups serving a variety of needs. The older person or the family could be encouraged to call to find a group that would fit their needs.

Retirement, Employee Assistance Programs, and Volunteer Work

In 1986, the American Association of Retired Persons found that only about 23% of employees over 40 were offered retirement planning by their employer. Employers who did offer this service were the larger companies. Today, however, with the baby boom generation beginning to plan for retirement, there has been an increase in preretirement planning across the economy (Atchley, 1991).

Health promotion activities and employee assistance programs (EAPs) in corporations have the goal to motivate their employees to make positive lifestyle changes. Many companies are finding that these programs are mutually beneficial in the long run to the employer and employees (Anspaugh, Hunter, & Mosley, 1995; Zarkin & Garfinkel, 1994).

It is estimated that between 38% and 41% of adults aged 60 and older participate in unpaid volunteer work and that the proportion of elders who volunteer is increasing. Motivations for volunteering include altruism, self-actualization, and desire for a meaningful life. Older volunteers tend to be of higher economic status, female, and in good health. In rural areas, elder volunteers serve their communities in such programs as home-delivered meals, food commodities distribution, chore services to the handicapped, and many other programs (Havir, 1991). Based on research and activity theory, which holds that the relationship between activity and life satisfaction is positive, participation in unpaid volunteer work was found to be positively related to life and retirement satisfaction in rural and urban retirees.

Religious Affiliations

It has been suggested that religiosity is highest in the oldest groups of the elderly population, especially those people who have severe health problems (Courtenay, Poon, Martin, Clayton, & Johnson, 1992). African American centenarians, in particular, attribute their survival to God (Segerberg, 1982). Church attendance by the younger age groups (65 and older) is also significant but may be more related to a cohort effect (i.e., going to church was an integral part of their growing up).

Being a member of a church group was found to have an association with a reduced mortality risk in the longitudinal Alameda County study (Kaplan & Haan, 1988). Churches are becoming more involved in providing wellness programs for their older members. Nurse members of congregations are conducting blood pressure screening after services for the older adults and also distributing pamphlets on healthy diets and healthier lifestyles. In Chicago, the archdiocese implemented a project called Friendly Visitor. This program was organized in several parishes with the explicit purpose of visiting isolated senior citizens. The visitor would sit down and talk with the older adult and through this visit assess the needs. These volunteers were professionally trained to assume this role of advocacy and practical assistance. This program was particularly successful in reaching minority elderly persons who were not involved in other programs for older adults (Atlas, 1985). In addition to assessing their health needs, these volunteers provided information and referral sources and helped them fill out forms to receive benefits for which they were eligible. These visitors were able to help the older minority back into active participation and interpersonal relationships.

Caregiver Education

In addition to the services for caregivers described earlier, many long-term care settings offer disease-specific education for the families of their residents. Education on the stages and progression of Alzheimer's disease seems to be helpful for residents' families and is an integral part of support groups offered to them by the facilities.

COMMUNITY REENTRY AFTER MEDICAL TREATMENT

Discharge Planning

Elder patients are moving quickly through the different medical systems and "shorter stays mean less time to educate the patient and family members about providing home care for patient needs, and less time to coordinate services from home health and community agencies" (Mamon et al., 1992, p. 157). Therefore, it is essential to provide adequate discharge planning for the return to the home or community.

Elder patients who are discharged to the home need different levels of support. Some return home requiring minimal or no support whereas others need social, medical, or rehabilitation support to remain in the community (Suter-Gut, Metcalf, Donnelly, & Smith, 1990). To prepare for home/community discharge the occupational therapist works with the treatment team for comprehensive discharge planning. The occupational therapist can be a patient advocate to help with the patient's transition home. Goals for home/community discharge planning include:

1. Communication and education with the patient, caregiver, or family members about the home living situation, assistive devices, and any home modifications that will help the elder remain at home. There is a tremendous need to provide elders with assistive devices and home modifications as approximately 23%

of elders in the community have difficulties with one or more activities of daily living (AARP, 1994). Assistive devices can help elders remain independent with activities of daily living. Examples of assistive devices are tools to help with dressing, grooming, and other daily living tasks (Aztell & Yasuda, 1993). The purpose of home modifications is "to adapt the physical environment to the diminishing physical capabilities of the elderly" (Gosselin, Robitaille, Trickey, & Maltais, 1993, p. 16). Home modifications may involve adapting the bathroom with equipment such as grab bars, tub seats, or elevated toilet seats that help make the living situation safer. Accessibility to the home and within the home can be improved by home modifications. For example, construction of a ramp can make a home wheelchair accessible. Adjusting the countertop height or removing cupboard doors can make a kitchen more accessible. Home modifications require therapeutic knowledge, awareness of community resources, and creative problem solving. The provision of home modifications can be limited by the family caregiver's or patient's resistance to change, expense, and landlord restrictions (Aztell & Yasuda, 1993). However, ultimately these suggestions enhance independence, increase safety, and help keep many elders in the community. Ideally, it is best to do a home visit prior to discharge to get a realistic picture of the home situation and possible adaptations needed when the patient returns home. However, this may wait if a home health occupational therapist will be working with the patient.

2. Written and verbal education about patient care with patient, family, or caregiver. This is especially important if the patient is going home without any additional therapy services. Communication about care should be both written and verbal to ensure maximal understanding. It is helpful to observe the family or caregivers working with the patient to ensure that they are providing care correctly and safely. In addition, if the patient is going to continue with home health, information about the patient's treatment plan should be shared with the home health agency and the occupational therapist who will be following the patient.

3. Suggestions for family or caregiver support. It is especially helpful in discharge planning for the occupational therapist and all members of the treatment team to be in tune with caregiver and family concerns. Often family members are not aware of the magnitude of caregiving until they are actually in the situation, or they may feel high anxiety if they perceive that their disabled elder family member was discharged too early or too quickly without providing them with adequate support (Murphy, 1988). A proactive approach to addressing caregiver needs and concerns may prevent future problems. The following is a brief discussion of caregiver needs and how to access community resources.

Elders often live with family members. Approximately 1.5 million to over 7 million households of elders include at least one caregiver (Stull, 1994). Family members provide 60% to 80% of elder care (Mahoney & Shippee-Rice, 1994). Caregivers take on the role for different reasons. Caregivers may feel "a sense of guilt or obligation, coupled with fear that no one else can provide quality care to a loved one" (Woodard, 1994, p. 18). In addition, "they may provide care out of a sense of affection and commitment to the elder, financial inability to hire outside help, close proximity to the elder, or because no other relative was willing or able to provide care" (Stull, 1994, p. 96).

Caregiving can be quite stressful emotionally, physically, and economically (Biegel, 1995; Sterneck, 1990; Stull, 1994). It can be perceived as a burden if it diverts energy from other family activities (Murphy, 1988). Caregiving can be especially difficult for those caring for elders with chronic conditions as providing care may be indefinite (Murphy, 1988). In particular, caring for an elder person with dementia who is uncooperative and displays disruptive behavior is stressful (Silliman & Sternberg, 1988). Caregiving can be a daily job with caregivers spending over six hours per day assisting the elder with instrumental and basic activities of daily living (Sterneck, 1990; Wykle, 1994).

Care of the elder is often delegated to a middle-aged daughter, wife, or daughter-in-law (Woodard, 1994; Wykle, 1994). This role can be especially stressful if the caregiver has additional employment and childcare responsibilities. Further stress can develop from the role shift of the elder parent becoming more dependent (Green, 1991).

Approximately one third of caregivers are over age 65 and 10% are over 75 (Sterneck, 1990; Wykle, 1994). Yet more than half of the caregivers over 75 have no paid assistance and many do not have informal assistance (Sterneck, 1990). Additionally, older caregivers are more frail and likely to suffer from chronic illnesses (Kim & Keshian, 1994; Wykle, 1994).

It is essential in discharge planning that family support services are discussed. These include, but are not limited to, local respite care services, informal support from church organizations, friends or neighbors, and financial assistance. Financial assistance can come from social service and some states provide tax breaks or direct financial support to caregivers (Biegel, 1995). Some area offices on aging offer volunteer support. Hospitals and organizations such as the American Heart Association provide family support groups.

Provision of appropriate referrals to community resources helps to optimize the chances that the patient can remain at home. The occupational therapist should learn the resources available in the community in order to provide maximal patient and family or caregiver guidance. Although community resources are considered to be important, many are not reimbursable and consequently patients may need to rely instead on informal support from family and friends (Mamon et al., 1992).

Table 2–4 provides general ideas for various community resources.

Table 2–4. Community Resources for Elders

Need	Description
General Information	• Local area office on aging • United Way • Public library • Hot lines: disease-related organizations or counseling • Referral sources for physicians and general medical questions • Senior centers
Assistance with Activities of Daily Living	• Meals on Wheels: program provides meals for homebound elders • Medical supply companies: many do free consultations about durable medical supplies • Community meal sites • Home health aides • Church resources • Strong family or support networks • Volunteer companions
Financial Needs	• State social services may have funding ideas • Local agencies may provide financial support for specific needs such as adapting a home • Church-affiliated support • Social Security office • Veterans Service office • Homestead Exemption Act: lowers house property tax for elder homeowners • States may provide tax supports and direct payment to caregivers
Mental Health	• Local hospitals and treatment programs • County mental health services • Alcoholics Anonymous

Table 2–4. Community Resources for Elders (Continued)

Need	Description
Patient Advocacy	• Better Business Bureau: for business-related problems • Area offices on aging • Law schools may provide free legal counseling • Legal Aid
Personal Safety	• Personal emergency response system: these devices enable elders to get help with the push of a button within the confines of their own home 24 hours a day • Neighborhood watch groups • Informal support of friends and neighbors • Adult Protection Services • Departments of Social Services: can provide subsidies for home heating and cooling
Respite	• Unaffiliated • Hospital • Church affiliated • Volunteers referred by some area offices on aging • Adult Day Care
Sensory Needs	• Services for the visually impaired and hearing impaired • Phone companies • Public libraries
Support	• Organizations for family and caregivers of patients with different diagnoses such as stroke, Alzheimer's disease, and multiple sclerosis • Support groups at hospitals

Table 2–4. Community Resources for Elders (Continued)

Need	Description
Transportation	• Local bus companies: many make accommodations for wheelchairs and other special needs • Department of Social Services: may provide financial assistance for transportation • Hospitals: may provide transportation • Handicap parking permits: County Driver's License Office • Refresher driving or safety course: AARP, local rehabilitation hospitals, local county department of motor vehicles • Taxi companies: may provide discounts for senior citizens
Volunteer Resources/Training	• Church • Hospice organizations • Office on Aging
Wellness Programs	Offered through elder programs, hospital programs, and local YMCAs; these include education, social exposure and exercise programs • Some offices on aging provide health maintenance services

Activities

1. In a brief essay, describe the differences between a medical model of treatment and a wellness and prevention orientation to service delivery. What are the roles of the occupational therapy practitioner in each method of service?

2. Define the following geriatric specialists:

   Geriatric Medical Doctor

   Geriatric Nurse Practitioner

   Gerontologic Clinical Nurse Specialist

   Geriatric Social Worker and Case Manager

   Geriatric Occupational Therapy Practitioner

   Geriatric Physical Therapist

   Geriatric Researcher

3. Describe the roles of the occupational therapy practitioner in the following settings:

   Acute Care Hospital

   Subacute Rehabilitation Facility

   Home Health Care

   Residential or Assisted Living Facility

   Senior Center

   Employee Assistance Program

4. What are some of the reasons that occupational therapy practitioners work primarily within a medical model of treatment?

5. Review a recent journal article about providing services to older adults (e.g., from *AJOT, Physical and Occupational Therapy in Geriatrics, Topics in Geriatric Rehabilitation*, etc.). Identify the orientation that the authors present, the setting where that service could be provided, and which professionals would provide those services.

References

Aavik, D. (1994, November 3). Measuring independence after injury. *OT Week, 44*(8), 18–19.

American Association of Retired Persons. (1994). *A profile of older Americans.* Washington, DC: Author.

American Occupational Therapy Association. (1987). *Guidelines for occupational therapy services in hospice.* Rockville, MD: Author.

American Occupational Therapy Association. (1991). *1990 member data survey.* Rockville, MD: Author.

Anderson, H. J. (1993, January 5). Geriatric services grow: Hospitals work together to fill gaps in continuum of care. *Hospitals, 67,* 31–33.

Anderson, K. N., Anderson, L. E., & Glanz, W. D. (1994). *Mosby's medical, nursing, and allied health dictionary* (4th ed.). St. Louis: Mosby.

Anspaugh, D. J., Hunter, S., & Mosley, J. (1995). The economic impact of corporate wellness programs: past and future considerations. *American Association of Occupational Health Nurses Journal, 43,* 203–210.

Atchley, R. C. (1991). *Social forces and aging: An introduction to social gerontology.* Belmont, CA: Wadsworth.

Atlas, F. (1985). *Programming for older minority group members* (unpublished report). Chicago, IL: Mayor's Office for Senior Citizens.

Aztell, L. A., & Yasuda, Y. L. (1993). Assistive devices and home modifications in geriatric rehabilitation. *Clinics in Geriatric Medicine, 9,* 803–821.

Barry, P. P. (1994). Geriatric clinical training in medical schools. *The American Journal of Medicine, 97,* 4A–8S–9S.

Benson, J. A. (1994). Educating the work force for geriatric care. *The American Journal of Medicine, 97,* 4A–3S–5S.

Biegel, D. (1995). Caregivers (family): Economic supports. In A. Romaine-Davis, J. Boondas, & A. Lenihan, (Eds.), *Encyclopedia of home care for the elderly* (pp. 98–102). Westport, CT: Greenwood.

Burton, J. R. (1994). The evolution of nursing homes into comprehensive geriatrics centers: A perspective. *Journal of the American Geriatrics Society, 42,* 794–796.

Conrad, K. J., Hanrahan, P., & Hughes, S. (1990). Survey of adult day care in the United States. *Research on Aging, 12,* 36–56.

Courtenay, B. C., Poon, L. W., Martin, P., Clayton, G. M., & Johnson, M. A. (1992). Religiosity and adaptation in the oldest old. *International Journal of Aging and Human Development, 34,* 47–56.

Cox, N. J., & Reifler, B. V. (1994). Dementia care and respite services program. *Alzheimer Disease and Associated Disorders, 8*(3), 113–121.

Creditor, M. C. (1993). Hazards of hospitalization of the elderly. *Annuals of Internal Medicine, 118*(3), 219–223.

Cristenson, M. (1983). Adaptations of the physical environment to compensate for sensory changes. In G. K. Gordon & R. Stryker (Eds.), *Creative long-term care administration* (pp. 293–228). Springfield, IL: Charles C. Thomas.

Ebersole, P., & Hess, P. (1994a). Achieving self-actualization through learning and creativity. In P. Ebersole & P. Hess (Eds.), *Toward healthy aging* (pp. 713–736). Baltimore: Mosby.

Ebersole, P., & Hess, P. (1994b). The development of gerontic nursing. In P. Ebersole & P. Hess (Eds.), *Toward healthy aging* (pp. 795–820). Baltimore: Mosby.

Ellis, N. B. (1986). The challenge of nursing home care. *The American Journal of Occupational Therapy, 40,* 7–11.

Elmore, T., & Smith, K. C. (1993, May 27). Patients win on the NRH team. *OT Week, 7*(21), 16–17.

Garfinkle, S. W. (1994). Staffing the subacute care facility. *Nursing Homes, 43,* 20–23.

Gill, H. S., & Balsano, A. E. (1994). The move toward subacute care: Key considerations for any nursing home wanting to make a go of it. *Nursing Homes, 43,* 9–11.

Gosselin, C., Robitaille, Y., Trickey, F., & Maltais, D. (1993). Factors predicting the implementation of home modifications among elderly people with loss of independence. *Physical and Occupational Therapy in Geriatrics, 12*(1), 15–27.

Granger, C. V., Ottenbacher, K. J., & Fiedler, R. C. (1995). The uniform data system for medical rehabilitation. *American Journal of Physical Medicine and Rehabilitation, 74,* 62–66.

Green. (1991). Midlife daughters and their aging parents. *Journal of Gerontological Nursing, 17,* 6–12.

Griffin, K. M. (1995). *Handbook of subacute health care.* Gaithersburg, MD: Aspen.

Havighurst, R. J., Neugarten, B. L., & Tobin, S. (1963). Disengagement, personality, and life satisfaction. In P. Hansen (Ed.), *Age with a future* (pp. 319–324). Copenhagen: Munksgaard.

Havir, J. (1991). Senior centers in rural communities: Potentials for serving. *Journal of Aging Studies, 5,* 359–374.

Heinold, J. W. (1984). The efficacy of smoking-cessation strategies: Does it vary with age? In R. Bosse, & C. Rose (Eds.), *Smoking and aging.* Lexington, MA: Lexington Books, D. C. Heath.

Hey, M. (1993). Nursing's renaissance: An innovative continuum of care takes nurses back to their roots. *Health Progress, 74*(8), 26–32.

Hickerson, M., & Gregoire, M. (1992). Characteristics of the nutrition provider in corporate and hospital wellness programs. *Journal of the American Dietetic Association, 92,* 339–341.

Hing, E. (1994, March 28). Characteristics of elderly home health patients: Preliminary data from the 1992 national home and hospice care survey. *Advance Data, 247,* 1–11.

Hirsch, C. H., Sommers, S. L., Olsen, A., Mullen, L., & Winograd, C. (1990). The natural history of functional morbidity in hospitalized older patients. *The Journal of the American Geriatrics Society, 38,* 1296–1303.

Hoenig, H. (1993). Educating primary care physicians in geriatric rehabilitation. *Clinics in Geriatric Medicine, 9,* 883–893.

Hoenig, J., Mayer-Oakes, S. A., Siebens, H., Fink, A., Brummel-Smith, K., & Rubenstein, L. V. (1994). Geriatric rehabilitation: What do physicians know about it and how should they use it? *Journal of the American Geriatrics Society, 42,* 341–347.

Hoffman, E. H., & Heller, J. (1994). The management challenge: Rehabilitation in a subacute environment. *Journal of Subacute Care 2,* 11–14.

Holland, A., & Tigges, K. N. (1981). The hospice movement: A time for professional action and commitment. *British Journal of Occupational Therapy, 44*(12), 373–376.

Jajich, C. L., Ostfeld, A. M., & Freeman, D. H. (1984). Smoking and coronary heart disease mortality in the elderly. *Journal of the American Medical Association, 252,* 2831–2834.

Joe, B. (1993, December, 9). Finding comfort and independence at home. *OT Week, 7*(47), 16–17.

Joe, B. (1994, August 18). Doing OT well. *OT Week, 8*(33), 15.

Joe, B. (1995, May 25). Proving rehab's value. *OT Week, 9*(21), 18–19.

Joint Commission on Accreditation of Healthcare Organizations. (1992). *Accreditation manual for home care (Vol.1 Standards)*. Oakbrook Terrace, IL: Author.

Joint Commission on Accreditation of Healthcare Organizations. (1995). *1995 Survey protocol for subacute programs*. Oakbrook Terrace, IL: Author.

Kaplan, G. A., & Haan, M. M. (1988). Is there a role for prevention among the elderly? Epidemiological evidence from the Alameda County Study. In M. G. Ory & D. Bond (Eds.), *Aging and health care: Social science and policy perspectives* (pp. 29–40). London & New York: Routledge.

Keating, H. (1992). Major surgery in nursing homes: Procedures, morbidity, and mortality in the frailest of the frail elderly. *Journal of the American Geriatrics Society, 40*, 8–11.

Keller, B. K., & Potter, J. F. (1994). Helping the elderly stay active: A technique for detecting disability in the primary care office. *Nebraska Medical Journal, 79*, 4–10.

Kielhofner, G. (1992). *Conceptual foundations of occupational therapy*. Philadelphia: Davis.

Kim, J. J., & Keshian, J. C. (1994). Old old caregivers: A growing challenge for community health nurses. *Journal of Community Health Nursing, 11*(2), 63–70.

Kropf, N. P., & Pugh, K. L. (1995). Beyond life expectancy: Social work with centenarians. *Journal of Gerontological Social Work, 23*, 121–137.

Krout, J. A. (1994). Changes in senior center participant characteristics during the 1980s. *Journal of Gerontological Social Work, 22*, 41–60.

Kurlowicz, L. H. (1994). Depression in hospitalized medically ill elders: Evolution of the concept. *Archives of Psychiatric Nursing, 8*(2), 124–36.

Leath, C., & Thatcher, R. (1991). Team managed care for older adults. A clinical demonstration of a community model. *Journal of Gerontological Nursing, 17*(7), 25–28.

Lindbeck-Perkins, S. (1993, March 4). Delivering mental health services at home: Giving clients freedom. *OT Week, 7*(9), 18–19.

Lowy, L. (1985). Multipurpose senior centers. In A. Monk (Ed.), *Handbook of gerontological services*. (pp. 274–301). New York: Van Nostrand Reinhold.

Mahoney, D. F., & Shippee-Rice. (1994). Training family caregivers of older adults: A program model for community nurses. *Journal of Community Health Nursing, 11*(2), 71–78.

Mamon, J., Steinwachs, D. M., Fahey, M., Bone, L. R., Oktay, J., & Klein, L. (1992). *Health Science Research, 27*(2), 155–173.

Menosky, J. A. (1995). Mental health services in the home health setting: Special considerations. In American Occupational Therapy Association, *Guidelines for occupational therapy practice in home health* (pp. 43–54). Bethesda, MD: Author.

Mokuau, N., & Fong, R. (1994). Assessing the responsiveness of health services to ethnic minorities of color. *Social Work in Health Care, 20*, 23–34.

Moon-Sperling, T., & Pinson, C. (1991, September). Implications of OBRA '87: Expansion of services and opportunities. *Gerontology Special Interest Newsletter, 14*(3), 1–2.

Morley, J. E. (1993). Geriatric medicine: A true subspecialty. *Journal of the American Geriatrics Society, 41,* 1150–1154.

Mosey, A. C. (1971). Involvement in the rehabilitation movement—1942–1960. *American Journal of Occupational Therapy, 25,* 234–236.

Murphy, K. E. (1988). The impact of home care on the family. *Physical Medicine and Rehabilitation: State of the Art Review, 2*(3), 327–339.

National Association for Home Care. (1994). *Basic statistics about home care 1994.* Washington, DC: Author.

National Hospice Organization. (1993, October). NHO *Newsline, 3,* 1–2.

National Hospice Organization. (1994). *The basics of hospice.* Arlington, VA: Author.

National Institute on Adult Daycare. (1990). *Adult day care.* Washington, DC: Author.

Omenn, G. S. (1990, Summer). Prevention and the elderly: Appropriate policies. *Health Affairs,* pp. 80–93.

Ozminkowski, R. J., & Branch, L. G. (1995). Home care use: Predictors. In A. Romaine-Davis, J. Boondas, & A. Lenihan (Eds.), *Encyclopedia of home care for the elderly* (pp. 224–229). Westport CT: Greenwood.

Parks, B. (1994). It's for seniors: An acute-care geriatric unit. *Nursing Management, 25,* 62, 64.

Petit, J. M. (1994). Continuing care retirement communities and the role of the wellness nurse. *Geriatric Nursing, 15,* 28–31.

Pizzi, M. (1992). Hospice: The creation of meaning for people with life-threatening illness. *Occupational Therapy Practice, 4,* 1–7.

Plotkin, D. A., & Wells, K. B. (1993). Partial hospitalization (day treatment) for psychiatrically ill elderly patients. *American Journal of Psychiatry, 150,* 266–271.

Polk, B. (1992, November 12). Developing rehab-specific CQI. *OT Week, 6*(45), 20–21.

Posner, B. M., Fanelli, M. T., et al. (1987). Position of the American Dietetic Association: Nutrition, aging, and the continuum of health care. *Journal of the American Dietetic Association, 87,* 344–347.

Pulliam, L. (1991). Client satisfaction with a nurse-managed clinic. *Journal of Community Health Nursing, 8,* 97–112.

Radosevich, D. M., Kane, R. L., Garrard, J., Skay, C. L., McDermott, S., Kepferle, L., Buchanan, J., & Arnold, S. (1990). Career paths of geriatric nurse practitioners employed in nursing homes. *Public Health Reports, 105,* 65–71.

Raffaele, S., & Zackowski, K. (1993, November 25). Stroke group sees patients and families as partners in rehab. *OT Week, 7*(47), 18–19.

Riley, M. (1983). Cancer and the life course. In R. Yancik, P. Carbone, W. Patterson, K. Steel, & W. Terry (Eds.), *Perspectives on prevention and treatment of cancer in the elderly.* New York: Raven.

Rodriguez, G. S., & Goldberg, B. (1993). Rehabilitation in the outpatient setting. *Geriatric Rehabilitation, 9,* 873–881.

Rogers, R. L., Meyer, J. S., Judd, B. W., & Mortel, K. F. (1985). Abstention from cigarette smoking improves cerebral perfusion among elderly chronic smokers. *Journal of the American Medical Association, 253,* 2970–2974.

Rothstein, J. M. (1992). The aged and the aging of physical therapy. *Physical Therapy, 72,* 166–167.

Segerberg, O. (1982). *Living to be 100: 1,200 who did and how they did it.* New York: Scribner's.

Shaughnessy, P. W., & Kramer, A. M. (1990). The increased needs of patients in nursing homes and patients receiving home care. *The New England Journal of Medicine, 322,* 21–27.

Silliman, R. A., & Sternberg, J. (1988). Family caregving: Impact of patient functioning and underlying causes of dependency. *Gerontologist, 28*(3), 377–381.

Silverman, P. R. (1980). *Mutual help groups: Organization and development.* Beverly Hills, CA: Sage.

Singleton, G. W. (1994). Transitioning to subacute: The keys to success. *Nursing Homes, 43,* 16–18.

Soares, H. H., & Rose, M. K. (1994). Clinical aspects of case management with the elderly. *Journal of Gerontological Social Work, 22,* 143–156.

Smith, J. M., & Sorrell, V. (1989). Developing wellness programs: A nurse-managed stay well center for senior citizens. *Clinical Nurse Specialist, 3,* 198–202.

Smyer, T., & Hillman, M. (1991). The public library system. Social services resource for the geriatric population. *Journal of Psychosocial Nursing Mental Health Services, 29,* 22–25.

Stahl, D. A. (1994). Subacute care: The future of health care, *Nursing Management, 25,* 34, 36, 38–40.

Sterneck, J. G. (1990). Family care giving: What price love? *The Journal of Long-Term Care Administration, 18*(2), 16–21.

Stone, R. J. (1995). Home care policy. In A. Romaine-Davis, J. Boondas, & A. Lenihan (Eds.), *Encyclopedia of home care for the elderly* (pp. 220–224). Westport, CT: Greenwood.

Strumpf, N. E. (1994). Innovative gerontological practices as models for health care delivery. *Nursing & Health Care, 15,* 522–527.

Stryker, R. (1983). The fallacy of comparing nursing homes to hospitals. In G.K. Gordon & R. Stryker (Eds.), *Creative long-term care administration* (pp. 14–22). Springfield IL: Charles C. Thomas.

Stull, D. E. (1994). Caregivers (family). In A. Romaine-Davis, J. Boondas, & A. Lenihan (Eds.), *Encyclopedia of home care for the elderly* (pp. 95 98). Westport, CT: Greenwood.

Suter-Gut, D., Metcalf, A. M., Donnelly, M.A., & Smith, I.M. (1990). Post-discharge care planning and rehabilitation of the elderly surgical patient. *Clinics in Geriatric Medicine, 6,* 669–683.

Teitelman, J. L. (1982). Eliminating learned helplessness in older rehabilitation patients. *Physical and Occupational Therapy in Geriatrics, 9*(2), 3–9.

Thiers, N. (1993, September, 9). Hospice care: helping bring life a full circle. *OT Week, 7*(36), 14–15.

Thiers, N. (1994, June 9). The proliferation of home care. *OT Week, 8*(23), 18–19.

Tibbitts, C. (1960). *Handbook of social gerontology.* Chicago: University of Chicago Press.

Timmreck, T. C. (1989). Subacute care in long-term-care facilities. *The Journal of Long-Term-Care Administration, 17,* 14–17.

Toliver, J. C., & Banks-Scott, P. M. (1987). Exercise: The outcomes of a program for elderly clients. *Journal of National Black Nurses' Association, 2,* 30–37.

Tresch, E. D., Duthie, E. H., & Gruchow, H. (1989). Coping with DRGs—A nursing home's experience. *American Journal of the Medical Sciences, 298,* 309–313.

U.S. Department of Health and Human Services. (1987). *Analysis of the environment for the recruitment and retention of registered nurses in nursing homes.* Washington, DC: U.S. Government Printing Office.

U.S. Department of Health and Human Services. (1990). *Healthy people 2000: National health promotion and disease prevention objectives.* Washington, DC: Public Health Service.

U.S. House of Representatives. (1992). *Shortage of health care professions caring for the elderly: Recommendations for change.* Select Comm. on Aging, U.S. House of Representatives, 102nd Congress, Comm. Pub. no. 102-915. Washington, DC: U.S. Government Printing Office.

Vladeck, B. C. (1989). Long-term care for the elderly: The future of nursing homes. *Western Journal of Medicine, 150,* 215–220.

Walsh, G. G. (1994). Myths & facts ... about subacute care units. *Nursing, 24,* 17.

Weiss, J. (1995). Universities for the second phase of life: Counseling, wellness, and senior citizen center programs. *Journal of Gerontological Social Work, 23,* 3–24.

Weissert, W. G., Elston, J. M., Bolda, E. J., Cready, C. M., Zelman, W. N., Sloane, P. D., Kalsbeek, W. D., Mutran, E., Rice, T. H., & Koch, G. G. (1989). Models of adult day care: Findings from a national survey. *Gerontologist, 29,* 640–650.

Williams, D. (1994, September, 8). Making safety a priority. *OT Week, 8*(36), 16–17.

Williams, L. S., & Lowenthal, D. T. (1995). Clinical problem-solving in geriatric medicine: Obstacles to rehabilitation. *Journal of the American Geriatrics Society, 43,* 179–183.

Wimo, A., Mattson, B., Adolfsson, R., Eriksson, T., Nelvic, A. (1993). Dementia day care and its effects on symptoms and institutionalization— A controlled Swedish study. *Scandinavian Journal of Primary Healthcare, 11,* 117–123.

Woodard, K. (1994, December 8). Lightening the load of caregivers. *OT Week, 8*(49), 18–19.

Woodard, K. (1995, February, 2). The elderly find hope in hospice. *OT Week, 9*(5), 16–17.

Wykle, M. L. (1994). The physical and mental health of women caregivers of older adults. *Journal of Psychosocial Nursing, 32*(3), 41–42.

Young, J. A., & Youngstrom, M. J. (1995). Teamwork, personnel issues, and supervision in the home health setting. In American Occupational Therapy Association, *Guidelines for occupational therapy practice in home health* (pp. 15–28). Bethesda, MD: Author.

Zarkin, G. A., & Garfinkel, S. A. (1994). The relationship between employer health insurance characteristics and the provision of employee assistance programs. *Inquiry, 31,* 102–114.

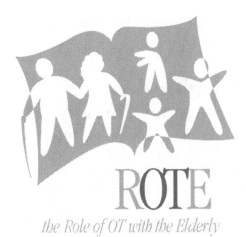

the Role of OT with the Elderly

Occupational Therapy Profession: Organizing Traditions
Section 1. Introduction: From Practical Responses to Theoretical Organization

K. Oscar Larson, MA, OTR

Abstract

The author provides a review of the philosophical base and guiding principles of occupational therapy and relates these principles to work with elderly individuals.

Introduction

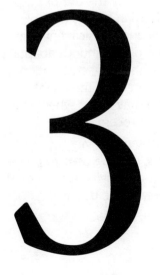

Occupational therapy, as a profession, developed from a tradition of responding to social demands of different generations (Hinojosa, 1996). From the early decades of this century, occupational therapy practitioners have responded to the health issues of people with psychiatric, chronic, and war trauma-related illnesses and injury (Quiroga, 1995). The profession has demonstrated great flexibility by adapting to new challenges as society's demographics and perspectives changed. Advances in psychiatric medications and neurology, decreases in infant and child mortality rates, and an increase in traumatic injury survival during the 1950s to 1970s have spurred growth in the profession as occupational therapy practitioners expanded knowledge and treatment in cognition, sensory integration, and assistive technology.

The 1970s brought a realization that the members of the demographic baby boom bubble would be rising in age and surviving longer. Practitioners have adapted again, expanding into areas of long-term care, home health and wellness, and environmental design. The original series of ROTE workshops and text (Davis & Kirkland, 1986) attest to the interest in information about working with an aging population. Other texts have furthered practitioners' study of gerontic occupational therapy (Bonder & Wagner, 1994; Cutler-Lewis, 1979, 1989; Keirnat, 1991).

With these developments within the profession and within the specialty of gerontic occupational therapy has come the challenge to organize how occupational therapists view and carry out their practice. This chapter will draw upon the body of knowledge in occupational therapy to identify how the following apply to gerontic occupational therapy: philosophy; conceptual models of practice and frames of reference; domain of concern; legitimate tools of practice; roles of the occupational therapist, registered (OTR), and

certified occupational therapy assistant (COTA); and ethics.

Philosophy of Occupational Therapy

Philosophical concepts are those ideas and beliefs held by the profession that cannot be tested by scientific means. Philosophy guides the practitioner by codifying her or his assumptions about health, the individual, and society. Philosophy can direct the practitioner, researcher, and scholar toward certain areas of scientific exploration by establishing the values of the profession. Philosophy closely links with ethics to establish the standards, boundaries, and sanctions of practice.

Three sets of philosophical statements are shown in the boxes (American Occupational Therapy Association [AOTA], 1979; Fidler & Bristow, 1992; Mosey, 1986). Primary to each of these statements is the belief that occupation, or purposeful activity, is an inherent part of the human condition, and when achieved may enhance the quality of a person's life. Adaptation, in order to pursue

The Philosophical Base of Occupational Therapy

Man is an active being whose development is influenced by the use of purposeful activity. Using their capacity for intrinsic motivation, human beings are able to influence their physical and mental health and their social and physical environment through purposeful activity. Human life includes a process of continuous adaptation. Adaptation is a change in function that promotes survival and self-actualization. Biological, psychological, and environmental factors may interrupt the adaptation process at any time throughout the life cycle. Dysfunction may occur when adaptation is impaired. Purposeful activity facilitates the adaptive process.

Occupational Therapy is based on the belief that purposeful activity (occupation), including its interpersonal and environmental components, may be used to prevent and mediate dysfunction, and to elicit maximum adaptation. Activity as used by the occupational therapist includes both an intrinsic and a therapeutic purpose.

Source: American Occupational Therapy Association, 1979, p. 785.

Guiding Principles and Philosophy of Patient Care

Principle I: The attitudes, values, and expectations of staff significantly influence the outcomes of interventions (p. 12).

Principle II: The interrelationship of mind and body is an especially significant concept in designing services for the elderly (p. 13).

Principle III: A multidisciplinary, collaborative, approach is essential (p. 13).

Principle IV: Achievement of the highest possible level of independent functioning in individually relevant activities of daily living is the primary focus of treatment and rehabilitation (p. 14).

Principle V: Independent functioning of the elderly is supported and more readily sustained in an environment that accommodates their physical, sensory, cognitive, and perceptual limitation (p. 15).

Principle VI: A sense of competence, personal integrity, and motivation is enhanced in an environment in which positive feedback and verification of individual achievement and contribution are integral elements of administrative, clinical, and interpersonal policies and behaviors (p. 15).

Principle VII: An environment that exemplifies, in its daily operations, the values of individual autonomy, open communication, and collaborative decision making, maximizes the potential of patients and staff (p. 16).

Source: Fidler & Bristow, 1992.

Philosophical Assumptions

1. Each individual has the right to a meaningful existence; to an existence that allows one to be productive; to experience pleasure and joy; to love and be loved; to live in surroundings that are safe, supportive, and comfortable.

2. Each individual is influenced by stage-specific maturation of the species, the social nature of the species, and the cognitive structure of the species.

3. Each individual has inherent needs for work, play, and rest that must be satisfied in a relatively equal balance.

4. Each individual has the right to seek his or her potential through personal choice within the context of some social constraints.

5. Each individual is only able to reach his or her potential through purposeful interaction with the human and non-human environment.

6. Each individual is only able to be understood within the context of his or her environment of family, community, and cultural group.

7. Occupational therapy is concerned with promoting functional independence through intervention directed toward facilitating participation in major social roles (occupational performances) and the development of the physical, cognitive, psychological, and social skills (performance components) that are fundamental to these roles. The extent to which intervention is focused on occupational performances or performance components is dependent on the needs of a particular client at any given point in time.

Source: Mosey, 1986, p. 6.

occupations, is seen as a life-long process. Achieving functional independence is seen as a goal for occupational therapy. What is purposeful activity? How does an individual adapt? When does a person achieve functional independence?

Occupation

Occupation may be inherently individual. Although we occupy much of our time with commonly understood tasks (e.g., self-care, home management, work, and leisure), the specific type, style, and organization of those tasks will be idiosyncratic for each person. Each older adult has had a lifetime of experiences that have shaped what activities she or he pursues and the way these are carried out, as well as why she or he defines particular activity as purposeful. One person may view job-related tasks as purposeful and therefore maintain a work role until disability or death prevents him or her from carrying out that occupation. Another person may view cooking for a large family as purposeful and adjust to a two-member household by inviting family and friends over for meals on a regular basis. Another may view work and cooking as laborious chores and prefer pursuing leisure and dining out.

Occupation may be socially defined. Again, older adults have spent 60, 70, 80, or more years aging within relationships. They have learned from parents, siblings, teachers, religious leaders, community leaders, famous personalities, and commercial marketing campaigns. Their interests and tastes for certain occupations may have developed within the contexts of those relationships. For example, consider musical tastes. Someone currently 90 years old may have come of age around World War I. This person may

relish ragtime jazz and think of dances at speakeasies and park band stands. A person around 70, coming of age in World War II, may enjoy big band music, recalling Roseland and the Coconut Grove dance halls. A 50-year-old person (who is aging too!), coming of age during the Vietnam War, may like rock 'n' roll and remember Woodstock and the Summer of Love. For each individual, the purpose in the activity of listening to music may be shaped by the social trends at influential times of his or her life.

Pathology may interfere with someone's occupation. Yet, having an illness or injury may not prevent someone from pursuing her or his desired occupations. The relationship between pathology and occupation is a very difficult one to analyze because of the subtle nuances that make a particular activity purposeful to a specific individual and the variety of responses that people have to illness or injury. For instance, two people have diabetes and peripheral vascular disease that resulted in below the knee amputations. One person enjoyed an active lifestyle, including hiking in the mountains. Until that person has healed from the surgery, been fitted for a prosthesis, and developed enough strength, coordination, and endurance to walk and hike, he or she will be prevented from pursuing hiking as an occupation. The second person enjoys watching classic movies. This person has cable TV at home and is quite content to transfer to a favorite easy chair and use the remote control to turn on American Movie Classics.

Conversely, someone's inability to act in a purposeful manner may result in pathology. It is possible to have difficulty occupying oneself without having a specific illness. Again, two people experience difficulty with the purposeful task of trying new recipes to prepare meals. Although neither finds cooking purposeful anymore, the first person continues to cook simple, routine meals. The second experiences discouragement and frustration, is unable to enjoy eating, loses all appetite, and becomes dehydrated and malnourished. As a result, the emergency medical technicians take this person to the hospital because of hyponatremia and delirium.

Because the purpose of activity depends upon personal beliefs and values, what the client and occupational therapy practitioner consider purposeful activity may be the same or different. For instance, most occupational therapy practitioners value healthy behaviors and believe that smoking cigarettes will be detrimental to health. The practitioner would not consider smoking as part of a purposeful activity. (This general trend is evident in the number of health care facilities that restrict smoking inside the building). A 70-year-old client who began smoking during World War II may see smoking to be part of a purposeful activity such as visiting with friends at the Veterans of Foreign Wars (VFW) Hall. Again, the conflict is not about whether smoking cigarettes may worsen the client's health, but between the two sets of values. The issue is whether to stop smoking to improve personal health but not be able to enjoy time with friends, versus continuing to smoke, potentially shortening life, but enjoying what time remains.

The occupational therapy practitioner may assist the individual by identifying what is purposeful activity for that person, within social roles, and assisting that person in carrying out that occupation. This assessment and intervention process is complex because of the numerous biological,

psychological, and social factors that influence how people perceive their experiences and choose to live their lives. This also raises the question about what degree of involvement we should pursue in our clients' lives. When does consultation become control? When does advocacy become intrusion? When does persuasion become coercion?

ADAPTATION

Adaptation is a life-long, developmental process. Many developmental theorists have focused on the physical, cognitive, psychological, and social development of infants, children, and adolescents. As outlined in chapter 1, some theorists have extended their continua of development to include adult and older adult periods. Other theorists have concentrated on a specific period of aging or developmental issue, such as retirement or bereavement. As occupational therapy practitioners, we assume that a person continues to change and adapt throughout his or her life as part of the developmental process.

This assumption is based on our belief that people have the ability to adapt. In viewing the aging person's ability to adapt, we make additional assumptions. The older adult will adapt in a manner similar to other situations in life. For instance, when someone becomes homebound by illness or frailty, the practitioner might inquire about other life experiences during which the person had restricted mobility, such as after a skiing accident. Did the person rally friends and family for assistance after the ski accident? Did the person make gadgets that helped manipulate things needed in the environment? Was the solitude and distance from other responsibilities at home and work enjoyable? Answers to each of these questions direct the therapist in the type of intervention that would fit the person's prior adaptation style, such as utilizing social supports, adaptive equipment, and enjoying time alone.

Yet, if the person has demonstrated difficulty adapting to changes and demands, how vulnerable might that person be to adapting poorly with aging? For example, an older man has recently received a diagnosis of prostate cancer. The oncology team prepares him for treatment, explaining the potential complications of urinary retention and metastasis of cancer if he does not have the procedure, or impotence if he does. The patient experiences much ambivalence. He postpones the procedures several times, but then calls the medical office to reschedule. He has experienced periods of his life when his sense of masculinity and immortality have been challenged: when his wife divorced him and when his father died of lung cancer. In both of those prior situations, he became depressed, withdrawn, and was unable to function in work and home management tasks. Now when both his sense of masculinity and immortality have been threatened, he experiences anxiety and indecision that prevent him from managing his health.

Another situation in which one would question whether the aging person continues to have the ability to adapt is when that person has cognitive decline. A hallmark symptom of dementia is the person's difficulty or inability to process new information. In this situation, the practitioner believes that the environmental setting can assist or hinder someone in adapting. A living situation that requires frequent adjustments to new information may not promote adaptation for the person. For example, streets with traffic and stores that frequently move merchandise may become beyond the person's ability to attend to the stimuli or problem solve where to find needed items. In contrast, living situations that consolidate resources and reduce unnecessary distractions may facilitate the person's ability to adapt. A planned community in which housing, shopping, banking, medical, social, and religious activities are accessible to the person without having to drive or travel far may allow the person with some cognitive decline or dementia to live in the community with some assistance and avoid placement in an institutional setting.

Occupational therapists who assess the person's community and home situations believe that social and environmental interventions can facilitate someone's process of adaptation. In the first example about the homebound man, the practitioner might work with the patient and social worker to inform his social supports about what type of assistance they could provide. Adaptive equipment and environmental adaptations, such as lowered countertops and ramps at outside entrances, may allow him to have access to work areas at home and local transportation services. The practitioner might help him to identify tasks that he enjoys doing by himself to occupy his time alone, such as using the Internet, with which he is familiar from working on computers, to research his family genealogy.

FUNCTIONAL INDEPENDENCE

Different professions define functioning according to the domain of concern of that profession. Medical and biological sciences are interested in the cellular functioning of the organism. Physical therapists are interested in the anatomical and physiological functioning of the body. Occupational therapists are interested in the person's ability to function in purposeful activity. Social workers and public health professionals are interested in the person's ability to function within social and community systems.

In terms of the older adult with an illness such as Parkinson's disease, the doctor would be concerned with diagnostic tests and medications, the physical therapist with the effects of the illness on the person's neuromuscular coordination as these affect movement, the occupational therapist with how the illness affects the person's ability to carry out tasks, and the social worker with what community resources are available to the person. Two issues arise here:

1. When communicating, each professional must realize that others may use an abstract word, *functioning*, in many different ways, and therefore should clarify what is meant by the term.

2. Each professional will have some degree of overlap with others in the domains of concern (this issue will be explored in more detail later in this chapter).

An occupational therapy practitioner views how someone functions in the contexts of activities, environmental settings, and relationships. To continue with the previous example of someone with Parkinson's disease, the practitioner would need to determine what activities the person does, wants to do, or needs to do as part of the daily routine. These occupations might include self-care tasks, home management, work, or leisure tasks. Dysfunction could include an inability to carry out prior and desired occupations, as well as the inability to carry out tasks that meet survival, safety, social, and self-actualization needs. The Parkinson's disease may have progressed to the point at which the person needs ambulation devices to walk. The effort required to walk and stand while doing tasks, such as toileting, dressing, and preparing meals, may be too great for the person. The potential cognitive decline associated with later stages of Parkinson's disease may interfere with the person's ability to initiate and organize new and familiar tasks.

Functioning occurs in an environmental setting. The occupational therapist may evaluate the person's living situation and identify potential barriers. The person with Parkinson's disease who has difficulty walking because of a shuffling gait may need throw rugs and 1/2-inch door thresholds removed from the home in order to move from room to room. The bathroom and kitchen may need lower countertops and grab bars that allow the person to sit while using the shower or sink. The closet may need doors to be removed and the closet bar lowered so that the person can more easily reach the clothes. For the person to go into the community, accessible transportation, curb cuts, and automatic opening doors may make a difference in determining whether the person can function in work, shopping, religious, and recreational activities.

Functioning occurs in the context of someone's relationships. The person with Parkinson's disease may need to rely on family, friends, and community supports. The person's prior relationships and ability to develop new relationships may affect his or her functioning. If this person has established and nurtured relationships over the years, there may be many people willing to take on responsibilities such as providing transportation, running errands, doing some housecleaning, and providing companionship. Someone who has preferred a more solitary lifestyle or developed only a few friendships may have difficulty functioning when physical or cognitive decline requires reliance on others. That person may have few existing supports and few social skills to endear potential service providers to him or her. How often have occupational therapists encountered someone in an acute hospital setting after the patient "fired" the home care attendants or refused to allow community-based professionals to provide services at home? This brings up the other half of this section's title: independence.

Just as *functional* is an abstract term with several possible definitions, so is *independence*. A nurse might consider a patient to be independent when the patient can manage medications without assistance (Mettler & Kemper, 1993). A psychologist might consider a person to be independent with a score within levels 1, 2, or 3 on the Brief Cognitive Rating Scale and Global Deterioration Scale for Assessment of Primary Degenerative Dementia (Painter, 1993; Reisberg & Ferris, 1988; Reisberg, Ferris, De Leon, & Crook, 1982; Sclan & Reisberg, 1992,). An occupational therapist might consider a person to be independent with a score of 3 on the Kohlman Evaluations of Living Skills (Thomson, 1992). In regard to assessment of self-care, Rogers and Holm (1994) defined independence as follows: "A rating of independence means that patients can do a task by themselves....

"Independence-dependence ratings may also connote that a task is completed within reasonable or unreasonable time, or without or with technical aids, or safely or unsafely, or in a normal or abnormal manner" (p. 188). Baum (1991) defined independence as "having access to using the necessary devices and human helpers in order to perform the tasks of daily living" (p. 790).

Two issues arise from these definitions:

1. How do occupational therapists and their clients view their functioning on a continuum from independence to dependence?

2. To what degree is independence a matter of completing the tasks without assistance versus using one's available resources to get tasks done?

In response to both of these questions, some practitioners have begun to promote the concept of interdependence (Brown & Gillespie, 1992). In this perspective, working with the person with Parkinson's disease, the practitioner would be less concerned with whether the person was independent in bed mobility, transferring, using a walker, and finding the toilet in the middle of the morning. Rather, the practitioner would be concerned with how the person interacted with his or her social supports to accomplish daily tasks. Does the person have a spouse or home aides to assist with mobility and toileting (as well as other daily tasks)? Is the person able to express specific needs and elicit necessary assistance? Is the person able to return a benefit to the other people, such as companionship, shared interests, wisdom, knowledge, and memories of the years? Under an independence-dependence dichotomous perspective, the practitioner may not consider the social contracts and exchanges that occur in the process of getting a task done. Under an interdependence perspective, the context of the relationship fosters the completion of the tasks.

With this in mind, the occupational therapy practitioner views someone's degree of interdependence as related to the demands and supports of the environment and people around. For the person with Parkinson's disease, a supportive spouse, family members, or home care providers may be both the link that offers assistance with ambulation around the home and the link to community resources. This link may occur when they drive the person to church or to the shopping mall or senior center. This link may occur when they contact architects and contractors to remodel the person's home for accessibility. This link may occur when they prepare meals and double check medication supplies.

Independence may be highly valued or even desired by some people. A conflict may arise between the person and practitioner when the person:

1. Does not view the tasks that the therapist has suggested to be important for independence; or

2. Values having the assistance of others.

These differences in values may occur because of culture or socioeconomic experience, and the secondary gain of being independent or dependent. The person may have lived in a cultural background in which younger generations are expected to care for elders. The practitioner who encourages the aging grandparent to do tasks may become frustrated that the person and the family do not follow up on recommendations. The person who has lived at an economic level that allowed for hired help to do house cleaning and meal preparation may be baffled by the practitioner who suggests baking muffins and making a cup of tea as a cooking safety evaluation. The aging person who has lived alone for many years after divorce, raised children, and worked in a career may resist assistance from the home health practitioner, seeing the practitioner as an intruder and an affront to independence. The person who wants to be cared for by others may not carry out tasks for which he or she has the strength, organization, and skills because then support services will be removed.

Persons' satisfaction with their degree of independence may relate more to their ability to complete tasks that they value and that meet the demands of their environmental and social situations, rather than to prescribed lists of self-care, home management, work, and leisure tasks. When assessing and promoting functional independence and interdependence, the occupational therapy practitioner should consider multiple factors that relate to the person doing relevant tasks. These factors will be discussed further in the section on domain of concern.

References

American Occupational Therapy Association. (1979). The philosophical base of occupational therapy. *American Journal of Occupational Therapy, 33,* 785.

Baum C. (1991). Identification and use of environmental resources. In C. Christiansen & C. Baum (Eds.), *Occupational therapy: Overcoming human performance deficits* (pp. 789–802). Thorofare, NJ: SLACK.

Bonder, B. R., & Wagner, M. B. (1994). *Functional performance in older adults.* Philadelphia: Davis.

Brown, K., & Gillespie, D. (1992). Recovering relationships: A feminist analysis of recovery models. *American Journal of Occupational Therapy, 46,* 1001–1005.

Cutler-Lewis, S. (1979). *The mature years: A geriatric occupational therapy text.* Thorofare, NJ: SLACK.

Cutler-Lewis, S. (1989). *Elder care in occupational therapy.* Thorofare, NJ: SLACK.

Davis, L. J., & Kirkland, M. (1986). *The role of the occupational therapist with the elderly.* Rockville, MD: American Occupational Therapy Association.

Fidler, G. S., & Bristow, B. (1992). *Recapturing competence: A system's change for geropsychiatric care.* New York: Springer.

Hinojosa, J. (1996). Practice makes perfect. *O.T. Practice, 1*(1), 34–38.

Keirnat, J. M. (1991). *Occupational therapy and the older adult: A clinical manual.* Gaithersburg, MD: Aspen.

Mettler, M., & Kemper, D. W. (1993). Self-care and older adults: Making health care relevant. *Generations, 17*(3), 7–10.

Mosey, A. C. (1986). *Psychosocial components of occupational therapy.* New York: Raven Press.

Painter, J. (1993). Cognitive impairment in the elderly. *Physical and Occupational Therapy in Geriatrics, 11*(3), 27–42.

Quiroga, V. A. M. (1995). *Occupational therapy: The first 30 years, 1900 to 1930.* Bethesda, MD: American Occupational Therapy Association.

Reisberg, B., Ferris, S. H., De Leon, M. J., & Crook, T. (1982). The global deterioration scale for assessment of primary degenerative dementia. *American Journal of Psychiatry, 139,* 1136–1139.

Reisberg, B., & Ferris, S. H. (1988). Brief cognitive rating scale (BCRS). *Psychopharmacology Bulletin 24,* 629–636.

Rogers, J. C., & Holm, M. B. (1994). Assessment of self-care. In B. R. Bonder & M. B. Wagner (Eds.), *Functional performance in older adults* (pp. 181–202). Philadelphia: Davis.

Sclan, S. G., & Reisberg, B. (1992). Functional assessment staging (FAST) in Alzheimer's disease: Reliability, validity, and ordinality. *International Psychogeriatrics, 4*(2), 55–69.

Thomson, L. K. (1992). *The Kohlman evaluation of living skills* (3rd ed.). Rockville, MD: American Occupational Therapy Association.

Section 2. Conceptual Models of Practice and Frames of Reference

K. Oscar Larson, MA, OTR

Abstract

The author covers conceptual models of practice and frames of reference for applying theoretical information in clinical practice.

Introduction

Both Kielhofner (1992) and Mosey (1992) have argued that we must organize the body of knowledge of occupational therapy. Each has presented a slightly different approach for organizing the theoretical concepts that occupational therapy practitioners may use. Kielhofner described conceptual models of practice, arranging many of the ideas used by practitioners into compatible groupings. Mosey recommended developing frames of reference as a way to apply theoretical information in clinical practice. This section will discuss how each approach defines and applies conceptual models of practice and frames of reference. Some examples will be given, although this section is intended to be an overview. The reader is encouraged to consider these ideas throughout later chapters of this text.

Conceptual Models of Practice

For Kielhofner, conceptual models of practice are one of three elements in the organization of a profession's body of knowledge. At the core of the profession is the paradigm, roughly similar to the profession's philosophy, as described earlier. Built around this paradigm are the conceptual models of practice. Outside of these are the related knowledge of the profession and other professions. Each element influences the others. For instance, the basic values and assumptions of the paradigm provide the boundaries in which the profession may develop conceptual models of practice. The theoretical ideas on which conceptual models of practice may be organized come from the area of related knowledge. In the other direction, new related knowledge may spur the growth of new conceptual models of practice, and changes within the conceptual models of practice may challenge the profession's paradigm, resulting in changes to core values and assumptions.

In terms of gerontic occupational therapy, belief in the value of independence provides one reason for utilizing biomechanical principles in rehabilitation of someone after a stroke. Through development of range of motion, muscle strength, and coordination, the person may be able to perform occupations more independently. Much of the theoretical information on which biomechanical conceptual models of practice are developed come from related knowledge from disciplines and professions such as biology, neuroscience, and physical therapy. This related knowledge has also influenced the biomechanical conceptual model of practice and occupational therapy's paradigm. With the exponential growth in knowledge about neurology, many treatment protocols that were developed during the late 1960s and 1970s became quite reductionistic. This led to the use of and debate over enabling activities and physical agent modalities. In turn, this

Components of a Conceptual Model of Practice

1. The interdisciplinary conceptual base

2. Theoretical arguments about order (i.e., organization and function) in the area of concern; disorder (i.e., dysfunction) in the area of concern; and therapeutic intervention (i.e., planned preservation and/or change of the order of the phenomena with which the model is concerned)

3. Technology for application (e.g., assessment protocols, instruments, and treatment methods)

4. Empirical scrutiny of the model (i.e., research that tests theoretical arguments and demonstrates how the model works in practice)

Source: Kielhofner, 1992, p. 18.

Types of Conceptual Models of Practice

1. Biomechanical Model

2. Cognitive-Disabilities Model

3. Cognitive-Perceptual Model

4. Group Work Model

5. Model of Human Occupation

6. Motor Control Model

7. Sensory Integration Model

8. Spatiotemporal Adaptation

Source: Kielhofner, 1992.

has provoked challenges in occupational therapy's paradigm, some promoting more reductionistic clinical approaches and others more holistic views (Gilfoyle, 1984; Hubbard, 1991; Sachs & Labovitz, 1994).

The conceptual models of practice should be familiar to most occupational therapy practitioners. Those who have studied any of these conceptual models of practice will note that the conceptual bases develop from interdisciplinary sources of knowledge. Some of the theoretical concepts have been gathered from within the profession and others from related disciplines and professions. This is particularly important to acknowledge when working

with older adults, because the occupational therapy practitioner will most likely be working as a member of an interdisciplinary team. Occupational therapy has much to gain from research conducted in related fields, and occupational therapy's body of knowledge has much to offer to the interdisciplinary team and the conceptual models that other professions may develop to guide their practice. It would be arrogant to believe that we had some exclusive right to some aspect of gerontology and ignorant not to delve into our colleagues' experiences.

A second component of a conceptual model of practice is that the model defines what is functional and dysfunctional, and what therapeutic interventions may be made in order to decrease dysfunction. A conceptual model of practice should not just describe a situation or problem, but should give the clinician direction as to what to do about that problem. For instance, an occupational therapist might be quite skilled at using assessment tools to evaluate a person's cognitive abilities. The therapist might identify the person's cognitive level according to the Allen Cognitive Level (ACL) test (Allen, 1985). The therapist might describe what tasks the person may be able to do using the Kohlman Evaluation of Living Skills (KELS; Thomson, 1992) or the Assessment of Process and Motor Skills (AMPS; Fisher, 1993; Nygard, Bernspang, & Fisher, 1994). However, if the therapist does not make some assertion about why this information is useful, how it can be used to set treatment goals, or what type of intervention may help this person, then the therapist is not utilizing the assessments as part of a conceptual model of practice. In this example, the therapist might be working within the cognitive disabilities model to evaluate and assist an older adult with dementia to identify a structured living situation and daily routine that promote the person's ability to function in his or her occupations.

In order to implement the conceptual model of practice, the practitioner must have access to the technology to put the concepts into practice. The therapist must have protocols that define how evaluations are conducted as well as the instruments that will give pertinent data. A number of assessment tools that are currently available for occupational therapy practitioners to use with aging adults will be described in Module 3 of this text. Once the therapist has completed

the evaluation and made recommendations, it is important to have access to the methods for carrying out that treatment. Again, methods of intervention will be described in later chapters of this text. While reading, consider with which type of conceptual model of practice they most closely align.

Finally, a conceptual model of practice should be tested. We need to not only describe and assert that our interventions work, we need to demonstrate the efficacy of our work. This is particularly keen at this time of cost containment and treatment justification. Rogers & Holm (1994) have written eloquently on this topic. An additional concern in testing our conceptual models of practice, as gerontic occupational therapy practitioners, is that they be tested with older adults. Interventions that work well with other age groups, may not be effective as one ages. Therefore, when reading the literature or setting up studies ourselves, we should not forget to review the demographics to determine whether the subjects fit our client group.

With this in mind, review the eight conceptual models of practice to consider whom these might serve and where one might utilize them. This review will be cursory, but should start the reader in thinking about the organization of the knowledge that she or he has acquired in courses and work experience.

BIOMECHANICAL MODEL

This model may be most familiar to occupational therapy practitioners who work within medical institutions and agencies. The focus is on musculoskeletal activity and pathology that may interfere with movement while performing occupations. Diagnosis and symptom reduction may be primary, with the assumption that once the disease has remitted and symptoms are reduced, the person will be able to resume desired tasks. Common diagnoses might include orthopedic injuries and disease (e.g., total hip fractures, osteoporosis), cardiopulmonary disease (e.g., myocardial infarction, congestive heart failure, emphysema), soft tissue injury (e.g., burns), tendon and ligament damage (e.g., tears, contractures), connective tissue disease (e.g., arthritis), and autoimmune diseases (e.g., cancer). Oddly enough, although many of these diagnoses are more prevalent in aging adults than in young adults, many practitioners who view themselves as "physical disabilities" specialists do not also view themselves as "geriatric" specialists.

COGNITIVE DISABILITIES MODEL

Claudia Allen has championed this conceptual model over the past 15 years. Although her initial research developed out of work with people who experienced chronic psychiatric illnesses (Allen, 1982), many of her ideas have been applied to older adults with depression and dementia (Allen, 1985; Wilson, Allen, McCormack, & Burton, 1989), and CVA (Thomas, Hicks, & Johnson, 1994). Practitioners working in home care, assisted living facilities, or long-term care may be quite familiar with the principles in the cognitive disabilities model. This model for evaluation and intervention assumes that the person may benefit from properly structured environments, routines, and tasks assistance. In contrast to many medical and rehabilitation models that emphasize progression and improvement, this model accepts that the person has some degree of limitation, but can still function with specific intervention.

Moreover, if intervention is not provided, the person will become dysfunctional more rapidly.

COGNITIVE-PERCEPTUAL MODEL

This model focuses on the processes of perception and cognition related to how a person responds to the environment to complete occupations. The interdisciplinary base derives information from neuroscience, neuropsychology, and fields concerned with the development of motor control. Cognitive-perceptual dysfunction occurs when the brain is damaged, such as during a cerebral vascular accident. Two approaches to treatment exist. Remedial training occurs when the practitioner presents tasks that assist in reorganizing the impaired central nervous system functions. For instance, dressing training and bathtub transfer training will not only teach the person how to don clothes or get onto a tub bench with a hemiparesis, but will provide sensory stimuli that will activate new neural pathways to increase coordinated muscle action. In the second approach, the functional or adaptive approach, the practitioner accepts that the cognitive-perceptual dysfunction is permanent. The practitioner assists the person to compensate for dysfunction and to adapt the environment, thus allowing the person to be more active in occupations.

GROUP WORK MODEL

Anyone who performs occupations in a social relationship may benefit from the concepts of group process. Although practitioners working in psychiatry with patients experiencing depression, bipolar illness, and adjustment disorders may be most aware of the group work involved in therapy, many other situations involve social interactions. Patients in acute care hospitals, rehabilitation centers, sub-acute rehabilitation units, and long-term care may interact in groups, even if they do tasks in a parallel group setting in the same clinic. Patients seen in the home setting may be functioning as part of a family group, and therefore influenced by the expectations and interactions of family members. Clients served in adult day treatment programs, senior centers, assisted living facilities, or congregate housing situations may do tasks together as a group and be affected by others. These tasks may be leisure oriented or focused on home management and self-care tasks. For instance, if a person attends a senior center or community activity at a retirement apartment, she or he may be encouraged to do more physical activity if other group members enjoy exercising or walking or square dancing. However, if the group members tend to be more sedentary or solitary, the activities may include more movies or spectator sports. Part of the role of the occupational therapy practitioner is to monitor the relationships and themes of the group and to bring up topics and tasks that direct the group toward the goals of the group, whether that is specifically a group to resolve problems or a group to prevent potential problems.

MODEL OF HUMAN OCCUPATION

This model applies general system theory (Kielhofner & Burke, 1980; von Bertalanffy, 1968) to how someone functions in daily tasks. The primary concerns are a person's performance of tasks, volition to do tasks, and habits in social roles. Events in a person's life and changes in environment may affect how that person carries out the daily routine. For an older adult, this model can be applied broadly, ranging

from how a person responds to retirement, to gradual declines in strength and sensory perception, or to traumatic illness or injury. The practitioner may intervene by providing tasks and environments that allow the person to use existing performance and to develop new habits. For instance, for the person facing retirement, the practitioner could guide the person in reviewing life roles and interests in order to select alternative tasks to replace work tasks. For a person experiencing physical changes, the practitioner might provide information about tools (adaptive equipment) that can be used while doing tasks, or environmental changes that can compensate for diminished strength and sensory perception (e.g., lowered countertops, reduced glare for lighting, etc.). For the person who has experienced a traumatic illness or injury, the practitioner might set up tasks that the person can do to reestablish skills in performing tasks.

MOTOR CONTROL MODEL

This model consists of four treatment approaches that have been developed to remediate problems of movement after brain trauma: the Rood approach (Rood, 1956), Bobath's neurodevelopmental treatment (Bobath, 1978), Brunstrom's movement therapy (Brunstrom, 1970), and proprioceptive neuromuscular facilitation (Voss, Ionta, & Meyers, 1985). Patients who have experienced a CVA are most likely to receive treatment from this model.

SENSORY INTEGRATION MODEL

This model attends to the organization of sensory information in the CNS and the effect that sensory input, especially at subcortical levels, has on a person's performance of occupations.

This model has evolved primarily for child development use.

SPATIOTEMPORAL ADAPTATION

Again, this model has been developed primarily with concern about child development and the effects of illness and injury on maturation of motor skills.

Frames of Reference

Mosey (1986) outlined three general types of frames of reference: analytic, developmental, and acquisitional. Mosey (1992) refined her method for organizing the body of knowledge of occupational therapy, emphasizing the development and use of frames of reference as guidelines for practice. A frame of reference consists of four elements:

1. Theoretical base of concepts and postulates

2. Function-dysfunction continua

3. Behaviors and physical signs indicative of function and dysfunction

4. Postulates regarding change.

The *theoretical base* consists of concepts and postulates. The concepts label and define the phenomena that are important in the frame of reference. The postulates explain the relationships between the concepts. Together, these guide the occupational therapist in identifying clinical problems, selecting intervention methods, and explaining why intervention works.

The *function-dysfunction* continua should be organized around the major concepts of the frame of reference. These continua give the therapist a means of measuring to what degree the person's behavior is functional.

The *behaviors and physical signs* indicative of function and dysfunction are the increments along each continuum. This acknowledges that some behaviors are more desired than others, allowing the practitioner to demonstrate improvement over the course of therapy. Of concern is where the threshold between functioning and not functioning exists along the continua.

Finally, the *postulates regarding change* are the explanations about how therapy will work. Therapy assumes that not only can occupational therapists accurately describe a problem, but they can do something about the problem (otherwise, they would be diagnosticians, not therapists). The postulates regarding change also allow clinicians and scholars to test the frame of reference for reliability and validity.

In contrast to Kielhofner's approach of collecting similar practice models together under established labels in the occupational therapy literature, Mosey proposed three categories of frames of reference, emphasizing the method of change inherent in the theoretical base.

Analytic frames of reference are based on theories from psychology. *Developmental frames of reference* are based on theories about human development and maturation (see chapter 1). *Acquisitional frames of reference* are based on learning theories. In their purest forms, the frames of reference would be targeted to specific functional problems of the client. Often, in actual practice, the practitioners will use concepts and postulates from more than one type of frame of reference. For example, when working with someone recovering from a CVA, the practitioner will be using postulates from learning theories (e.g., repetition) to develop motor skills, but might also be using postulates from analytic theories (e.g., grieving process) in adapting to the loss of skills. Also of note, there may be several frames of reference that provide guidance for intervention with a specific clinical problem. The existence of multiple frames of reference does not mean that one is correct and the others in error, but that the therapist has several ways of approaching the clinical situation.

Analytic frames of reference deal with the meaning of activity for the person. Someone will be dysfunctional when unable to tolerate or resolve conflicts between ideas, beliefs, feelings, and values about life and personal experiences. For aging adults, these conflicts often revolve around existential concerns about growing older, productivity, accomplishment and failure, their place in society, continuation and loss of relationships, and death and dying. Change occurs when the person is able to explore the conflicts and integrate the intrapsychic dimensions into a view of life. For aging adults this may occur through acceptance of past and anticipated events. This may occur in philosophical (e.g., "I've been healthy all my life. It's my turn to be sick"), spiritual ("Soon I'll be in a better place"), or practical terms ("I've talked with my kids about the estate"). The therapist would be concerned with the meaning of activities and with designing environments that provoke the client to become aware of these conflicts and find a sense of resolution. This process could occur while working in bereavement support groups, working with someone experiencing depression, guiding someone in learning compensatory skills, or designing living facilities for older adults.

Developmental frames of reference focus on the physical, social, and personal maturation of the aging person. Dysfunction may be related to part of the developmental process, when the person experiences injury or illness that is not inherently part of development, and when the person does not continue to develop within the parameters of the developmental theory. Change occurs when the aging person is able to resume the developmental process or achieve expected milestones. These frames of reference will have to view the complex interaction between the biological, social, and personal aspects of an individual's maturation.

Practitioners in all types of settings will need to consider the development of the client, although the length of the therapeutic interaction may affect the degree of intervention that the practitioner may be able to apply. As one might anticipate, developmental frames of reference generally need to be in place over a period of time. Practitioners in an acute care hospital may provide sensitivity about developmental issues, while the primary focus of treatment may be on diagnosis and symptom resolution. Practitioners in rehabilitation facilities and home health care may see the patient over a few weeks or months. This would be a more appropriate setting for addressing the resumption of the person's developmental processes. Practitioners working in hospice settings should be keenly aware of the developmental processes of their clients as these relate to the person's process of dying in comfort and with dignity. Practitioners working in the community, such as at senior centers, assisted living facilities, adult education institutions, or wellness and prevention programs, will be concerned with facilitating their client's maturation through environmental design, programming, and case management.

Acquisitional frames of reference, most prevalently used by occupational practitioners from acute care to rehabilitation to community settings, are concerned with learning skills. This learning may occur:

1. In response to an illness or injury that impedes the person's ability to function (e.g., CVA, myocardial infarction, depression)

2. To prevent loss of function when the person has a progressive illness (e.g., cancer, dementia, diabetes)

3. To prevent injury or illness from developing (e.g., community education about falls, nutrition, health screenings, etc.).

For most patients and clients, acquisitional frames of reference are pragmatic and focused on the specific functional skills that the person wants to learn. These frames of reference fit nicely into managed care and clinical pathway types of protocols. (For example, on day 1 post surgery for total hip replacement, patient will be shown tools for dressing and bathing, and on day 2, patient will sit at edge of bed and receive instruction on using reacher, sock aid, etc.)

Of concern though, are those patients who appear to lack the ability or motivation to learn, have different expectations about therapy (for example, the patient may expect the practitioner to put on the patient's shoes rather than teach the patient how to put them on), have a social support network that has different values than the practitioner, will not follow through on learning objectives, or simply do not appear to "get it" within the usual number of visits. In these situations, the therapist may need to consider a different acquisitional frame of reference (e.g., working within the person's social support system to identify what outcomes they would consider functional and dysfunctional) or may need to utilize a different type of frame of reference before addressing the learning objectives (e.g., using an analytic frame of reference to address the motivational conflict before continuing with prosthetic training for someone with peripheral vascular disease and an amputation).

References

Allen, C. K. (1982). Independence through activity: The practice of occupational therapy (psychiatry). *American Journal of Occupational Therapy, 36,* 731–739.

Allen, C. K. (1985). *Occupational therapy for psychiatric diseases: Measurement and management of cognitive disabilities.* Boston: Little, Brown.

Bobath, B. (1978). *Adult hemiplegia: Evaluation and treatment.* London: William Heihemann Medical Books.

Brunstrom, S. (1970). *Movement therapy in hemiplegia.* New York: Harper and Row.

Fisher, A. G. (1993). The assessment of IADL motor skills: An application of many faceted Rasch Analysis. *American Journal of Occupational Therapy, 47,* 319–329.

Gilfoyle, E. M. (1984). Eleanor Clark Slagle lectureship, 1984: Transformation of a profession. *American Journal of Occupational Therapy, 38,* 575–584.

Hubbard, S. (1991). Toward a truly holistic approach to occupational therapy. *British Journal of Occupational Therapy, 54,* 415–418.

Kielhofner, G. (1992). *Conceptual foundations of occupational therapy.* Philadelphia: Davis.

Kielhofner, G., & Burke, J. (1980). A model of human occupation, part one: Conceptual framework and content. *American Journal of Occupational Therapy, 34,* 572–581.

Mosey, A. C. (1986). *Psychosocial components of occupational therapy.* New York: Raven Press.

Mosey, A. C. (1992). *Applied scientific inquiry in the health professions: An epistemological orientation.* Bethesda, MD: American Occupational Therapy Association.

Nygard, L., Bernspang, B., & Fisher, A. G. (1994). Comparing motor and process ability of persons with suspected dementia in home and clinic settings. *American Journal of Occupational Therapy, 48,* 689–696.

Rogers, J. C., & Holm, M. B. (1994). Accepting the challenge of outcome research: Examining the effectiveness of occupational therapy practice. *American Journal of Occupational Therapy, 48,* 871–876.

Rood, M. (1956). Neurophysiological mechanisms utilized in the treatment of neuromuscular dysfunction. *American Journal of Occupational Therapy, 10*(4, part 2), 220–225.

Sachs, D., & Labovitz, D. R. (1994). The caring occupational therapist: Scope of professional roles and boundaries. *American Journal of Occupational Therapy, 48,* 997–1005.

Thomas, K. S., Hicks, J. J., & Johnson, O. A. (1994). A pilot project for group cognitive retraining with elderly stroke patients. *Physical and Occupational Therapy in Geriatrics. 12*(4), 51–66.

Thomson, L. K. (1992). *The Kohlman evaluation of living skills* (3rd ed.). Rockville, MD: American Occupational Therapy Association.

von Bertalanffy, L. (1968). General systems theory: A critical review. In W. Buckley (Ed.), *Modern systems research for the behavioral scientist.* Chicago: Aldine.

Voss, D. E., Ionta, M. K., & Meyers, B. J. (1985). *Proprioceptive neuromuscular facilitation: Patterns and techniques* (3rd ed.). New York: Harper and Row.

Wilson, D. S., Allen, C. K., McCormack, G., & Burton, G. (1989). Cognitive disability and routine task behaviors in a community based population with senile dementia. *Occupational Therapy Practice,1*(1), 58–66.

Section 3. Domain of Concern

K. Oscar Larson, MA, OTR

Abstract

The author discusses occupational therapy's domain of concern for older adults.

Introduction

A domain of concern of a profession is the area in which that profession has expertise and may provide assistance to someone. By striving to define occupational therapy's domain of concern for older adults, this section intends to identify what aspects of human experience are within the realm of intervention by occupational therapy practitioners. Up front, we must acknowledge that domains of concern are constantly evolving, with details being refined and new phenomena being added or deleted. The purpose of this section is to identify at this point in the profession's development what is considered to be within its domain of concern. Future authors, researchers, and practitioners should challenge and revise this definition!

The Uniform Terminology for Occupational Therapy, 3rd ed. (American Occupational Therapy Association, 1994), outlined in Appendix A, is the national organization's attempt to categorize, label, and define the domain of concern for occupational therapy. The reader should notice the breadth of ideas covered within the three main categories of performance areas, performance components, and performance contexts. Also, the reader should notice that the uniform terminology does not include every aspect of human experience. This is important in understanding the construction of a domain of concern and the congruence with other professions' domains of concern.

Concerning the construction of a domain of concern, the profession is essentially asking the question, "In what areas do we have expertise and some potential effect?" In this manner, occupational therapy is reviewing its literature, practice, and history to see what it is that occupational therapists do well. Thus, phenomena that have not been addressed may not be present, or at least not thoroughly defined, in this document. Therefore, some practitioners may find that what they do does not seem to fit easily into one of these labels, which does not mean, necessarily, that they are practicing outside the domain of concern of occupational therapy. However, those practitioners should be reviewing what they do to see how they might articulate it within the present uniform terminology and how they might include their areas of practice into future revisions.

Concerning the relationship toward other professions' domains of concern, occupational therapy practitioners should be aware that the uniform terminology is not mutually exclusive of other professions' domains of concern. Occupational therapy does not have some inherent ownership of some aspect of human experience. In fact, as the reader may know from practical experience, many aspects of practice overlap with other professions. The range of responses to these overlaps go from "turf battles" within agencies and state licensure laws to cooperation among professions acknowledging each other's areas of expertise. The most common discussions about overlap concern occupational therapy, physical therapy, and recreation therapy.

Occupational and physical therapy overlap in many of the performance components. Occupational and recreation therapy overlap in the performance area of play or leisure activities and many of the performance components. Additionally, other professions that are not traditionally grouped together in rehabilitation departments, such as nursing and social work, have overlaps with occupational therapy's stated domain of concern. When working with older adults, as part of a geriatric team, I advocate a cooperative, integrative approach, allocating responsibilities according to the professionals' expertise. Because of the complex combination of sensorimotor, psychosocial, and environmental challenges that the aging adult experiences (see chapter 4), the geriatric team serves the person best with a variety of perspectives that different professionals can provide.

As a final note about developing the uniform terminology, some have advocated for, and questioned the omission of, terminology used more widely within the international community of health care providers. Specifically, Nieuwenhuijsen (1995) lamented that the World Health Organization's (1980) International Classification of Impairments, Disabilities and Handicaps (ICIDH) was not incorporated into the uniform terminology revision. The chair of the Commission on Practice (COP; Hinojosa, 1995) responded, stating that although AOTA advocates the use of WHO definitions, those definitions have been constructed for different reasons than the uniform terminology, and those definitions are not consistently compatible with the labels that our profession has developed. COP continues to study how these two sets of definitions may be coordinated, but at this time the resolution has not been found.

Performance Areas

For aging adults, all three major performance areas, activities of daily living, work and productivity, and play and leisure activities, continue to be of interest. The stereotype of older adults being retired, with lots of leisure time and few work activities may only hold true for some people. Rather, occupational therapy practitioners working with older adults should be aware of the diversity of lifestyles that their clients live. Some may continue working regularly into their 70s and 80s. Others may take early retirement, enjoying more leisure time or substituting other work tasks, such as part-time work, a job that they always wanted to pursue, adult education, or volunteer work.

Unless some major event has precipitated major changes in the aging person's lifestyle (e.g., retirement, illness or injury, loss of a spouse, family, or friends), the person's daily routine is likely to maintain continuity with prior periods of life. Therefore, occupational therapy practitioners should be inquisitive about the aging person's prior lifestyle. Checking off a box "homemaker" or "retired" on a form gives the geriatric treatment team little information or direction in how to approach the person who has 60, 70, or 80 years of experiences. Home-makers who raised two children or seven children; stayed home, or worked part time, or carried out community service volunteering; or lived in an urban area or rural farming community may have very different styles of approaching tasks and responding to services offered by professionals.

Also, the practitioner should be sensitive to how the client defines certain tasks. For instance, an older adult who regularly spends time caring for grandchildren may consider this a work task or a leisure task. One person may view grooming and hygiene as an important part of the daily routine, while another would rather dispense with all that fussing and get into doing a valued leisure or work task. Again, while approaching the older adult with labels and definitions in mind, occupational therapists should listen and observe carefully how each individual carries out daily tasks and allow flexibility in describing these observations.

The reality of cost containment and length of stay statistics in certain settings often restricts how thoroughly the occupational therapy practitioner can delve into evaluating the person's daily routine. When the practitioner in an acute care setting has possibly three to five sessions of 15 to 30 minutes to evaluate and intervene, and the emphasis of treatment is to remediate or compensate for symptoms of an illness, the practitioner is not likely to have the time to review every performance area in detail. On the one hand, a streamlined screening procedure may help to identify quickly the target areas of intervention, but may also develop a mindset that does not consider the broader implications of the illness or injury. Certainly, basic ADL, such as toileting and eating, may be the most essential tasks for someone to return home with family assistance and home health care. However, the therapist should keep other performance areas in mind to identify whether these areas should also be addressed. For instance, a 73-year-old woman had a total hip replacement and was referred to occupational therapy for "ADL evaluation and training." When the practitioner

demonstrated various mobility precautions and tools, the woman indicated that she would find a reacher useful, but did not want a sock aid or dressing stick. Her husband, who was present at the treatment sessions, would be able to help her with toileting, bathing, and dressing. Her concern was how soon she could get into her MG Midget (manual transmission) in order to drive down to their country house to see the change of seasons. Because she was the primary driver in the family, the inability to don socks and shoes was less of a concern than her inability to hop in the car and go off for the weekends!

Performance Components

Looking over the list of performance components, the reader may notice that some are routinely familiar and others vaguely reminiscent of a third semester college course. As Kielhofner (1992) has noted, during the 1970s and 1980s, occupational therapy practitioners became quite reductionistic and often focused on specific performance components. "Physical disabilities," "sensory integrative," or "psychosocial" therapists tended to address certain components while disregarding other components that appeared less central to the problem at hand. For the gerontic occupational therapy practitioner, it is imperative to consider a wide range of performance components both in problem identification and resolution. Often the aging adult may experience deficits in more than one component of functioning, and the interaction of several components may complicate the problem.

For instance, the home health occupational therapist of a geriatric assessment team receives a referral to evaluate a man's ability to function in his home environment. The neighbors have noticed that he has been wandering around the apartment complex more and appears to be losing weight. In meeting with the man, talking with neighbors and family members (with the client's permission), the therapist identifies several potential problems that may require further evaluation and intervention. Sensorimotor components include decreased hearing and vision, confusion in figure ground and spatial relations, diminished stereognosis in the left hand, and diminished muscle tone and strength of the left upper and lower extremity. Cognitive components include deficits in orientation (oriented to person and place only), short-term memory deficits, and difficulty with spatial operations and problem solving. Psychosocial components include loss of interests, changes in social conduct (as noticed by the neighbors), and difficulty coping with the death of his spouse six months ago. The therapist's observations identify a number of deficits in performance components and suggest that the man should receive further evaluation for potential medical etiology of these deficits. Potential medical explanations for the behavior could include a mild right hemispheric CVA or cancerous tumor, delirium related to malnutrition and dehydration, depression, or deconditioning related to visual and auditory sensory loss and subsequent withdrawal from daily tasks. Potential social explanations for the behavior could be an atypical grief reaction, social isolation related to the death of his spouse, and sensory deficits, or withdrawal from his daily routine.

Performance Contexts

Although the concepts included in performance contexts are familiar to practitioners, the designation of a spe-

cific category is new for the uniform terminology. These issues are broader than the performance areas and components. The interventions for these contexts will not be easily carried out in the isolation and confinement of institutions and agencies. The practitioner will most readily use these ideas in regard to discharge planning and community reentry. Also, occupational therapy practitioners working in wellness, preventive health care, and advocacy will find these ideas useful, as they often address the systems issues that begin a decline into ill health and dependency upon a health care system.

Concerning discharge planning, occupational therapy practitioners will be familiar with the "problem" and the "revolving door" patient. In these situations, the difficulty is that the person has achieved the anticipated goals for treatment in the hospital, rehabilitation facility, or home health care agency, but cannot or will not easily move out of the system. The social worker expresses frustration that the patient cannot be safely discharged home because of lack of social supports to assist the person at home, whether with ADL, taking medications correctly, or finding satisfaction with his or her situation. Or, after repeated attempts at mobilizing the person to return to the community, the person soon returns to the emergency department and reenters the medical system with similar or new problems.

Many of these dilemmas revolve around the allocation of the individual's, family's, and society's resources. One woman wants to live at home, attend outpatient rehabilitation appointments, and go to social activities at the senior center. However, she does not "qualify" for or cannot afford subsidized transportation services, and therefore remains at home until she is too ill to care for herself. A man can no longer live alone at home and has no family living in the area. The social worker arranges for transfer to a nursing home, but because he has no financial resources and has only Medicaid assistance, he must wait for a "Medicaid" bed to open up (e.g., be vacated by someone else) before he can be transferred to long-term care. A woman, after raising four children as a single parent, feels distraught that they have "abandoned" her, moving out of the area, not writing or phoning her, and not letting her see her grandchildren. She experiences recurrent depression that her life has not had the rewards that she expected (e.g., lifelong marriage, grateful children, and golden years spent with children and grandchildren). She returns to the emergency department regularly with various somatic complaints and is admitted several times each year for depression and physical conditions. On each admission, she becomes cheerful and active once around familiar staff and surroundings. Whenever staff prepare for discharge, she becomes sullen and threatens suicide.

Because most of these performance context issues occur at the systems levels, occupational therapy practitioners should be aware of the systems in which their clients live their lives. At times, the practitioner may be able to make an intervention within the system, such as connecting a client to a volunteer organization for social support. At other times, the practitioner may need to work to change the social systems that result in or perpetuate dysfunction in aging adult lives, such as working with the independent living and universal design movements to reduce environmental barriers for people of all ages and abilities.

Appendix A.
Uniform Terminology for Occupational Therapy

I. Performance Areas

  A. Activities of daily living

    1. Grooming

    2. Oral hygiene

    3. Bathing/showering

    4. Toilet hygiene

    5. Personal device care

    6. Dressing

    7. Feeding and eating

    8. Medication routine

    9. Health maintenance

    10. Socialization

    11. Functional communication

    12. Functional Mobility

    13. Community Mobility

    14. Emergency response

    15. Sexual expression

  B. Work and productive activities

    1. Home management

     a. Clothing care

     b. Cleaning

     c. Meal preparation

     d. Shopping

     e. Money management

     f. Household maintenance

     g. Safety procedures

    2. Care of others

    3. Educational activities

    4. Vocational activities

     a. Vocational expression

     b. Job acquisition

     c. Work or job performance

     d. Retirement planning

     e. Volunteer participation

  C. Play or leisure activities

    1. Play or leisure exploration

    2. Play or leisure performance

II. Performance Components

  A. Sensorimotor components

    1. Sensory

     a. Sensory awareness

     b. Sensory processing

      (1) Tactile

      (2) Proprioceptive

      (3) Vestibular

      (4) Visual

      (5) Auditory

      (6) Gustatory

      (7) Olfactory

     c. Perceptual processing

      (1) Stereognosis

      (2) Kinesthesia

      (3) Pain response

      (4) Body scheme

      (5) Right-left discrimination

      (6) Form constancy

      (7) Position in space

      (8) Visual-closure

      (9) Figure ground

      (10) Depth perception

      (11) Spatial relations

      (12) Topographical orientation

    2. Neuromusculoskeletal

     a. Reflex

     b. Range of motion

     c. Muscle tone

     d. Strength

     e. Endurance

     f. Postural control

     g. Postural alignment

     h. Soft tissue integrity

    3. Motor

     a. Gross coordination

     b. Crossing the midline

c. Laterality

d. Bilateral integration

e. Motor control

f. Praxis

g. Fine coordination/dexterity

h. Visual-motor integration

g. Oral-motor control

B. Cognitive integration and cognitive components

   1. Level of arousal

   2. Orientation

   3. Recognition

   4. Attention span

   5. Initiation of activity

   6. Termination of activity

   7. Memory

   8. Sequencing

   9. Categorization

   10. Concept formation

   11. Spatial operations

   12. Problem solving

   13. Learning

   14. Generalization

C. Psychosocial skills and psychological components

   1. Psychological

     a. Values

     b. Interests

     c. Self-concept

   2. Social

     a. Role performance

     b. Interpersonal skills

     c. Self-expression

   3. Self-management

     a. Coping skills

     b. Time management

     c. Self-control

III. Performance Contexts

A. Temporal aspects

   1. Chronological

   2. Developmental

   3. Life cycle

   4. Disability status

B. Environmental aspects

   1. Physical

   2. Social

   3. Cultural

Source: American Occupational Therapy Association, 1994.

References

American Occupational Therapy Association. (1994). Uniform terminology for occupational therapy (3rd ed). *American Journal of Occupational Therapy, 48*, 1047–1054.

Hinojosa, J. (1995). Letters to the editor: Author's response. *American Journal of Occupational Therapy, 49*, 570–571.

Keilhofner, G. (1992). *Conceptual foundations of occupational therapy.* Philadelphia: Davis.

Mosey, A. C. (1992). *Applied scientific inquiry in the health professions: An epistemological orientation.* Bethesda, MD: American Occupational Therapy Association.

Nieuwenhuijsen, E. R. (1995). Letters to the editor: Why is AOTA not using the ICIDH terminology? *American Journal of Occupational Therapy, 49*, 570.

World Health Organization (1980). *International classification of impairments, disabilities, and handicaps: A manual of classification relating to consequences of disease.* Geneva: Author.

Section 4. Legitimate Tools of Practice

K. Oscar Larson, MA, OTR

Abstract

The author discusses legitimate tools for use by occupational therapists in working with elderly persons.

Introduction

Legitimate tools of practice are the methods by which occupational therapy practitioners effect change (Mosey, 1992). Often these tools are the tangible objects that practitioners use, such as splints, adaptive equipment, crafts, or ultrasound, and that become identified with the profession. Yet, the reader should analyze her or his practice beyond the concrete manifestations of change to identify the process of change and methods, tangible and abstract, that assist the client in meeting the goals of treatment.

Returning to the philosophy of occupation again, the use of purposeful activity, or occupation, is the core legitimate tool for occupational therapy. The use of occupation can be divided into three major forms:

1. Analysis and synthesis

2. The nonhuman environment

3. Human interactions.

Each of these will be defined and described in terms of providing treatment for older adults.

Occupation: Analysis and Synthesis

Activity analysis and synthesis are two processes in which the occupational therapist identifies the important components of a task (analysis) and determines how those components can be used to achieve therapeutic goals (synthesis). To define what components are relevant to analyze and synthesize in a task, the therapist must refer back to a conceptual model of practice or frame of reference. Without some guideline for identifying which components are important, the therapist risks over-including, randomly selecting, or neglecting relevant behaviors. In any case, the therapist will not target specific and useful behaviors to identify functional deficits and plan for treatment. Because activity analysis and synthesis should be organized on a conceptual base, no all-encompassing, definitive list is sufficient. The therapist should become familiar with those conceptual models of practice and frames of reference frequently used to determine which components of task performance to observe and manipulate. AOTA's uniform terminology, discussed in the section on domain of concern, is a useful generic taxonomy listing many aspects of task performance. Each performance area, component, and context certainly will need much elaboration for a specific situation.

When working with aging adults, the occupational therapist should keep in mind that the aspects of functioning to be analyzed and synthesized should cover a broad spectrum in addition to the narrower focus of the specific diagnosis on the referral. For instance, a patient is referred to the occupational therapist on the pulmonary rehabilitation team because of deconditioning from pneumonia and chronic obstructive pulmonary disease (COPD). Although the core emphasis of the evaluation and intervention may be on how the person's strength and endurance affect completion of ADLs, the therapist should make a number of other observations.

In performance areas, the therapist should analyze the range of roles that the person wants or needs to perform and the demands of the tasks involved in those roles. Does the person don pullover sweatsuits or need ironed blouses and skirts? Does the person cook frozen dinners in the microwave or prefer meals made from fresh ingredients? Does the person have work or caregiving responsibilities? Does the person find satisfaction in low energy leisure tasks or desire to be more active?

In regard to performance components, the person may have many deficits other than decreased strength and endurance that affect functioning. Some may be related to other disease processes and may need attention during the pulmonary rehabilitation process or afterward. Is the person's vision and hearing diminished, thereby interfering with the ability to understand and follow through with instruction for exercises and energy conservation? Does the person have cognitive deficits that interfere with learning and carry over from one session to another, as well as after-care planning? Does the person feel depressed and lack the energy to become engaged in treatment?

Finally, the performance context can profoundly affect the patient's recovery and follow through with treatment. Does the person's physical environment present too many barriers or does it promote functioning in daily tasks? Does the person's cultural background value perseverance and support of people with chronic illness? Does the person have a supportive social network to help with transportation to outpatient follow up appoint-

ments, support groups, and other desired activities?

By taking this broader perspective, the occupational therapist can synthesize the functional assets and deficits into a treatment plan that will address both the specific referral diagnosis, as well as other aspects that affect functioning with that diagnosis. In the example of the person with pneumonia, work has great significance to the person and returning to the work setting may be an important goal once the person has recovered sufficiently from the pneumonia and become stable with a portable oxygen unit. The occupational therapist might notice symptoms of depression affecting task performance and recommend an evaluation by the psychiatrist. The person may indicate that the home environment is accessible, being on one level, but live alone. This person will have to be able to arrange taxi service or drive independently in order to follow up on outpatient treatment and resume part-time work. Coordinating with the social worker, the occupational therapist suggests contacting the local taxi company to arrange for discounted fares offered to senior citizens and people with disabilities. By analyzing and synthesizing the specific components related to the diagnosis and broader components of the patient's task performance, the occupational therapist increases the probability of a successful and sustained outcome.

Occupation in the Nonhuman Environment

The nonhuman environment includes all elements that have material or organic existence, but are not defined as human. Searles (1960) explored the concept of the nonhuman environment and its effect on growth and development. Of particular interest to occupational therapists are the ways in which the nonhuman environment can be manipulated to achieve a desired change. Occupational therapy practitioners commonly use five aspects of the nonhuman environment as tools:

1. The physical environment

2. Devices for positioning

3. Adaptive equipment and assistive technology

4. Adapted activities

5. Physical agent modalities.

Physical environments are the places in which we live, work, and carry out daily tasks. The range of environments can be narrow, such as in the case of the person with weakness from Stage IV cancer who lives on the ground floor of a house because of weakness and pain and receives hospice care at home. The range of environments can be broad, such as the case of the person who has received rehabilitation after an MI and returns to home and work. This person must be able to negotiate the home and office environments, the streets and highways to commute to work, parking lots and stores to run errands, and a variety of indoor and outdoor settings to engage in desired leisure tasks, whether square dancing, golfing, or attending a football game.

The occupational therapy practitioners may use the physical environment by designing or adapting the environment to allow the person to function in occupations. From a prevention perspective, the practitioner would work as a design consultant to eliminate barriers. From a rehabilitation perspective, the practitioner would analyze the client's abilities and the environmental and task demands, and

then make recommendations about adapting the environment to allow the person to do tasks with the greatest ease. Areas in geriatric practice in which occupational therapy practitioners may utilize the physical environment could include:

1. Senior centers, retirement residences, assisted living facilities, and long-term care facilities

2. Consultations with government offices, businesses, retailers, and entertainment establishments in connection with the Americans with Disabilities Act (ADA)

3. Acute care and rehabilitation facilities working on discharge planning

4. Home health care agencies where the practitioner may work with the client in the actual community environment.

Devices for positioning include splints, bed and chair cushions, etc. that correctly align the body or a body part. The alignment may prevent further dysfunction (e.g., a resting hand splint for someone with a flaccid hemiparesis or arthritis) or promote correct movement (e.g., a wedge cushion and foot rest that position someone in an upright posture in order to eat a meal from a lap tray). These devices and their purposes are generally not familiar to the patients or other staff members not involved in rehabilitation. Therefore, the occupational therapy practitioner's role in using devices for positioning include constructing and arranging the device and training caretakers in how to correctly use the device. Some devices can actually lead to iatrogenic problems if used incorrectly (e.g., pressure areas and skin breakdown).

Adaptive equipment and assistive technology are familiar objects to occupational therapy practitioners, though often foreign to clients. However, consumer demand for tools and gadgets to make tasks easier to do is growing. This demand can be seen in the exponential growth in the variety of tools being developed and marketed through catalogues and the availability of products in home health stores, drug stores, home improvement stores, and department stores. Some products may use simple mechanical principles, such as lever handles on sinks and doors to help someone with arthritis use these devices more easily. Other products may use more complex electronic systems, such as computer programs that monitor schedules for medications and ADL, and control lights and security systems for someone with mild dementia. Both low tech and high tech tools may allow the person to remain at home and in the community independently or with some degree of assistance with family, volunteers, and professionals. The occupational therapist intervenes by analyzing the person's skills, the demands of the physical environment and task, and the equipment options. In addition to physical skills, the practitioner should be aware of the person's ability and desire to learn how to use the tool. Too often, equipment ends up in a closet or behind furniture when the person lacks the ability to carry over new learning or does not desire to try something new.

Adapted activities often accompany adaptive equipment and assistive technology. Essentially, the person needs to learn how to do the desired task differently. As with adaptive equipment and assistive technology, the client's ability to accept the need to adapt to change can influence how invested he or she will be in developing new task skills. Energy conservation techniques are examples of adapted activities. The person might do tasks sitting down, plan out the steps of the task, and place frequently needed supplies in readily accessible drawers and cabinets. The person may continue to carry out grooming, dressing, home management tasks, work, or leisure tasks, but with reduced energy expenditure. Clients who have chronic illnesses, such as COPD, CHF, arthritis, or cancer, might benefit from adapting how they do tasks. Clients recovering from acute illnesses, such as MI, CVA, depression, or hip fracture, might benefit from using adapted activities during their recovery period, as well as incorporating some adapted activity principles to prevent future problems.

Physical agent modalities have become accepted within occupational therapy as adjunctive activities (McGuire, 1992). The proponents of occupational therapy practitioners using physical agent modalities acknowledge that they are not inherently purposeful activities, but can be used to enable the client to subsequently perform occupations (Pedretti et al., 1992). The practitioner should pursue adequate training and continuing education to maintain competency in the use of specific physical agent modalities. Physical agent modalities that are frequently used by occupational therapy practitioners include fluidotherapy, paraffin wax, hot and cold packs, ultrasound, contrast baths, whirlpool, functional electrical stimulation/neuromuscular electrical stimulation (FES/NMES), and transcutaneous electrical nerve stimulation (TENS; Taylor & Humphry, 1991). These may be administered in inpatient settings to remediate acute episodes of an illness, or in outpatient or home health care settings to continue treatment or prevent recurrence of acute symptoms. Some patients may be able to learn to use some physical properties, either for self-administration, or to incorporate into other activities (e.g., a hot shower for someone with arthritis as part of the morning warm up before doing range of motion exercises and then daily tasks).

Occupation in Human Interactions

The element of human interaction is essential in the therapy process. If clients had access to all the material resources described as the nonhuman environment and knowledge of how to use those resources, there might be little need for occupational therapy. Granted, some people are able to browse through catalogues of adaptive equipment and select out useful tools. Some people develop compensatory skills to complete ADL without having completed a rehabilitation program. Some people find that swimming three times each week and soaking in the jacuzzi helps maintain muscle strength and reduce fatigue of arthritic joints. However, many people have never considered how to adapt to illness or injury. Occupational therapy practitioners intervene through human interaction in two ways:

1. Dyadic and

2. Group educational situations.

In considering the educational process, whether in dyadic pairs or groups, the practitioner must consider the differences between teaching and learning. The role of the teacher (occupational therapy practitioner) is to be the person with expert knowledge both in the content of the subject and the process of how to convey that information to the learner (patient or client). The role of the learner is to be interested in the topic and receptive to the experiences that the teacher will provide in order to learn.

The practitioner should be aware of the locus of control in the educational experience. For instance, does the setting promote authority and power in the practitioner to guide and direct the patient? Acute care and rehabilitation centers are more likely to work in a practitioner-directed mode, as the practitioner identifies the patient's assets and deficits, develops treatment plans related to the diagnosis and dysfunction, and documents progress toward goals. In contrast, does the setting utilize self-directed learning, placing the authority and power in the client to select goals, topics, and educational methods? Community-based practices might utilize more of a client-directed mode in which the therapy occurs in a naturalistic setting and clients have more decision-making authority in whether to initiate or sustain the learning. Both methods have benefits and risks as far as the achievement of the client's and practitioner's roles and objectives.

DYADIC EDUCATION

Dyadic teaching and learning may occur when two people interact. This may occur in a formal manner, such as when an occupational therapist receives a referral and meets with the person to complete assessment tools, evaluates the person's ability to function, and then works toward therapeutic goals. This may occur informally when a patient works with several staff members and develops an attachment to one particular member. The patient may bestow a special degree of authority on this therapist, listening and following directions and suggestions while disregarding other's ideas. In these situations, a keen therapy team may utilize those attachments by allowing that team member to assist the patient with the more difficult aspects of treatment (e.g., pain management, discharge planning and termination of treatment, etc.). Of equal concern is when the patient and practitioner develop too strong an attachment, such that the benefits of therapy become jeopardized (e.g., the patient rejects all other staff members' assistance or the patient refuses to terminate treatment because of fear of losing the support of the practitioner).

Because isolation and loneliness can be a major problem for many aging people, the dyadic relationship has some inherent features that may encourage the client to become engaged in therapy. Therapy becomes a place of human contact. The practitioner becomes a source of solace and reassurance, especially when the body becomes frail or ill, and social supports may become distant. Many aging adults will seek and be satisfied with existing supports in their communities: families, friends, or clergy. However, when physical or psychological discomfort becomes too complex or intolerable for the person, he or she may perceive the problem as a somatic problem and seek medical attention.

The practitioner should also consider the person's early learning experiences about human contact and aging. When today's 60-, 70-, and 80-year-old adults were growing up, cellular phones were not something that one might see someone else using; computers did not exist, let alone E-mail and the Internet; video camcorders did not record the last family reunion; television did not bring the latest sitcom, natural disaster, or war into the living room.

In the 1910s, 1920s, and 1930s, many of today's aging adults may have lived in rural communities where local newspapers brought the news weekly, wireless radios reported the national and international news, film newsreels showed scenes of the times, and an automobile might carry the family to church or a community event. Those living in urban areas might not have had access to transportation to travel far from their neighborhoods. In either case, large families and extended families made up a greater percentage of an older person's social contacts. Today, in addition to the potential geographical distance of families scattered across counties and states, the aging adult has an onslaught of vicarious relationships waiting to consume time and attention. Even if the older adult has family and friends to call or write, she or he has much access through tabloid newspapers and television to the personal lives of famous film, music, and business personalities.

In the diagnosis, symptom reduction, and outcome-oriented atmosphere of health care today, the dyadic relationship of practitioner and patient may become quite focused around the immediate problem at hand. Although this reductionistic approach may work efficiently for patients with very specific health issues and treatment goals, for many aging adults, health and social problems have multiple layers and ramifications.

An example of a focused situation might be the person who comes to the hospital for a total hip replacement. This person receives preoperative instruction in pain management and wound healing from the nurses, mobility and body mechanics from the physical therapist, and adaptive equipment and joint projection in ADL from the occupational therapy practitioner. Postsurgery treatment includes practicing the information provided earlier and referral to subacute care rehabilitation or home health care.

An example of a multiple issue situation is another person who receives a total hip replacement. However, this woman has lived alone for six months since her husband died. She has a history of depression and appears to have decompensated while grieving her loss. She has difficulty retaining information that practitioners provide her because of her decreased attention span. In addition to the osteoarthritis in her hip, she has arthritis in her knees and hands. She is unable to manipulate a reacher and dressing stick because of ulnar deviation and pain in her hands.

In the former situation, the dyadic educational experience appears to be straightforward. The occupational therapy practitioner provides the person with information, tools, and experiences to try out those tools. In the later situation, the dyadic educational experience will not fit as easily into a reductionistic approach. The practitioner must address social, psychological, and sensorimotor aspects of the woman's ability to function after her hip surgery.

One approach to the dyadic relationship is to allow time to establish a rapport with the client and to identify that person's perspective on the situation. This requires listening to themes that the client brings up, allowing the person to talk about subjects that do not immediately appear related to the referral diagnosis, and asking a broad range of questions. In the second situation described earlier, the practitioner may need to allow the woman to talk about the effects of her husband's death on her ability to carry out daily tasks and responsibilities. Hearing stories about her grieving may not appear to be related to her hip fracture, but listening to how she copes with changes may. Does she have other social supports who will be able to help her when she returns home? Does she sto-

ically bear the intense emotions required to overcome challenges? Does she become withdrawn or reject help from others? The answers to these types of questions may affect discharge planning. Some information may need to be passed on to other professionals, such as suggesting a psychiatric evaluation for depression and antidepressant medications, or a social work evaluation for home care services.

GROUP EDUCATION

Group teaching and learning occur when people gather for some common experience. The leadership style may vary from formally appointed leaders, such as an instructor, to more self-directed groups in which a facilitator initiates and occasionally guides the subject around which the group focuses, to leaderless groups, such as support groups in which the leadership rotates among members, formally or informally. Group formats may vary from highly intellectualized, such as illness prevention lectures, to instructional courses on range of motion exercises or stress management techniques, to experiential events, such as a holiday celebration in which spontaneous social interaction is the desired goal. Group topics may change frequently, such as a guest lecture series, have a routine course, such as a stroke rehabilitation group in which activity of the group changes as the group progresses, or be consistent, such as a daily exercise session. The leadership style, format, and topic of the group should relate to the people assembled for the group.

Group education may not work in every setting in which occupational therapists practice. People referred to occupational therapy may not have common areas of interest related to their reason for referral. In an acute hospital, the practitioner's caseload may include a dozen different diagnoses, or the clients may be at different points of their recovery and not working on similar goals. An additional restriction on group work is reimbursement. Some provisions in third-party payer contracts may not reimburse for treatment when the practitioner gathers several patients at once to work on common tasks. These issues should be identified according to the practitioner's specific treatment environment.

Of course, participation in a group requires that each member be able to relate at some level, not necessarily the same level, to the group. People with very limited orientation, organization, or impulse control may not benefit from or help a group situation. The occupational practitioner should evaluate in what type of group the members can participate. The practitioner should determine whether the person's condition is stable (in which case the group may need to be graded to accommodate his or her ability), or has a prognosis for improvement (in which case the person may become better able to join in after some time).

Providing educational experiences in groups offers a number of benefits that cannot be gained in individual or dyadic situations. Given the limited number of occupational therapists and certified occupational therapy assistants available and the limited number of sessions allowed, group education may offer efficient use of time. Should the practitioner have three or four clients with similar functional deficits, treatment goals, and utilizing similar intervention techniques, the group setting allows the practitioner to see all at once. Examples of these types of groups include teaching and practicing:

1. Energy conservation techniques in home management skills to clients with COPD

2. Self-range of motion for clients who have had a CVA

3. Cueing and task breakdown skills to caregivers of people with dementia

4. Retirement planning strategies for employees through an Employee Assistance Program.

Also, the practitioner might organize the group to meet divergent goals when the skills of some group members can compensate for deficits of others. For instance, in an assisted living facility, senior center, or long-term care facility, members who are more mobile and alert could prepare a snack and tea in the afternoon for other clients who could then join in a reminiscence session.

A second benefit of the group setting is the dynamics that occur when people interact. Many aging adults resist identifying with other people of similar age or physical status. When the person remains distant from the group, she or he can defend her or his sense of identity by claiming to be different and usually healthier than "those old folks in wheelchairs." However, the cost of this defense may be the loss of social supports by failing to continue or to establish relationships. When a person does integrate into the group, whether at a volunteer job, senior center, or activity time in the long-term care facility, that person can begin to develop a sense of identity with and connection to others who are experiencing similar challenges in life. Older adults may first direct their attention toward somatic or physical concerns. However, behind many of these lists of aches and pains, or wheelchairs and walkers, are issues about loneliness, loss of abilities, and changes in self-image.

A third benefit of group situations is shared learning. When the group has existed over a period of time, group members can begin to develop cohesion, aligning with other group members. Because each group member has a different learning style and amount of recall later, interaction of group members allows collective repetition, reinforcement, and retention. One group member misses or forgets certain information, while another may be able to remind or guide the first person through the procedure. In addition to the practical aspects of shared learning (e.g., learning to do leisure tasks without the use of a hemiparetic arm), group members can learn about each other, reinforcing their interdependence (e.g., learning to remind a group member where the group meets).

Additional Considerations

Legitimate tools of practice in gerontic occupational therapy span a wide range from activity analysis and synthesis, using the nonhuman environment and using human interactions. Practitioners should be aware that these tools are not exclusively the property or ownership of occupational therapy. Occupational therapists have borrowed tools from other professions, and other professions are interested in what occupational therapists use to intervene. This raises the question of how occupational therapists differentiate themselves from those in other professions. I recommend practitioners consider not just what they use as tools, but how and why they use these tools. Other professions may use similar tools, but for different purposes. At this point, each profession should return to the review

of the domain of concern to identify the situations in which legitimate tools may be used.

A related issue is how to determine what are not legitimate tools of practice for occupational therapy, and specifically what are tools of occupational therapy but not for gerontic specialization. An obvious example of a tool that is not legitimate for occupational therapy practitioners to use is the prescription and administration of medications. Medications can have a profound and beneficial effect on how someone functions. However, occupational therapists generally ascribe these tools to physicians and nurses. If readers review the domain of concern, they will notice that the action of the medication does not work on any performance area, component, or context that occupational therapy defines as its concern. Medication acts upon biological and chemical processes that are within the domains of concern of medicine and nursing.

A second restriction upon use of a tool is training and competency of the practitioner. Although basic education provides the entry-level practitioners with specific skills to practice, and knowledge of where to develop additional skills, the practitioner must take the initiative to seek training in the specific tools to use within a specific position. This may include continuing education, graduate, or postgraduate education. For working with aging adults, the practitioner may need to develop additional skills in neurodevelopmental treatment, dementia assessments, environmental adaptation, or bereavement counseling.

As a final note, practitioners must acknowledge that tools continue to evolve because of changes in technology, changes in social values and priorities, and changes in clientele. Occupational therapists should avoid two fallacies in considering new technology:

1. Discarding established tools for new ideas

2. Resisting new tools because they are different.

Rather, they should explore the possible utility of tools that assist in meeting the ultimate goal of providing better intervention to clients. And, the profession should consider the ease or difficulty of educating practitioners to become competent in using these tools. I hope that by the next revision of this text, occupational therapy's toolbox will have grown larger still!

References

McGuire, M. J. (1992). Position paper: Physical agent modalities. *American Journal of Occupational Therapy, 46,* 1090–1091.

Mosey, A. C. (1992). *Applied scientific inquiry in the health professions: An epistemological orientation.* Bethesda, MD: American Occupational Therapy Association.

Pedretti, L. W., Smith, R. O., Hammel, J., Rein, J., Anson, O., & McGuire, M. J. (1992). Use of adjunctive modalities in occupational therapy. *American Journal of Occupational Therapy, 46,* 1075–1081.

Searles, H. F. (1960). *The nonhuman environment.* New York: International Universities Press.

Taylor, E., & Humphry, R. (1991). Survey of physical agent modality use. *American Journal of Occupational Therapy, 45,* 924–931.

Section 5.
OTR and COTA Roles and Collaboration

K. Oscar Larson, MA, OTR

Abstract

The author provides an overview of the roles performed by OTRs and COTAs in gerontic practice.

Introduction

Occupational therapists, registered (OTRs) and certified occupational therapy assistants (COTAs) frequently work together in settings where older adults receive services. The Occupational Therapy Roles document, approved by the Representative Assembly in 1993 (American Occupational Therapy Association [AOTA], 1993) is the most explicit description of the variety of roles that practitioners may perform. This document speaks in general terms and does not directly address roles and relationships in gerontic occupational therapy practice. This section will outline the primary roles that OTRs and COTAs may perform, with examples relating these roles to gerontic practice. The reader should consider these roles when reading other sections of this text.

The roles document describes five aspects of a role:

1. Major functions
2. Scope of role
3. Key performance areas
4. Supervision
5. Qualifications.

Some roles are specifically for OTs or COTAs, although many can be performed by both OTRs and COTAs who possess the education, skills, and legal qualifications (see Table 3–1).

Three skill levels and three supervision levels are described, with roughly entry-level practitioners receiving close supervision, intermediate-level practitioners receiving routine or general supervision, and advanced-level practitioners receiving minimal supervision. OTRs and COTAs working in collaboration should be particularly sensitive to the degree of supervision provided and needed in the geriatric setting. Given the allocation of scarce resources today, it is common for a setting to hire COTAs to perform many of the daily work functions, while OTRs consult at several facilities throughout the course of the work week. This arrangement may work well with intermediate and advanced-level practitioners, but may jeopardize the quality of care when entry-level practitioners and new supervisors are developing their professional skills.

Common Skills and Responsibilities

The OTR and COTA practitioners share many common practice skills and responsibilities, according to each practitioner's level of competency. The OTR retains the role of supervisor and ultimately has professional, ethical, and legal responsibility for her or his own behavior as well as that of other OTRs and COTAs supervised. Both practitioners can be involved in gathering data from assessment, while the OTR is responsible for interpreting that data in an evaluation and developing relevant treatment goals and plans. This division works well in the long-term care, rehabilitation, or community setting where the COTA may have the primary contact with the client. The COTA can complete assessments in areas of competence, gathering the data that the OTR utilizes to direct further treatment. Because of the OTR's greater knowledge of theoretical approaches to treatment, it is important that the OTR analyze and provide direction for treatment, rather than rationalize the temptation to rubber-stamp documentation assembled by the COTA. Whether in supervisory meetings, in-service training, or encouragement of continuing educational programming, the OTR should accept responsibility to stimulate the COTA's interest in developing knowledge and skills.

In settings where the OTR and COTA work as co-therapists, such as with some neurodevelopmental treatment (NDT) techniques or group sessions, the practitioners should develop a synergy of action. One practitioner should take primary leadership for the specific technique or session, while the other provides support for safety and reinforcement. For instance, while promoting normal muscle tone and movement patterns during an NDT treatment, the OTR may take the role

Table 3–1. OTR and COTA Roles

Role	OTR	COTA
Practitioner-OTR	X	
Practitioner-COTA		X
Educator	X	X
(Peer, Consumer)		
Fieldwork Educator		
(Practice Setting)		
Fieldwork I	X entry level	X entry level
Fieldwork II	X 1 year's experience	
(OT or OTA)		
(OTA only)		X 1 year's experience
Multiple Students	X 3 years' experience	X 3 years' experience
Supervisor	X 2 or 3 years' experience; 1 year if supervising COTA	X 2 or 3 years' experience; COTA may supervise a COTA if OTR also supervises
Administrator	X 3 to 5 years' experience	
(Practice Setting)		
Consultant	X	X

continued on next page

Table 3–1. OTR and COTA Roles (Continued)

Role	OTR	COTA
Fieldwork Coordinator (Academic Setting)	X	X
Faculty	X PhD preferred, MS or MA recommended	X MS or MA preferred, BS or BA recommended
Program Director (Academic Setting)		
Technical Level	X MS or MA preferred, 3 years' experience in practice and academic settings	
Professional Level	X PhD preferred, MS or MA recommended, 5 years' experience in practice and academic settings	
Post-Professional	X PhD, 5 years' experience in practice and academic settings	
Researcher/Scholar	X	X
Entrepreneur	X 3 years' experience	X 3 years' experience

Source: American Occupational Therapy Association, 1993.

of guiding the patient with verbal instructions and tactile cues, while the COTA positions equipment or provides additional biomechanical support. In an activity group setting to promote socialization among patients experiencing depression, the COTA may take formal leadership by setting up the tasks and directing the patients to become involved in the task. The OTR may take a supportive role, adding additional cues and encouragement, while also analyzing the group processes to interpret the actions of patients and give feedback to the COTA about facilitating the recovery of the patients.

The OTR and COTA can work together with elements of the nonhuman environment. The OTR may design a treatment plan that requires fabrication of splints, ordering and education in the use of adaptive equipment or home modifications, or staff education in the use of a positioning device. The OTR can review these interventions with the COTA, who can implement the plans (assuming competency in these techniques). The OTR can reevaluate the progress after a sufficient period of time. In this type of collaboration, the OTR and COTA should jointly meet with the client at the initiation of treatment to familiarize the older client with the members of a treatment team. For older adults, who may be inundated with dozens of health care professionals doing tests, procedures, and daily care, keeping track of who does what can be quite overwhelming. Taking a few minutes to familiarize the person with the OTR–COTA team can ease the transition for OTR evaluation to COTA intervention.

Peer and consumer education is an area rich for exploration by OTRs and COTAs. Two current trends provide opportunities for practitioners to become more involved in education:

1. Cross-training
2. Consumers' interest in managing their own health.

Toward the former, many facilities are concerned with utilizing staff as efficiently as possible. As discussed earlier, many aspects of different professions' domains of concern and legitimate tools of practice may overlap. Most facilities cannot afford the specialist who cannot carry out multiple roles within professional and educational abilities. Within rehabilitation departments this may mean developing skills in physical medicine, psychiatry, and gerontology. Interdepartmentally, this may mean considering what nursing, occupational therapy, physical therapy, and social work have in common and developing skills in shared areas so that staff can complement each other in treatment teams. The debate should not be whether nursing or OT owns ADL, whether OT or PT owns modalities, or whether OT or social work owns community resources, but who on the team has the rapport with the patient and the skills to complete the task. Some areas where OTRs and COTAs could provide peer education might include fall safety, positioning devices, ADL training, transfers and ambulation, social interactions, leisure task pursuits, home modifications, and access to community resources.

With the increase in education and awareness of being able to control their health, aging adults are seeing themselves as consumers of health care services. Settings and events where preventive health care practices are presented offer many opportunities for OTRs and COTAs to provide education to consumers. These settings might include health fairs or wellness lecture series sponsored by hospitals or health maintenance organizations, guest lectures at senior centers, synagogues, churches, mosques, or civic organizations, or demonstration workshops at home improvement centers or gardening clubs. Topics for displays, posters, or lectures might include preparing for retirement, maintaining health and fitness, home modifications, adapting roles after losses, adapting to physical and sensory changes, accessing community resources, preventing accidents, driver safety in aging, or caring for aging parents. Obviously, both this list of settings and topics could be expanded.

Fieldwork Education

Fieldwork education provides the practitioner with opportunities to develop skills in gerontic occupational therapy, as well as developing future practitioners with a sensitivity and awareness of gerontic practice. Currently, fieldwork sites are becoming more scarce, especially in the areas of psychiatry and nontraditional practice settings. The gerontic practitioner may offer experiences not only in physical medicine, but also mental health and community practice. As the seasoned practitioner knows well, even when the diagnosis and reason for referral lists a physical problem such as a hip fracture, deconditioning, or COPD, key factors in accomplishing treatment goals are helping the client to have the motivation to improve and working with secondary depression or cognitive changes.

Obstacles to developing student fieldwork programs include isolation, contract relationships with a facility, and nontraditional work sites. Certainly the lone occupational therapy practitioner working for a facility will have to have a degree of initiative to present to the administration and establish a training program. However, having students allows that practitioner to have more professional contact. Practitioners in these situations should consider continuing education and resources from AOTA and state and local associations to help develop a training program for OTRs or COTAs. Practitioners who work for contract agencies will need to collaborate with both their employers and the facilities to which they are sent. A persuasive factor for training students is the increased visibility of the contract agency to future employees. Of course, the agency should consider the implications of increased need for supervision for entry-level employees, should students seek employment with the agency after completing fieldwork experiences. As more practitioners work outside the traditional hospital or long-term care setting, practitioners should consider developing fieldwork programs that introduce students to a wider variety of practice settings. Home health care and adult day treatment programs in the community are settings that carry over traditional occupational therapy practices into different practice environments. Entrepreneurial practitioners with private practices and consulting businesses would offer different experiences to students who have similar interests in applying their skills. Those in nontraditional settings may wish to consider prerequisite fieldwork experiences, such as having completed two prior fieldwork II programs, to ensure that students have developed basic skills before exploring new horizons in occupational therapy practice.

Administrative and Consultant Roles

The role of administrator is reserved for the OTR. An administrator will have responsibility for program development and supervision of staff. Occupational therapists working in the capacity should consider how to incorporate the collaboration of OTR and COTA practitioners for efficiency and economy. In settings where many clients are aging, but staff do not consider themselves to be gerontic specialists, the administrator can use supervisory sessions, in-service, and continuing education to direct the staff in developing identities as specialists in gerontology and other areas, to overcome stereotypes and fears that inhibit identification as gerontic specialists, and to enhance staff's skills in working with the wide range of health care issues of aging people. This may include subscribing to geriatric journals and AOTA's *Gerontology Special Interest Section Newsletter* and including texts about gerontology in the staff library.

The role of consultant is an area with much potential use by OTRs and COTAs, depending on their competency and ambition. Those pursuing the role of consultant may need to step out on their own accord, whether developing a consultant role within a current work site or developing a private practice. Those who wish to work within an existing employment setting should consider what degree of contact they have with aging patients and where within the facility they might expand their role as consultants. This approach may be particularly useful in larger acute care and long-term-care facilities or community agencies.

For instance, the practitioner might allot time to join interdisciplinary rounds on units where occupational therapy services are not frequently or efficiently utilized. The practitioner, although not directly working with clients, may be able to give advice to current line staff or even begin to develop a pool of referrals. If the facility has an existing geriatric specialty team, the practitioner should consider becoming a member of that team, collaborating with medical and social work staff. More formally, the gerontic occupational therapy consultant may offer ideas for program development, evaluation, and physical environmental design before construction or remodeling. These consultations may take place over a long period of time, such as when programs are developed, marketed, and evaluated, or at specific meetings, such as explaining to housekeeping how high-gloss tile floors can contribute to injury when older adults with low vision cannot perceive the difference between a wet floor and a well-buffed floor.

Consultants working in private practice may contract with existing or developing facilities for program development and environmental design. Contract agencies may be in the private sector, such as assisted living facilities, hospitals, and long-term care facilities, architectural design companies or home improvement centers; or the public sector, such as area agencies on aging, locally owned recreational programs, accessibility review committees, and so on. Entrepreneurially spirited consultants may need to consider developing a mix of on-going direct patient care cases and consultation contracts for the sake of cash flow. A consultation project may have an attractive fee, but that fee may be many months or years from collection depending on the legal design of the contract.

Academic and Entrepreneurial Opportunities

Academic settings offer experienced practitioners opportunities to expand upon their knowledge and pass on their skills to future practitioners. With the expansion and development of schools at the technical and professional level, practitioners can become involved in education by being guest lecturers, hosting labs, coordinating fieldwork site contracts and assignments, and serving as adjunct faculty.

Practitioners who wish to pursue teaching full time should consider additional education, especially in the field of adult education. This might include graduate and postgraduate level degree work. For the geriatric specialist, educational opportunities might also include lecturing or designing courses for related professions, such as nursing, physical and recreation therapy, or social work, or for gerontology programs. Of concern in occupational therapy education and literature is the isolating habit of occupational therapy educators staying among themselves. With the emphasis on interdisciplinary cooperation, educators may need to explore expansion into other departments and curriculums. The educator working in this capacity should have a strong sense of professional identity as an occupational therapy practitioner as well as a geriatric specialist.

For practitioners with entrepreneurial ambitions, gerontic occupational therapy offers many opportunities. Private practices may be developed to offer services in most traditional and community practice settings. An OTR is more likely to be able to work in a sole-proprietor situation, whereas a COTA will need to collaborate with an OTR because of requirements for supervision and the OTR's evaluation skills. Many OTRs who have set out to develop private practices have soon found the need to hire additional staff to service contracts that develop.

When an OTR or COTA seeks employment from an entrepreneurial OTR, this work relationship may be different from seeking employment from larger facilities or agencies. For instance, contracts may be time limited and end once the project is completed. Contract employees may work in a variety of settings throughout the course of a work week, thereby meeting the demand for occupational therapy services in settings that do not warrant full-time employment. The hours worked may not fit into the usual Monday through Friday, 8 to 5 format. The independent practitioner will need to be much more responsive to the customer's expectations and requests. Early morning, evening, and weekend work hours may substitute or supplement the usual work week. Similarly, the pace of work may be different, in that there may be periods of much activity as contracts and referrals come in and periods of slow activity between assignments. Practitioners should anticipate these business cycles and consider how to use the nonrevenue-generating days effectively for program development, marketing calls, and exploration of new business opportunities.

In regard to entrepreneurial practice, practitioners should consider how they may use their skills in jobs outside of occupational therapy. The role document addresses the current realm of practice within the profession. However, some practitioners may find that they develop skills or opportunities to work in positions that are not specifically directed to occupational therapy, and certainly not reimbursable under current definitions of occupational therapy practice.

These situations are likely to appeal to the advanced, experienced practitioner. Some might explore political roles, such as involvement in local, state, and national offices; school boards; advocacy groups; consumer boards; and lobbying. Others might be drawn to the private sector to work in design, research, and development. For older adults this could be very beneficial in regard to universal design in architecture, product packaging design (e.g., medication containers that are grandchild proof, but usable by aging adults with arthritis, low vision, and mild dementia), and adaptive equipment design. Others might be interested in working in public relations and marketing departments. With ADA and the graying of America, advertising agencies and departments are attempting to reach people of all abilities and ages using products. This has ranged from a woman in a wheelchair talking about her sexy new sports car with adaptive driving devices, to grandparents heading out for a road trip while their children worry about whether mom and dad forgot to pay the electric bill, to 90-year-old baseball stars playing softball to sell tennis shoes.

In any discussion about practice and competency, one must consider the ethical implications. The final section of this chapter will review ethics related to gerontic occupational therapy practice.

Reference

American Occupational Therapy Association. (1993). Occupational therapy roles. *American Journal of Occupational Therapy, 47,* 1087–1099.

Section 6. Ethical Issues and Gerontic Occupational Therapy Practice

Beverly P. Horowitz, DSW, OTR/L

Abstract

The author provides an overview of values and ethics in gerontic practice and a discussion of ethical dilemmas that gerontic occupational therapists may face.

Introduction

Gerontic occupational therapy practice focuses on services to heterogeneous older adults who present with a wide range of medical diagnoses and occupational dysfunctions in a variety of settings. Despite the many differences between older individuals seen in occupational therapy and the kinds of services provided, occupational therapy gerontic practice seeks to support maximum independence of older adults by addressing the "biopsychosocial origins of older adults' occupational dysfunctions" (Rogers, 1986, p. 119). Although occupational therapy treatment goals are similar to those for younger individuals (Rogers, 1986), many of our older patients challenge our knowledge and skills differently than younger patients, given the high incidence of multiple diagnoses and complex medical and social histories (Becker & Kaufman, 1988; Collopy, 1988; Gutheil, 1994; Kiernat, 1991).

Complex histories and social needs, multiple diagnoses, and frequent functional impairments of many older clients add to the complexity involved in occupational therapy treatment planning. Clinical reasoning and decision making typically need to balance multiple client concerns and needs, and often family concerns and needs, with appreciation of gender issues and how culture, religion, and ethnicity may influence client values and concerns. In addition, the added reality of frailty, often combined with decreased physical and mental capabilities, further complicate these issues, requiring occupational therapists to be especially attentive to bioethical concerns and frequent ethical dilemmas that occur in practice (Archea et al., 1993; Crabtree, 1991a; Halper, 1978; Kiernat, 1991; Libow, 1993; Moody, 1992).

Commonly, clinical situations arise that require occupational therapists to make decisions that involve values and ethical decision making, so that they need to ask questions of themselves, gather relevant information, identify problems, consider possible alternatives, and finally, determine how to proceed (Purtilo, 1993). The specific situation may be relatively mundane, such as whether to disclose medical information to a patient's family member without specific approval from the patient, or it may involve the complexities that are often encountered with home care treatment of individuals with Alzheimer's disease or those slowly recovering from a CVA relative to the need to distinguish the treatment goals for our patient from those of caregivers and family members (Baum, 1991; Purtilo, 1993). Ethical decision making may also include larger institutional organizational issues. These may include the rationing of scarce services (Callahan, 1987; Kapp, 1988) and methods of allocation of resources, including principles of equity and justice (Purtilo, 1993), the role of third party payers and health care, and how reimbursement affects provision of occupational therapy services (Cassidy, 1988; Howard, 1991; Neuhaus, 1988), including the different tiers of medical care, often reflecting an individual's insurance and socioeconomic status (Friedman, 1986) or the special challenges involved when an occupational therapist witnesses incompetent or unethical professional behavior by colleagues or supervisors (Purtilo, 1993).

Ethical dilemmas pose difficulties for all health care providers. Although clinicians typically use their own values to help guide their decisions, occupational therapy's history and values offer a framework to help occupational therapists choose a course of action. Occupational therapists' heritage and work with disabled people to help them maximize their capabilities, particularly socially devalued populations (i.e., mentally ill and developmentally disabled persons), and their shared values regarding client self-determination and appreciation for the relationships between efficacy, self-esteem, and competency can help guide their clinical practice and professional relationships with aged clients (Lewis, 1989; Trombly, 1996). The following section will discuss how professional values, including the *Code of Ethics*, can assist and support occupational therapists when they are faced with ethical dilemmas in clinical practice.

Values and Ethics in Gerontic Practice

Although all of us have our own particular beliefs and personal values, we are also influenced by principles that guide us in our relationships with people, or "morality." These personal values, often coupled with religious perspectives, support our concepts of morality. Ethics is defined by Purtilo (1993) as "a systematic reflection on and analysis of morality" (p. 6).

Ancient philosophers and the major religions have struggled with issues related to values and morality, and we continue to struggle with these same concerns. Ethical theories and principles thus have developed with the growth of civilization. Two major ethical theories include the deontological and the teleological. Deontology can best be summarized as a duty-driven theory that is strongly identified with the philosopher Immanuel Kant (1724–1804), who held that individuals have basic dignity and are entitled to respect because they are human. This position supports the view that a person's actions need to be based on moral obligation or "duty" and that his or her behavior or conduct can be distinguished as following moral, or correct ways of behavior versus immoral, incorrect conduct, regardless of the consequences that result from such behavior. Teleological ethics are less concerned with correct conduct than with the consequences of actions. They are often identified with "utilitarianism," whose basic principle has commonly been simplified into the following—the end justifies the means—and with philosophers John Stuart Mill (1806–1873) and Jeremy Bentham (1748–1832), who were opponents of deontology and emphasized the attainment of successful results for the greatest number (Bailey & Schwartzberg, 1995; Kyler-Hutchison, 1988; Purtilo, 1993).

These ethical theories undergird many of our ethical perspectives today and provide a foundation for understanding the elements of ethics, including the concepts of duty, fidelity, beneficence, veracity, justice, and rights, including principles of autonomy and self-determination. Duty commonly refers to a person's obligations and commitments; fidelity denotes faithfulness and often entails meeting professional expectations; beneficence refers to doing good; and veracity refers to being truthful. The concept of justice includes multiple meanings, from that of fairness, to the method of distributing benefits or goods (distributive justice), the concept of compensatory justice, to "compensate" individuals for past wrongs, and that of impartial or procedural justice to support fairness and impartiality. Similarly, the concept of rights is complex and multifaceted. Historically, rights were considered "properties of individuals" (Purtilo, 1993, p. 25) to be protected; more recently some rights have been defined as legal entitlements by government, often with assigned monetary value. Within bioethics, rights are often viewed in the context of a uniquely human claim to self-determination or autonomy (Brock, 1987; Shapiro & Spece, 1981). This is a major focus of many of the discussions and debates today as occupational therapists struggle to integrate therapy with the realities and dilemmas of daily practice (Moody, 1992). Differences between intellectual ethical dilemmas and those rooted in situations that confront occupational therapists daily often demand the substitution of negotiated compromise rather than adherence to the "tyranny of principles" (Moody, 1992, p. 10).

Historically, the occupational therapy profession grew out of the Moral Treatment Movement with its belief in the inherent dignity of individuals, particularly those devalued because of mental illness, or developmental or physical disability, combined with occupational therapy's belief in the value of human engagement in meaningful, self-directed life tasks (Cynkin & Robinson, 1990; Howard, 1991; Townsend, 1993). Although practice has evolved with changing social and health care needs and technological advances, current theoretical foundations for practice continue to support occupational therapists' early professional beliefs and values. Occupational therapy's leaders continue to emphasize the need to promote empowerment and self-efficacy to support all individuals, including the aged, to increase competency in their individual life roles, including support for personal independence in individual tasks that support successful life roles (Cynkin & Robinson, 1990; Rogers, 1986; Trombly, 1995). At the same time, the profession acknowledges the importance of culture and individual meaning for successful occupational therapy interventions, particularly for older client populations (Kielhofner, 1992; Kiernat, 1991; Occupational Therapy Commission on Practice, 1993).

Professional codes of conduct are written by professions to enunciate shared values and establish a basis for evaluating professional activities (Wenston, 1987). Current professional codes typically emulate the ancient physicians' Hippocratic Oath and also look to the paradigmatic professions of law, medicine, and clergy to establish ethical codes of conduct. Although this section focuses on ethics related to gerontic occupational therapy practice, there appear to be relationships between professional conduct and established codes of ethics, which extend as far back as the Hippocratic Oath. In addition to promoting shared values, codes of ethics are also seen by some ethicists as exclusionary business mechanisms that socialize members of the profession through shared values and ideals while regulating professional behaviors and entry in the profession (Peterson, 1987). Although these aspects of medical code ethics are self-serving, the historical presence of so many codes of ethics across so many cultures seems to demonstrate a common need for such social pronouncements to enunciate a shared professional ethos as well as to inform society of the physician's ethical values and duties, thereby clarifying expectations of the medical professional (Reich, 1976). Without legal sanction, such codes are a means for professions to regulate member behaviors, although separate current licensure laws are the only means of legally regulating professional actions.

Thus, in this long tradition, the Occupational Therapy *Code of Ethics* (American Occupational Therapy Association [AOTA] 1994b) is the occupational therapy profession's vehicle for espousing shared values to guide ethical conduct. It includes six principles that address the following :

1. Concern for the welfare of clients
2. Respect for the rights of clients
3. Compliance with policies of the profession and laws regulating practice
4. Compliance with laws and policies that guide the profession
5. Public information to provide accurate information to clients to support professional integrity and quality services to clients
6. Professional conduct.

In 1993, AOTA charged its Standards and Ethics Committee to write a document that would more fully describe the attitudes and shared values of the occupational therapy profession. Seven core values and attitudes were described including:

1. Altruism, reflected in commitment and dedication to others
2. Equality and impartiality
3. Freedom, including professional independence and the commitment to freedom of choice for all people

4. Justice, including the multiple principles of fairness, equity, and legal ramifications of justice
5. Dignity, valuing each person's uniqueness
6. Truthfulness
7. Prudence and the values of discipline, discretion, and vigilance (Standards and Ethics Commission of the American Occupational Therapy Association, 1993).

Both the Occupational Therapy *Code of Ethics* (Code of Ethics) and the professional "core values and attitudes" serve to promote the ideals of occupational therapy to guide occupational therapists in clinical practice and in their dealings with colleagues and the larger social environment of which they are a part. They also serve to provide a basis for appreciating the common values of other professionals. Within gerontic practice specifically, occupational therapists' support of individual autonomy and independence is similar to many current views of gerontologists who increasingly have addressed both the need to maximize individual independence and autonomy, and the importance of promoting the quality of life for the older person (Collopy, 1988; Gurland, 1992; Moody, 1983, 1992). In this way, the *Code of Ethics* promotes values that encourage relationships with like-minded professionals who share occupational therapists' interests in supporting wellness, independence, and quality of life for older persons.

Gerontic Occupational Therapy Practice, Ethics, and Legal Issues

Although codes of ethics speak to values and guide professional conduct and behavior, they generally are weak in their ability to sanction members.

Licensure is a state function that regulates the practice of an occupation, setting individual state standards for professional practice to both protect consumers and maintain limits on who is able to advertise and perform specific occupations. In the early 1900s few occupations were licensed, but by the 1970s, licensure was seen as a means to regulate many occupations including health-related occupations. Puerto Rico established licensure for occupational therapists in 1968; New York and later Florida became the first states to enact licensure in 1975. As of 1995, 41 jurisdictions licensed occupational therapists; 39 jurisdictions licensed certified occupational therapy assistants (COTAs); 3 states registered occupational therapists and COTAs; 5 states certified occupational therapists; 4 states certified COTAs; and 3 jurisdictions used trademark law to regulate occupational therapy. Only Colorado does not have any form of state regulation for occupational therapy, and Rhode Island, Virginia, and Colorado do not regulate occupational therapy assistants (AOTA, 1995; Gray, 1993).

Both the *Code of Ethics* and professional credentialing by AOTA are organizational methods of promoting professional standards but do not have legal authority or sanctions as established by law. Licensure, on the other hand, defines the legal parameters of a profession in a particular state. For occupational therapy, this definition establishes a legally sanctioned scope of practice, including the types of modalities and treatment techniques that can legally be used in each state and requirements regarding referral or physician prescription for treatment. Licensure also sets specific requirements for entry into the profession in that state, defines professional misconduct, and establishes a mechanism for disciplining licensed professionals who

engage in unprofessional conduct, including both ethical misconduct and practice that extends beyond the proscribed legal definition and parameters of the profession.

Occupational therapists are legally required to adhere to professional standards of conduct established by each state for licensed professionals, but are also ethically bound to uphold the standards of practice and values of occupational therapy and the *Code of Ethics*. To support the *Code of Ethics*, AOTA socializes members to support and espouse these standards and this professional code. AOTA also has formal procedures reserved to the American Occupational Therapy Certification Board (AOTCB) Disciplinary Action Committee to investigate complaints and violations and discipline members through reprimand, censure, suspension, or revocation of professional certification (Gray, 1993). However, state licensure and disciplinary mechanisms have greater power than professional organizational enforcement proceedings, given their governmental power to censure, suspend, or revoke an individual's license and ability to practice. Membership in a licensed profession thus requires members to be knowledgeable about professional ethics and standards for practice as well as defined standards for professional conduct and their legally recognized scope of practice in the state in which they choose to practice. This can vary from one state to another.

In addition to licensure, the health care environment includes multiple federal, state, and local laws and regulations, as well as organizational policies and procedures. As licensed professionals, occupational therapists are expected and ethically bound to comply with all appropriate regulations and laws that impact upon their practice. In gerontic practice, occupational therapists need to be knowledgeable about multiple federal and state programs and policies, as well as laws and regulations regarding professional practice. The major federal and state programs that provide services and benefits to older persons include Medicare, Medicaid, need-based income support programs including Supplemental Social Security, Food Stamps, Veterans' Administration programs, senior citizen community programs, and services offered through local offices of the aged. Many localities offer additional services for senior residents including chore services and reductions in local property taxes for low-income seniors. Medicare and Medicaid provide reimbursement for occupational therapy for most older clients or patients and require adherence to specific regulations, including specific documentation requirements for patient evaluation, progress notes, and discharge plans. The Omnibus Reconciliation Act of 1987 (OBRA '87) requirements for participating skilled nursing homes requires occupational therapists to understand the Minimum Data Set (MDS), the required assessment tool, the Resident Assessment Protocol (RAP) or care plan, and how to support quality of care including the definition of restraints in order to work toward reduced use of restraints to support restraint-free environments for nursing home residents (Moon-Sperling & Crispen Pinson, 1991). OBRA '87's focus on maximizing the quality of life for nursing home residents additionally has supported increased attention to the overall well-being of such residents and greater appreciation of the importance of individual autonomy and self-determination (Crabtree, 1991c). This is in keeping with both ongoing discussion and debate about how best to support patients' rights in all settings, how to maximize autonomy for aged

patients, particularly those in skilled nursing facilities (Hofland, 1994; Zuckerman, 1994), and increased consumer knowledge and dialogue with providers of health care services and activism for quality care.

Passage of the Americans with Disabilities Act (Public Law 101–336) in 1990 (ADA), represents antidiscrimination legislation to provide equal rights protection in the areas of employment in both private sector and municipal, state, and federal government, public accommodations, transportation, and telecommunication for the promotion of equal opportunities for persons with disabilities (Bailey & Schwartzberg, 1995), and has broad implications for occupational therapists who work with older adults in all settings. ADA may be seen as a tool to deal with some common problems to support equal opportunities for those who have disabilities, be they physical or cognitive, and to prevent discriminatory administrative policies, for example, when admission to a nursing home is based primarily on diagnosis. It also serves to protect individuals against retaliation for complaints regarding discrimination (Gottlich, 1994).

Although there is much general knowledge about ADA, it is important to understand that ADA includes the following titles: Title I, Employment; Title II, Public Services and Transportation; Title III, Public Accommodations and Services Operated by Private Entities; Title IV, Telecommunications; Title V, Miscellaneous Provisions on compliance procedures. This 1990 legislation requires both public and private agencies to provide equal opportunity for disabled people to participate in society. Knowledge of this civil rights legislation empowers disabled persons of all ages to seek equal access and reasonable accommodation for their disability to increase use of general community services and activities, and to reject discrimination on the basis of disability, physical or cognitive. Disabled older persons dwelling in the community find transportation to be a major stumbling block in keeping physician appointments or getting involved in community activities. Title II prevents discrimination in public transportation, supporting mechanisms that enable disabled individuals reasonable access to public transportation, with paratransit systems being but one option for compliance. Similarly, access to public accommodations (Title III) is a concern for many individuals and families and may limit decisions to travel or visit with family members in other communities. Appreciation of the meaning of ADA enables occupational therapists to educate patients about how this legislation supports greater access and opportunities to use public accommodations (Jacobs, 1992; Reed, 1992), while acknowledging that there still is a long road ahead in fulfilling the mandates of ADA. Although there is much discussion about the limited successes of ADA, knowledge of this legislation combined with advocacy and networking can only assist the goals for maximum independence through advocacy for increased opportunities for community engagement.

Despite many societal barriers to equal opportunities for disabled persons, the American business community, in addition to governmental agencies, has worked to increase access to many services. Awareness of the individual community's resources enables occupational therapists to support their patients' individual interests to participate in the arts, recreation, and civic activities with a realistic understanding of the kinds of reasonable accommodations that they can expect. For example, in regard to travel, wheel-

chair-accessible hotel rooms are not uncommon in large hotel chains. These rooms often have "auxiliary aids" such as grab bars and bath seats, as well as accommodations for individuals with visual or hearing disabilities, to comply with ADA and support equal access to all goods and services for consumers. Grocery shopping, a daily living task, has traditionally been difficult for many older individuals with mobility limitations or reduced endurance. ADA (Title III) has supported numerous types of reasonable accommodations in many large supermarkets, including provision of motorized scooters and assistance with shopping activities such as carrying packages to the person's car upon request. However, often an individual needs to know to request such assistance. Older patients or clients have lived the majority of their adult lives during a time when disabled individuals were not expected to fully participate in social activities. It is occupational therapists' responsibility to develop collaborative rehabilitation goals with them that include providing them with information to support realistic community reintegration and involvement. Such involvement is only possible when occupational therapists are informed professionals, knowledgeable about the community's resources and programs and about legislation established to promote independence and quality of life.

OBRA '87 and ADA provide occupational therapists with long-needed tools to increase quality care for nursing home residents and promote equal opportunities and community reintegration for many community-dwelling older clients with disabilities. Although OBRA '87 did not change Medicare reimbursement for occupational therapy, it mandates comprehensive resident assessments and care plans that require evaluation of multiple areas related to functional capabilities, including cognitive loss and dementia, visual function, communication, activities of daily living functional potential, rehabilitation potential, psychosocial well-being, activities, falls, nutritional status, and physical restraints.

These federally mandated assessments and care plans provide a vehicle for referral to rehabilitation services, including occupational therapy, and treatment planning that addresses individual treatment needs as well as organizational rehabilitation programming for long-term support of rehabilitation goals and quality care (Moon-Sperling & Crispen Pinson, 1991). Gerontic practice's concerns with "the biopsychosocial" origins of dysfunction combine many aspects of practice, such that occupational therapists use clinical skills to treat orthopedic conditions and neurological impairments, provide cognitive rehabilitation for those recovering from CVA or head injury, and provide hand rehabilitation, as well as treatment for individuals with psychosocial disorders. Among older adults, depression is a common problem that is often unrecognized and undertreated in nursing home settings (Rovner et al., 1991). Rehabilitation services that relate to occupational therapy may include psychosocial programs for residents dealing with bereavement or programs that support empowerment and self-efficacy, relaxation programs, mealtime programs, exercise and fitness programs, daily living skill programs, and patient or family education programs, particularly for those planning to return to home. Although individual restorative treatment needs to be provided by occupational therapists and certified occupational therapy assistants to qualify for most third-party reimbursement, specialized reha-

bilitation programs are often developed by and supervised by occupational therapists and other rehabilitation team members but are carried out by nursing aides given funding constraints. To ensure successful programs of all kinds requires a commitment to rehabilitation goals by administration and all departments and a coordinated team approach that stresses in-service education and values the efforts of all team members (Kiernat, 1991).

Knowledge of regulations, legislation, and legal issues surrounding practice and patient care is the responsibility of all therapists. The regulations involved may relate to specific rehabilitation and civil rights issues, documentation requirements for third-party payers and billing issues, referral issues and prevention of conflicts of interest in the highly privatized health care industry, legal definitions of practice and the use of physical agent modalities, or the rights of patients regarding informed consent and the right to refuse treatment. Occupational therapists traditionally have been employed in institutional settings with primary involvement in the clinical treatment of patients. Because of marked changes in the health care industry, increasing numbers of therapists are working more independently in home care, nursing homes, outpatient settings, private offices or community-based agencies, with fewer opportunities for peer interactions and supervision. This has coincided with increased attention to the role of ethics and patient's rights in our aging society, the growth of managed care plans, and increased consumerism. As larger numbers of therapists work more autonomously in increasingly complex health care environments, legal and related ethical issues once primarily the responsibility of supervisory staff are now the responsibility of most clinicians. Consequently, just as occupational therapists need clinical skills and tools for evaluations and patient treatment, they also need skills and tools to effectively navigate through the increasingly regulated, legalistic, and privatized health care environment.

However, how do we differentiate the unethical from the illegal? In many situations there are no clear lines between the two. Illegal activity is usually unethical by violating the shared values of the profession; however, unethical behavior may not necessarily violate specific regulations or laws. Thus, what most clearly distinguishes unethical from illegal conduct is whether an individual violated a specific law, knowingly or unknowingly. Unethical activities, on the other hand, occur when a therapist's conduct violates a professional code of ethics, specifically the *Code of Ethics* for occupational therapists, occupational therapy assistants, and occupational therapy students.

Examples of unethical activities include practice beyond the scope of one's expertise, a violation of Principle 3, regarding competence; inaccurate representation of one's certification for specific types of treatment, a violation of Principle 5, regarding providing accurate information; or a professional relationship between an employer and therapist that does not inform the employer about the laws and regulations that apply to occupational therapy practice, a violation of Principle 4, that speaks to compliance with laws and regulations (AOTA, 1994a; Evert, 1993). In each of these examples, the therapist did not necessarily violate a particular law, but certainly violated the ethical standards of the profession regarding competence, provision of accurate public information, and compliance with laws and regulations.

Therapists reported to the profession to be engaging in unethical behavior can be investigated by the profession as discussed earlier. However, legal sanctions, including fines, monetary penalties, or suspension or revocation of a state license to practice occupational therapy can only result from governmental disciplinary proceedings for conduct or activity that violates a particular law. Professional disciplinary proceedings for licensed professionals are the responsibility of each state's licensing board (Kyler-Hutchison, 1994).

Ethics and legal issues additionally relate to documentation responsibilities. Health care professionals, including occupational therapists, deal with legal medical documents on a daily basis, often focusing only on the medical implications of these records with limited attention to the ethical and legal implications of chart records. Occupational therapists review many client records daily, document treatment, cosign progress notes, and routinely communicate with other professionals, often in different settings to effect appropriate discharge and continuity of services. The legal and ethical issues involved in these daily activities are sometimes acknowledged, but given occupational therapists' focus on clinical practice and the pace of clinical practice, ethical and legal implications are often overshadowed by patient treatment needs, unless specific ethical or legal questions or dilemmas arise.

Therapists recognize the client record as a confidential medical record, but they also need to appreciate the fact that any disclosure of medical information both ethically and legally requires patient consent. Ethically, therapists are bound to keep all information they learn about their patients confidential, with the patient's understanding that this information needs to be appropriately shared with the physician for the best medical care. Consultation with other team members to coordinate patient care and treatment planning is accepted practice because admission to a rehabilitation program carries with it the understanding that rehabilitation professionals utilize a team approach for optimal patient treatment. However, disclosure of confidential information to anyone, even team members, who have no professional need for such information, regardless of position, or to outside agencies, including physicians or therapists, requires specific approval from the patient, with written releases the accepted method of documenting consent (Kornblau, 1992; Purtilo, 1993; Welles, 1986). Although this procedure is followed for legal reasons, ethically it protects individual privacy, thus supporting individual autonomy.

Ethical dilemmas periodically also result when therapists are provided with information that is not relevant to treatment needs, particularly information that is potentially detrimental to the patient's best interests or relates to illegal activities. Although occupational therapists have a responsibility to patients, in addition, they have a responsibility to the referring or prescribing physician who is also responsible for the authorized treatment. Given the responsibility to do no harm and to protect the confidential nature of the information occupational therapists learn from and about their patients (Principles 1 and 6 of *Code of Ethics*), great care needs to be taken in evaluating a course of action regarding this type of information. The type of action taken may depend upon the nature of the information; for example, information about a problem in the distant past, or past illegal activities, has a very different

meaning with different ramifications than information concerning present behaviors or activities, especially ones that could cause harm to the patient or others. Sometimes discussion with the patient can clarify the meaning of this information, and the therapist can encourage the patient to get counseling to resolve the problem. More commonly, problems are not remedied easily, and therapists grapple with ethical principles to help guide them and weigh the best course of action, but this does not have to be a solitary endeavor. Opportunities exist in most locales and areas of practice for dialogue with other professionals to support the most informed, wisest course of action. The ethical decision-making process can be aided by fellow team members, a supervisor, or other colleagues. Therapists can also utilize the resources of AOTA at the local, state, or national level to aid this process while appropriately maintaining client privacy and confidentiality.

From another perspective, documentation is an inherent part of routine practice. A therapist's signature on patient records, including patient attendance forms, notes, discharge reports, and so on is typically required organizationally and by third-party payers. However, to attest to the accuracy of documentation carries with it legal significance. Therapists who are employed in agencies where policy requires them to procedurally sign off on progress notes or billing documents with little direct oversight may run the risk of validating inaccurate information. Although some human errors occur and are often noted during retrospective chart reviews, audits are routinely conducted in health care facilities for multiple purposes, one purpose being to distinguish human error from fraudulent claims. Therapists unfamiliar with the fraud and abuse provisions of the Medicare and Medicaid laws, for example, can find themselves facing civil and criminal charges and being responsible for restitution, or facing severe fines. The most severe penalty for fraud is a maximum of 5 years in federal prison (Kornblau, 1992).

Recent reports of overcharges for occupational therapy services in nursing homes by the General Accounting Office (GAO) in 1995 (Kyler-Hutchison, 1995) may represent ethical violations of the AOTA *Code of Ethics* (Principle 1 in regard to financial exploitation) if therapists were knowledgeable and responsible for such billing. The ethical issues, however, are complicated when nursing home administrators or other employers engage therapists and then overcharge for their occupational therapy treatment sessions, thereby promoting a negative image for occupational therapists. These 1995 reported overcharges, however, were apparently not illegal due to legal loopholes in Medicare's payment rules (Kyler-Hutchison, 1995). Nevertheless, they were destructive to occupational therapy's image because they can erode relationships with the public and damage occupational therapy's reputation with the very governmental agencies that are the primary third-party payers for most of the profession's older patients. Although therapists always have recourse to report unethical and illegal conduct to appropriate professional and governmental agencies, it is also beneficial to consider proactive methods to protect our individual professional reputations. Some strategies may include the following:

1. Establishing a dialogue with the employer early on to be knowledgeable about billing practices for occupational therapy services, given their implications for occupational therapy's professional reputation

2. Developing assertiveness by individual occupational therapists to effectively communicate professional values, ethics, and legal responsibilities to employers

3. Establishing personal guidelines to help therapists individually choose employers who maintain high ethical standards, given the envious position of being in demand in a wide variety of settings throughout the country.

Legal and ethical issues can also arise in regard to provision of consultation services or supervision of others including certified occupational therapy assistants (COTAs). The *Code of Ethics* and AOTA's *Guide to Classification of Occupational Therapy Personnel* provide guidelines for such supervisory relationships (AOTA, 1993, 1994b). However, given the need to provide generic information, these documents can only have limited specificity. For example, The Guide for Supervision of Occupational Therapy Personnel describes supervision as a "process" and a "mutual undertaking between the supervisor and the supervisee" to promote "quality occupational therapy" (AOTA, 1994a, p. 1). The *Code of Ethics* (Principle 3) adds the need for "appropriate supervision" as defined in AOTA guidelines, or state laws, regulations, and institutional policies (AOTA, 1994b, p. 3). Thus, these guidelines are necessarily general and cannot provide clear direction in day-to-day decision making. Although ethical obligations in these areas may be subject to interpretation, legal responsibilities are usually much clearer. By cosigning a note, the supervisory therapist acknowledges legal responsibility for the reported treatment and for the ramifications of that treatment in case of ill effects of treatment, as well as responsibility for the accuracy of the note (Bailey & Schwartzberg, 1995).

Occupational therapy consultants additionally need to understand the ramifications of advertising themselves as experts in a particular area of practice, and the legal responsibilities involved if they advise a consultee to do something that results in injury or damage to a patient. Provision of inaccurate information, failure to provide proper and complete information, or the use of poor professional judgment with subsequent damage can open a therapist up to malpractice litigation (Kornblau, 1992).

From a different perspective, there are also ethical and legal issues surrounding patient referrals, especially in our privatized health care environment in which there are so many interrelationships between health care agencies and providers, including relationships among hospitals, home care agencies, and physicians, employed therapists and outpatient facilities, and private rehabilitation offices (Relman,1991). Potentials for conflict of interest and compromised consumer decision making increase when there is a financial relationship between the referral source and the service provider or when the clinician stands to profit from the referral (Crabtree, 1991b). Given the currently financially stressed health care environment, potential for conflict of interest is great, and occupational therapists need to appreciate the short-term effects of conflict of interests on professional autonomy, including its impact upon their patient's freedom to exercise their options for continued therapy, as well as the long-term effects on the profession and its reputation.

Conflicts of interest may result when therapists are asked to encourage referrals to a colleague who is starting a new practice and needs "business," or when they are discouraged from making referrals to a well-regarded outpatient facility in preference to an out-patient department with financial ties to their medical staff. Even the way in which therapists present referral information has potential ethical implications given the fiduciary, or confidential, relationships with their patients built upon confidence and trust (Crabtree, 1991b; Kutchins, 1991). The *Code of Ethics* (Principle 5, regarding ethical behavior) recognizes this ethical issue and states: "Occupational therapy personnel shall not disclose any affiliations that may pose a conflict of interest" (AOTA, 1994b, p. 3). The legal implications of such conflicts of interest, particularly if they include financial benefit to the referring therapist, such as fee-splitting, have potentially more serious implications. The line between unethical and illegal behaviors may appear grey to some, but participation in defined illegal activities has more serious consequences including potential charges against the therapist, governmental disciplinary procedures, and permanent loss of the therapist's state license to practice occupational therapy.

Additionally, as discussed, occupational therapists' relationships with their clients or patients are built upon trust, established during a time when many patients or clients are ill and often vulnerable. Patients or clients, as well as colleagues, expect therapists to make appropriate recommendations in the patient's best interests when planning to discharge patients to home or a skilled nursing home, decisions often made based upon collective professional judgments. When there is fair competition and more than one option to choose from, those therapists providing inpatient services can provide patients with information about options for further occupational therapy and encourage them to choose settings and therapists who provide services that best meet their individual needs. Decision making may commonly consider the provider's participation in a managed care plan, location, provision of transportation, the impression made by the facility after a visit, or the reputation of the facility or clinician. But frequently, occupational therapists are asked for their professional opinion about the rehabilitation facility and its therapists. The expectation is that the occupational therapist's recommendation reflects professional autonomy and judgment, as opposed to one biased by economic or professional gain.

The relationships between care issues, ethical considerations, and the need for therapists to be knowledgeable about regulations and documentation is explored further in chapter 7, "Restoring Occupational Performance." This chapter focuses on special considerations when restoring occupational performance, including sections on geriatric rehabilitation in general, home health care and long-term care and the evaluation process, treatment planning, discharge planning and follow-up, and care issues and ethical considerations related to documentation.

Implications of Biases, Values, and Ethics for Practitioners and the Profession

Although occupational therapists may like to believe that their values and education protect them from engaging in ageism and prejudice regarding the health care, rehabilitation, and social support needs of older patients, they are members of this society and some individuals hold such biases. The success of Social Security and Medicare legislation was due in part to society's "compassionate stereo-types" of seniors as a "deserving" disadvantaged group with special claim to age-based benefits. Today, given the very successes of such legislation coupled with the economic stability of some older persons resulting from pensions and related investments, there is a new backlash and increasing scapegoating of the aged for many of our economic problems (Minkler, 1984). Increasing social dialogue regarding the utility and legitimacy of age-based programs needs to be juxtaposed to the very real demographic changes in the United States and throughout the industrialized world, with implications for many of our conceptions regarding older persons' social roles and life passages (Atchley, 1993; Binstock, 1994; Callahan, 1987, 1989; Friedan, 1993; Moody, 1993).

Occupational therapists are influenced by the discourse of the times, but need to differentiate stereotypes, images, politics, and ideology from research and data that finds older Americans to be a heterogeneous mix of individuals, with persons of color, older women, and the very-aged (over 80 years old) to have statistically the fewest financial resources (Estes, Gerard, & Clarke, 1984; Fahey & Holstein, 1993; Friedan, 1993; Lowy, 1985). Although some patients or clients have enjoyed successful lives, parented healthy children, succeeded in their occupations and careers, and received quality health care, enabling them to reach old age with successful life histories, others more commonly have enjoyed youth and the joys of family but have also known hardships. These may have been related to family stresses, poverty, illness, or disability, or for others discrimination and inequalities resulting from racism or sexism. Appreciation of individual histories, experiences, culture, ethnicity, and values is invaluable in assisting therapists to determine the most appropriate evaluations and their interpretation, and in developing collaborative treatment plans with patients. Additionally, therapists are ethically bound to maintain professional relationships in order to provide quality services equitably to patient or clients based upon their current situation and needs, regardless of individual background, or social or financial status (AOTA, 1994b). Clinical practice thus is often the setting in which situational ethical decisions are made, sometimes fraught with tensions resulting from a need to appreciate the influences of culture and ethnicity on clients or patients, while therapists seek to follow their professional obligations to treat all individuals regardless of differences due to race, ethnicity, age, sex, disease, handicap, or religious or economic status. The relevance of culture, individual habits and familiar routines, and family interactions and capabilities to occupational therapy practice is explored further in chapters 6, 7, 10, and 11.

Ethical dilemmas are often complicated when therapists deny their personal biases and those prejudices commonly voiced in the society and in their facility, including biases against frail older persons (Anderson & Glesnes-Anderson, 1987; Kiernat, 1991). These are exacerbated by scarce resources, shortages of occupational therapists and rehabilitation professionals, competition between patient groups for services and resources, and conflicts between concerns for designated "patients" and concerns for their caregivers. Regardless of ethical perspectives, current demand for health care services, including occupational therapy services, exceeds the supply and often our ability to equitably distribute medical services (Reitemeier & Brody, 1988). Situational ethical decision making occurs within a facility

regardless of a therapist's consciousness whenever the therapist reviews records to determine the priority status of individuals for direct treatment, find less expensive consultative treatment or services, and determine who will and who will not receive treatment or services. In addition to physician referral, treatment determinations may be based upon diagnosis and prognosis, as well as issues related to discharge status, family pressures, and reimbursement issues (Bailey & Schwartzberg, 1995; Friedman, 1986). This may become an ethical issue in subacute rehabilitation programs within skilled nursing facilities when discharge to home is often dependent upon improvement in ADL capabilities, and limited resources require staff to triage patients based upon their discharge plans. Such treatment plans are often dependent upon patient resources, including finances and social supports, as opposed to specific medical justification. This dilemma can be couched in utilitarian, teleologic perspectives that seek "the greatest good for the greatest number" versus the deontologic perspective that requires action based on the morality, or correctness of one's decision, and ultimately requires us to address complex issues of equity and equality as well as justice in health care (Bailey & Schwartzberg, 1995; Binstock, 1994; Cassidy, 1988; Crabtree, 1991a; Daniels, 1987; Purtilo, 1993).

This same complex mix of biases, values, and ethical issues arises in regard to treatment of the chronically ill aged individual. Given limited resources, how should services be allocated for aged individuals with chronic disease such as chronic obstructive pulmonary disease, Parkinson's disease, or rheumatoid arthritis, versus individuals post fracture, or those recovering from a recent CVA, or carpal tunnel surgery? Should allocation decisions be made based upon strict principles of equality, with referral date the basis for scheduled therapy, or should principles of equity, or fairness, be applied using the individual's multiple medical needs to prioritize entry into the therapy program? Although these are difficult theoretical questions, reality increases their difficulty. Additionally, to what extent should family members engage in the treatment process, or participate in what Crabtree (1991a, p. 343) called a "partnership model" to support some degree of autonomy for those individuals who have difficulty expressing their wishes and needs?

These real-life questions are difficult, much more so than academic questions and concerns about ethical decision making within an intellectual dialogue. Each specific ethical dilemma is also distinct with an individual history that challenges therapists to formulate decisions tailored to the specific needs of each person and situation. Nevertheless, despite the difficulty inherent in the process occupational therapists must engage in the difficult ethical decision-making process. Their professional responsibility requires this given both their shared ethical values and specialized expertise about the rehabilitation needs of their patients and the benefits occupational therapy can provide for them (Brody & Morrison, 1992; Bruckner, 1988; Crabtree, 1991a).

These ethical dilemmas have implications for our profession as well as for our patients and individual clinicians. As discussed earlier, Health Care Financing Administration (HCFA) findings of overcharges for occupational therapy in nursing homes (Kyler-Hutchison, 1995) negatively reflect on the profession. It is hoped that these findings represent a minority of unethical billing practices, because abuses in any profession have the potential to destroy public confidence in the profession as well as interfere with relationships between third-party payers of all sorts, including Medicare, Medicaid and growing numbers of managed care providers.

Growing opportunities in alternative practice, including opportunities as consultants to community-based recreation and wellness centers, industry, day programs, assisted living centers, and so on are in part based upon the public's knowledge of occupational therapists' skills and positive interactions between the profession and the public. But how can occupational therapists best promote occupational therapy and their professional skills? Why does any adult community center decide to hire an occupational therapy consultant and how do private practitioners convince managed care organizations to include them in their provider network? Although carefully researched outcome studies most assuredly can demonstrate the value of occupational therapy for aged patients with particular diagnoses and degrees of impairment or disability, positive interactions between occupational therapists and patients, families, colleagues and third-party payers provide positive images of the profession. Positive experiences with occupational therapists can demonstrate their expertise in promoting independence, or more broadly stated in the words of Polatajko, "enabling living" (Townsend, 1993, p. 176) and corresponding quality of life for patients (Kiernat, 1991; Rogers, 1986). However, negative associations and interactions often make even stronger impressions. Although there are few immutable principles regarding ethics and health care, one principle is clear: professionals are accorded privileges by society given their unspoken compact with society to promote the welfare of individuals receiving medical services (Principle 1, AOTA *Code of Ethics*; AOTA, 1994b). Ignorance, disregard, and violation of this unwritten compact, even by a small minority of occupational therapy practitioners endangers all of us, especially at this time of financial constraints and uncertainty in a changing health care environment.

Activities

1. Describe how the philosophical ideas of occupation, adaptation, and functional independence relate to older adults.

2. What are some similarities and differences between conceptual models of practice and frames of reference? Review recent journals (e.g., *AJOT, Physical and Occupational Therapy in Geriatrics, Topics in Geriatrics*, etc.) to identify an article that describes the application of either a conceptual model of practice or frame of reference.

3. What is the purpose of a profession's domain of concern? To better understand occupational therapy's domain of concern with older adults, read a journal article or chapter of a book that describes an aspect of an older adult's life. Identify the performance areas, components, and contexts that this reading highlights.

4. Three types of legitimate tools of practice were described in the text: analysis and synthesis, the nonhuman environment, and human interaction. Write a brief essay describing each of these tools, giving examples of each, and identifying how the occupational therapy practitioner can coordinate these tools in practice.

5. Describe how an OTR and COTA can collaborate in the following settings: home health care, skilled nursing facility, senior center, and acute care hospital.

6. What are some basic differences between deontological and teleological ethics? How might these different approaches influence an occupational therapy practitioner's view of treatment?

7. What are the differences between ethical and legal principles? How might these differences affect an occupational therapist whose actions in practice have violated an ethical principle but not a legal statute?

8. Describe the six ethical principles adopted by the Representative Assembly of AOTA in 1994.

References

American Occupational Therapy Association. (1993). Guide to classification of occupational therapy personnel. In *Reference manual of the official documents of the American Occupational Therapy Association* (5th ed., pp. vii.3–vii.18). Rockville, MD: Author. (Original work published 1986).

American Occupational Therapy Association. (1994a). 1994 guide for supervision of occupational therapy personnel. In *Addenda to the reference manual of the official documents of the American Occupational Therapy Association, Inc.* (5th ed., pp. 1-4). Rockville, MD: Author.

American Occupational Therapy Association. (1994b). 1994 occupational therapy code of ethics. In *Addenda to the reference manual of the official documents of the American Occupational Therapy Association, Inc.* (5th ed., pp. vii.1–vii.2). Rockville, MD: Author. (Replaced 1988 *Code of Ethics*).

American Occupational Therapy Association. (1995). *1995 annual conference and exposition licensure information, Denver, Colorado.* Bethesda, MD: Author.

Americans With Disabilities Act of 1990. (Public Law 101–336), 42 U.S.C. 12101.

Anderson, G., & Glesnes-Anderson, V. (Eds.). (1987). *Health care ethics.* Rockville, MD: Aspen.

Archea, C., McNeely, E., Martino-Saltzman, D., Hennessy, C., Whittington, F., & Myers, D. (1993). Restraints in long term care. *Physical and Occupational Therapy In Geriatrics, 11*(2), 3–23.

Atchley, R. (1993). Critical perspectives on retirement. In T. Cole, W. A. Achenbaum, P. Jakobi, & R. Kastenbaum (Eds.), *Voices and visions of aging* (pp. 3–19). New York: Springer.

Bailey, D., & Schwartzberg, S. (Eds.). (1995). *Ethical and legal dilemmas in occupational therapy.* Philadelphia: F.A. Davis.

Baum, C. (1991). Addressing the needs of the cognitively impaired elderly from a family policy perspective. *American Journal of Occupational Therapy, 45*(7), 594–606.

Becker & Kaufman. (1988). Old age, rehabilitation, and research. *The Gerontologist, 4*(28), 459–467.

Binstock, R. (1994). Old-age-based rationing: From rhetoric to risk? *Generations, 18*(4), 37–43.

Brock, D. (1987). Informed consent. In D. VanDeVeer & T. Regan (Eds.), *Health care ethics* (pp. 98–126). Philadelphia: Temple University Press.

Brody, S., & Morrison, M. (1992, winter). Aging and rehabilitation: Beyond the medical model. *Generations,* 23–26.

Bruckner, J. (1988). Behind the curtain of silence: Ethical dilemmas in rehabilitation. In J. Monagle & D. Thomasma (Eds.), *Medical ethics: A guide for health professionals* (pp. 111–121). Rockville, MD: Aspen.

Callahan, D. (1987, August 15). Limiting health care for the old. *The Nation,* 125–127.

Callahan, D. (1989). Aging and the ends of medicine. In J. Arras & N. Rhoden (Eds.), *Ethical issues in modern medicine* (pp. 533–539). Mountain View, CA: Mayfield Publishing.

Cassidy, J. (1988). Access to health care: A clinician's opinion about an ethical issue. *American Journal of Occupational Therapy, 42*(5), 295–299.

Collopy, B. (1988). Autonomy in long term care: Some crucial distinctions. *The Gerontologist, 28*, 10–17.

Crabtree, J. (1991a). Ethical dilemmas and the older adult. In J. Kiernat (Ed.), *Occupational therapy and the older adult* (pp. 338–351). Gaithersburg, MD: Aspen.

Crabtree, J. (1991b). Five freedoms of autonomy. *Gerontology Special Interest Section Newsletter, 14*(1), 1–2.

Crabtree, J. (1991c). The effect of referral for profit on therapists' and clients' autonomy and fair competition. *American Journal of Occupational Therapy, 45*(5), 464–466.

Cynkin, S., & Robinson, A. (1990). *Occupational therapy toward health through activities*. Boston: Little, Brown.

Daniels, N. (1987). Justice in health care. In D. VanDeVeer & T. Regan (Eds.), *Health care ethics* (pp. 290–321). Philadelphia: Temple University Press.

Estes, C., Gerard, L., & Clark, A. (1984). Women and economics of aging. In M. Minkler & C. Estes (Eds.), *Readings in the political economy of aging* (pp. 209–225). Amityville, NY: Baywood.

Evert, M. (1993). Competency: Ethical issues and dilemmas. *American Journal of Occupational Therapy, 47*(6), 487–489.

Fahey, C., & Holstein, M. (1993). Toward a philosophy of the third age. In T. Cole, W. A. Achenbaum, P. Jakobi, & R. Kastenbaum (Eds.), *Voices and visions of aging* (pp. 241–257). New York: Springer.

Friedan, B. (1993). *The fountain of age*. New York: Simon & Schuster.

Friedman, E. (1986). Two tiers of care: The unthinkable meets the inevitable. In E. Friedman (Ed.), *Making choices: Ethics issues for health care professionals* (pp. 71–75). Chicago: American Hospital Publishing.

Gottlich, V. (1994). Protection for nursing facility residents under the ADA. *Generations, 18*(4), 43–48.

Gray, M. (1993). The credentialing process in occupational therapy. In S. Ryan (Ed.), *Practice issues in occupational therapy* (pp. 307–314). Thorofare, NJ: SLACK.

Gurland, B. (1992, June). Quality of life: A motivating force in assessment. In *Multidimensional assessment and quality of life for the elderly*. Presented at Columbia Presbyterian Medical Center, New York, NY.

Gutheil, I. (Ed.). (1994). *Work with older people; challenges and opportunities*. New York: Fordham University Press.

Halper, T. (1978). Paternalism and the elderly. In S. Spiker, K. Woodward, & D. Tassel (Eds), *Aging & the elderly* (pp. 321–339). Highlands, NJ: Humanities Press.

Hansen, R. (1994). Ethical considerations for the consultant. In E. Jaffe & C. Epstein (Eds.), *Occupational therapy consultation* (pp. 622–633). St. Louis: Mosby YearBook.

Hofland, B. (1994). When capacity fades and autonomy is constricted; a client-centered approach to residential care. *Generations, 18*(4), 31–37.

Howard, B. (1991). How high do we jump? The effect of reimbursement on occupational therapy. *American Journal of Occupational Therapy, 45*(10), 875–882.

Jacobs, K. (1992). Integrating the Americans With Disabilities Act of 1990 into client intervention. *American Journal of Occupational Therapy 46*(5), 445–449.

Kapp, M. (1988). Forcing services on at-risk adults: When doing good is not so good. *Social Work in Health Care, 13*(4), 1–13.

Kielhofner, G. (1992). *Conceptual foundations of occupational therapy.* Philadelphia: F. A. Davis.

Kiernat, J. (1991). The rewards and challenges of working with older adults. In J. Kiernat (Ed.), *Occupational therapy and the older adult* (pp. 2–11). Gaithersburg, MD: Aspen.

Kornblau, B. (1992). Legal issues in occupational therapy consultation. In E. Jaffe & C. Epstein (Eds.), *Occupational therapy consultation* (pp. 594–622). St. Louis: Mosby YearBook.

Kutchins, H. (1991). The fiduciary relationship: The legal basis for social workers' responsibilities to clients. *Social Work, 36*(2), 106–113.

Kyler-Hutchison, P. (1988). Ethical reasoning and informed consent in occupational therapy. *American Journal of Occupational Therapy, 42*(5), 283–294.

Kyler-Hutchison, P. (1994). Unethical and illegal; what's the difference. *Occupational Therapy Week, 8*(24), 8.

Kyler-Hutchison, P. (1995). Overcharges affect public view of OTs. *Occupational Therapy Week, 9*(22), 10–11.

Lewis, S. L. (1989). *Elder care.* Thorofare, NJ: SLACK.

Libow, L. (1993, April 30). Doing the right things...? (Introduction). Grappling with ethical dilemmas in geriatric long term care. Paper presented at the New York Academy of Medicine, New York.

Lowy, L. (1985). *Social work with the aging* (2nd ed.). New York: Longman.

Minkler, M. (1984). Blaming the aged victim. The politics of retrenchment in times of fiscal conservatism. In M. Minkler & C. Estes (Eds.), *Readings in the political economy of aging.* Amityville, NY: Baywood.

Moody, H. (1983). Ethical dilemmas in long term care. *Journal of Gerontological Social Work, 5*(1 & 2), 97–111.

Moody, H. (1992). *Ethics in an aging society.* Baltimore: Johns Hopkins Press.

Moody, H. (1993). What is critical gerontology and why is it important? In T. Cole, W. A. Achenbaum, P. Jakobi, & R. Kastenbaum (Eds.), *Voices and visions of aging* (pp. xv–3). New York: Springer.

Moon-Sperling, T., & Crispen Pinson, C. (1991). Implications of OBRA '87: Expansion of services and opportunities. *Gerontology Special Interest Section Newsletter, 14*(3), 1–2.

Neuhaus, B. (1988). Considerations in clinical reasoning: The impact of technology and cost containment. *American Journal of Occupational Therapy, 42*(5), 288–295.

Occupational Therapy Commission on Practice. (1993). Position paper: Purposeful activity. *American Journal of Occupational Therapy, 47*(12), 1081–1082.

Omnibus Budget Reconciliation Act of 1987 (Public Law 100–203), 1819, 42 U.S.C. 1395(i)–3.

Peterson, S. (1987). Professional codes and ethical decision making. In G. Anderson & V. Glesnes-Anderson (Eds.), *Health care ethics* (pp. 321–329). Rockville, MD: Aspen.

Purtilo, R. (1993). *Ethical dimensions in the health professions* (2nd ed.). Philadelphia: Saunders.

Reed, K. (1992). History of federal legislation for persons with disabilities. *American Journal of Occupational Therapy, 46*(5), 397–416.

Reich, W. (Ed.). (1976). *Encyclopedia of bioethics*. New York: Free Press.

Reitemeier, P., & Brody, H. (1988). Treatment refusal for economic reasons. In J. Monagle & D. Thomasma (Eds.), *Medical ethics: A guide for health professionals* (pp. 285–291). Rockville, MD: Aspen.

Relman, A. (1991). The health care industry, where is it taking us? *New England Journal of Medicine, 325*(12), 854–859.

Rogers, J. (1986). Roles and functions of occupational therapy in gerontic practice. In L. Davis & M. Kirkland (Eds.), *The role of occupational therapy with the elderly* (pp. 117–123). Rockville, MD: American Occupational Therapy Association.

Rovner, B., German, P., Brant, L., Clark, R., Burton, L., & Folstein, M. (1991). Depression and mortality in nursing homes. *Journal of the American Medical Association, 265*(8), 993–996.

Shapiro, M., & Spece, R. (1981). *Bioethics and law*. St. Paul, MN: West.

Standards and Ethics Commission of the American Occupational Therapy Association. (1993). Core values and attitudes of occupational therapy practice. *American Journal of Occupational Therapy, 47*(12), 1085–1086.

Townsend, E. (1993). 1993 Muriel Driver lecture: Occupational therapy's social vision. *Canadian Journal of Occupational Therapy, 60*(4), 174–184.

Trombly, C. (Ed.). (1995). *Occupational therapy for physical dysfunction*. Baltimore: Williams and Wilkins.

Trombly, C. (Ed.). (1996). *Occupational therapy for physical dysfunction* (4th ed.). Baltimore: Williams and Wilkins.

Welles, C. (1986). Ethics and the older adult. In L. Davis & M. Kirkland (Eds.), *The role of occupational therapy with the elderly* (pp. 189–193).

Rockville, MD: American Occupational Therapy Association.

Wenston, S. (1987). Applying philosophy to ethical dilemmas. In G. Anderson & V. Glesnes-Anderson (Eds.), *Health care ethics* (pp. 22–33). Rockville, MD: Aspen.

Zuckerman, C. (1994). Clinical ethics in geriatric settings. *Generations, 18*(4), 9–13.

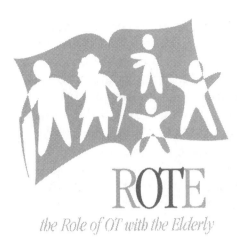

ROTE

the Role of OT with the Elderly

Older Adults: Living Lives

Joan C. Rogers, PhD, OTR, FAOTA
K. Oscar Larson, MA, OTR

Abstract

The authors present a framework for analyzing older adults' lives utilizing terminology from the World Health Organization and the American Occupational Therapy Association.

Introduction

Besides understanding the development of gerontology and gerontic occupational therapy, we must consider how aging adults are living their lives when we ponder how to provide services to them. This chapter will provide an overview of how older adults experience the later years of their lives. In exploring this theme, we will try not to limit the discussion to problems and deterioration, but instead will try to provide a perspective of function and dysfunction. Although some aging adults will experience disease, inability to do tasks, loss of roles, and isolation, many will remain healthy, continue to carry out desired activities as part of lifelong and new roles, and approach their deaths with the support and comfort of family, friends, and caretakers. To organize this chapter, older adults' lives will be viewed in terms of their ability to function in performance components, performance areas, and performance contexts.

The occupational therapy practitioner who views an aging person's life will be keenly concerned with how the person functions. Unfortunately, occupational therapy practitioners do not agree on the precise meaning of function. One practitioner may speak of muscle function, another of shoulder func-

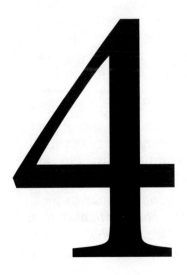

tion, a third of cooking function, and a fourth of homemaker function. If each of these practitioners were to conduct a functional assessment of the same patient, they would each assess different aspects of human performance, and there would be little or no overlap in their descriptions of the patient's functional performance.

Rehabilitation theorists have attempted to clarify the meaning of function by viewing chronic health conditions as a multidimensional experience. The conceptual model endorsed by the International Classification of Impairments, Disabilities, and Handicaps (ICIDH) and the World Health Organization (WHO) (1980), for example, distinguishes among four concepts—pathology, impairment, disability, and handicap.

Pathology is a disruption of normal body systems or processes. It includes acquired medical diagnoses, such as cerebral vascular accident, myocardial infarction, and emphysema; and psychiatric diagnoses, such as schizophrenia and depression. Pathologic conditions related to age-associated decrements (e.g., presbycusis and reduced energy) and environmental deprivation (e.g., failure to thrive and disuse syndrome) also are experienced at this level. If a pathology cannot be cured or is only controlled, impairments result.

Impairment refers to the loss or abnormality of an anatomic, physiologic, cognitive, or emotional structure or function. Examples of impairment include restricted range of motion, inability to think abstractly, visual-perceptual dysfunction, and poor self-concept (WHO, 1980). If an impairment is severe, the ability to perform one's daily functions might be restricted. Impairments are concerned with function of body parts, systems, or processes in isolation. By contrast, a *disability* is concerned with the integrated func-

tioning of the entire person that is required to accomplish tasks, interactions, and other human behaviors. Examples of a disability are problems in feeding, driving, using a tape recorder, playing bingo, and communicating effectively with a bank teller.

Tasks form the basis of social roles (e.g., worker, homemaker, grandparent, or religious participant). If task disabilities are severe, social role performance can become impaired and the person will no longer be able to enact roles satisfactorily. The experience of pathology at this level is referred to as *handicap*. A handicap can reflect a lack of opportunity to perform a socially expected role, as well as the inability to do so. For example, the person recovering from a CVA can become proficient in home management tasks, but because family members may not permit them to perform these tasks, they are rendered handicapped.

Thus, according to the WHO conceptual model, function can be evaluated in terms of pathology, impairment, disability, or handicap. Although this taxonomy implies a cause-and-effect relationship, it should be recognized that not every pathologic condition results in impairment, not every impairment results in disability, and not every disability results in handicap. Also, the model can be bidirectional. Failure to participate in social roles, for example, can result in sufficient inactivity to cause disability (e.g., diminished task skills) and impairments associated with generalized deconditioning. The WHO model helps occupational therapy practitioners appreciate that functional consequence occurs at three levels: impairment, disability, and handicap.

The *Uniform Terminology for Occupational Therapy, third edition,* (American Occupational Therapy Association, 1994) provides a compendium of occupational therapy concepts (see chapter 3, Appendix A of this text). It also implies a conceptual hierarchy analogous to that of the WHO model. The *Uniform Terminology* includes the following concepts: performance components, performance areas, and performance contexts. Each notion is further conceptualized along a continuum of dysfunction to function. The notions of dysfunction in the components of performance, areas of performance, and contexts of performance, are similar to the WHO concepts of impairment, disability, and handicap, respectively.

As discussed in chapter 3 of this text, the delimitations of the *Uniform Terminology* concepts and WHO concepts are similar but not exactly the same. The purpose for developing the two taxonomies has neither the same intent nor the same utility. Uniform Terminology was designed to articulate occupational therapy's domain of concern, WHO ICIDH was designed to organize research data. *Uniform Terminology* considers continua of functional to dysfunctional behaviors, whereas WHO ICIDH considers only dysfunction in each area. Also, therapists, scholars, and researchers within occupational therapy and the larger field of rehabilitation are debating how to coordinate these two sets of concepts. The arguments are not yet resolved and beyond the scope of this text. With these uncertainties in mind, however, this chapter will seek to continue this debate by considering the parallel concepts diagramed in table 4–1 when discussing the lives of older adults.

The first section of this chapter will consider the level of the performance components. As one ages, how does health or impairment affect the person's ability to function in the sensorimotor, cognitive, and psychosocial components? The second section will review the level of performance areas. As one ages, how does task ability or disability affect the person's ability to function in activities of daily living, work or productivity, and leisure areas? The final section will analyze the level of performance contexts. As one ages, how does the fulfillment of social roles or experience of handicaps affect functioning in the physical, cultural, and social environments?

Table 4–1. Uniform Terminology and WHO ICIDH Concepts

Uniform Terminology Concepts	WHO ICIDH Concepts
(Continua from function to Dysfunction)	(Areas of Dysfunction Only)
—	Pathology
Performance Component	Impairment
Performance Area	Disability
Performance Context	Handicap
Source: AOTA, 1994	Source: WHO, 1980

References

American Occupational Therapy Association. (1994). Uniform terminology for occupational therapy (3rd ed.). *American Journal of Occupational Therapy, 48,* 1047–1054.

World Health Organization. (1980). *International classification of impairments, disabilities, and handicaps: A manual of classification relating to consequences of disease.* Geneva: Author.

Section 1. Health and Impairment: The Performance Context

Linda L. Levy, MA, OTR/L, FAOTA

Abstract

The author reviews normal and pathological changes in aging.

Introduction

The aging process is difficult to define because it connotes three distinct phenomena: the biological capacity for survival, the psychological capacity for adaptation, and the sociological capacity for the fulfillment of social roles (Birren & Renner, 1977). Within each of these developmental spheres, older adults are presented with developmental challenges that occur at different times and different rates. For example, a 60-year-old who is unable to establish intimate relationships would be considered young in terms of psychological age. A still-employed 70-year-old would be considered young in terms of social age. Conversely, a 50-year-old with high blood pressure would be considered older in terms of biological age. As a result, growing old is not age-specific. There are vast variations in biological, psychological, and social aging, which are only roughly related to one's chronological age. Aging, then, is best conceptualized in terms of one's health and diverse psychological and sociological functional capacities rather than by one's chronological age. This perception is aptly expressed by the adage "You are only as old as you feel."

At the same time, it cannot be overemphasized that any of the challenges presented by aging are approached by individuals whose life experiences have provided them with a rich and complex variety of adaptive capacities and coping mechanisms. As a result, it would be inaccurate to characterize any but a broad and heterogeneous view of normal aging, or normal older adult functioning. Older adults vary more in patterns of normal functioning than do individuals at any other stage in the life span. One of the few generalizations that researchers are willing to make is that older adults tend to become less like each other and more like themselves; that is, they become increasingly individualistic as they age. With an appreciation of the tremendous variability that exists among older adults, we can begin to explore the biological, cognitive, and psychological challenges presented by the aging process.

Biological Changes in Older Adults

The biological changes that occur with aging are a continuation of the decline that, most researchers agree, begins when physical maturity is reached, at approximately age 18 to 22. It is not yet possible to distinguish which changes are a result of aging (those determined by heredity), and which result from a variety of environmental and physical factors (i.e., nutrition, obesity, physical activity, smoking, environmental toxins, and economic advantage) or disease. It may well be that conditions thought to be part of normal aging are in fact related to lifestyle and environment. For example, heart and vascular diseases are uncommon in populations that eat no meat and little fat, and cataract formation appears to be related to the degree of exposure to ultraviolet B radiation (sunlight) (Mattox, Wu, & Schuman, 1995). Nor is there a clear line between what is considered normal aging and what constitutes disease. What are referred to as aging processes could well be the sum effect of a large number of very slowly evolving disease processes (Manton, 1989; T. F. Williams, 1993). For example, arteriosclerosis and demineralization of bone are regarded as expressions of aging until they progress to a point where they lead to diseases such as heart attacks, strokes, or osteoporosis; how the point of transition is identified is not clear. Researchers also are beginning to suspect that there might be a continuum between the brain lesions in aging and those in Alzheimer's disease (VonDras & H. T. Blumenthal, 1992). And, we know that death in advanced old age, in the absence of disease, is rare. Evans characterizes the difficulty this way: "To draw a distinction between normal aging and disease is to separate the undefined from the undefinable" (quoted in Blumenthal, 1993, p. 1272; Evans, 1988, p. 57).

Biogerontologists define aging as a failure to maintain homeostasis under conditions of physiological stress, which is associated with a decrease in viability and an increase in vulnerability of the individual (Comfort, 1979; Evans, 1988). In their view, aging is related to the deteriorative physiological effects on homeostatic reserve capacity associated with the passage of time. Indeed, the diminishing ability to respond to stress and return to the pre-stress level, for example, a decrease in homeostatic capacity, is one of the most consistently documented aging changes. Although there is little change in homeostatic mechanisms under resting conditions, the rate of readjustment to normal equilibrium after stress is slower in older adults than in their younger counterparts. For example, the capacity of the kidneys for removing waste, the ability to maintain body temperature during exposure to heat or cold, and the efficiency of blood sugar regulation decrease with age. Similarly, when an older adult develops an infection, the body temperature does not rise as rapidly or as markedly as in younger people and, once raised, it takes longer to return to normal. The stressors that disrupt these processes either can be physical (a virus or exercise) or psychosocial (fear or loss of spouse). In either case, with advancing age the capacity for homeostasis gradually declines, and the range of adjustment to stressors becomes smaller and narrower. Accordingly, biological aging results in increased vulnerability to environmental conditions. Biological aging also results in progressive physiological changes in every major organ system.

Before we address these diverse biological changes, there are a number of issues to keep in mind. First, it should be emphasized that, within individuals, biological changes occur at different times and rates in different organs, tissues, and cells. For example, an individual might experience marked arthritis or severe visual loss despite excellent cardiovascular function. And, within different individuals, these changes occur at vastly different times and rates. For example, visible signs of aging such as graying can occur at age 30 in one individual and at age 70 in another.

Second, while some biological aging occurs naturally in body organs, biochemical pathways, musculoskeletal systems, and the central nervous system, the health and physical abilities of most older adults do not precipitously decline, nor are the changes severe enough to interfere seriously with activities of daily living. Most older adults function well enough to meet all the demands of daily life, at least until well into late adulthood. This is because the human body is endowed with elaborate compensation systems and a vast amount of reserve function despite the changes that aging can bring. For example, as little as 60% of vital lung capacity is sufficient for most daily activities; an individual can survive with less than half of the liver, fractions of stomach and intestines, one lung, and one kidney (Shock, 1974). As will be discussed more fully in the next section of this text on disability and performance areas, survey data of community residents reveal that limitations in activities of daily living are experienced by only 23% of the population over the age of 65. Furthermore, these difficulties are experienced by 14% of those between ages 65 and 74, 29% of those between 75 and 84, and 34% of those 85 years and older (National Center for Health Statistics [NCHS], 1995; U.S. Senate, 1991). As a result, even the majority of older adults who live into their 80s (66%) do so without experiencing difficulties in carrying out major tasks and without significant changes in their normal functioning caused by biological aging. And yet, 85% of older adults over 65 years of age experience at least one chronic condition, with multiple chronic conditions such as arthritis, hypertension, and hearing impairments commonplace (NCHS, 1995). The clear implication is that despite the probability of chronic impairments, impairments do not necessarily lead to disabilities. Most older adults have developed adaptive strategies that enable them to lead well-functioning lives. At the same time, it becomes apparent that criteria such as absence of disease are not useful when addressing the question of what it means for older adults to be healthy. The more important consideration is the effect that

a given impairment has on an individual's ability to maintain function and quality of life. This is a perspective that was well-recognized nearly four decades ago by the World Health Organization in this statement: "Health in the elderly is best measured in terms of function" (WHO, 1959, p. 3).

Finally, it should be recognized that there is not necessarily a direct cause-and-effect relationship between the degree of structural impairment within an organ and the presence of impaired function or disease. For example, researchers are finding the phenotypic lesions (amyloid) of Alzheimer's disease in all brains after age 65 (VonDras & H. T. Blumenthal, 1992), leading to the speculation that these lesions could be an aging phenomenon—not a disease. That fact notwithstanding, it cannot be assumed that the existence of a biological change necessarily leads to a commensurate decline in function.

Having considered these issues, we can begin to provide an overview of age-related biological changes that have particular relevance to occupational therapists working with older adults. Biological changes can be grouped into two categories:

1. Gradual progressive physiological changes in various organ systems

2. Specific diseases that are more common in older adults.

As suggested earlier in this section, these categories are not necessarily mutually exclusive. Researchers are beginning to view progressive changes related to age and major disease entities that present in older adults as related to each other in subtle and complex ways (Brody & Schneider, 1986; M. E. Williams, 1984; T. F. Williams, 1993). For purposes of this discussion, emphasis is given to biological changes that most directly affect sensorimotor performance components and occupational performances; therefore, the content is selective. For a more comprehensive discussion of this vast and complex topic, the reader is referred to Hazzard, Andres, Bierman, and Blass (1990); Brocklehurst (1985); Saxon and Etten (1987); and Reichel (1995).

SENSORY CHANGES

Vision

For most people, the aging process leads to a slow but steady decrease in visual efficiency. Specifically, it produces the following effects:

1. A reduced visual acuity
2. A steadily decreasing power of accommodation (the ability to focus)
3. A reduced capacity to adjust to changes in illumination (dark adaptation)
4. A decreased resistance to glare
5. A shift in color vision.

As might be expected, there is a consequent increase in defective vision. For example, the NCHS (1995) reported that defective visual acuity of 20/50 or poorer (with visual correction) increases from 0.7% at 35 to 45 years, to more than 14% at 65 to 74 years. Consequently, older adults are more than 20 times as likely to suffer impairment that limits such activities as reading and driving than are middle-aged adults. By age 70, the probability of suffering significant visual defects increases to 92% (reviewed in Schieber, 1992). The magnitude of the overall change in visual acuity has been calculated as a 300% decrease (Gittings & Fozard, 1986). Visual decline in advanced age has been associated with many unmet needs of older adults, such as housekeeping, grocery shopping, and food preparation, and with physical and emotional disabilities (Branch, Horowitz, & Carr, 1989). It

also contributes to disorientation and behavioral deterioration (O'Neil & Calhoun, 1975).

The physiological changes accounting for deteriorating vision involve multiple structures: the lens, the cornea, the sclera, the vitreous humor, the retina, the pupil, and the exterior structures.

Lens. The lens of the eye begins to lose elasticity in the mid-40s and progresses with aging. Because the lens must adjust to view near and distant objects clearly, the increased rigidity has a detrimental effect on both the ability to focus (acuity) and the speed of focusing. The visual clarity of near objects is particularly affected. The lens is normally under some tension and thereby flattened, creating a natural tendency for distant vision. Less lens elasticity interferes most with the bulging of the eye needed for near vision (accommodation). As a result, most older people are not able to focus well on near objects and experience presbyopia, or farsightedness. Bifocal eyeglasses minimize the need for the lens of the eye to change shape and usually can correct this deficit. Without glasses, however, older people usually cannot see objects or people who are closer than an arm's length. The oft-bemoaned expression, "My arms aren't long enough anymore," refers to the difficulty older adults experience with print or small detail unless it is held at a distance.

As the pliability of the lens is decreasing, the lens is developing opacities that reduce its transparency. The lens continues its cellular growth throughout life. New cellular layers constantly are being added to the outer segment of the lens, exerting increased pressure on the inner layers. Without any direct blood supply to the nucleus of the lens, cells at the center atrophy and harden. Waste products are not removed and opacities develop (Mattox, Wu, & Schuman, 1995).

In addition to presbyopia, other practical visual problems develop. The thickening of the lens and the increasing light scatter (from the reduced transparency and the opacities) result in decreased light transmission through the lens. As a result, middle-aged and older adults require much more illumination than younger adults do to maintain the same degree of visual discrimination. The increase in light scatter within the eye can be an even more serious problem in environments lacking proper brightness control, because older adults experience a marked increase in sensitivity to visual glare. Glare produces a painful overload problem, induced by too much illumination that scatters light within the eye and blurs the retinal image. Glare problems can develop from either direct or indirect sources. Direct glare occurs when light reaches the eye directly from its source (e.g., sunlight shining into a darker room). Indirect glare occurs when the light rebounds off another surface and reflects into the eye (e.g., light, intensified, as it is reflected off highly polished floors, plastic-covered furniture, and chrome wheelchairs). Both conditions can create ambulation hazards (Mezey & Grisso, 1989). The problem with glare is compounded by the fact that older people need much more illumination (or more intense illumination) to complete most tasks. The goal of lighting for older adults, then, is to achieve a balance between getting enough light into the eye and preventing the immobilizing and hazardous effects of glare. Note also that depth perception declines with increasing lens opacity as well (Tideiksaar & Kay, 1986).

Another age-related change in the lens is that it undergoes an increased yellowing because of waste products (protein pigments) that accumulate. As a result, color vision is altered. Older adults can more easily discriminate colors at the upper end of the visual spectrum (yellow, orange, and red) than colors at the lower end (violet, blue, and green). Dark colors (navy, brown, and black), and pastel colors (blues, yellows, and pinks) become especially difficult to distinguish. By old age, color sensitivity over the entire spectrum has declined markedly: Older adults near the age of 90 are unable to identify the color of more than 50% of objects presented (Weale, 1988). The oldest older adult can best distinguish between the colors red and white.

Cataracts. Cataracts are present when the clear lens within the eye opacifies, producing a milky white appearance. The process begins at the periphery of the lens, gradually spreading to the central portion. Functionally, older adults with cataracts have hazy or blurred vision, and difficulty with glare. Some degree of lens clouding is present in 95% of the population over 65 years of age (NCHS, 1995). The high incidence of cataracts in the later years raises the question of whether the process of cataract formation represents an exaggeration of the normal aging of the human lens. Yet there is evidence that cataract formation is precipitated by unprotected exposure to ultraviolet B radiation (sunlight) (Mattox, Wu, & Schuman, 1995).

Cataract surgery (lens extraction) is the only treatment for cataracts at this time. It is the most frequently performed operation in the United States among older adults, accounting for 12% of the Medicare Part B Budget (NCHS, 1995). It also is one of the most successful surgical procedures: about 95% of postoperative older adults regain excellent vision (Abrams, Beers, Berkow, & Fletcher, 1995).

Cornea. The second change in visual structure involves the cornea, which becomes less translucent and takes on a smoky appearance with progressive age. As a result, light transmission is even more compromised and light scattering even more pronounced. More illumination is needed to produce a satisfactory image on the retina. There also is a change in the curvature of the cornea, which often flattens with age. This produces astigmatism, which further distorts depth perception and the perception of the relationship between objects (Abrams et al., 1995).

Directly behind the cornea lies the aqueous, a fluid continually in flux, that nourishes and cleanses the lens. *Glaucoma* occurs when there is obstruction of aqueous fluid outflow. Intraocular pressure (pressure in the aqueous) increases, which eventually results in "hardening" of the eye; hardening reduces blood flow to the optic nerve and the retina and leads first to loss of peripheral vision and visual fields, and eventually to blindness. Typically, glaucoma begins in midlife, progresses slowly, and impairs functional vision until its progression is slowed by medical or surgical intervention. Glaucoma affects approximately 3% of individuals over the age of 65 (NCHS, 1995), and accounts for 10% of all cases of blindness in the United States (Abrams et al., 1995). Intraocular pressure has been associated with hypertension.

Sclera. Another change in structure is that the scleral tissue loses water and increases its fatty deposits, causing a yellow cast and decreased opacity. This permits stray light to enter the eye, and images wash out, necessitating more striking color contrasts for adequate visual discrimination.

Vitreous humor. With advancing age, the vitreous humor tends to shrink, causing traction on the retina. It also becomes more liquid, and exhibits an increase in densities called "floaters," which are described by older

adults as black spots floating within the field of vision. They are annoying and distracting.

Retina. The retina also changes in the aging eye. Both arterial and venous occlusion can occur in retinal blood vessels (see cardiovascular changes below). This can result in "spotty" fields of vision; portions of objects become indistinct if their image falls on a blind spot in the retina. Vascular insufficiencies also can result in a reduced blood supply to the retina, with consequent metabolic deficiencies and cell loss. One consequence of these changes is a gradual decrease in the size of the visual field, requiring the individual to scan the environment to attain peripheral vision. Another consequence is an increase in the size of the macular blind spot (the source of pigmentary changes located in the center of the retina) that can only be compensated for by increased magnification. The retina also becomes less sensitive to low levels of illumination. The receptors themselves require almost 50% more light in order to respond to a visual stimulus. Dark adaptation, the ability to adjust vision when moving from high to low levels of illumination, is compromised. The time required to adapt increases with age, and the ability to adapt to dark decreases. Walking from sunlight into a darker hallway can produce blindness for a period. Consequently, older adults need to avoid lighting extremes in their environments (Mezey & Grisso, 1989).

Several diseases can affect the retina, including macular degeneration and diabetic retinopathy. *Macular degeneration* is the most common cause of vision loss and the leading cause of blindness in older adults. Age-related macular degeneration rises with advancing age, from 6% in older adults between the ages of 65 and 74 to 20% in those 75 and over (NCHS, 1995). It results from the degenerative neuronal changes that are secondary to a compromised blood supply that occurs in the retina with advancing age. These degenerative changes are most pronounced in the central macula, the area of the retina responsible for sharp central vision. Older adults with this condition report decreased central vision, changes in color perception, and loss of fine-detail discrimination. For most older adults, sufficient peripheral vision is retained to assist in mobility, but not enough for activities such as reading or watching television. *Diabetic retinopathy* occurs in older adults with long-term, poorly controlled diabetes, and affects 3% of adults over the age of 85 (NCHS, 1995). Blood vessels in the eye rupture, and the blood prevents light rays from getting to the retina. This produces scotoma, or blind spots, in the central visual fields. Repeated bleeding can bring about partial or complete blindness. Retinal detachment also can occur when scar tissue forms near the retina and detaches it from the eye. When diagnosed at its earliest stages, it can be treated with laser therapy.

Pupil. The pupil of the eye is affected by the aging process as well. There is a general reduction in pupil diameter and a decrease in maximum pupillary opening, which further limits the amount of light reaching the retina. The effects of this miosis, as it is called, are most evident at low and intermediate illumination levels. Less light is able to reach the retina, and the eye requires more time to adapt to changes in illumination. Older people require 30 to 40 minutes to achieve full dark adaptation and never achieve the same degree of dark adaptation as younger people (Mezey & Grisso, 1989). Unfortunately, devices to compensate for the loss of either pupillary or retinal ability to adjust to light are not available, and the practical difficulties that

arise can be considerable. In particular, falls can occur. Archea (reported in Fozard & Popkin, 1978) found that most falls occurred on the step at the top of the landing where daylighted windows preceded darkened stairs. A similar circumstance occurs when an older adult is driving at night: The driver must be able to adapt rapidly to the headlights of an oncoming car and then recover to see the dark road. A decreased ability to make these adjustments is one of the reasons older adults avoid night driving.

Exterior structures. Finally, the exterior structures of the eye are affected as people age. Changes in the upper and lower eyelids can result in irritation of the cornea and conjunctiva. Muscle weakness results in a decreased ability to rotate the eye upward and can contribute to a relatively common outward deviation of the eyeball, known as exotropia. There are losses in fat padding around the socket, causing the eyes to sink back into their sockets and contributing to the decreased visual field experienced by older adults (Kallman & Vernon, 1987). In addition, there is a tendency for the eyelids to droop (ptosis), which further narrows the field of vision. Some older people also experience a reduction in tear formation, causing dryness and irritation. And yet, tear overflow also can occur because of impaired drainage of the ductal system.

Hearing

Hearing loss is the third most prevalent chronic condition of older adults. It affects about 33% of all older adults between 65 and 74, and about 75% of those between 75 and 79 (Fozard, 1990; NCHS, 1995). Although the ability to detect high-frequency sound is affected, most decreases in auditory acuity are relatively slight during the early and middle years. Thereafter, decrements accelerate. As aging advances, the ability to hear progressively lower frequencies declines to the extent that, by age 65, 50% of the male population and 30% of the female population suffer a hearing loss significant enough to interfere with social interaction (Plomp, 1978). The incidence of deafness increases from 3% at age 55, to 15% at age 75. Nursing home surveys report that 85 to 90% of residents experience serious hearing impairment (for a review, see Schieber, 1992).

Age-related losses in hearing are called *presbycusis*. These losses primarily involve degenerative changes in the cochlea (the primary neural receptor for hearing), and result in impaired discrimination (the ability to identify words), impaired tone threshold (high-tone hearing loss), and impaired higher frequency thresholds (difficulty hearing in noisy environments). Note that older adults experience the most difficulty hearing under what are termed masking conditions. Masking occurs when a sound is obscured or rendered inaudible by other sounds. In general, a sound must be 10 decibels louder than the background noise to be heard. Masking presents specific difficulty when one is trying to understand high-frequency (speech) sounds against a noisy background (Dubno, Dirk, & Morgan, 1984). Audiometric findings aside, the individual's ability to hear a conversation is of primary importance, and it can depend on the ability to separate a voice from background noise.

Four types of presbycusis have been identified (Abrams et al., 1995):

1. Sensory presbycusis, associated with degeneration of the basal end of the organ of Corti, appears in middle age and is manifested by a loss in high-frequency hearing. It might not have a significant effect on functional hearing because normal speech frequencies do not seem to be affected.

2. Neural presbycusis is associated with progressive degeneration of the auditory neurons in the auditory pathways of the cochlea. The onset of this type occurs late in life and is characterized by losses in speech discrimination but not in pure tone thresholds. The problem with this presbycusis is not necessarily an inability to hear: the person continues to hear tone, but cannot understand what he or she hears. Consequently, older adults frequently ask others to repeat what they say or to speak more distinctly or louder. Unfortunately, amplification does not help because it amplifies distorted, unintelligible sounds.

3. Metabolic presbycusis results from the atrophy of blood vessels in the wall of the cochlea, probably as a result of arteriosclerotic vascular changes. This leads to deficiencies in the bioelectric and biochemical properties of the lymph fluids that supply energy to the sensory organs. It results in a relatively uniform reduction in pure tone sensitivity for all frequencies and is accompanied by "recruitment," an abnormally rapid increase in loudness as the sound intensity increases.

4. Mechanical (or cochlear conductive) presbycusis is associated with a stiffening of the basilar membrane, which interferes with the vibratory mechanics of the cochlear duct. This condition leads to increasing hearing loss from low to high frequencies that could well affect the ability to understand speech. High-frequency consonants such as z, s, g, f, and t become increasingly difficult to hear. As a result, an older adult with this kind of presbycusis would hear /ip/, /ing/, /on/, /un/, and /ime/ instead of /zip/, /sing/, /gone/, /fun/, and

/time/. Vowel sounds usually are louder and lower in frequency and tend to be more easily understood than consonant sounds. Lowering the voice can sometimes help the older adult discriminate the tones of high-frequency sounds.

Hearing loss is considered the most devastating of the sensory losses because, even more than visual loss, it isolates older adults from their environment. It interferes most obviously with social interaction, for example, over the telephone and in conversation. It also significantly affects an individual's sense of safety and security. In addition, it negates some of the more aesthetic and orienting characteristics of human existence that tend to be undervalued until they are missing, such as the sound of music, birds, wind, rain, and children playing.

The extent to which a hearing loss interferes with social interaction depends on the extent of the loss. Yet, even at best, communicating with a hearing impaired person is frustrating and time-consuming for both parties, often requiring that the message be repeated several times before it is understood. At the same time, hearing loss often is associated with a sense of suspicion in dealings with other people, or even overt paranoia (Cooper, 1976; Fozard, 1990; Hyams, 1982), because inaccurately heard comments can be taken personally. A relationship between depression and hearing loss has been established (O'Neil & Calhoun, 1975). In addition, Oyer and Oyer (1978) found increased fatigue, vulnerability, irritability, tension, depression, and negativism, as consequences of age-related hearing loss.

Taste and Smell

With age, the decline in the ability to taste sweet substances is pro-

nounced, and older people might consume increasing amounts of sugar to compensate for this deficit. The threshold for salt also is increased; thus more salt is necessary to achieve baseline taste sensations (Mezey & Grisso, 1989).

Age-related changes in taste correlate with a gradual decrease both in the number of papillae and in the number of taste buds per papilla; as many as two thirds of the papillae become atrophic in old age (Bartoshuk et al., 1986). These changes also might correlate with a progressive reduction in the neurons found in taste centers in the cortical centers of the parietal lobe (see central nervous system changes below). There also is a reduction in saliva flow that comes with aging, which can aggravate an already dulled sense of taste.

Studies of olfactory acuity are somewhat contradictory. There are suggestions that the sense of smell is not seriously affected by age alone, but also by other factors associated with age. The current view is that age-related decline in the ability to smell is probably caused by a combination of changes in the olfactory tracts and bulb, cellular degeneration in the parietal lobe of the brain (both of which parallel changes in the central nervous system, discussed below); and, in some cases, nerve damage, nasal polyps, or nasal mucus membrane changes exacerbated by smoking (Mezey & Grisso, 1989).

Somatosensory System

Data that describe age-related changes in the somatosensory system is limited. Evidence to date indicates that aging is accompanied by declines in sensitivity to light touch, pinprick sensation, deep pain perception, position sense, and vibratory sensation (Imms & Edholm, 1981; Wolfson et al., 1985).

Consistent evidence documents that vibratory sensation declines with age, and that sensation in the lower extremity is more affected by aging than the upper extremity. Microscopically, a loss of the number and integrity of peripheral receptors and nerve fibers is thought to account for these alterations (Bolton, Winkelmann, & Dyck, 1966; O'Sullivan & Swallow, 1968; Sabin & Venna, 1984; Takahashi, 1966; see also peripheral nervous system changes below). These changes are thought to raise the sensitivity thresholds for pain, temperature, perceived movement, and to increase the risk of thermal and mechanical injury (Kenney, 1989).

Vestibular System or Balance

The vestibular system in older adults demonstrates a loss of sensory receptor organs and their supporting structures. Studies indicate an age-related 20% decline in hair cells of the saccule and utricle, and a 40% reduction in hair cells in the semicircular canals (Ochs et al., 1985; Oosterveld, 1983; Paparella & Shumrick, 1991).

There is evidence of age-related unsteadiness in standing or walking (Briggs, Gossman, Birch, Drews, & Shaddeau, 1989), increased postural sway (Abramson & Lovas, 1988; Hayes et al., 1985; Kirshen et al., 1984; Maki, Holliday, & Fernie, 1991; Sheldon, 1963), and onset of a wide-based compensatory gait "senile gait disorder," Koller, Glatt, & Fox, 1985). Righting responses (Cape, 1978) and balancing synergies also deteriorate with age (Woollacott, Shumway-Cook, & Nashner, 1986). These changes are more pronounced in inactive than active older adults (Rikli & Busch, 1986).

Presbyastasis is the term used to describe age-related disequilibrium when no other pathology is noted

(Kennedy & Clemis, 1990). Wyke (1979) postulated that age-related disequilibrium is affected by degeneration of the mechanoreceptors of the spinal apophyseal joints, secondary to cervical spondylosis (see joint changes below). The consequences of disequilibrium are compounded by reductions in vision and position sense (see above), as well as by changes in muscle strength, blood pressure, and central nervous system processing (see below). As a result, older adults are at increased risk for falls in response to slight or routine losses of balance (Duncan & Studenski, 1994; Wild, Nayak, & Isaacs, 1987).

MUSCULOSKELETAL CHANGES

Bones

Loss of skeletal mass is a normal, and at times disabling, consequence of aging. Bone mass in both men and women reaches a peak in the 40s and thereafter begins to erode, leading to a slow but inexorable decline at a rate of about 5% per year. The more metabolically active trabecular bone (forming the internal latticework) is lost more rapidly than cortical bone (forming the outer shell). All told, women lose about 35% of their cortical bone and as much as 50% of their trabecular bone mass; men lose about 20% and 35%, respectively, of the masses (Riggs, 1991). The strength of the skeleton and the ability of the bone to withstand trauma without fracture is directly related to the amount of bone in the skeleton.

Osteoporosis is defined as "an age-related disorder characterized by decreased bone mass (osteopenia) and increased susceptibility to fracture in the absence of other recognizable causes of bone loss" (National Institutes of Health, 1986, p. 1). To some extent, osteoporosis is a part of normal aging. It occurs when bone mass declines to a universal "fracture threshold," the point at which bones can break if they are exposed to mild stress. This point occurs at two standard deviations below the ideal peak bone mass for a 30-year-old, which reflects a reduction of approximately 30% of total bone mass. Each standard deviation below peak bone density doubles fracture risk.

About 50% of all women reach the fracture threshold, and thus have osteoporosis, by age 65; about 20% of men reach the threshold by age 70 (Riggs & Melton, 1986, 1992). The first outward signs of osteoporosis (back pain, dorsal kyphoscoliosis [dowager's hump], and declining height secondary to multiple vertebral crush fractures) usually occur about 5 years after reaching the fracture threshold. Eventually, seemingly benign actions, such as coughing or picking up a bag of groceries, can cause fractures. The majority of fractures occur in the neck of the femur (located at the hip), and these cause more deaths and disability than all other osteoporotic fractures combined (NCHS, 1995). Vertebrae, pelvis, and distal forearm (Colles's fracture) also are common locations for fractures in older adults.

The major cause of age-related bone loss is not known. Several factors, however, are associated with a greater risk of osteoporosis, either because they influence the peak bone mass achieved or because they accelerate the rate of bone loss. Factors that reduce initial bone mass include gender (female), race (White or Asian), nutritional status (a diet low in calcium and excessive alcohol and caffeine consumption), and insufficient physical activity (specifically, weight-bearing exercise). Factors that accelerate bone loss are menopause (estrogen deficiency), heavy alcohol use, smoking, prolonged immobility (secondary to any disease that markedly reduces mobility, such as rheumatoid arthritis), and long-term use of corticosteroids (frequently prescribed for older adults with rheumatoid arthritis, polymyalgia rheumatica, asthma, and skin diseases). Modest gains in bone density can significantly reduce fracture risk, and there are medications that can help achieve this goal. These include estrogen (appropriate only for women), injectable calcitonin (Calcimar™), and the recently approved alendronate (Fosamax™). There also are indications that exercise can slow the rate of bone loss and might even help increase bone density (J. Blumenthal et al., 1991; Dalsky, 1988; Simkin et al., 1987).

Joints

As people age, the cartilage tissues that line the joints decline in cell number, metabolic activity, and function. Cartilage contains no blood vessels, and depends on the blood supply of the synovium (the tissue that produces joint fluid) for nutrients. Blood supply decreases with age (see cardiovascular changes below). The cartilage tissues lose collagen as a result of enzymatic degradation. They become dehydrated, more fibrous, and show signs of degeneration, which reduces their ability to protect the ends of the bones from repetitive stress. In places, the cartilage splits, and the bone underneath produces extra calcium and thickens, thus enlarging the joint. This process also results in a proliferation of bony outgrowths, known as osteophytes (crepitus), in those areas. As a result, degenerative joint disease, known as osteoarthritis, occurs in and around many joints of the body. Note also that cartilage deterioration contributes to what is characterized as normal shrinkage with age. It is estimated that men shrink about 1 inch and women shrink about 2 inches as a result of osteoporotic collapse of the spine and thinning and deterioration of vertebral cartilage disks (Kauffman, 1987).

Osteoarthritis involves gradual deterioration and a slow onset of pain and disfigurement as the cartilage is worn away and the bones rub together. The ligaments that allow the joint its full range of motion are weakened and the joint becomes deformed and unstable. Ultimately, the joints are damaged to such an extent that subluxation or fusion can occur. In the usual form of osteoarthritis, the joints involved are the knees, the hips, the distal meta-carpels of the fingers and thumb (Herbeden's nodes), the joints around the base of the thumb, the base of the big toe, the lower cervical spine, and the lumbrosacral spine. When osteo-arthritis extends to the neck and the back, it is known as *cervical* or *spinal spondylosis* (or stenosis), respectively. In these conditions, the osteophytes can compress the spinal cord and peripheral nerves and produce additional neurological dysfunction (myelopathy) superimposed on the osteoarthritis. Early symptoms of *cervical spondylosis* include numbness and tingling of the fingers and difficulty with fine motor tasks. As the condition progresses, there may be mild weakness in the legs and decreased sensation in the feet. Cervical spondylosis has been reported in over 80% of adults over the age of 55 (Wyke, 1979). *Spinal spondylosis* frequently occurs in the lumbar spine and causes pain, numbness, and weakness in the buttocks, thighs, or legs on standing or walking, which often is relieved by sitting. Both conditions are treated by surgical decompression of the spinal cord.

The major cause of osteoarthritis is unknown, although age is considered to be the leading factor in the breakdown of cartilage and tissue. When it extends to the weight-bearing joints (most typically the knees), it becomes the leading cause of physical disability in older adults, surpassing coronary artery disease (NCHS, 1995; U.S. Senate, 1991). By age 65, 50% of older adults have impairments from osteoarthritis, and 80 to 90% demonstrate radiographic changes. By age 75, more than 80% of older adults are significantly affected (Schumacher, Klippel, & Koopman, 1993). Obesity is emerging as a predisposing factor in the development of the disease, especially in osteoarthritis of the hip and knee. The major problems are joint pain (mainly with activity, but also at rest), stiffness, and reduced mobility. Although the anatomical changes of osteoarthritis can only be managed with surgery (arthroscopy, osteotomy, or total joint arthroplasty), joint functioning often can be improved with strengthening exercises, anti-inflammatory medications, analgesics, modalities (heat, paraffin, interferential electrical stimulation), and adaptive devices. Note also that, by impeding mobility, osteoarthritis can exacerbate other conditions (heart disease, hypertension, and diabetes) that might otherwise be prevented or treated by physical activity.

Muscles

A universal finding in aging is slowly progressive muscle-wasting and decline in strength, known as sarcopenia. In healthy young adults, 10% of body weight is bone, 30% is muscle, and 20% is adipose tissue. By age 75, about 8% is bone, 15% is muscle, and 40% is adipose tissue (Evans, 1995a). Muscle mass has decreased by half because of a reduction in the number and diameter of slow twitch (type I) and fast twitch (type II) muscle fibers and also a reduction in the size of each alpha-motor neuron. The fast twitch fibers, responsible for speed and power, appear to be more affected than the slow twitch fibers, which are responsible for endurance. To some extent, muscle mass is replaced by fat content between muscle fibers and connective tissue (fibrin) deposits. Age-related reductions in muscle mass are directly related to age-related reductions in muscle strength (Evans, 1995a). Isometric contraction force is 20% lower by age 60 and 50% lower by age 80 compared with younger adults (Evans, 1995a; Hurley, 1995). Data from the Framingham study demonstrated significant relationships between decline in strength and ADL-IADL function (Jette, Branch, & Berlin, 1990). This study also revealed that 40% of 60-year-old women and 70% of 70-year-old women were unable to lift 10 pounds. In addition, reduced muscle strength has been implicated as a precipitant to institutionalization (Fisher, Pendergast, & Calkins, 1991).

Not all muscles show the same degree of decline with aging. Age-related change appears earlier in lower extremity flexor muscles than in other muscle groups, and is more pronounced in lower extremity than in upper extremity muscle groups (Evans, 1995; Frontera, Hughes, & Evans, 1991). Older adults also are at risk for an accelerated loss of muscle mass during any acute illness that restricts mobility. When restricted to bed, healthy older adults lose muscle mass and strength at a rate of about 5% per day (Jones, 1984; Payton & Poland, 1983). Geriatricians estimate that for each day of bed rest, 2 weeks of reconditioning are necessary to return to baseline functioning. Overall, the effects of deconditioning are accentuated in older people (Bortz, 1982; Harper & Lyles, 1988; Lentz, 1981; Reddy, 1986; Siebens, 1990).

There is ample evidence that age-related muscle changes might be prevented by physical exercise. A number of studies demonstrate the value of exercise in maintaining muscle strength and physical function well into the 80s and 90s (Evans, 1995b; Rogers & Evans, 1992; McCartney, Hicks, Martin & Webber, 1995; Simonsick et al., 1993; Tseng, Marsh, Hamilton, & Booth, 1995). Even structural changes of the muscles (increases in fast twitch [type II] muscle fibers) have been documented following formal exercise programs in older adults (Frontera, Meridith, O'Reilly, Knuttgen, & Evans, 1988). In addition, landmark studies by Fiatarone et al. (1990, 1994) and Fisher (1991) with frail nursing home residents provided evidence that high-intensity weight training results in significant improvements in muscle strength, size, balance, bone density, functional mobility, and mood, even up to the age of 96. In fact, a 10-week strengthening program for frail older adults resulted in a 100% increase in strength (Fiatarone et al., 1990). These findings suggest that muscle strength can be improved or maintained in frail older persons using a low-level, mildly progressive strength training program.

Muscle diseases that occur predominantly in older adults, albeit infrequently, include *polymyalgia rheumatica* and *polymyositis*. Polymyalgia rheumatica is characterized by weakness, pain, and stiffness occurring in the proximal muscles, particularly in the upper extremities. Treatment in the majority of patients is with steroids, and it appears to be self-limiting. The average duration of the disease is 1 year. The pathophysiology of this disease is unclear. Polymyositis, an inflammation of the muscles, is considered an autoimmune disorder primarily because of its association with systemic lupus erythematosus. It presents with shoulder and hip girdle weakness, skin rash, and joint or muscle pain and progresses over weeks or months rather than years. It too is treated with steroids.

Cardiovascular System

HEART

In the heart, aging is accompanied by several structural and functional changes in the absence of any identifiable pathology. It also is accompanied by an increased incidence of cardiac disease.

Structural changes include the following:

1. The muscle fibers of the heart are surrounded by collagen that grows progressively stiffer, and less elastic. As more collagen accumulates in and around muscle fibers and valves, the valves thicken and become more rigid, and the relative proportion of muscle drops.

2. The heart muscle becomes fattier (accumulating amyloid deposits), and both heart mass and volume increase.

3. There is left ventricle hypertrophy, probably as an adaptive mechanism to maintain wall stress.

4. Coronary arteries lose elasticity (see vascular changes below).

5. The electrical conduction system shows change: The pacemaker cells of the ventricles, responsible for producing heartbeats, become infiltrated with connective tissue and fat, producing an increasingly high incidence of sino-atrial and atrio-ventricular node dysfunction (dysrhythmias).

These changes produce differences in the mechanism by which the heart responds to the need for increased blood supply during activity. In younger individuals, the need for an increased blood supply to meet metabolic demand is met through an increase in heart rate. The aging heart, however, contracts more slowly and relaxes more slowly after each contraction. As a result, the maximum heart rate gradually decreases as does the ability to increase the heart rate sufficiently to meet metabolic demand. In older adults, demand for an increased blood supply is met by increasing the volume of blood pumped with each heartbeat to compensate for the decreased maximum heart rate. Resting heart rate is not notably affected by age.

Functional changes, then, include decreases in the maximum heart rate (from approximately 190 in a person's 20s, to 130 in the 70s, as estimated by subtracting a person's age from 220); decreases in myocardial contractibility (the strength and force of each cardiac contraction); decreases in stroke volume (the volume of blood pumped during each contraction); and decreases in cardiac output at rest (the overall amount of blood pumped by the heart to the rest of the body each minute). In addition, the heart's weaker pumping of blood combined with less efficient vascular function (see section on the vascular system) result in a reduced supply of blood to various organs. The extent varies by organ site: in the kidney, blood supply could decrease by 50%, and in the brain, by 15% to 20%.

Normally these changes do not result in disease. The aging heart can generate adequate cardiac output to provide necessary blood and nutrients when the body is at rest, or while a person is engaged in regular day-to-day activities. Under conditions of physiological stress, physical exercise, or disease, however, the heart's pumping ability appears unable to provide an adequate supply of oxygenated blood to meet the needs of the peripheral tissues—especially the muscles. This diminished supply of oxygenated blood is commonly believed to be a major cause of what older adults experience as early fatigue, limited endurance, decreased work capacity, and gradually reduced exercise tolerance. (An alternative view, proposed by Evans [1995a], is that decline in work capacity and exercise tolerance is related more significantly to decreased lean muscle mass than to decreased cardiac function.) Thus, even fit older adults might report that activities such as walking, climbing stairs, and carrying objects are unduly demanding.

Age need not necessarily result in a decline in work capacity or exercise tolerance. There is considerable evidence that conditioning programs can improve functional capacity, maximize cardiovascular reserve capacity, and might even forestall functional cardiac decline (Frontera & Evans, 1986; Larson & Bruce, 1987; Morley & Reese, 1989; Posner, Gorman, Klein, & Woldow, 1986; Renlund & Gerstenblith, 1987; Shephard, 1986). Specifically, exercise has been shown to improve cardiac function, increase cardiac contractility and pumping action, decrease pulse rate, increase artery size, reduce clotting, and improve blood pressure.

VASCULAR SYSTEM

Two major changes in the blood vessels also occur with age. First, blood vessels thicken and lose as much as 50% of their elasticity. This decrease in elasticity results in increases in blood vessel diameter and vessel wall rigidity or "stiff" arteries, commonly known as arteriosclerosis. When artery walls stiffen, they do not readily expand when filled with blood. Increased resistance in the blood vessel forces the heart to pump harder, resulting in an elevation of systolic blood pressure. Baroreflex sensitivity (blood pressure control mechanisms) declines with increased blood pressure (McGarry, Laher, & Fitzgerald, 1983), which, paradoxically perhaps, increases the risk for sudden drops in blood pressure (orthostatic hypotension), particularly in response to postural position changes. This can induce vertigo (dizziness), syncope (fainting), and falls.

Second, atherosclerotic plaques develop, consisting of calcium deposits, fatty material, clotting factors, platelets, and other cells and cellular components. Atherosclerotic changes result in a narrowing of the arteries, reduced blood flow, decreased oxygen supply to tissues (ischemia), and a tendency toward arterial occlusion. Atherosclerosis (the buildup of plaques on the walls of the arteries) is the most common form of arteriosclerosis (the hardening and thickening of the walls of the arteries), and is regarded by some as the universal disease of aging (Bierman, 1985). It also is the major cause of hypertension in older adults. Note that hypertension, in turn, further damages blood vessel walls.

Hypertension is defined as the sustained elevation of the mean arterial blood pressure. It is usually a "silent disease" and yet it is a significant concern. Hypertension is present in 40% of older adults, is the second most prevalent chronic condition among older adults, and is the single greatest risk factor for heart disease, stroke, kidney failure, peripheral vascular disease, and vascular dementia in people over age 65 (U.S. Senate, 1991). At the same time, there is consistent evidence that control of hypertension significantly reduces cardiovascular death, congestive heart failure, and stroke. For example, treating hypertension has helped reduce the incidence of fatal stroke in the United States by almost 60%, and fatal myocardial infarction by almost 50% (Abrams et al., 1995).

Whether systolic blood pressure increases as an inevitable consequence of aging is unknown (diastolic blood pressure generally is stable with advancing age). Although a number of studies have shown that aging is associated with an increase in systolic blood pressure, more recent studies have suggested that systolic pressure tends to remain stable in older adults who live in isolated, less technologically developed societies (Whelton & Klag, 1989). In addition, atherosclerotic coronary artery disease is largely considered an inevitable concomitant of aging. Evidence is mounting, however, that suggests that the effect of lifestyle on cardiovascular function (level of physical activity, diet, smoking, and alcohol use) might be greater than that of aging (Goleman & Gurin, 1993).

CARDIOVASCULAR DISEASE

Cardiovascular diseases, including coronary artery disease (CAD) and *cerebral vascular accident* (CVA), are a major cause of disability and the leading cause of death in older Americans, killing more than 50% of those 65 and older (NCHS, 1995). CAD alone accounts for 43% of all deaths, whereas stroke accounts for 9% of all deaths. By age 65, 30% of older adults have some form of heart disease (NCHS, 1995).

The most important form of cardiovascular disease in aging is *coronary artery disease,* also known as *ischemic heart disease.* The prevalence and severity of coronary artery disease increase dramatically with age. The increase is greater in men than in women and reaches a peak between one's 60s and 70s. The prevalence reaches 60% for both men and women in their 80s and thereafter (U.S. Senate, 1991). Coronary artery disease occurs when atherosclerotic plaques narrow the coronary arteries by 50% or more and the blood supply to the heart muscle becomes inade-

quate to meet metabolic demands, creating myocardial ischemia. There are four clinical syndromes: angina pectoris, cardiac arrest, myocardial infarction, and heart failure.

At first, myocardial ischemia causes *angina pectoris,* which means literally pain in the chest. The most common type of angina presents as midsternal chest pain that occurs on exertion and subsides when the older adult rests or takes a nitroglycerine tablet. Nitroglycerine dilates the coronary arteries and increases blood flow to the heart muscle. Coronary artery bypass grafting often is used to replace the atherosclerotic vessel and staves off more severe symptoms of heart disease for about 10 years.

More severe and prolonged myocardial ischemia can result in a heart attack. This event can be manifested as either cessation of normal cardiac contractions, called cardiac arrest, or an actual necrosis of heart muscle, termed a myocardial infarction. *Cardiac arrest* occurs when an arrhythmia produced by prolonged myocardial ischemia disrupts the pumping of the ventricles. The most devastating arrhythmia is an uncoordinated quivering of the ventricles, called ventricular fibrillation. This is the most common cause of cardiac arrest and sudden death in patients with coronary artery disease. Death takes place when too much of the heart tissue has been destroyed to sustain life. Cardiac arrest also is the most common cause of sudden unexpected death in older adults outside the hospital (NCHS, 1995). A *myocardial infarction* occurs when blood flow to the coronary arteries is insufficient to sustain the heart muscle, and some heart muscle is destroyed. The infarct is associated with severe chest pain and often with shock and collapse. Complications of myocardial infarct include arrhythmia, heart failure, thrombolytic complications (deep vein or mural thrombi), and irreversible damage to the heart structure.

Heart failure results whenever the heart is no longer able to pump adequate blood to the tissues for respiration and metabolism. Rapid failing of the heart, as happens when a large portion of the muscle undergoes infarction, is called acute heart failure. In most cases, however, cardiac failure develops slowly and insidiously, with multiple silent (asymptomatic) coronary events that can damage small amounts of cardiac tissue. The heart tries to compensate for its inability to supply adequate blood to the tissues by beating faster and harder. In the process, it undergoes structural change, which is termed cardiac remodeling. Cardiac remodeling leads to enlargement of the left ventricle, thinning of the ventricular wall, ultimately progressing to chronic heart failure, specifically, failure of one or both of the heart's ventricles. The term *congestive heart failure* (CHF) is used when referring to chronic heart failure, because the most prominent characteristic of chronic heart failure is the congestion of tissues (edema) caused by an accumulation of blood and fluid resulting from the heart's inability to pump adequate blood in a forward direction (Abrams et al., 1995).

Congestive heart failure is the only cardiovascular disease that is increasing in incidence and prevalence. The reason is that improved treatment for heart attack, one of the major risk factors for CHF, is producing a growing number of survivors, many of whom have significant heart damage and go on to develop CHF. Currently, it is the most common diagnosis in hospitalized older adults (NCHS, 1995).

The second most significant cardiovascular disease in aging is *CVA*, or stroke. Stroke is the third most common form of death in the United States as well as most other industrialized countries, surpassed only by heart disease and cancer, and it is the second most common cause of death for those over age 85 (NCHS, 1995). Stroke also is a leading cause of serious disability, and a major contributor to late-life dementia (vascular dementia). About 72% of stroke victims are 65 or older. For people over 55, the incidence of stroke more than doubles in each successive decade (NCHS, 1995). One third of stroke survivors remain permanently disabled and need continued supportive services (Gresham, Therese, Wolf, & McNamara, 1979). The probability of death within the first 30 days of experiencing a stroke is 20% to 30% (Posner, Gorman, Klein, & Woldow, 1986).

The term *stroke* is used to designate any brain tissue injury resulting from reduced cerebral perfusion as an effect of atherosclerosis. Reduction in blood flow reduces available oxygen and can result in temporary deficits or permanent brain damage. Strokes are divided into two major types: ischemic and hemorrhagic. Lack of blood supply (infarct/ischemia) and leakage of blood outside the damaged vessels (hemorrhage) both cause anoxic damage to nervous tissue. Of the two types, ischemic strokes occur much more frequently than hemorrhagic strokes, and account for 80% of all strokes (Caplan, 1988). The neurological deficits that result depend on where the blood supply was lost, how widespread the damage was, and how well the body restores the blood supply. The most common residual impairments include hemiplegia, aphasia, dysarthria, apraxia, paraphasia, bilateral planning deficits, unilateral visual-perceptual neglect, and homonymous hemianopsia.

The term *transient ischemic attack,* or TIA, is used to designate a minor stroke, or temporary interference with the blood supply to the brain. The symptoms occur rapidly and can last up to 24 hours, although most last for less than 30 minutes. Symptoms depend on which part of the brain was affected and can include temporary nausea, fleeting blindness in one eye, hemiparesis, aphasia, dizziness, double vision, sudden severe headache, unsteadiness, or sudden falls. The main distinction between TIAs and stroke is the short duration of the symptoms and the lack of permanent neurological damage. Clearly, TIAs are a warning that blood supply and oxygen are temporarily insufficient; all prospective studies show dramatically increased stroke risk in older adults who have had one or more TIAs (Friedman, 1995). Hence, detection of TIAs is essential so that medical treatment and precautions can be initiated.

Vascular dementias result from the additive effects of multiple small strokes (infarcts), which produce a loss of brain tissue. The location of the vascular damage is an important factor in determining whether stroke patients develop dementia; vascular dementia is more likely when a blood vessel in the back of the brain is damaged. Vascular dementia occurs more often in older adults with hypertension (with resultant cerebral infarctions), and generally can be prevented with control of blood pressure. Emboli from the heart or elsewhere within the vascular system also cause vascular dementias. The incidence of the disease parallels that of strokes (NCHS, 1995).

Vascular dementia usually presents with a progression of symptoms, each with an abrupt onset, often in association with a neurological incident. This produces deficits that give the appearance of preserved areas of ability along with other neuropsychological and neurological deficits. In general, no particular pattern of deficits emerges.

Often emotional control is impaired, but there is relative preservation of the personality. Sudden changes in symptoms are thought to reflect new infarctions. Although it is characterized by the same cognitive deficits as dementia of the Alzheimer's type, the signs of abrupt onset, step-by-step deterioration, fluctuating course, and emotional lability are specific to vascular dementia (American Psychiatric Association, 1994).

Nervous System

CENTRAL NERVOUS SYSTEM

Various anatomic and physiological changes are seen in the brain with age. Anatomic changes in the brain include a decrease in the number of cells and nerve fibers in certain portions of the brain, and a slight decrease in brain weight. Studies have shown a loss of neurons varying from 20% to 50% in areas of the cerebral cortex, the cerebellum (involved with balance, muscle tone, and fine motor coordination), and in the hippocampus (involved with some aspects of memory function). The areas of the brain that show the greatest loss of neurons with normal aging are the frontal lobe (the area of cognition), the superior area of the temporal lobe (the main auditory area), the occipital area (the visual area), and the prefrontal gyrus (the major sensorimotor area of the parietal lobe). Fewer losses occur in deeper brain structures. Within the nerve cells, there can be a significant reduction in the complexity of the cell structure, resulting from a loss in the number, density, and length of dendrites, and some shrinkage and distortion of the cell body. Overall, brain weight gradually declines (about 10%) from age 20 to age 90 but, as indicated, this decline appears in a few specific places rather than overall.

Atrophy of the cerebral cortex usually is moderate in healthy older people, as compared with more extensive loss of cells in older adults with dementia. In addition, cerebral ventricles can enlarge three to four times from the 30s to the 90s. From age 30 to 70, the blood flow to the brain decreases by 15% to 20%. There is a slowing of response to stimuli as measured by electroencephalogram (EEG), perhaps as a symptom of reduced blood supply from aging arteries. Evidence to date, however, demonstrates no direct correlation between structural changes and cognitive function (Kolb & Whishaw, 1990; Abrams et al., 1995).

Other changes in the brain include deposits of the aging pigment lipofuscin in nerve cells, deposits of the aging protein amyloid in blood vessels and cells, the appearance of senile plaques (microscopic lesions composed of dying axon terminals and dendrites surrounding a core of amyloid), and neurofibrillary tangles (strands of neurofibrous proteins that become tangled and disorganized). These can compromise neuronal function by obstructing the flow of cytoplasm and neurotransmitters from cell bodies into the axons and dendrites. Consequently, transmission of information from one neuron to another becomes slower with advancing age (Kolb & Whishaw, 1990).

There also are age-related changes in neurotransmitter uptake and metabolism. Concentrations of neurotransmitters generally decline, and are more pronounced in the dopaminergic than the cholinergic or noradrenergic systems. Although the significance of reduced neurotransmitter levels is not completely understood, abnormally low levels of some transmitters can be associated with functional changes (for example, low acetylcholine levels in Alzheimer's disease, and low dopamine

levels in Parkinson's disease). Conversely, the activity of other enzymes, such as monoamine oxidase, might increase.

Certain properties of the brain can mitigate these adverse changes. First is a property called redundancy, that is, many more nerve cells exist than are needed. Second, compensatory mechanisms can appear if the brain is damaged. For example, when speech centers in the dominant hemisphere are damaged, the nondominant hemisphere can compensate and speech function can return. Finally, it is likely that more plasticity at the nerve cell level exists than was previously recognized. Studies have shown two simultaneous processes in the aged brain: a gradual deterioration and dying off of nerve cells, and compensatory lengthening and increasing of the number of dendrites in the remaining nerve cells (Buell & Coleman, 1979). It even has been suggested that this proliferation of dendritic branches may result in a net gain in the density of synapses with increasing age (Scheibel, 1996). This implies a possible repatterning of the aging nervous system (Abrams et al., 1995), which likely is a biological mechanism to preserve function.

PERIPHERAL NERVOUS SYSTEM

A number of age-related changes in the peripheral nervous system have been documented (Sabin & Venna, 1984), including age-related declines in peripheral receptors (Bolton, Winkelmann, & Dyck, 1966) and in afferent nerve fibers (O'Sullivan & Swallow, 1968; Takahashi, 1966). Some studies have reported a gradual decline in nerve conduction velocity at approximately 0.4% per year starting at age 20 (Dorfman & Bosley, 1979; Downie & Newell, 1961), whereas other studies reported no significant change in sensory and motor conduction velocity

(Merchut & Toleikis, 1990). Hence, the data on this issue are equivocal. We do know that older adults consistently demonstrate slower reaction times (see cognitive changes, next section). We also know that reaction-time tasks measure a very complex response pattern. The pathways involved include central nervous system processing, afferent nerve pathways, and the effector organ (muscles); sensory stimuli and cognitive function are also involved.

Alzheimer's disease is the leading cause of cognitive impairment in older adults (NCHS, 1995) and, by some estimates, the fourth leading cause of death in the United States (Abrams et al., 1995). Alzheimer's disease is not listed separately as a cause of death in vital statistics. It is a chronic neurodegenerative disorder of undetermined cause characterized by cognitive impairments, particularly memory impairment, accompanied by impairments in abstract thinking, judgment, language, the ability to carry out familiar movements, and changes in mood, personality, and behavior. Myoclonus and epilepsy also can occur. Alzheimer's disease typically progresses through stages from mild memory loss, through significant cognitive impairment, to very serious confusion and the loss of ability to carry out any activities of daily living. The mean survival for older adults with the disease is about 8 years, with a range of 1 to 20 years. The prevalence is slightly higher in women than men. It is strongly associated with age, affecting 3% of people age 65 to 74, 18% of people aged 75 to 84, and 47% of people over the age of 85 (U.S. Senate, 1991). It also is the disease most feared by older adults. (For a comprehensive discussion of this disease, see chapter 2, section 2.)

Alzheimer's disease appears to result from a degenerative process that is characterized by a loss of cells from the cerebral cortex (especially frontal, parietal, and medial temporal regions), hippocampus, and subcortical structures, with a concomitant enlargement of the ventricular system. The cortex becomes shrunken or atrophied, losing as much as one third of its volume as the disease progresses; the limbic system undergoes even more severe degenerative changes. Significant EEG slowing occurs by the middle stage of the disease. Senile plaques and neurofibrillary tangles play an important role in the disease. Although both occur with normal aging, they are far more prevalent in older adults with Alzheimer's disease. Specific neurotransmitter deficiencies also are found, primarily with reduced levels of acetylcholine, but also with serotonin, dopamine, somatostatin, and norepinephrine. As indicated earlier, there are arguments that Alzheimer's disease might represent an acceleration of normal aging changes; this is because normal aging is associated with decrements in some neurotransmitters and cholinergic activity as well as some of the neuropathological findings of Alzheimer's disease (Brody & Schneider, 1986; Blumenthal, 1993).

Parkinson's disease is the second-most common degenerative disease of the nervous system, after Alzheimer's disease. The incidence increases with age, peaking at age 75. It is a progressive neurodegenerative disease characterized by rigidity, bradykinesia (slowing in initiation and speed of movement), and tremor, resulting in disturbances of speech, gait, and coordination. It is associated with an average survival of about 14 years.

Parkinson's disease results from loss of dopaminergic neurons and development of Lewy bodies (abnormal neuronal cytoplasmic filaments) in the substantia nigra part of the basal ganglia. With normal aging, there is a less dramatic, but nevertheless apparent, loss of dopaminergic neurons in the same nucleus. This finding has led to speculation that Parkinson's disease too might reflect an accelerated aging process. As neurons in the substantia nigra degenerate, they no longer are able to transmit dopamine to the striatum. Normally, the two opposing neurotransmitters, dopamine (which exerts an inhibitory function) and acetylcholine (which exerts an excitatory function) in this structure are in balance. When dopamine is depleted, acetylcholine becomes hyperactive, producing the hypokinetic rigidity characteristic of Parkinson's disease (Kolb & Whishaw, 1990).

Older adults with Parkinson's disease respond to treatment with levadopa (L-dopa), which is converted within the brain into dopamine and helps to reestablish neurotransmitter balance. In addition, drugs that block acetylcholine (such as amantadine) might help reduce symptoms. There is, however, no therapy that slows the progression of the disease. Depression and some cognitive impairment occur in a large percentage of older adults with Parkinson's disease; in addition, dementia afflicts about 30% of older adults with the disease (Friedman, 1995).

Respiratory System

Aging affects not only the physiological functions of the lungs (ventilation and oxygen or carbon dioxide exchange) but also the ability of the lungs to defend themselves. The specific biological mechanisms responsible for these changes are unclear. For example, it is not known whether the progressive decline in pulmonary function is a result of exposure to environmental toxins such as air pollution and cigarette smoke, or from progressive declines in respiratory reserves related to aging itself.

Age-related changes in ventilation and gas exchange result primarily from changes in compliance of the lungs and the chest wall. At about age 55, respiratory muscle mass (including the diaphragm) decreases and strength begins to wane. The end of the ribs calcifies to the breastbone, stiffening the chest wall. Hence, when older adults breathe, their chests expand less and they take in less air than younger people do. This weakened outward muscular force and the increased stiffness of the chest wall are counterbalanced by a loss of elastic recoil of the lung tissue, the principal mechanism of normal expiration. The loss of elastic recoil in the lungs is thought to result from damage to the elastic fibers, which reduces airway diameter, increases resistance to airflow, and reduces alveolar surface area (they become shallower, narrower, and expand less with every breath). In addition, air can become trapped in the alveoli, which eventually contributes to their collapse, resulting in fewer, less efficient sacs and a reduced amount of oxygen getting into the blood. The increased outward pull of the stiffer chest wall, combined with the reduced ability of the lung to pull inward, results in inefficient breathing. It also results in an increase in total lung capacity, functional residual capacity, and residual volume (the amount of residual air left in the lungs after each breath) (Sherman & Skovrinski, 1995; Abrams et al., 1995).

The consequence of these aging changes is an overall decrease in the functional ability of the lungs to move air in and out. Progressive declines are seen in vital capacity (the volume of air that the lung can hold after a normal inspiration), the rate of air flow (the forced expiratory volume in one second), and the efficiency of gas exchange (also secondary to vascular changes cited above). From age 29 to 80, vital capacity declines linearly; the vital capacity of a 65-year-old is about 77% of that of a 25-year-old. Residual capacity increases—from about 20% of total lung capacity at age 20 to 35% at age 60. In addition, there is a 10% to 15% decrease in the oxygen content of the blood. As a result, an older adult must move more air in and out of the lungs to attain the same amount of oxygen as a younger person. Metabolic rate also is reduced. Functional consequences include distressed breathing, especially during exercise, and a reduced ability to breathe deeply. Respiratory changes may also lead to a decreased capacity to cough (and subsequent aspiration), increasing susceptibility to respiratory complications of surgery and pneumonia (Sherman & Skovrinski, 1995).

Despite these changes, it has been noted that if the cardiovascular and neuromuscular systems are relatively free from disease, then the progressive changes in functional status will consist primarily of a loss of reserve capacity without obvious functional limitations (Keltz, 1984; Larson & Bruce, 1987; Naughton, 1982). It also has been demonstrated that regular exercise can improve cardiopulmonary fitness at any age. Training will increase oxygen consumption, enhance efficiency, and reduce vulnerability to future stressors (Keltz, 1984; Larson & Bruce, 1987; Naughton, 1982; Shephard, 1986).

Chronic obstructive pulmonary disease (COPD) is defined as chronic airway obstruction secondary to a number of diseases (including chronic bronchitis, emphysema, and asthma) that produce airway collapse or inflammation and result in airway bronchospasm or swelling, and excess mucus. Whether primarily a disease of bronchioles (chronic bronchitis) or of alveoli (emphysema), the pathological changes ultimately result in chronic airway obstruction (limited airflow through the lungs). The term COPD was introduced because these conditions often coexist. COPD is characterized by difficulty breathing and shortness of breath (dyspnea).

In the United States, these diseases are recognized in approximately 10% of the older adult population, and rank as the fourth leading cause of death and the second leading cause of disability (U.S. Senate, 1991). The most common contributor to COPD is smoking, the leading cause of chronic bronchitis and emphysema. The number of COPD cases is rapidly increasing (NCHS, 1995) as those who have spent a lifetime smoking grow older. These diseases typically develop insidiously and, because of the large reserve in lung function, do not produce significant symptoms until an advanced stage. When the disease is recognized, however, lung function often is severely compromised and the disease is largely irreversible.

In most COPD patients, the airways of the lungs have become permanently narrowed, walls between alveoli have been destroyed, and tissue has lost its elasticity and is stretched out of shape. The lung passages become inflamed and swollen, cilia are destroyed, and the mucus-producing glands hypertrophy, producing secretions that often are colonized with bacteria and that block the flow of air to and from the lungs. As a result, the lungs and the heart cannot provide sufficient oxygen to muscles to sustain normal levels of activity. Eventually, COPD leads to pulmonary insufficiency, right heart failure (cor pulmonale), and respiratory failure.

Bronchodilators, which open the air passages and make breathing easier, are commonly used to treat COPD.

Corticosteroids are used to reduce inflammation, and antibiotics might be needed to treat infection. The two principal objectives of pulmonary rehabilitation are to control and alleviate the symptoms and pathophysiological complications of respiratory impairment, and to teach older adults how to achieve optimum potential to carry out activities of daily living (American Association of Cardiovascular and Pulmonary Rehabilitation, 1993). Comprehensive rehabilitation programs contribute to improvements in quality of life by reducing the severity of dyspnea related to functional mobility and self-care (Ries, 1990; Rondinelli & Hill, 1988).

Sexual Function

Sexual change in aging is a process of gradual slowing: more time is needed to become sexually aroused and to reach orgasm. This is not necessarily considered an impairment, because it might enable a better response synchrony between the sexes, compared with that in earlier years when men responded more quickly than women. Although frequency of sexual intercourse generally decreases in older adults, satisfaction in sexual expression remains high for both partners (Shearer & Shearer, 1977; Alexander & Allison, 1995).

In men, changes include a decrease in sperm production and ejaculatory force. Testosterone levels decline only gradually, if at all. Men do not undergo a physiological climacteric and remain fertile until the end of life (Ludeman, 1981; Masters & Johnson, 1970). The prostate tissue is replaced by scar tissue. The gland enlarges, particularly around the urethra. Changes in the concentration of testosterone appear to cause the enlargement. A common concern of older men is their ability to maintain sexual potency. Impotence can occur

from time to time for a variety of reasons (stress, fatigue, tension, guilt, depression, illness, excessive drinking, or anxiety over performance). It usually is remediable and often is inaccurately attributed to aging (Abrams et al., 1995; Masters & Johnson, 1970).

In women, most sexual changes are associated with menopause, when estrogen production slows. This can produce vaginal dryness that can lead to irritation or pain, a change in vaginal shape (shortening and narrowing), less acidic vaginal secretions with a greater possibility of vaginal infections, cystitis because of a thinning of the vaginal walls, reduction in clitoral size, and a general diminution of muscle tone in vaginal and breast tissue (Masters & Johnson, 1970). Estrogen replacement therapy long has been used for menopausal symptoms and is effective in treating these changes as well.

Enlargement of the prostate, known as *benign prostatic hypertrophy*, occurs in the majority of older men. Because of its position around the urethra, enlargement of the prostate quickly interferes with the normal passage of urine from the bladder. If the condition is not surgically corrected by prostatectomy, it can lead to bladder infection or bladder and kidney damage.

Summary

This section has provided an overview of some of the more usual biological changes that occur as various body systems age and the major age-related diseases that compromise functional independence in older adults. Other chapters in this volume address mechanisms by which therapists can provide effective intervention for these conditions. It is likely that the discussion has created an impression of inevitable deterioration, loss of resiliency, and a trend toward lesser degrees of capacity or competence. Although there is some degree of reality to such an impression, it is just as important to remember the following:

1. Generalizations about biological change reflect an "average" and individual variability remains great.

2. The human body is endowed with systems for compensation and vast amounts of reserve capacity; hence, biological change does not necessarily mean loss of function.

3. Older adults retain their capacity to adapt to changing biological functions through years of accumulated experience (see Section 3, Adaptation and the Aging Adult).

4. Advances in medical science are providing mechanisms for compensation and remediation of a number of biological changes.

These factors enable the majority (77%) of older adults to maintain their ability to function effectively (NCHS, 1995) and their well-being, even with age-related impairment and the probability of some form of chronic disease. There is, however, still truth to the adage "Aging ain't for sissies!"

References

Abrams, W. B., Beers, M., Berkow, R., & Fletcher, A. (1995). *The Merck manual of geriatrics*. Whitehouse Station, NJ: Merck.

Abramson, M., & Lovas, P. (Eds.). (1988). *Aging and sensory change: An annotated bibliography*. Washington, DC: Gerontological Society of America.

Alexander, E., & Allison, A. (1995). Sexuality in older adults. In W. Reichel (Ed.), *Care of the elderly: clinical aspects of aging*. Baltimore: Williams and Wilkins.

American Association of Cardiovascular and Pulmonary Rehabilitation. (1993). *Guidelines for pulmonary rehabilitation programs*. Windsor, Ontario: Author.

American Psychiatric Association, (1994). *Diagnostic and statistical manual of mental disorders* (4th ed.). (DSM–IV). Washington, DC: Author.

Bartoshuk, L. M., Refkin, B., Markes, L. E., et al. (1986). Taste and aging. *Journal of Gerontology, 41*, 51–57.

Bierman, E. L. (1985). Aging and atherosclerosis. In R. Andres, E. L. Bierman, & W. R. Hazzard (Eds.), *Principles of geriatric medicine*. New York: McGraw Hill.

Birren, J., & Renner, V. (1977). Research on the psychology of aging: Principles and experimentation. In J. Birren & K. Schaie (Eds.), *Handbook of the psychology of aging*. New York: Van Nostrand Reinhold.

Blumenthal, H. T. (1993). The aging-disease dichotomy is alive, but is it well? *Journal of the American Geriatrics Society, 41*, 1272–1273.

Blumenthal, J., Emery, C., Madden, D., Schniebolk, S., Riddle, M., Cobb, F., Higginbotham, M., & Coleman, R. (1991). Effects of exercise training and bone density in older men and older women. *Journal of the American Geriatrics Society, 39*, 1065–1070.

Bolton, C., Winkelmann, R., & Dyck, P. (1966). A quantitative study of Meissner's corpuscles in man. *Neurology, 16*, 1–9.

Bortz, W. M. (1982). Disuse and aging. *Journal of the American Medical Association, 248*, 1203–1208.

Branch, L., Horowitz, A., & Carr, C. (1989). The implications for everyday life of incidents of self-reported visual decline among people over 65 living in the community. *Gerontologist, 29*, 359–366.

Briggs, R., Gossman, M., Birch, R., Drews, J., & Shaddeau, S. (1989). Balance performance among noninstitutionalized elderly women. *Physical Therapy, 69*, 748–756.

Brocklehurst, J. C. (1985). *Textbook of geriatric medicine and gerontology*, (3rd ed.). London: Churchill Livingstone.

Brody J. S., & Schneider, E. L. (1986). Diseases and disorders of aging. *Journal of Chronic Diseases, 39*, 871–876.

Brown, M., Sinacore, D., & Host, H. (1995). The relationship of strength to function in the older adult. *Journal of Gerontology, 50(A)*, 55–59.

Buell, S. J., & Coleman, P. D. (1979). Dendritic growth in the aged human brain and failure of growth in senile dementia. *Science, 206*, 854–856.

Cape, R. (1978). *Aging: Its complex management*. New York: Harper & Row.

Caplan, L. R. (1988). Stroke. *Clinical Symposia, 40*, 1–32.

Comfort, A. (1979). *The biology of senescence* (3rd ed.). New York: Elsevier.

Cooper, A. F. (1976). Deafness and psychiatric illness. *British Journal of Psychiatry, 129*, 215–226.

Dalsky, G. P. (1988). Weight bearing exercise training and lumbar bone mineral content in postmenopausal women. *Annals of Internal Medicine, 108*, 824–828.

Dorfman, L. J., & Bosley, T. M. (1979). Age related changes in peripheral central nerve conduction in man. *Neurology, 29*, 38–44.

Downie, A. W., & Newell, D. J. (1961). Sensory nerve conduction in patients with diabetes mellitus and controls. *Neurology, 11*, 876–892.

Dubno, J., Dirk, D., & Morgan, D. (1984). Effects of age and mild hearing loss on speech recognition and noise. *Journal of the Acoustical Society of America, 76*, 87–96.

Duncan, P., & Studenski, S. (1994). Balance and gait measures. In M. P. Lawton & J. A. Teresi (Eds.), *Annual review of gerontology and geriatrics, 14.* New York: Springer.

Evans, J. G. (1988). Aging and disease. In D. Evred & J. Whalen (Eds.), *Research and the aging population.* Chichester, UK: Wiley.

Evans, W. J. (1995a). Effects of exercise on body composition and functional capacity of the elderly. *Journal of Gerontology, 50(A)*, 147–150.

Evans, W. J. (1995b). What is sarcopenia? *Journal of Gerontology, 50(A)*, 5–8.

Fiatarone, M. A., Marks, E. C., Ryan, N. D., Meredith, C. N., Lipsitz, L. A., & Evans, W. J. (1990). High intensity strength training in nonagenarians: Effects on skeletal muscle. *Journal of the American Medical Association, 263*, 3029–3032.

Fiatarone, M. A., O'Neill, E. F., Ryan, N. D., Clements, K. M., Solaris, G. R., Nelson, M. E, Roberts, S. B., Kenhayias, J. J., Lipsitz, L. A., & Evans, W. J. (1994). Exercise training and nutritional supplementa-tion for physical frailty in very elderly people. *New England Journal of Medicine, 330*, 1769–1775.

Fisher, C. M., Pendergast, D. R., & Calkins, E. (1991). Muscle rehabilitation in impaired nursing home residents. *Archives of Physical Medicine and Rehabilitation, 72*, 181–185.

Fozard, J. L. (1990). Vision and hearing in aging. In J. E. Birren & K. W. Schaie (Eds.), *Handbook of the psychology of aging* (3rd ed.). New York: Academic Press.

Fozard, J. L., & Popkin, S. J. (1978). Optimizing adult development: Ends and means of an applied psychology of aging. *American Psychologist, 33*, 975–989.

Friedman, J. (1995). Neurologic diseases in the elderly. In W. Reichel (Ed.), *Care of the elderly: Clinical aspects of aging.* Baltimore: Williams and Wilkins.

Frontera, W. R., & Evans, W. J. (1986). Exercise performance and endurance training in the elderly. *Topics in Geriatric Rehabilitation, 2*, 17–31.

Frontera, W. R., Hughes, V. A., & Evans, W. J. (1991). A cross sectional study of upper and lower extremity muscle strength in 45–78 year old men and women. *Journal of Applied Physiology, 71*, 664–650.

Frontera, W. R., Meridith, C. N., O'Reilly, K. P., Knuttgen, H. G., & Evans, W. J. (1988). Strength training in older men: Skeletal muscle hypertrophy and improved function. *Journal of Applied Physiology, 64*, 1038–1044.

Gittings, N. S., & Fozard, J. L. (1986). Age related changes in visual acuity. *Experimental Gerontology, 21*, 421–433.

Goleman, D., & Gurin, J. (1993). *Mindbody medicine*. Yonkers, NY: Consumers Reports.

Gresham, G. E., Therese, P. F., Wolf, P. H., & McNamara, P. M. (1979). Epidemiologic profile of long term stroke disability: The Framingham study. *Archives of Physical Medicine and Rehabilitation, 60*, 487–492.

Harper, C. M., & Lyles, Y. M. (1988). Physiology and complications of bed rest. *Journal of the American Geriatrics Society, 36*, 1047–1054.

Hayes, K. C., Spencer, J. D., Lucy, S. D. et al. (1985). Age related changes in postural sway. In D. A. Winter, R. W. Norman, R. P. Wells, K. C. Hayes, & A. E. Patla (Eds.), *Biomechanics IX–A*. Champaign, IL: Human Kinetics.

Hazzard, W. R., Andres, R., Bierman, E. L., & Blass, J. P. (1990). *Principles of geriatric medicine and gerontology*. New York: McGraw-Hill.

Hurley, B. (1995). Age, gender, and muscular strength. *Journal of Gerontology, 50(A)*, 41–44.

Hyams, D. (1982). Psychological factors in rehabilitation of the elderly. *Gerontological Clinics, 11*, 129–134.

Imms, F. J., & Edholm, O. G. (1981). Studies of gait and mobility in the elderly. *Age and Aging, 10*, 145–156.

Jette, A., Branch, L., & Berlin, J. (1990). Musculoskeletal impairments and physical disablement among the aged. *Journal of Gerontology, 45*, 203–207.

Jones, R. H. (1984). Physiological basis of rehabilitation therapy. In T. F. Williams (Ed.), *Rehabilitation in the aging*. New York: Raven Press.

Kallman, H., & Vernon, M. (1987). The aging eye. *Postgraduate Medicine, 81*, 108–129.

Kauffman, T. (1987). Posture and age. *Topics in Geriatric Rehabilitation, 1*, 13–20.

Keltz, H. (1984). Pulmonary function and disease with aging. In T. F. Williams (Ed.), *Rehabilitation in the aging*. New York: Raven Press

Kennedy, R., & Clemis, J. D. (1990). The geriatric auditory and vestibular systems. *Otolaryngology Clinics of North America, 23*, 1075–1082.

Kenney, R. A. (1989). *Physiology of Aging—A Synopsis* (2nd ed.). Chicago: Year Book Medical Publishers.

Kirshen, A. J., Cape, R. D., Hayes, K. C., et al. (1984). Postural sway and cardiovascular parameters associated with falls in the elderly. *Journal of Clinical and Experimental Gerontology, 6*, 291–307.

Kolb, B., & Whishaw, I. (1990). *Fundamentals of human neuropsychology* (3rd ed.). New York: Freeman.

Koller, W. C., Glatt, S. L., & Fox, J. H. (1985). Senile gait: A distinct neurologic entity. *Clinics in Geriatric Medicine, 1*, 661–669.

Larson, E. B., & Bruce, R. A. (1987). Health benefits of exercise in an aging society. *Archives of Internal Medicine, 147*, 353–356.

Lentz, M. (1981). Selected aspects of deconditioning secondary to immobilization. *Nursing Clinics of North America, 16*, 729–737.

Ludeman, K. (1981). The sexuality of the older person: Review of the literature. *Gerontologist, 21*, 203–208.

Maki, B. E., Holliday, P. J., & Fernie, G. R. (1991). Aging and postural control: A comparison of spontaneous and induced sway balance tests. *Journal of the American Geriatrics Society, 38*, 1–9.

Manton, K. (1989). Life style risk factors. *Annals of the Academy of Political and Social Science, 503*, 72–88.

Masters, W. H., & Johnson, V. (1970). *Human sexual inadequacy*. Boston: Little, Brown.

Mattox, C., Wu, H., & Schuman, J. (1995). Ocular disorders of the aged eye. In W. Reichel (Ed.), *Care of the elderly: Clinical aspects of aging*. Baltimore: Williams and Wilkins.

McCartney, N., Hicks, A. L., Martin, J., & Webber, C.E. (1995). Long term resistance training to the elderly: Effects on dynamic strength, exercise capacity, muscle, and bone. *Journal of Gerontology, 50*, B97–B107.

McGarry, K., Laher, M., & Fitzgerald, D. (1983). Baroreflex activity in elderly hypertensives. *Hypertension, 5*, 763–765.

Merchut, M. P., & Toleikis, S. C. (1990). Aging and quantitative sensory thresholds. *Electromyographical Clinical Neurophysiology, 30*, 293–297.

Mezey, M., & Grisso, J. (1989). Preventing dependence and injury: An approach to sensory changes. In R. Lavizzo-Mourey, S. Day, D. Diserens, & J. Grisso (Eds.), *Practicing Prevention for the Elderly*. Philadelphia: Mosby.

Morley, J. E., & Reese, S. S. (1989). Clinical implications of the aging heart. *American Journal of Medicine, 86*, 77–86.

National Center for Health Statistics. (1995). *Trends in the health of older Americans, 1994*. (DHHS Pub. No. [PHS 95]–1414). Washington, DC: U.S. Government Printing Office.

National Institutes of Health. (1986). *National Institutes of Health consensus development conference on osteoporosis*. Washington, DC: Author.

Naughton, J. (1982). Physical activity and aging. *Primary Care, 9*, 231–238.

Ochs, A., Newberry, J., Lenhardt, M., et al. (1985). Neural and vestibular aging associated with falls. In J. E. Birren & K. W. Schaie (Eds.), *Handbook of the psychology of aging* (2nd ed.). New York: Von Nostrand Reinhold.

O'Neil, P. M., & Calhoun, K. S. (1975). Sensory deficits and behavioral deterioration in senescence. *Journal of Abnormal Psychology, 84*, 579–582.

Oosterveld, W. J. (1983). Changes in vestibular function with increasing age. In R. Hinchcliffe (Ed.), *Hearing and balance in the elderly*. Edinburgh: Churchill Livingstone.

O'Sullivan, D., & Swallow, M. (1968). Fiber size and content of the radial and aural nerves. *Journal of Neurology, Neurosurgery, and Psychiatry, 31*, 464–470.

Oyer, H. J., & Oyer, E. J. (1978). Social consequences of hearing loss for the elderly. *Allied Health and Behavioral Sciences, 2*, 123–138.

Paparella, M. M., & Shumrick, D. A. (Eds.). (1991). *Otolaryngology* (3rd ed.). Philadelphia: Saunders.

Payton, O. D., & Poland, J. L. (1983). Aging process: Implications for clinical practice. *Physical Therapy, 63*, 41–49.

Plomp, R. (1978). Auditory handicap of hearing impairment and the limited benefit of hearing aids. *Journal of the Acoustical Society of America, 63*, 533–549.

Posner, J. D., Gorman, K. M., Klein, H. S., & Woldow, A. (1986). Exercise capacity in the elderly. *American Journal of Cardiology, 57*, 52–58.

Reddy, M. P. (1986). A guide to early mobilization of bed-ridden elderly. *Geriatrics, 41*, 59–70.

Reichel, W. (1995). *Care of the elderly: clinical aspects of aging*. Baltimore: Williams and Wilkins.

Renlund, D. G., & Gerstenblith, G. (1987). Exercise and the aging heart. *Cardiology Clinics, 5*, 331–336.

Ries, A. (1990). Pulmonary rehabilitation. In B. Kemp, K. Brummel-Smith, & J. Ramsdell (Eds.), *Geriatric Rehabilitation*. Boston: College Hill Press.

Riggs, B. L. (1991). Overview of osteoporosis. *Western Journal of Medicine, 154*, 63–77

Riggs, B. L., & Melton, L. J. (1986). Involutional osteoporosis. *New England Journal of Medicine, 314*, 1676–1684.

Riggs, B. L., & Mclton, L. J. (1992). The prevention and treatment of osteoporosis. *New England Journal of Medicine, 327*, 620–627.

Rikli, R., & Busch, S. (1986). Motor performance of women as a function of age and physical activity. *Journal of Gerontology, 41*, 645–651.

Rogers, M. A., & Evans, W. J. (1992). Changes in skeletal muscle with aging: Effects of exercise training. *Exercise Sport Scientific Review, 20*, 65–102.

Rondinelli, R., & Hill, N. (1988). Rehabilitation of the patient with pulmonary disease. In J. DeLisa (Ed.), *Rehabilitation medicine: principles and practice*. Philadelphia: J. B. Lippincott.

Sabin, T. D., & Venna, N. (1984). Peripheral nerve disorders in the elderly. In M. L. Albert (Ed.), *Clinical neurology of aging*. New York: Oxford University Press.

Saxon, S. V., & Etten, M. J. (1987). *Physical change and aging* (2nd ed.). New York: Tiresias Press.

Scheibel, A.B. (1996). Structural and functional changes in the aging brain. In J. E. Birren & K. W. Schaie (Eds.), *Handbook of the psychology of aging*, (4th ed.). San Diego: Academic Press.

Schieber, F. (1992). Aging and the senses. In J. Birren, J. B. Sloane, & G. D. Cohen (Eds.), *Handbook of mental health and aging*. San Diego: Academic Press.

Schumacher, H. R., Klippel, J., & Koopman, W. (1993). *Primer on rheumatic diseases* (10th ed.). Atlanta: Arthritis Foundation.

Shearer, M. R., & Shearer, M. L. (1977). Sexuality and sexual counseling in the elderly. *Clinical Obstetrics and Gynecology, 20*, 197–210.

Sheldon, J. (1963). The effect of age on the control of sway. *Gerontological Clinics, 5*, 129–131.

Shephard, R. J. (1986). Physical training for the elderly. *Clinical Sports Medicine, 5*, 515–533.

Sherman, C., & Skovrinski, T. (1995). Pulmonary problems in the elderly. In W. Reichel (Ed.), *Care of the elderly: Clinical aspects of aging*. Baltimore: Williams and Wilkins.

Shock, N. (1974). Physiological theories of aging. In B. Rockstein (Ed.), *Theoretical aspects of aging*. New York: Academic Press.

Siebens, H. (1990). Deconditioning. In B. Kemp, K. Brummel-Smith, & J. Ramsdell (Eds.), *Geriatric rehabilitation*. Boston: College Hill Press.

Simkin, A. et al. (1987). Increased trabecular bone density due to bone loading exercises in postmenopausal osteoporotic women. *Calcified Tissue International, 40*, 59–63.

Simonsick, E. M., Lafferty, M. E., Phillips, C. L., Mendes De Leon, C. F., Kasl, S. V., Seeman, T. E., Fillenbaum, G., Herbert, P., Lemke, J. H. (1993). Risk due to inactivity in physically capable older adults. *American Journal of Public Health, 83*, 1443–1450.

Takahashi, J. (1966). A clinicopathologic study of the peripheral nervous system of the aged: Sciatic nerve and autonomic nervous system. *Journal of the American Geriatric Society, 21*, 123–133.

Tideiksaar, R., & Kay, A. (1986). What causes falls? A logical diagnostic procedure. *Geriatrics, 41*, 32–47.

Tseng, B., Marsh, D., Hamilton, M., & Booth, F. (1995). Strength and aerobic training attenuate muscle wasting and improve resistance to the development of disability with aging. *Journal of Gerontology, 50(A)*, 113–119.

U.S. Senate, Special Committee on Aging. (1991). *Aging America: Trends and projections, 1991*. Washington, DC: U.S. Government Printing Office.

VonDras, D., & Blumenthal, H. T. (1992). Dementia of the aged: Disease or atypical accelerated aging? Biopathological and psychological perspectives. *Journal of the American Geriatrics Society, 40*, 285–294.

Weale, R. (1988). Age and the transmittance of the human crystalline lens. *Journal of Physiology, 395*, 577–587.

Whelton, P. K., & Klag, M. K. (1989). Epidemiology of high blood pressure. In W. Applegate (Ed.), *Clinics in Geriatric Medicine*. Philadelphia: Saunders.

Wild, D., Nayak, U. S., & Isaacs, B. (1987). Description, classification, and prevention of falls in old people at home. *Rheumatology Rehabilitation, 20*, 153–159.

Williams, M. E. (1984). Clinical implications of aging physiology. *American Journal of Medicine, 76*, 1049–1054.

Williams, T. F. (1993). Aging versus disease: Which changes seen with age are the result of "biological aging"? In R. L. Sprott, R. W. Huber, & T. F. Williams (Eds.), *The biology of aging*. New York: Springer.

Wolfson, L. I., Whipple, R., Amerman, P., et al. (1986). Stressing the postural response: A quantitative method for testing balance. *Journal of the American Geriatrics Society, 34*, 845–850.

Woollacott, M. P., Shumway-Cook, A. T., & Nashner, L. M. (1986). Aging and postural control: Changes in sensory organization and muscular coordination. *International Journal of Aging and Human Development, 23*, 81–98.

World Health Organization, Regional Office for Europe. (1959). *The public health aspects of the aging population: Report of the advisory group*. Copenhagen: Author.

Wyke, B. (1979). Conference on the aging brain. *Age and Aging, 8*, 251–257.

Section 2. Cognition and the Aging Adult

Linda L. Levy, MA, OTR/L, FAOTA

Cognitive Changes in Older Adults

Most people experience detectable changes in cognitive function as they age (Kausler, 1991, 1994; Salthouse, 1991). The effects of these changes on occupational and daily life functioning are small. As is the case with all aging changes, cognitive changes do not occur uniformly in all persons or at given ages (Schaie, 1990). There is no reason to assume that all older adults undergo cognitive decline with age, even if some do. This section will provide an overview of the most consistently documented cognitive changes that accompany normal aging.

Memory

The most intensely studied cognitive process in aging is memory. Before we can identify the specific nature of changes that occur with age, it is important to review some basic concepts.

Memory is a complex phenomenon. It builds on attention (information needs to be attended to before it can be remembered), and includes the ability to learn information through any of the senses, to retain it for variable periods of time, and then to retrieve the information when it is needed. Memory and learning are difficult to differentiate. Learning involves the acquisition of new information whereas memory involves the retention of that information. Clearly, there can be no memory if learning has not occurred first.

A number of theoretical models have been proposed to explain how memory operates. Some of these models focus on the process of learning and memory; others focus on the structure of memory stores. Information-processing theorists (Best, 1989; Cerella, 1990) describe memory in terms of three basic processes that humans engage in when we try to learn and remember information: attending and taking in new information through the senses (learning-encoding), interpreting and retaining it for variable periods of time (storage), and then accessing the information when needed (retrieval). Structural information-processing theories focus on the ways in which information is stored and organized in the brain.

The most prominent structural theory (Atkinson & Shiffrin, 1968) proposes three distinct types of memory storage systems: sensory memory, primary (short-term) memory, and secondary (long-term) memory. According to this theory, information first must pass through sensory memory to reach primary memory, and then pass through primary memory to enter secondary memory. Notice that the theorists suggested that the terms *short-term memory* and *long-term memory* be relabeled *primary memory* and *secondary memory*, respectively, to avoid confusion with the more conventional use of these terms.)

Sensory memory is the initial momentary memory in which there is brief (merely .25 to 3 seconds) registration of uninterpreted sensory information, primarily in the visual and auditory memory stores. Information can be retrieved from sensory memory by attending to it, whereupon it is entered into the primary store. Primary memory has a very small capacity and is quite brief: It can hold up to 7 (plus or minus 2) items of information (Miller, 1956) for conscious processing, and can retain this material for up to 30 seconds. Units of information beyond 7 (plus or minus 2) are lost by displacement. An example of primary memory is remembering a telephone number long enough to dial it. If you need to remember the number for later use, then the number should be encoded in the form of concepts that can be recalled. Secondary memory stores information in terms of abstract symbols (primarily words), has unlimited capacity, retains information permanently, and requires that information be analyzed and organized for storage and retrieval at some later time. Information from secondary memory stores can be retrieved in two ways: recall or recognition. Recall requires search and retrieval of information from storage without using any orienting cues. Recognition requires information in storage to be matched with orienting cues. Clearly, recall is a more demanding test of retrieval than recognition: Recalling the name of the current Speaker of the House is more difficult than recognizing his name when it is presented along with several others.

Experimental data on memory demonstrate only slight changes in learning-encoding processes before age 65, after which there is noticeable decline. There is consistent evidence that older adults require more time and effort than younger people to learn-encode an equivalent amount of new information (Perlmutter et al., 1987; Poon, Fozard, Cermak, Arenberg, & Thompson, 1980; Poon et al., 1986). At the same time, learning-encoding can be enhanced by practice or repetition and by efforts to associate new information with already-stored information (Smith, 1980; Zachs, 1982). Additionally, there is evidence that many of the factors that put elders at

a disadvantage at this stage of information processing can be reversed so that ultimately there is minimal decline in the ability to learn (Gounard & Hulicka, 1977). Reversible factors include pace—allowing sufficient time for the older adult to respond—(Witte, 1975), diminished motivation—secondary to increased caution, response reluctance, increased anxiety, or disinterest in content—(Botwinick, 1967; Eisdorfer, 1968), reduced depth of information processing—skimming the material rather than subjecting it to more meaningful analysis—(Craik, 1977), decreased use of memory enhancing strategies—mnemonic devices such as visual images—(Rowe & Schnore, 1971), and sensory impairment—mitigated by compensatory strategies for visual and auditory deficits. Thus, although information-processing theorists propose a model of age-related changes in learning and memory performance based on decrements, they also suggest that these decrements can be compensated for.

Structural information-processing theorists have found age-related decrements in the sensory memory store (Craik, 1977; Craik & Jennings, 1992), although they are considered to be of limited practical importance. (The sensory memory store represents pure visual or auditory input and is likely to be adversely affected by sensory changes.) Similarly, age differences in primary memory are minimal (Craik, 1977; Craik & Jennings, 1992; Woods & Britton, 1985). As a result, we can expect that older adults will be able to attend to, perceive, and retain information within the normal span of 7 (plus or minus 2) items with little difficulty. The average memory span for words is 5. For digits, it is about 7 or 8.

It is at the level of secondary memory that significant age-related deficits have been documented. Beginning around age 50, older adults appear to have more difficulty with retrieval of information from secondary storage (Crook & West, 1990). Although they perform almost as well as their younger counterparts on recognition tests, older adults do not fare as well when using recall (no cue in the environment) to retrieve information. This deficit worsens over time (Albert, 1988; Craik & Jennings, 1992). The oft-bemoaned expression, "Why did I come into this room?" illustrates this difficulty. Curiously, very long-term memory (tertiary or remote memory) appears not to be affected until well after age 70 (Weingartner & Parker, 1984).

The difficulty with recall has been identified as a problem of retrieval rather than encoding or storage. This is because recall requires the individual to independently call up information that previously was organized and stored for future retrieval; recognition furnishes the individual with the item itself as an orienting cue to search memory and retrieve the information. In essence, the cues provided in recognition tests compensate for deficient retrieval strategies and provide a way to retrieve information that previously was stored. The implication here is that older adults who experience difficulty retrieving previously acquired information benefit from cues (Craik & Jennings, 1992). Compensatory cues can include the use of notes, lists, and calendars; redundant cuing (e.g., simultaneous oral and written instructions); and questions posed in recognition rather than in recall form (e.g., "Was your last appointment Monday or Wednesday?" rather than "When was your last appointment?")

This secondary memory deficit now is described as "age-related cognitive decline" (Caine, 1993), a condition characterized by concerns about diminished performance of desired life activities in otherwise healthy older adults. The term *age-related cognitive decline* has replaced the older terms *age-associated memory impairment* (AAMI) (Albert, 1988; Crook et al., 1986) and *benign senescent forgetfulness*. Such concerns can include problems remembering newly learned facts or names of new acquaintances, difficulties remembering tasks on a list, misplacing objects, forgetting telephone numbers, or forgetting what one intended to do minutes after deciding to do it. They are distinguished from dementia by their minor severity and by the fact that they do not significantly interfere with social or occupational functioning. Research is leading to the development of cognitive intervention strategies to help the older adult compensate for any adverse effects of age-related cognitive decline on daily life functioning (Crook et al., 1986; Kausler, 1989; Riley, 1995; Scogin, Storandt, & Lott, 1985; Willis & Schaie, 1994).

One final note: As is apparent from this discussion, mild forgetfulness (age-related cognitive decline) can be considered a part of normal aging, and given the current state of our knowledge is not a cause for undue concern. One recent study has presented disconcerting evidence that dementia may be one extreme on a continuum of cognitive decline (Brayne, Gill, Paykel, Huppert, & O'Connor, 1995). In contrast, moderate or severe memory difficulties (e.g., repeated or permanent forgetting of recent, personally relevant facts, the gist of conversations with significant others, or past knowledge and skills) are not normal and should be brought to the attention of a medical provider. Significant memory difficulty can indicate a major disease process, specifically a major depression or dementia (see previous and succeeding sections of this chapter; see also chapter 12, section 2), although those older adults who complain about their memory are more likely to be depressed than demented (Kahn et al., 1975; Thompson, Gong, Haskins, & Gallagher, 1987). Moderate to serious memory difficulties also can signal a medical problem, such as untreated hypertension, diabetes, anemia, thyroid dysfunction, infection, malnutrition, or, the most common cause of reversible memory impairment, adverse drug reactions or interactions (Perlmutter et al., 1987).

Speed of Information Processing and Reaction Time

One of the most consistent findings in the study of aging is that speed of information processing and reaction time declines with advancing age (Salthouse, 1985; Shock, 1985). This is found on a variety of experimental tasks ranging from the simple (how long it takes to press a button after a light goes on) to the complex (how fast a person can write). The decrement increases with the complexity of the task and response, and is more pronounced in tasks requiring psychomotor rather than verbal responses. Overall, the speed with which older adults perform such tasks decreases approximately 20% for simple tasks and can reach 50% or more for complex tasks (Cerella, 1990; Schaie & Willis, 1996). Most of the psychomotor slowness observed in very old age is probably a product of this decline.

The generalized slowing of information processing and reaction time does not appear to be primarily a function of peripheral nervous system factors—sensory acuity, speed of peripheral nerve conduction, or speed of movement after the response is initiated—(Botwinick, 1984). Rather, the general-ized slowing appears to reflect a basic change in the speed with which the central nervous system processes information. The cause for this slowing has been attributed to disruptions of connections within the neural network, which increases the time required to process information (Cerella, 1990). And yet there is evidence that average reaction times are faster among active older adults than among nonathletic younger adults (Spirduso & Clifford, 1978; Spirduso & MacRae, 1990; Woollacott, 1988), that reaction time is better in older adults who engage in physical activity than it is in those who are sedentary (Stelmach & Worringham, 1985), and that reaction times can be improved significantly by physical exercise (Botwinick, 1978; Emery, Burker, & Blumenthal, 1992; Stelmach & Worringham, 1985). Because exercise increases blood flow to the brain, increases the amount of oxygen in the blood, and might even affect the structure of neural tissue, these factors also are implicated in age-related changes in reaction time (Birren & Fisher, 1992; Birren, Woods, & Williams, 1980; Schaie & Willis, 1996).

Intelligence

One of the more controversial issues in gerontology is whether intelligence declines with age. Intelligence is not a unidimensional concept; it includes a variety of intellectual abilities (verbal, numerical, reasoning, spatial relations, and memory), and is extremely difficult to measure or even define. The most influential measure of global or general intelligence in use today is the Weschler Adult Intelligence Scale (WAIS). The WAIS includes a verbal scale and a performance scale, which are combined to assess IQ. As measured by the WAIS, IQ remains stable into the mid 50s or early 60s and thereafter decreases with advancing age, a finding that is consistent among studies (Hertzog & Schaie, 1988). And so, although debate continues about whether intelligence actually declines with age, there is general agreement that people perform worse on intelligence tests as they grow older.

It is important to take note, however, of the differential rates in decline and stability with advancing age seen in the various categories of intellectual ability on the WAIS. Specifically, the performance scale that measures the speed of copying a picture, for example, shows earlier and significant decline. The verbal scale, which measures information retention, vocabulary, and comprehension, remains fairly steady. The differences between these two scales has been found so often that the phenomenon is known as the "classic aging pattern" (Botwinick, 1978; Kausler, 1991).

There is a growing consensus that traditional intelligence tests are not an appropriate measure of intellectual functioning in older adults. The fact that speed of response is given great weight in these tests clearly puts older people at a disadvantage. There also are compelling arguments that declines demonstrated by the WAIS could reflect well-documented slowing of information processing and reaction time (reflecting biological changes of the central nervous system) rather than decline in intellectual ability (Salthouse, 1985; Schaie, 1989).

Horn and Cattell (1967) and Cattell (1963) offered one of the first theoretical explanations for this differential decline by proposing two general kinds of intelligence: crystallized and fluid. Fluid intelligence involves the mechanics of intelligence, such as memory capacity, speed of processing, efficiency of receptors, and elementary cognitive operations. It operates by the mechanics of information processing

and is believed to decline with increasing age. Crystallized intelligence involves the pragmatics of intelligence (Staudinger, Cornelius, & Baltes, 1989). It is measured by using tests of vocabulary, information, and mechanical knowledge, and reflects content-rich, pragmatic knowledge systems that have been acquired through years of education and acculturation. Crystallized intelligence is believed to remain stable or increase at least up to about age 70 (Kausler, 1991), and can show additional increase through self-directed learning and education (Hayslip & Sterns, 1979). These age trends are similar to the WAIS classic aging pattern, because the verbal scale deals primarily with crystallized intelligence and the performance scale emphasizes fluid intelligence.

The continuing debate about intelligence in aging has resulted in greater appreciation for the fact that conventional methods of measuring intellectual abilities have not always been sensitive to the skills actually used by older adults in everyday life. Increasingly, theorists argue that the intellectual functioning of older adults is more accurately assessed in the context of the social, cultural, and life-stage demands of older adulthood than by the youth-based standards of intellectual functioning (as measured by the WAIS). Labouvie-Vief (1985, 1989) argued that formal operational thinking is well suited to adolescence and young adulthood, when considering all options equally is desirable. By midlife and beyond, however, decisions must be made on the basis of prior commitments and appreciation of consequences for all real persons involved. From this perspective, cognitive maturity and adaptation are more relevant conceptualizations of intellectual capacity in older adulthood (Cornelius & Caspi, 1987; Schaie, 1990; Willis &

Baltes, 1980). This recognition is providing impetus to the development of new testing methods, such as age-relevant intelligence tests. Some of these efforts focus on assessing the practical intelligence required to carry out instrumental activities of daily living (IADL) independently (Diehl, Willis, & Schaie, 1995). Steps toward defining or measuring age-relevant intelligence are still in the early stages, but the effort holds promise.

Cognition and Health

An emerging body of literature is concerned with investigating the relationship between cognition and health and illness in older adults. The major hypothesis is that cognition in healthy older adults remains relatively intact, whereas cognition in those with chronic disease processes shows precipitous declines (Launer, Masaki, Petrovitch, Foley, & Havlik, 1995; Schaie, 1990). Empirical evidence lends support to this premise, particularly with reference to chronic disease processes such as hypertension, cardiovascular disease, and diabetes (Elias, Elias, & Elias, 1990; Elias, Wolf, D'Agostino, Cobb & White, 1993; Sands & Meredith, 1992; Schaie, 1990; Siegler & Costa, 1985), as well as with self-reported pain (such as osteoarthritis) (Parmelee, Smith, & Katz, 1993). In these studies, health consistently emerged as a more important variable in predicting cognitive decline than chronological age. The implication here is that changes in cognitive function (typically memory) might more usefully be viewed as potentially modifiable manifestations of disease. Further, medications that prevent subtle brain changes caused by hypertension, low blood pressure, and elevated blood sugar could have an important effect on the occurrence of cognitive impairment (Launer et al., 1995). Longitudinal studies demonstrate that older adults

experience a marked decline in IQ only a few years or months from death (Berkowitz, 1965; Kleemeier, 1962; Riegel & Riegel, 1972; Steuer, La Rue, & Blum, 1981). These observations have led to the terminal drop hypothesis, which proposes that time before death, rather than time since birth, predicts intellectual decline. In this view, there might be little or no cognitive decline until physical deterioration occurs in the final years of life. Observations that marked declines in verbal abilities predict imminent death lend support to this premise (Jarvik, 1962; Jarvik & Falek, 1963).

The corollary to the hypothesis of disease and cognitive decline with age is that the preservation of health might preserve cognitive abilities. Indeed, there is evidence that physical exercise is related to both the maintenance and improvement of cognition in older adults. Active older adults perform better on a variety of cognitive measures than their sedentary peers (Clarkson-Smith & Hartley, 1989; Stones & Kozma, 1989). Exercise also has been shown to improve memory performance (Hassmen, Ceci, & Backman, 1992; Dustman, Ruhling & Russell, 1984), even with the cognitively impaired (Powell, 1974; Diesfeldt & Diesfeldt-Groenendijk, 1977). An implication to be considered here is that the level of physical activity inherent in occupational therapy protocols itself might provide ancillary cognitive benefit.

Emerging findings about the relationship between health and cognition have additional implications for occupational therapy. Given the preponderance of chronic disease within rehabilitation settings, it is probable that older adults will experience more than the usual level of age-related cognitive change. Because rehabilitation protocols typically require that patients learn new procedures, carry over learning from one day to the next, and retain these gains after returning home, it is likely that older adults will benefit from approaches that help compensate for age-related cognitive change. The following are some compensatory approaches to use:

1. Present new information more slowly.

2. Provide more response time when presenting new information.

3. Allow individuals to set their own pace or provide self-paced instructional materials, if possible. This often means reducing content in a given time period to offer greater clarity, specificity, and depth.

4. Present information orally and visually at the same time. Written material assists in learning when it is very similar to what is being taught orally.

5. Repeat information to increase information storage.

6. Associate new information with known information to improve retention.

7. Instruct individuals in the use of various mnemonic techniques (e.g., visual images, verbal associations) that can be used to organize material for storage.

8. Increase the rehearsal of information to be committed to memory.

9. Encourage thinking aloud (Giambra & Arenberg, 1980) to determine if principles taught are being applied correctly, and to provide for rehearsal and repetition of new information.

10. Present information using methods that compensate for the potential sensory problems of older adults (e.g., increased intensity, glare-free lighting; large-print instructional materials; lowered voice pitch).

These findings also open the possibility that age is an indirect indicator of physical disease or health problems that can influence cognitive performance (Ferrucci et al., 1993). As a result, age-related cognitive change might not be inevitable and could represent an underlying pathological process of some kind (Salthouse, 1989). Indeed, there is evidence that some older adults show no decline in test scores even into their 90s (Jarvik, 1988). It might well be that healthy older adults who maintain an active physical and intellectual life will show little or no loss of cognitive abilities unless they are confronted with serious disease.

Summary

Although controversy and debate continue in the area of cognition and aging, some general conclusions appear to be warranted by the available evidence. It appears that many cognitive functions do not begin to decline until the mid-50s or into the 60s, especially those functions involving verbal ability, and the declines tend to be small. There are important exceptions, however, with regard to response speed, psychomotor skills, and certain aspects of memory, wherein declines are mild, but are more significant. And so, although losses in some cognitive abilities are probable with increasing age or pathology, they are not likely to interfere with daily relationships and function, nor are they likely to significantly affect quality of life. Impairment sufficient to compromise these areas suggests a disease process such as depression or dementia (see next section).

At the same time, there is evidence that some functional competencies might actually increase with aging (e.g., crystallized intelligence). And there is promising evidence that, in the absence of disease, cognition may remain relatively stable throughout the later years.

References

Albert, M. S. (1988). Cognitive function. In M. S. Albert & M. B. Moss (Eds.), *Geriatric Neuropsychology*. New York: Guilford.

Atkinson, R. C., & Shiffrin, R. M. (1968). Human memory: A proposed system and its control processes. In K. Spence & J. Spence (Eds.), *The psychology of learning and motivation (Vol. 2)*. New York: Academic Press.

Berkowitz, B. (1965). Changes in intellect with age: IV. Changes in achievement and survival in older people. *Journal of Genetic Psychology, 107*, 3–14.

Best, J. B. (1989). *Cognitive Psychology*. St. Paul: West Publishing.

Birren, J., & Fisher, L. (1992). Aging and slowing of behavior: Consequences for cognition and survival. In T. Sonderegger (Ed.), *Psychology and aging: Nebraska symposium on motivation, 1991*. Lincoln, NE: University of Nebraska Press.

Birren, J. E., Woods, A. M., & Williams, M. V. (1980). Behavioral slowing with age: Causes, organization, and consequences. In L. W. Poon (Ed.), *Aging in the 1980's*. Washington, DC: American Psychological Association.

Botwinick, J. (1967). *Cognitive processes in maturity and old age*. New York: Springer.

Botwinick, J. (1978). *Aging and behavior*, (2nd ed.). New York: Springer.

Botwinick, J. (1984). *Aging and behavior: A comprehensive integration of research findings*. New York: Springer.

Brayne, C., Gill, C., Paykel, E., Huppert, F., & O'Connor, D. W. (1995). Cognitive decline in an elderly population—A two wave study of change. *Psychological Medicine, 25*, 673–683.

Caine, E. D. (1993). Should aging-associated cognitive decline be included in DSM–IV? *Journal of Neuropsychiatry and Clinical Neuroscience, 5*, 1–5.

Cattell, R. B. (1963). The theory of fluid and crystalline intelligence. *Journal of Educational Psychology, 54*, 1–22.

Cerella, J. (1990). Aging and information-processing rate. In J. E. Birren & K. W. Schaie (Eds.), *Handbook of the psychology of aging* (3rd ed.). New York: Academic Press.

Clarkson-Smith, L., & Hartley, A. A. (1989). Relationships between physical exercise and cognitive abilities in older adults. *Psychology and Aging, 4*, 183–189.

Cornelius, S. W., & Caspi, A. (1987). Everyday problem solving in adulthood and old age. *Psychology and Aging, 2*, 14–153

Craik, F. I. (1977). Age differences in human memory. In J. E. Birren & K. W. Schaie (Eds.), *Handbook of the psychology of aging*, Cincinnati: Van Nostrand Reinhold.

Craik, F. I., & Jennings, J. (1992). Human Memory. In F. Craik & T. Salthouse (Eds.), Chichester, England: Wiley.

Crook, T., Bartus, R. T., Ferris, S. H., Whitehouse, P. J., Cohen, G. D., & Gershon, S. (1986). Age-associated memory impairment: Proposed diagnostic criteria and measures of clinical change—Report of a National Institute of Mental Health Work Group. *Developmental Neuropsychology, 2*, 261–265.

Crook, T. H., & West, R. L. (1990). Name recall performance across the adult life span. *British Journal of Psychology, 81*, 335–349.

Diehl, M., Willis, S., & Schaie, K. W. (1995). Older adults competence: Observational assessment and cognitive correlates. *Psychology and Aging, 10,* 478–491.

Diesfeldt, H., & Diesfeldt-Groenendijk, H. (1977). Improving cognitive performance in psychogeriatric patients: The influence of physical exercise. *Age and Aging, 6,* 58–64.

Dustman, R., Ruhling, R., & Russell, E. (1984). Aerobic exercise training and improved neuropsychological function of older individuals. *Neurobiology and Aging, 5,* 35–42.

Eisdorfer, C. (1968). Arousal and performance: Experiments in verbal learning and tentative memory. In G. A. Tallend (Ed.), *Human aging and behavior.* New York: Academic Press.

Elias, M. F., Elias, J. W., & Elias, P. K. (1990). Biological and health influences on behavior. In J. E. Birren & K. W. Schaie (Eds.), *Handbook of the psychology of aging* (3rd ed.). New York: Academic Press.

Elias, M. F., Wolf, P. A., D'Agostino, R. B., Cobb, J., & White, L. (1993). Untreated blood pressure is inversely related to cognitive functioning: The Framingham Study. *American Journal of Epidemiology, 138,* 353–364.

Emery, C., Burker, E., & Blumenthal, J. (1992). Psychological and physiological effects of exercise among older adults. In K. W. Schaie (Ed.), *Annual review of gerontology and geriatrics.* New York: Springer.

Ferrucci, L., Guralnik, J., Marchionni, N., Costanzo, S., Lamponi, M., & Baroni, A. (1993). Relationship between health status, fluid intelligence, and disability in a non-demented elderly population. *Aging, Clinical and Experimental Research, 5,* 435–443.

Giambra, L., & Arenberg, D. (1980). Problem solving, concept learning, and aging. In L. W. Poon (Ed.),

Aging in the 1980s. Washington, DC: American Psychological Association.

Gounard, B. R., & Hulicka, I. M. (1977). Maximizing learning efficiency in later adulthood: A cognitive problem-solving approach. *Educational Gerontology: An International Quarterly, 2,* 417–427.

Hassmen, P., Ceci, R., & Backman, L., (1992). Exercise for older women: Training method and its influences on physical and cognitive performance. *European Journal of Applied Physiology, 64,* 460–466.

Hayslip, B., & Sterns, H. L. (1979). Age differences in relationships between crystallized and fluid intelligence in problem solving. *Journal of Gerontology, 34,* 404–414.

Herzog, C., & Schaie, K. W. (1988). Stability and change in adult intelligence: Simultaneous analysis of longitudinal means and covariance structures. *Psychological Aging, 3,* 122–130.

Horn, J. L., & Cattell, R. B. (1967). Age differences in fluid and crystallized intelligence. *Acta Psychobiologica, 26,* 107–129.

Jarvik, L. F. (1962). Biological differences in intellectual functioning. *Vita Humana, 5,* 195–203.

Jarvik, L. F. (1988). Aging of the brain: How can we prevent it? *Gerontologist, 28,* 739–747.

Jarvik, L. F., & Falek, A. (1963). Intellectual stability and survival in the aged. *Journal of Gerontology, 18,* 173–176.

Kahn, R., Zarit, S., Hilbert, N., et al. (1975). Memory complaint and impairment in the aged. *Archives of General Psychiatry, 32,* 1569–1573.

Kausler, D. H. (1989). Impairment in normal memory aging: Implications of laboratory evidence.

In G. C. Gilmore, P. J. Whitehouse, & M. R. Wycle (Eds.), *Memory, aging, and dementia.* New York: Springer.

Kausler, D. H. (1991). *Experimental psychology, cognition, and human aging* (2nd ed.). New York: Springer.

Kausler, D. H. (1994). *Learning and memory in normal aging.* San Diego: Academic Press.

Kleemeier, R. W. (1962). Intellectual change in the senium. *Proceedings of the Social Statistics Section of the American Statistical Association, 1,* 290–295.

Labouvie-Vief, G. (1985). Intelligence and cognition. In J. E. Birren & K. W. Schaie (Eds.), *Handbook of the psychology of aging* (2nd ed.). New York: Van Nostrand Reinhold.

Labouvie-Vief, G. (1989). Cognitive functioning in the middle years. In S. Hunter & M. Sundel (Eds.), *Midlife myths: Issues, findings, and implications.* Newbury Park, CA: Sage.

Launer, L., Masaki, K., Petrovitch, H., Foley, D., & Havlik, R. (1995). The association between midlife blood pressure levels and late-life cognitive function. *Journal of the American Medical Association, 274*(23), 1846–1851.

Parmelee, P. A., Smith, B., & Katz, I. R. (1993). Pain complaints and cognitive status among elderly institution residents. *Journal of the American Geriatrics Society, 41,* 517–522.

Perlmutter, M., Adams, C., Berry, J., Kaplan, M., Person, D., & Verdonik, F. (1987). In K. W. Schaie & K.W. Eisdorfer (Eds.), *Annual review of gerontology and geriatrics, 7.* New York: Springer.

Poon, L. W., Fozard, J. R., Cermak, L. S., Arenberg, D., & Thompson, L. (Eds.). (1980). *New directions in memory and aging.* Hillsdale, NJ: Erlbaum.

Poon, L. W., Gurland, B., Eisdorfer, C., Crook, C., Thompson, T., Kasniak, A., & Davis, K. (Eds.). (1986). *Handbook for the clinical assessment of older adults.* Washington, DC: American Psychological Association.

Powell, R. (1974). Psychological effects of exercise on the psychiatric state of institutionalized geriatric mental patients. *Journal of Gerontology, 29,* 157–161.

Riegel, K., & Riegel, R. (1972). Development, drop, death. *Developmental Psychology, 6,* 306–319.

Riley, K. P. (1995). Bridging the gap between researchers and clinicians: Methodological perspectives and choices. In R. L. West & J. Sinott (Eds.), *Everyday memory and aging: Current research and methodology.* New York: Springer.

Rowe, E. J., & Schnore, M. M. (1971). Item concreteness and reported strategies in paired associate learning as a function of age. *Journal of Gerontology, 26,* 470–475.

Salthouse, T. A. (1985). Speed of behavior and the implications for cognition. In J. E. Birren & K. W. Schaie (Eds.), *Handbook of the psychology of aging* (2nd ed.). New York: Van Nostrand Reinhold.

Salthouse, T. A. (1989). Age-related changes in basic cognitive processes. In M. Storandt & G. R. VandenBos (Eds.), *The adult years: Continuity and change.* Washington, DC: American Psychological Association.

Salthouse, T. A. (1991). *Theoretical perspectives on cognitive aging.* Hillsdale, NJ: Erlbaum.

Sands, L. P., & Meredith, W. (1992). Intellectual functioning in late midlife. *Journal of Gerontological and Psychological Science, 47,* 81–84.

Schaie, K. W. (1989). Perceptual speed in adulthood: Cross sectional and longitudinal studies. *Psychology and Aging, 4,* 443–453.

Schaie, K. W. (1990). Intellectual development in adulthood. In J. E. Birren & K. W. Schaie (Eds.), *Handbook of the psychology of aging* (3rd ed.). New York: Academic Press.

Schaie, K. W., & Willis, S. (1996). *Adult Development and Aging,* (4th ed.). Harper Collins: New York.

Scogin, F., Storandt, M., & Lott, R. (1985). Memory skills training, memory complaints, and depression in older adults. *Journal of Gerontology, 40,* 562–568.

Shock, N. W. (1985). Longitudinal studies of aging in humans. In C. E. Finch & E. L. Schneider (Eds.), *Handbook of the biology of aging,* (2nd ed.). New York: Van Nostrand Reinhold.

Siegler, I. C., & Costa, P. T. (1985). Health behavior relationships. In J. E. Birren & K. W. Schaie (Eds.), *Handbook of the psychology of aging* (2nd ed.). New York: Van Nostrand Reinhold.

Smith, A. (1980). Age differences in encoding, storage, and retrieval. In L. W. Poon, J. R. Fozard, L. S. Cermak, D. Arenberg, & L. Thompson (Eds.), *New directions in memory and aging.* Hillsdale, NJ: Erlbaum.

Spirduso, W. W., & Clifford, P. (1978). Replication of age and physical activity effects on reaction and movement time. *Journal of Gerontology, 33,* 26–30.

Spirduso, W. W., & MacRae, P. G. (1990). Motor performance and aging. In J. E. Birren & K. W. Schaie (Eds.), *Handbook of the psychology of aging* (3rd ed.). New York: Academic Press.

Staudinger, U., Cornelius, S., & Baltes, P. (1989). The aging of intelligence: Potentials and limits. *Annals of the American Academy of Political and Social Science, 503,* 43–59.

Stelmach, C. E., & Worringham, C. J. (1985). Sensorimotor deficits related to postural stability: Implications for falling in the elderly. In T. S. Radebaugh et al. (Eds.), *Clinics of geriatric medicine.* Philadelphia: Saunders.

Steuer, J., LaRue, A., & Blum, J. (1981). "Critical loss" in the eighth and ninth decades. *Journal of Gerontology, 36,* 211–213.

Stones, M. J., & Kozma, A. (1989). Age, exercise, and coding performance. *Psychology and Aging, 4,* 190–194.

Thompson, L., Gong, V., Haskins, E., & Gallagher, D. (1987). Assessment of depression and dementia during the later years. In K. W. Schaie (Ed.), *Annual review of gerontology and geriatrics, 7.* New York: Springer.

Weingartner, H., & Parker, E. (1984). *Memory Consolidation.* Hillsdale, NJ: Erlbaum.

Willis, S., & Baltes, P. (1980). Intelligence in adulthood and aging: Contemporary issues. In L. W. Poon (Ed.), *Aging in the 1980's.* Washington, DC: American Psychological Association.

Willis, S., & Schaie, K. W. (1994). Cognitive training in the normal elderly. In F. Forette, Y. Christen, & F. Boller (Eds.), *Cerebral plasticity and cognitive stimulation.* Paris: Fondation Nationale de Gerontologie.

Witte, K. L. (1975). Paired-associate learning in young and elderly individuals as related to presentation rate. *Psychological Bulletin, 82,* 975–985.

Woods, R. T., & Britton, P. G. (1985). *Clinical psychology with the elderly.* Rockville, MD: Aspen.

Woollacott, M. J. (1988). Response preparation and posture control: Neuromuscular changes in the older adult. *Annals of the New York Academy of Science, 51*(5), 42–53.

Zachs, R. T. (1982). Encoding strategies used by young and elderly adults in a keeping track task. *Journal of Gerontology, 37,* 203–207.

Section 3. Adaptation and the Aging Adult

Linda L. Levy, MA, OTR/L, FAOTA

Psychological Adaptation

Psychological aging refers to older adults' capacities for adaptation to the demands of biological changes and changing environments during their life span (Birren & Renner, 1977). Adaptation is defined as the process of meeting one's biological, psychological, and social needs under recurrently changing circumstances. Clearly, the process of aging is characterized by continual adaptation in the face of biological, psychological, and sociological challenges.

As detailed earlier, normal aging affects all physiological processes and provides significant challenges to adaptation. Visual impairment can lead to loss of self-esteem and restriction in activity. Hearing impairment can lead to increased anxiety at not understanding, and heightened suspiciousness. A blunted sense of taste and smell can adversely affect appetite. Perceptual-motor slowing can constrain efficiency in accomplishing desired activities. Decreased strength and cardiopulmonary functioning can limit mobility and independence. Forgetfulness can arouse fears of dementia. At the same time, the majority of older adults struggle with the consequences of one or more chronic illnesses.

Alterations other than somatic changes also affect the lives of older adults. They sustain important emotional losses (by relocation or death) of significant others—spouse, children, friends, relatives, associates, and colleagues. Changes in roles, such as those caused by retirement, affect the lives of many (these are detailed in section 5 of this chapter). In addition to facing loss of income and a secure daily routine, older adults in retirement often suffer a loss of prestige and identity, given the highly prized work ethic of the American cultural value system (Ekerdt, 1986). Hence, aging is accompanied by serious challenges to adaptation—in health, physical abilities, social networks, and roles. All older adults experience at least some stressors that are inimical to their well-being.

Despite the presence of significant problems, older adults are by no means destined to live unfulfilled, unsatisfying lives. The view of old age as a time of stress and despair is not supported by systematic research. In fact, most older adults maintain their well-being, function at positive levels, and report positive life satisfaction (Baltes & Baltes, 1990; Butt & Beiser, 1987; Gatz & Hurwicz, 1990; Ryff, 1989). To emphasize the overall well-being of older adults and to recount their exposure to potentially damaging experiences is not the contradiction it might at first appear. The explanation lies in the resources that older adults have developed to adapt to the changing demands and conditions of their lives, and that enable them to maintain well-being in the face of evolving and difficult circumstances (Baltes & Baltes, 1990; Pearlin & Skaff, 1995). Optimal aging has been described as an adaptive process wherein older adults are selective in their efforts and use alternative strategies and activities to compensate for the losses that aging can bring (Baltes & Baltes, 1990; Carstensen, 1992). The following will provide an overview of adaptive resources that have most consistently been identified to date in the literature: coping strategies, social support, and one's sense of control. In addition, very recent work by Clark et al. (1996) is beginning to document a broad range of adaptive strategies used by older adults to maintain well-being. This work also will be considered here.

COPING STRATEGIES

Coping strategies are strategies that individuals develop to prevent, avoid, or control emotional distress. There are a wide variety of coping strategies, representing conscious, learned ways of confronting problematic situations, as well as unconscious strategies, commonly known as defense mechanisms. To a large extent, coping operations are established very early and persist throughout life (Costa & McCrae, 1989).

Three functions of coping have been identified: managing situations that give rise to the stressors, managing the meaning of the problematic situations, and managing the stresses that result from the situation (Pearlin & Schooler, 1978). Age differences have been found in the types of strategies that individuals tend to use (see Aldwin, 1994, for a review of this research) that are considered to reflect the changes in types of stressors that individuals face at different life stages. Specifically, older people are less likely to direct their coping efforts toward managing a difficult situation through problem-solving (Lazarus, Averell, & Opton, 1974), a coping strategy that regards stressful situations as problems to be resolved by appropriate action (e.g., "I came up with a couple of solutions to the problem," or "I made a plan of action and followed it"). Instead, older adults are more likely to employ strategies for managing meaning and controlling symptoms of stress—functions that collectively are referred to as emotion-focused coping (Lazarus, Averell, & Opton, 1974; Lerner & Gignac, 1992). Here, the individual tries to achieve an emotional acceptance of the existing situation, or attempts to put the issue out of his or her mind, perhaps with the aid of defense mechanisms, such as "Well, maybe I am not too well off, but what can you expect from someone my age," or, "I looked for the 'silver lining.'" (Chiriboga, 1992; Folkman, Lazarus, Pimley, & Novacek, 1987; Martin, Carstensen, Tamsky, Wright, & Pellegrini, 1992; Meeks, Carstensen, Tamsky, Wright, & Pellegrini, 1989; Quayhagen & Quayhagen, 1982). As indicated, these age-related differences in coping strategies appear to reflect changes in the types of stressors facing older adults (McCrae, 1982, 1984). Older adults might rely on emotional-focused coping more often than their younger counterparts because they must contend more often with stressful situations that cannot be resolved successfully by a direct action or problem-solving approach, such as frailty, irreversible loss, or chronic health concerns (Folkman et al., 1987; Kahana, 1992; Koenig, George, & Siegler, 1988). Given these types of stressors, emotion-focused coping is more likely to be the adaptive solution.

There are two types of emotion-focused coping strategies that older adults tend to use. The first involves a restructuring of priorities. Problems arising around activities, relationships, or aspirations that are highly valued can result in considerable distress. One way to minimize the effect of stressors arising within an important life domain is to move the domain to a position of reduced importance, such as reconsidering the value placed on physical strength or one's place in society (Krause, 1994; Peck, 1968). A second strategy is positive comparison. Although people of all ages use their own age group as a frame of reference for self-evaluation, this strategy is particularly common among older adults. Older adults tend to describe their lives and problems in light of what is to be normally expected at their location in the life course (Lerner & Gignac, 1992; Prohaska et al., 1987), and are reassured to know that their difficulties are shared by others in their networks, especially others of similar age (Brandstadter & Baltes-Gotz, 1990; Pearlin & Skaff, 1995). An example is, "Even if I am bad off, there are many whose health is worse."

SOCIAL SUPPORT

Perhaps the most important resource is social support, a moderating influence that appears to be particularly beneficial to people facing problems that are resistant to individual coping efforts (Hansson & Carpenter, 1994; Pearlin & Skaff, 1995; Zarit, Pearlin, & Shaie, 1993). The concept of social support as an important resource is particularly useful for health professionals because it can be improved, even as many stressors cannot be prevented.

Social support is both formal and informal. It can be defined as follows:

1. The roles and attachments of individuals and groups of individuals within the social network, such as spouse, children, siblings, neighbors, colleagues, friends, who are available to the older adult.

2. The frequency of social interactions or the actual number of times the older individual speaks in person or by telephone with members of the social network.

3. The perceived social support or the subjective evaluation by the older adult of his or her dependable social network, ease of interaction with the network, sense of belonging to the network, and sense of intimacy with network members.

4. The instrumental support of concrete and observable services provided to the older adult by the social network, such as food preparation, transportation, or nursing services (Blazer, 1994).

The mechanisms by which social support buffers the individual from the challenges of aging are not fully understood. Cassell (1976) suggested that feedback, information, and guidance enable the older adult to understand and adapt to an ever-changing social network. Cohen (1988) suggested that social interaction can provide older adults with a more positive view of themselves, which in turn can affect feelings of mastery and control; see below (Sarason, Sarason, & Pierce, 1989). Emotional support also can minimize the effect of reduced mastery or control that older adults might experience (Berkman, 1983; Cohen, 1988). Social support can be of instrumental help as well. For instance, transportation to grocery stores and medical facilities can be provided.

Social support is paramount to the mental health of older adults. Those who are part of a supportive network are less likely to be depressed, especially when faced with illness and limitations (Zarit et al., 1993). Cobb (1976) found that older adults who believe they are loved, esteemed, and mutually obligated to a support system have better coping mechanisms. In addition, social support from family and friends is associated with lower death rates at any age (Berkman & Syme, 1979; House, Landis, & Umberson, 1988; Pilisuk & Parks, 1986). The absence of social support is considered a risk factor for morbidity and mortality in older adults that rivals the effects of well-established health risk factors such as smoking, obesity, and hypertension (House, Landis, & Umberson, 1988).

SENSE OF CONTROL

The third resource is control, the sense people have regarding their ability to exercise control over the important circumstances of their lives. As with coping and social support, a sense of control can serve as a buffer against the stressors associated with aging (Cohen & Edwards, 1989; Rodin, 1986; Ryff, 1989). To the extent that individuals can make decisions about their activities, the nature of their participation in these activities, the sequencing of activities, and the pace of activities, they are better able to adapt (Rodin, 1986). When they perceive themselves to lack control, older adults experience what Seligman (1975) has aptly termed "learned helplessness": they are more passive, depressed, less satisfied with their lives, and perform less well. They also could be at increased risk for illness or death.

Evidence that a sense of control is strongly related to health comes from a landmark study investigating the effects of enhanced responsibility and decision making on the physical and psychological well-being of nursing home residents (Langer & Rodin, 1976). The residents in the experimental group were given a variety of decisions to make—for example, meal schedules, activity preferences, and movie choices—to enhance their feelings of control. They also were given a choice of caring for plants. Residents in the control group were cared for as usual by the staff, which involved dependency and minimal decision making or choices, and were given plants that the staff took care of. After 3 weeks, the experimental group demonstrated significant improvements on measures of alertness, affect, and life satisfaction. Even more impressive, a follow-up study 18 months later revealed that only half as many in the experimental group as in the control group had died. At the same time, the experimental group continued to demonstrate better psychological and physical health (Rodin & Langer, 1977). What this experiment revealed was that even increasing control over apparently mundane matters can have dramatic effects. It also suggested that any event that depletes or diminishes control could undercut health.

In reviews of the literature that have emerged since this study, Rodin (1986, 1989) and others (Rowe & Kahn, 1987) have argued that the relationship between control (as a coping mechanism) and health strengthens with age (Rowe & Kahn, 1987). In this view, older adults are particularly vulnerable to loss of perceived control in life and consequently are increasingly susceptible to illness.

There is consistent evidence that a sense of control serves as an effective buffer mitigating the impact of stressors (Cohen & Edwards, 1989; Krause & Stryker, 1984; Wheaton, 1983), although little is known about how it enables older adults to sustain well-being in the face of these stressors. One explanation is that a sense of control by itself helps to reduce the threat of difficult life situations; to the extent that one feels in control of stressful conditions, one is less likely to feel victimized by them (Pearlin & Skaff, 1995). Research on the construct of health locus of control supports the hypothesis that individuals with higher levels of perceived control take greater responsibility for meeting their health needs (Wallston & Wallston, 1982). It also has been proposed that the sense of control frees people to cope actively and to mobilize social support in their own behalf (Brandstadter & Baltes-Gotz, 1990; Folkman, 1984; Krause, 1986). This literature also underscores what should now be considered a guiding principle for intervention in the lives of older adults. Intervention should never undermine an older adult's sense of control, lest it undermine physical and psychological health. Instead, it should empower and enable older adults to maintain a sense of control over their circumstances.

LIFE DOMAINS AND ADAPTIVE STRATEGIES

In their efforts to identify components of well-being in later life, Clark and associates (1996) have documented older adults' subjective perceptions regarding life domains (areas of personal importance), as well as adaptive strategies used to cope with challenges presented within each domain. The researchers identified life domains on the basis of interview data, and provided typologies of adaptive strategies associated with each domain (see table 4–2).

Table 4–2. Life Domains and Adaptive Strategies

Grave illness and death—spirituality. Confrontation of sickness, dying, and death in terms of their implications for meaning in life and the spiritual dimensions of one's being.
1. Strengthening one's personal relationship with God (e.g., through praying, reading the Bible, attending church)
2. Preparing for one's own death (e.g., developing the proper mental attitude toward death, composing a will)
3. Talking to others about death and dying
4. Choosing not to worry about catastrophic illness or death
5. Avoiding close relationships with others to minimize the pain of dying.

Health maintenance. Concern with avoiding illness and maintaining or enhancing one's physical health.
1. Complying with general health knowledge (e.g., maintaining a proper diet, staying active, exercising)
2. Seeking formal medical assistance (e.g., visiting doctors and complying with their recommendations
3. Maintaining a positive mental attitude toward health.

Mobility maintenance. Concern with one's capacity to physically get around.
1. Promoting one's generalized or future ability to be physically mobile (e.g., walking to maintain one's physical capacity to remain mobile in the future)
2. Using public or private transportation (e.g., car, bus, taxi)
3. Using situational contextual cues to maximize one's potential to be physically mobile (e.g., waiting for a nice day before going on a shopping trip, allowing one's stomach to settle before walking).

Personal finances. Attention to personal income, budgeting, and financial decisions.
1. Planning and adhering to a budget
2. Avoiding unnecessary expenditures and items (e.g., not buying a pet)
3. Engaging in informal money-making or saving ideas (e.g., selling one's meal tickets)
4. Taking advantage of formal money making opportunities that extend to seniors (e.g., receiving payment for jury duty).

Table 4–2. (continued)

Personal safety. Concern with threats to one's physical well-being such as crime and violence, physical disaster, and personal mishaps.
1. Maintaining oneself in a safe physical location (e.g., avoiding dangerous neighborhoods, staying inside, choosing to reside in a low crime district)
2. Using the protective advantage of other people (e.g., going out with other people as opposed to alone, engaging in crime watch networks with other residents)
3. Making use of general preventive measures (e.g., concealing one's purse when outside, exercising earthquake preparedness, staying alert, practicing self-defense).

Psychological well-being and happiness. Concern with living a satisfying and happy life.
1. Keeping active by engaging in worthwhile activities (e.g., spiritual activities, visiting with one's family)
2. Using formal professional services to remain happy or well (e.g., seeking psychiatric help to avoid depression)
3. Maintaining a proper, positive state of mind (e.g., avoiding feeling sorry for oneself).

Relationships with others. Attention to issues surrounding contact with one's family, pursuing friendships, coping with loneliness, and dealing with interpersonal conflict.
1. Making use of formal gatherings to meet and interact with others (e.g., being a member of a club)
2. Treating other persons in such a way as to foster positive relationships with them
3. Reaching out to family and friends
4. Resorting to alternate channels to furnish substitutes when human friendship is not available (e.g., buying a pet, owning a teddy bear, reading a book)
5. Avoiding others to prevent the negative aspects of social life (e.g., refusing to open up to nonworthwhile persons, attempting to limit one's relationships to a circle of close friends).

Source: Clark, F., Carlson, M., Zemke, R, Frank, G., Petterons, K., et al. (1996). *Life domains and adaptive strategies of a group of low-income, well older adults*. AJOT, 50, pp. 106–107.

This delineation of adaptive strategies, subjectively derived, and connected to the achievement of highly valued life goals, constitutes a major step in documenting the broad range of strategies that older adults are using to meet the challenges presented by the aging process. It also provides welcome guidance in conceptualizing how occupation might best serve to mediate major stressors experienced by older adults in their daily lives.

Summary

Adaptation in later life requires individual initiative in maintaining mental, physical, and social functioning in the face of numerous stressors and inevitable losses. As indicated in previous sections, there is strong evidence that many of the losses attributed to aging, such as cognitive decline and physical deterioration, are preventable and might even be reversible by individual effort (Rowe & Kahn, 1987). Even losses that are irreversible (e.g., health, reserve capacity, roles, significant others) can, however, be mitigated by adaptive coping mechanisms, including mechanisms that enable one to restructure personal meaning and those that enable one to retain some sense of control over one's circumstances. In addition, social resources within the family, the neighborhood, and the community are important buffers and moderators of the stressors of later life.

There is yet much to learn about how older adults respond successfully to the normal stresses of later life. Clark and associates (1996) are making ground breaking contributions to this effort through research that directly asks older adults about their problems and how they handle them; from this, data have emerged that are beginning to identify the role and the nature of adaptive strategies used by older adults to minimize the effects of problems that challenge their ability to lead independent and fulfilling lives. It is nonetheless clear that adaptation to aging is a dynamic process in which older adults confront the stressors and challenges of aging not as passive victims, but as actors drawing on resources gleaned from years of accumulated experience (Featherman, Smith, & Peters, 1990; George, 1987). Successful aging reflects the ability of the older adult to adapt to those stressors, and at the same time to maintain life satisfaction and well-being.

References

Aldwin, C. M. (1994). *Stress, coping, and development: An integrative perspective*. New York: Guilford.

Baltes, P. B., & Baltes, M. B. (1990). Psychological perspectives on successful aging: The model of selective optimization and compensation. In P. B. Baltes & M. B. Baltes (Eds.), *Successful aging: Perspectives from the behavioral sciences.* (pp. 1–34). New York: Cambridge University Press.

Berkman, L. F. (1983). The assessment of social networks and social support in the elderly. *Journal of the American Geriatrics Society, 31,* 743–749.

Berkman, L. F., & Syme, S. L. (1979). Social networks, host resistance, and mortality: A nine year follow-up study of Alameda County residents. *American Journal of Epidemiology, 109,* 186–204.

Birren, J., & Renner, V. (1977). Research on the psychology of aging: Principles and experimentation. In J. Birren & K. Schaie (Eds.), *Handbook of the psychology of aging.* New York: Von Nostrand Reinhold.

Blazer, D. G. (1994). *Intervention strategies for emotional problems in later life*. Northvale, NJ: Aronson.

Brandstadter, J., & Baltes-Gotz, B. (1990). Personal control over development and quality of life perspectives in adulthood. In P. B. Baltes & M. B. Baltes (Eds.), *Successful aging: Perspectives from the behavioral sciences* (pp. 197–224). New York: Cambridge University Press.

Butt, D. S., & Beiser, M. (1987). Successful aging: A theme for international psychology. *Psychology and Aging, 2,* 87–91.

Carstensen, L. L. (1992). Selectivity theory: Social activity in life-span context. In K. W. Schaie (Ed.), *Annual review of gerontology and geriatrics.* New York: Springer.

Cassell, J. (1976). The contribution of the social environment to host resistance. *American Journal of Epidemiology, 104,* 107–115.

Chiriboga, D. A. (1992). Paradise lost: Stress in the modern age. In M. L. Wykle, E. Kahana, & J. Kowal (Eds.), *Stress and health among the elderly.* New York: Springer.

Clark, F., Carlson, M., Zemke, R., Frank, G., Patterson, K., et al. (1996). Life domains and adaptive strategies of a group of low-income, well older adults. *American Journal of Occupational Therapy, 50,* 99–108.

Cobb, S. (1976). Social support as a moderator of life stress. *Psychosomatic Medicine, 38,* 300–304.

Cohen, S. (1988). Psychosocial models of the role of social support in the etiology of physical disease. *Health Psychology, 7,* 269–297.

Cohen, S., & Edwards, J. (1989). Personality characteristics as moderators of the relationship between stress and disorder. In R. Neufeld (Ed.), *Advances in the investigation of psychological stress.* New York: Wiley.

Costa, P., & McCrae, R. (1989). Personality continuity and the changes of adult life. In M. Storandt & G. VandenBox (Eds.), *The adult years: Continuity and change* (pp. 45–77), Washington, DC: American Psychological Association.

Ekerdt, D. (1986). The busy ethic: Moral continuity between work and retirement. *Gerontologist, 26,* 239–244.

Featherman, D., Smith, J., & Peters, J. (1990). Successful aging in a post-retired society. In P. B. Baltes & M. B. Baltes (Eds.), *Successful aging:*

Perspectives from the behavioral sciences, 50 (p. 93). Cambridge, England: Cambridge University Press.

Folkman, S. (1984). Personal control and stress and coping processes. *Journal of Personality and Social Psychology, 46,* 839–852.

Folkman, S., Lazarus, R., Pimley, S., & Novacek, J. (1987). Age differences in stress and coping. *Psychology and Aging, 2,* 171–184.

Gatz, M., & Hurwicz, M. (1990). Are old people more depressed? Cross sectional data on Center for Epidemiological Studies depression scale factors. *Psychology and Aging, 5,* 284–290.

George, L. (1987). Adaptation. In G. Maddox (Ed.), *The encyclopedia of aging* (pp. 5–7). New York: Springer.

Hansson, R. O., & Carpenter, B. N. (1994). *Relationships in old age: Coping with the challenge of transition.* New York: Guilford.

House, J. S., Landis, K. R., & Umberson, D. (1988). Social relationships and health. *Science, 241,* 540–545.

Kahana, E. (1992). Stress research and aging: Complexities, ambiguities, paradoxes, and promise. In M. L. Wykle, E. Kahana, & J. Kowal (Eds.), *Stress and health among the elderly.* New York: Springer.

Koenig, H., George, L., & Siegler, I. (1988). The use of religion and other emotion-regulating coping strategies among older adults. *Gerontologist, 28,* 303–310.

Krause, N. (1986). Stress and coping: Reconceptualizing the role of locus of control beliefs. *Journal of Gerontology, 41,* 617–622.

Krause, N. (1994). Stressors in salient social roles and well-being in later life. *Journal of Gerontology, 49,* 137–148.

Krause, N., & Stryker, S. (1984). Stress and well-being: The buffering effect of locus of control beliefs. *Social Science Medicine, 18,* 783–790.

Langer, E., & Rodin, J. (1976). The effects of choice and enhanced personal responsibility for the aged: A field experiment in an institutional setting. *Journal of Personality and Social Psychology, 34,* 191–198.

Lazarus, M. P., Averell, J. R., & Opton, E. M. (1974). The psychology of coping: Issues of research and assessment. In C. V. Coelho, D. A. Hamburg, & J. E. Adams (Eds.), *Coping and adaptation.* New York: Basic Books.

Lerner, M. J., & Gignac, M. A. (1992). Is it coping or is it growth? A cognitive-affective model of contentment in the elderly. In L. Montada, S. Filipp, & M. J. Lerner (Eds.), *Life crises and experience of loss in adulthood.* Hillsdale, NJ: Erlbaum.

Martin, P., Poon, L., Clayton, G., Lee, H., Fulks, J., & Johnson, M. (1992). Personality, life events, and coping in the oldest-old. In L. W. Poon (Ed.), *The Georgia Centenarian Study.* Amityville, NY: Baywood.

McCrea, R. R. (1982). Age differences in the use of coping mechanisms. *Journal of Gerontology, 37,* 454–460.

McCrae, R. R. (1984). Situational determinants of coping responses: Loss, threat, and challenge. *Journal of Personality and Social Psychology, 46,* 919–928.

Meeks, S., Carstensen, L., Tamsky, B., Wright, T., & Pellegrini, D. (1989). Age differences in coping: Does less mean worse? *International Journal of Aging and Human Development, 28,* 127–140.

Pearlin, L., & Schooler, C. (1978). The structure of coping. *Journal of Health and Social Behavior, 19,* 2–21.

Pearlin, L., & Skaff, M. (1995). Stressors and adaptation in late life. In M. Gatz (Ed.), *Emerging issues in mental health and aging*. Washington: American Psychological Association.

Peck, R. (1968). Psychological development in the second half of life. In B. Neugarten (Ed.), *Middle age and aging*. Chicago: University of Chicago Press.

Pilisuk, M., & Parks, S. (1986). *The healing web: Social networks and human survival*. Hanover, NH: University Press.

Prohaska, T. R., Keller, M. L., Leventhal, E. A., et al. (1987). Impact of symptoms and aging attribution on emotions and coping. *Health Psychology, 6*, 495–514.

Quayhagen, M. P., & Quayhagen, M. (1982). Coping with conflict: Measurement of age-related patterns. *Research on Aging, 4*, 364–377.

Rodin, J. (1986). Aging and health: Effects on the sense of control. *Science, 233*, 1271–1276.

Rodin, J. (1989). Sense of control: Potentials for intervention. *Annals of the Academy of Political and Social Science, 504*, 29–42.

Rodin, J., & Langer, E. (1977). Long-term effects of a control relevant intervention with the institutionalized aged. *Journal of Personality and Social Psychology, 35*, 897–902.

Rowe, J., & Kahn, R. (1987). Human aging: Usual and successful. *Science, 237*, 143–149.

Ryff, C. D. (1989). Beyond Ponce de Leon and life satisfaction. *International Journal of Behavioral Development, 12*, 35–55.

Sarason, I. G., Sarason, B. R., & Pierce, G. R. (Eds.). (1989). *Social support: An interactional view*. New York: Wiley.

Seligman, M. (1975). *Helplessness: On depression, development, and death*. San Francisco: Freeman.

Wallston, K., & Wallston, B. (1982). Who is responsible for your health? The construct of health locus of control. In G. S. Sanders & J. Suls (Eds.), *Social psychology of health and illness*. Hillsdale, NJ: Erlbaum.

Wheaton, B. (1983). Stress, personal coping resources, and psychiatric symptoms. *Journal of Health and Human Behavior, 24*, 208–229.

Zarit, S. H., Pearlin, L. I., & Shaie, K. W. (Eds.). (1993). *Caregiving systems: Formal and informal helpers*. Hillsdale, NJ: Erlbaum.

Section 4.
Mental Disorders in Aging Adults

Linda L. Levy, MA, OTR/L, FAOTA

Mental Disorders in Older Adults

Mental disorders in older adults are the result of three patterns of development: An individual can develop a mental disorder early in life and grow old; an individual can grow old and develop a mental disorder; or, an individual can be exposed to a variety of stressors earlier in life that eventually lead to the development of a mental disorder in later life (Gatz, Kasl-Godley, & Karel, 1996). Mental illness is not part of normal aging. The majority of older adults are in good mental health cognitively, emotionally, behaviorally, and spiritually. Nonetheless, older adults are at somewhat greater risk than younger groups for the development or recurrence of mental health problems. Nearly one out of five suffer from mental health problems serious enough to warrant intervention.

Approximately 22% of older adults suffer from a mental disorder (Park, Cavanaugh, Smith, & Smyer, 1993), with the highest rates (typically 50% or more) among the institutionalized elderly (Burns et al., 1988; Rovner et al., 1990). Dementias and depression are the most frequent problems of older adults in both the community (Myers et al., 1984; Rabins, 1992) and nursing home settings (Lair & Lefkowitz, 1990; National Center for Health Statistics [NCHS], 1993). Suicide among older adults is a significant concern, particularly for those who lack social support and are isolated. Another concern is alcohol abuse. Each of these will be discussed briefly to provide a framework for understanding some of the most common challenges to the mental health of older adults.

DEMENTIA

Dementia, a generally progressive and irreversible impairment of cognition and functional ability, increases in prevalence with age. Of Americans over age 65, about 5% have severe dementia, and 15% have mild to moderate dementia. Of Americans over age 80, about 20% have severe dementia (Schneck, Reisberg, & Ferris, 1982). In long-term care settings, dementias are the most frequently diagnosed clinical problem: at time of admission, approximately one half of all nursing home residents suffer from dementia (NCHS, 1993).

Dementias are classified according to their suspected cause (American Psychiatric Association [APA], 1994). These include degenerative (Alzheimer's disease, Pick's disease); vascular (multiple strokes); infectious (AIDS, neurosyphilis); toxic (alcohol, drugs, heavy metal exposure); or metabolic (thyroid disease, vitamin B-12 deficiency). The vast majority (about 60%) of all cases of dementia are caused by Alzheimer's disease. Between 10% and 15% result from vascular causes. An additional 10% to 20% are caused by a combination of Alzheimer's and vascular diseases. A smaller percentage (4%) results from alcoholism, trauma, and all other causes (Clarfield, 1988; Wells, 1977). And although not yet prevalent, there is increased awareness of the AIDS-dementia complex.

About 10% to 15% of older adults who exhibit symptoms of dementia have potentially treatable, reversible conditions (Arnold & Kumar, 1993).

Treatable conditions include systemic disorders, such as heart disease, renal disease, and congestive heart failure; endocrine disorders such as hypothyroidism; vitamin deficiency; medications; and major mental disorders, most notably, depression (pseudodementia), mentioned later.

Older adults presenting with changes in mental status that are relatively recent are not suffering from dementia. Dementia is characterized by the gradual deterioration of intellectual function, memory, or cognitive ability over a period of months to years. An older adult who presents with acute confusion, disorientation, behavioral alterations, and an altered level of consciousness (e.g., diminished clarity or awareness of the environment) is likely to be suffering from delirium (Inouye et al., 1990). Delirium reflects a widespread derangement of cerebral metabolism, and is considered a medical emergency. When it occurs, there should be an urgent search for the acute medical illness or other profound physiological change that produced it. Delirium can result from almost any physical ailment or drug problem (e.g., heart attack, dehydration, urinary tract infection, pneumonia, fecal impaction, pulmonary embolism, gastrointestinal hemorrhage) and many types of drug intoxication and withdrawal. It affects 30% to 40% of older adults admitted to hospitals; it is all too often unrecognized in nursing home settings, where it can coexist with dementia. Delirium is a powerful predictor of increased mortality among hospitalized older adults, and appears to be the final pathway through which many diseases express themselves (National Institute of Mental Health, 1993; Tune, 1991).

In the event of an irreversible dementia, the primary degenerative process is, as yet, untreatable. Nonetheless, rehabilitation can reduce morbidity and improve func-tion (Chiu & Smith, 1990; Gottlieb, 1990; Larson, Reifler, Featherstone, & English, 1984; Levy, 1992; Rovner, 1994). Rehabilitative efforts for dementia are tertiary in nature. The intent is to prolong preservation of retained capacities, prevent excess disability, improve short-term functional outcomes, and ease the burdens of caregiving activities. Dementia affects not just the older adult, but also the spouse or caregiver of that individual. Caregivers (often older adults themselves) experience high rates of depression, anxiety, exhaustion, burnout, and other problems, which also need to be addressed (Zarit, Orr, & Zarit, 1985). Further information on irreversible dementia is contained in chapter 4, section 2. For a comprehensive discussion on rehabilitation, the reader is referred to chapter 12, section 2.

DEPRESSION

Depression is the most frequently occurring mental disorder in later life; approximately 15% of all older adults experience clinically significant depression (National Institutes of Health [NIH] 1992). Older adults at highest risk for the disorder are those hospitalized with medical illness and those in nursing homes (Koenig & Blazer, 1992). More than 64% of nursing home residents experience depressive symptoms (Lair & Lefkowitz, 1990).

Depression is a heterogeneous condition that includes cases that are recurrences of illnesses that began in earlier adulthood as well as those whose initial onset is in later life. Early onset patients are likely to have mood disorders in their families, whereas those with late onset more commonly suffer from chronic medical or neurological illnesses (Caine, 1994). Late onset depression is viewed as an age-related disorder.

Although depression is a treatable disorder, it is underrecognized and undertreated in older adults (Callahan & Wolinsky, 1995; NIH, 1992). The recognition and treatment of depression often are complicated by multiple coexisting chronic conditions. Cultural stereotypes about aging can make the diagnosis even more difficult: Health care providers and patients themselves often conclude, inaccurately, that depression is a normal consequence of physical illness, social and economic problems, or aging itself.

Criteria for the diagnosis of depression are those contained within the *Diagnostic and Statistical Manual of Mental Disorders, 4th Ed.* (APA, 1994). These criteria include either depressed mood or loss of interest or pleasure, and four of the following associated symptoms: change in appetite; insomnia or hypersomnia; observed psychomotor agitation or retardation; fatigue or loss of energy; feelings of worthlessness or guilt; concentration or decision-making difficulties; and suicidal attempts, ideation, or recurrent thoughts of death. Hence, depressive syndromes can present in a variety of ways, depending on the combination of symptoms present. And yet, there is increasing evidence that depression in older adults could be qualitatively different from depression in middle-aged adults (Benedict & Nacoste, 1990). Depressed older adults often deny being depressed and do not report feelings of sadness or dysphoria. They are more likely to present with nonspecific somatic complaints (e.g., pain, ill-defined dyspnea, or constipation), memory or concentration problems, or apathy, than with a depressed mood (Benedict & Nacoste, 1990; Kasniak & Allender, 1985; Salzman & Shader, 1979). The vegetative signs of weight loss, sleep disorder, or altered libido can be absent, or can be attributed incor-rectly to normal aging or to a concomitant of medical illness. Once recognized, depressive symptoms respond positively to treatment (Folks & Kinney, 1991; Koenig & Blazer, 1992); nearly 60% of older adults suffering from late onset depression improve significantly (National Advisory Mental Health Council, 1993).

There is a well-established association between depression in older adults and chronic disease. At the same time, it is important to recognize that depression can be a cause, as well as a result, of disability. Mossey, Knott, & Craik (1990) found that depression significantly undermines rehabilitation outcomes; older adults who were depressed when hospitalized for a hip fracture were less likely to be ambulatory and independent a year later than nondepressed older adults with comparable injuries. There also is evidence that depression increases the disability associated with conditions as diverse as Alzheimer's disease, Parkinson's disease, stroke, rheumatoid arthritis, myocardial infarction, and chronic obstructive pulmonary disease, even after controlling for the severity of the underlying illnesses (for a review, see Reynolds, Schneider, Lebowitz, & Kupfer, 1994; Robinson & Rabins, 1989; and Starkstein & Robinson, 1993). Other consequences of depression include nutritional deficits, increased sensitivity to pain, increased sensitivity to drug side effects, increased use of health care services, and increased mortality.

Cognitive impairment in depressed older adults is referred to as the dementia syndrome of depression (previously known as pseudodementia), a treatable disorder often confused with dementia. It occurs in about 15% of depressed older adults (NIH, 1992). Discriminating between dementia syndrome of depression and true dementia is difficult. In dementia syndrome of depression, deficits in attention and concentration are variable; and, when uncertain, older adults are likely to say, "I don't know." There also is weight loss, often a past history of depression, and a more sudden onset of symptoms. By contrast, intellectual performance deficits are usually global in true dementia; and, when uncertain, patients are likely to confabulate (Rabins, Merchant, & Nestadt, 1984).

Depression in older adults also can be associated with the medications used for treating common medical conditions. These either can induce depression, aggravate preexisting depression, or produce depression-like symptoms (Salzman, 1992). Drugs most frequently associated with depressive symptomatology include antihypertensives, digoxin, steroids, oral hypoglycemics, anticonvulsants, cytotoxic agents, and all central nervous system depressants, such as barbiturates, neuroleptics, opiates, and especially, alcohol (NIH, 1992). When the offending drugs are eliminated or less psychotoxic drugs are substituted, the depression usually improves with no additional treatment.

Similarly, there are a number of neurological, endocrine, nutritional, and metabolic disorders that can result in depressive-like symptoms in older adults (Ban, 1984; Robinson & Rabins, 1989). After the underlying medical cause of the depression is recognized and treated, the depression usually remits. These disorders can include neurological conditions such as multiple sclerosis, normal pressure hydrocephalus, and temporal lobe tumors; endocrine conditions such as hypothyroidism, adrenal insufficiency, and hyperparathyroidism; and metabolic disorders with an associated decrease in sodium, potassium, or both. In addition, the effects of fever, viral illness, dehydration, decreased cardiac output, and hypoxia can also mimic depres-

sive-like symptoms (Ouslander, 1984). Further information on depression in older adults is contained in chapter 12, section 2 of this text.

SUICIDE

Suicide is one of the top 10 causes of death among older adults. Older adults commit 21% of all suicides, a rate substantially higher than the 13% rate for the population as a whole (U.S. Senate, 1991). Older White men are at the highest risk (Conwell, 1994; Koenig & Blazer, 1992). As disturbing as these statistics are, it is likely that they underestimate the magnitude of the problem. Suicide is rarely listed as the actual cause of death on death certificates in older adults, even when it is suspected. Instead, death is attributed to frailty, coexisting chronic disease, or advanced age. In addition, suicide rates in older adults also fail to take into account indirect or passive suicide (e.g., refusing to eat or drink, stopping medications, drug overdose, single-car accidents). Explanations offered for the high rates of suicide among older adults include access to more lethal methods for committing suicide (i.e., firearms); living alone, which can delay discovery; chronic medical problems; fear of Alzheimer's disease; organic mental dysfunction, which impairs judgment or the ability to generate alternative options; and greater premeditation about the action (Frierson, 1991; Koenig & Breitner, 1990; Richardson, Lowenstein, & Weissberg, 1989).

Depression is a long-acknowledged risk factor for suicide. Given the high risk of suicide in this population, it is essential that expression of suicidal ideation lead those involved to respond and make intensive efforts to treat the depression. As indicated earlier, however, depression is notoriously under-recognized and undertreated in older adults. This is poignantly illustrated by a study that found more than 75% of older adults who committed suicide had visited a primary care physician within the month before their deaths (Miller, 1978; Rabins, 1992). Recent evidence demonstrates that as many as 50% of depressed older adults are not diagnosed as depressed by their primary care physicians (Butler & Lewis, 1995). And yet, suicide is the most preventable cause of death in older adults (Gottlieb, 1993).

ALCOHOL ABUSE

Alcohol abuse in later life often is hidden and, consequently, overlooked. Most older adults are retired and do not have work problems caused by alcohol use, they often live alone, and they usually drink in the privacy of their homes and thus are less likely to be disruptive in public or arrested for driving while intoxicated (Schonfeld & Dupree, 1990; Shipman, 1990). Nonetheless, the National Institute on Alcohol Abuse and Alcoholism estimates that as many as 10% of older adults suffer from alcoholism (Jinks & Raschko, 1990). A disproportionately small number of older adults with alcoholism receive treatment for it, despite the fact that treatment in older adults can be twice as effective as in younger persons (Shipman, 1990; Stultz, 1984).

Older adults with alcohol dependence usually are medically ill (primarily with liver disease), and are divorced persons, widowers, or men who never married. They typically present with falls, confusion, poor personal hygiene, malnutrition, depression, or the effects of exposure. Research indicates that there are two types of alcohol abusers: an early onset group (before age 40), and a late onset group. The late onset group makes up 33% of all abusers (Atkinson & Kofoed, 1983; Schonfeld & Dupree, 1990). With this later group, the stresses of late life, including loss of a loved one and chronic illness, seem to increase the level of dependence (Horton & Fogelman, 1991; Zimberg, 1983).

A major concern in substance abuse with older adults is that a given amount of alcohol results in a higher blood alcohol level and quicker intoxication for an older adult than for a younger adult because of age-related changes (such as decreased lean body mass and lower body water content, decreased kidney and liver function). Accordingly, the amount of alcohol necessary to cause dependence is much lower in older adults than in younger adults; and organs and tissues can be damaged by smaller quantities of alcohol. In addition, prescription and over-the-counter medications can intensify the effects of alcohol, leading to more rapid intoxication and intensifying the dangers associated with alcohol use (Willenbring & Spring, 1990). The consequences of excessive drinking among older adults are serious. Nutritional deficiencies are common because alcohol inhibits the absorption of many nutrients (vitamins, minerals) necessary to support essential body functions. In older adults, these effects often are seen at very low levels of consumption. Years of excessive drinking also can lead to liver disease, cancer (especially of the mouth, larynx, and esophagus), and cardiovascular problems (e.g., cardiomyopathy, stroke, hypertension).

Summary

The fact that sound mental health is the norm for older adults underscores the importance of recognizing and effectively treating mental health problems. Too often, symptoms of mental disorder are overlooked as inevitable to the aging process. Failure to diagnose and appropriately treat mental disorders of later life significantly limits the potential for well-being, exacerbates physical illness, constrains rehabilitation, endangers independent living, and might even lead to premature death. Treatment can improve function, autonomy, and enable older adults to experience vital and satisfying lives.

References

American Psychiatric Association. (1994). *Diagnostic and statistical manual of mental disorders* (4th ed.). Washington, DC: Author.

Arnold, S., & Kumar, A. (1993). Reversible dementias. *Medical Clinics of North America, 77,* 215–230.

Atkinson, R., & Kofoed, L. (1983). Alcohol and drug abuse in old age: A clinical perspective. *Substance-Alcohol Actions Misuse, 3,* 353–356.

Ban, T. (1984). Chronic disease and depression in the geriatric population. *Journal of Clinical Psychiatry, 45,* 18–23.

Benedict, K. B., & Nacoste, D. B. (1990). Dementia and depression: A framework for addressing difficulties in differential diagnosis. *Clinical Psychology Review, 10,* 513–537.

Burns, B. J., Larson, D. B., Goldstrom, I. D., et al. (1988). Mental disorders among nursing home patients: Preliminary findings from the National Nursing Home Survey. *International Journal of Geriatric Psychiatry, 3,* 27–35.

Butler, R. N., & Lewis, M. I. (1995). Late-life depression: When and how to intervene. *Geriatrics, 50,* 44–57.

Caine, E. (1994). Clinical and diagnostic heterogeneity in depression in late life. In L. S. Schneider, C. F. Reynolds, B. D. Lebowitz, & A. Friedhoff (Eds.), *Diagnosis and treatment of depression in late life: Results of the NIH consensus development conference.* Washington, DC: American Psychiatric Press.

Callahan, C. M., & Wolinsky, F. D. (1995). Hospitalization for major depression among older Americans. *Journal of Gerontology, 50(A),* M196–M202.

Clarfield, A. M. (1988). The reversible dementias: Do they reverse? *Annals of Internal Medicine, 109,* 476–486.

Conwell, Y. (1994). Suicide in the elderly. In L. S. Schneider, C. F. Reynolds, B. D. Lebowitz, & A. Friedhoff (Eds.), *Diagnosis and treatment of depression in late life: Results of the NIH consensus development conference.* Washington, DC: American Psychiatric Press.

Folks, D. G., & Kinney, F. C. (1991). Consultation-liaison in the general hospital. In J. Sadavoy, L. W. Lazarus, & L. F. Jarvik (Eds.), *Comprehensive review of geriatric psychiatry.* Washington, DC: American Psychiatric Press.

Frierson, R. (1991). Suicide attempts by the old and the very old. *Archives of Internal Medicine, 151,* 141–144.

Gatz, M., Kasl-Godley, J., & Karel, M. (1996). Aging and Mental Disorders. In J. E. Birren & K. W. Schaie (Eds.), *Handbook of the psychology of aging* (4th ed.), San Diego: Academic Press.

Gottlieb, G. (1990). Rehabilitation and dementia of the Alzheimer's type. In S. Brody & L. G. Paulson (Eds.), *Aging and rehabilitation II: The state of the practice.* New York: Springer.

Gottlieb, G. (1993). Statement prepared for the *Mental Health and Aging Forum, Special Committee on Aging* (Serial No. 103–10). Washington, DC: U.S. Government Printing Office.

Horton, A., & Fogelman, C. (1991). Behavioral treatment of aged alcoholics and drug addicts. In P. A. Wisocki (Ed.), *Handbook of clinical behavior therapy with the elderly client.* New York: Plenum.

Inouye, S. K., van Dyck, C. M., Aleissi, C. A., Balkin, S., Siegal, A. P., & Horwitz, R. I. (1990). Clarifying confusion: The confusion assessment method. A new method for detecting delirium. *Annals of Internal Medicine, 113,* 941–948.

Jinks, M., & Raschko, R. (1990). A profile of alcohol and prescription drug abuse in a high-risk community-based elderly population. *The Annals of Pharmacotherapy, 24,* 971–975.

Kasniak, A. W., & Allender, J. (1985). Psychological assessment of depression in older adults. In G. M. Chaisson-Stewart (Ed.), *Depression in the elderly: An interdisciplinary approach.* New York: Wiley.

Koenig, H. G., & Blazer, D. G. (1992). Mood disorders and suicide. In J. E. Birren, R. B. Sloane, & G. D. Cohen (Eds.), *Handbook of mental health and aging* (2nd ed.). San Diego: Academic Press.

Koenig, H. G., & Breitner, J. C. (1990). Use of antidepressants in medically ill older patients. *Psychosomatics, 31,* 22–31.

Lair, T., & Lefkowitz, D. (1990). *Mental health and functional status of residents of nursing homes and personal care homes* (DHHS Pub. No. PHS 90–4370). Washington, DC: U.S. Department of Health and Human Services.

Larson, E. B., Reifler, B. V., Featherstone, H. J., & English, D. J. (1984). Dementia in elderly outpatients: A prospective study. *Annals of Internal Medicine, 100,* 417–423.

Levy, L. L. (1992). The use of the cognitive disability frame of reference in rehabilitation of cognitively disabled older adults. In N. Katz (Ed.), *Cognitive rehabilitation: Models for intervention in occupational therapy.* Boston: Andover Medical Publishers.

Miller, M. (1978). Geriatric suicide: the Arizona study. *Gerontologist, 18,* 495–499.

Mossey, J., Knott, K., & Craik, R. (1990). The effects of persistent depressive symptoms on hip fracture recovery. *Journal of Gerontology, 45,* M163–M168.

Myers, J., Weissman, M., Tischler, et al. (1984). Six month prevalence of psychiatric disorders in three communities. *Archives of General Psychiatry, 41,* 959–970.

National Advisory Mental Health Council. (1993). Health care reform for Americans with severe mental illnesses: Report of the National Advisory Mental Health Council. *American Journal of Psychiatry, 150,* 1447–1465.

National Center for Health Statistics. (1993). *Chartbook on health data on older Americans, 1992* (DHHS Pub. No. [PHS] 93–1413). Washington, DC: U.S. Government Printing Office.

National Institutes of Health. (1992). Diagnosis and treatment of depression in late life (Reprinted from NIH Consensus Development Conference Consensus Statement 1991). *Journal of the American Medical Association, 268,* 1018–1024.

National Institute of Mental Health. (1993). Mental health and aging: Scientific discoveries and prospects. (Fact Sheet). Rockville, MD: Author.

Ouslander, J. G. (1984). Physical illness and depression in the elderly. *Journal of the American Geriatrics Society, 30,* 593–599.

Park, D., Cavanaugh, J., Smith, A., & Smyer, M. (1993). *Vitality for life: Psychological research for productive aging.* Washington, DC: Public Policy Office, American Psychological Association.

Rabins, P. V. (1992). Prevention of mental disorder in the elderly: Current perspectives and future prospects.

Journal of the American Geriatrics Society, 40, 727–733.

Rabins, P., Merchant, A., & Nestadt, G. (1984). Criteria for diagnosing reversible dementia caused by depression. *British Journal of Psychiatry, 144*, 488–492.

Reynolds, C. F., Schneider, L. S., Lebowitz, B. D., & Kupfer, D. (1994). Treatment of depression in the elderly: Guidelines for primary care. In L. S. Schneider, C. F. Reynolds, B. D. Lebowitz, & A. Friedhoff (Eds.), *Diagnosis and treatment of depression in late life: Results of the NIH consensus development conference*. Washington, DC: American Psychiatric Press.

Richardson, R., Lowenstein, S., & Weissberg, M. (1989). Coping with the suicidal elderly: A physician's guide. *Geriatrics, 9*, 43–51.

Robinson, R., & Rabins, P. (1989). *Aging and clinical practice: Depression and coexisting disease*. New York: Igaku-Shoin.

Rovner, B. (1994). What is therapeutic about special care units?: The role of psychosocial rehabilitation. *Alzheimer's Disease and Related Disorders, 8*(1), 355–359.

Rovner, B., German, P., Broadhead, J., et al. (1990). The prevalence and management of dementia and other psychiatric disorders in nursing homes. *International Psychogeriatrics, 2*, 13–24.

Salzman, C. (1992). *Clinical Geriatric Psychopharmacology* (2nd ed.). Baltimore: Williams and Wilkins.

Salzman, C., & Shader, R. I. (1979). Clinical evaluation of depression in the elderly. In A. Raskin & L. F. Jarvik (Eds.), *Psychiatric symptoms and cognitive loss in the elderly: Evaluation and assessment techniques*. Washington, DC: Hemisphere.

Schneck, M. K., Reisberg, B., & Ferris, S. H. (1982). An overview of current concepts of Alzheimer's disease. *American Journal of Psychiatry, 139*, 165–173.

Schonfeld, L., & Dupree, L. (1990). Older problem drinkers: Long term and late-life onset abusers. *Aging, 361*, 5–8.

Shipman, A. (1990). Outreach to elder alcoholics works, *Aging, 361*, 18–21.

Starkstein, S., & Robinson, R. (1993). *Depression in neurologic disease*. Baltimore: Johns Hopkins University Press.

Stultz, B. M. (1984). Preventive care for the elderly. *Western Journal of Medicine, 141*, 832–845.

Tune, L. E. (1991). Postoperative delirium. *International Psychogeriatrics, 3*, 325–332.

U.S. Senate, Special Committee on Aging. (1991). *Aging America: Trends and projections, 1991*. Washington, DC: U.S. Government Printing Office.

Wells, C. E. (1977). *Dementia* (2nd ed.). Philadelphia: F. A. Davis.

Willenbring, M., & Spring, W. (1990). Evaluating alcohol use in elders. *Aging, 361*, 22–27.

Zarit, S., Orr, N., & Zarit, J. (1985). *The hidden victims of Alzheimer's disease: Families under stress*. New York: University Press.

Zimberg, S. (1983). Alcohol problems in the elderly. *Journal of Psychiatric Treatment and Evaluation, 5*, 515–528.

Section 5. Ability and Disability: The Performance Areas

Joan C. Rogers, PhD, OTR, FAOTA

Abstract

This section focuses on the integrated use of biologic, psychologic, and social abilities in task performance areas—activities of daily living, work and productive activities, and leisure activities. Task performance will be explored from three distinct but interrelated perspectives. The first perspective examines time use in late life, whereas the second perspective highlights specific task abilities and disabilities. In the third perspective, the enactment of roles is explored. These three perspectives provide a comprehensive picture of change and stability in task performance in the daily lives of older adults. Changes in task performance can readily be attributed to the age-related and disease-associated impairments discussed in the prior section. This section concludes with a discussion of the maintenance of competence, which is essential for understanding adaptation in late life.

Daily Living in Late Life

Activities are organized in regard to time and space. One goal of occupational therapy intervention is to assist clients in developing a healthy balance of activities for daily living—productive activities, leisure activities, and rest. Meyer (1922) proposed that occupational therapy view time use as a means of capturing the essential qualities of daily life. Slagle (1922) applied Meyer's proposal in her habit-training program, which capitalized on normal time use as a powerful force for organizing human behavior. Kielhofner (1977) further developed the concept of temporal adaptation and called for the reintroduction of time-use strategies into occupational therapy practice. Understanding how people use their time thus becomes a prerequisite for knowledge-based practice.

How do older adults spend their time? This question assumes particular salience in late life for several reasons. First, the reduction or termination of work time stimulates interest in how time that was previously occupied by work is now used. Second, although American society has norms for other age strata, it has few expectations concerning time use by older adults. In fact, some have labeled the post-work years as the "roleless" role. Third, the youth orientation of American society is accompanied by a devaluation of old age. This youth orientation can influence the opportunities that older adults have to fully participate in the mainstream of American society, as well as the willingness of society to channel resources and services to foster this integration. The manner in which older adults come to resolve the issues surrounding increased free time, lack of age-graded role expectations, and societal devaluation is reflected in their daily lives. This renders the examination of their time use a valuable tool for understanding their personal well-being.

Activities can be categorized as obligatory and discretionary. Obligatory activities are necessary for survival and include caring for one's personal needs and living environment as well as working to obtain the funds to pay for needed resources (Moss & Lawton, 1982). In terms of the occupational therapy uniform terminology, obligatory activities encompass the performance areas of activities of daily living, work, and productive activities (AOTA, 1994). Participation in discretionary activities is voluntary. These activities are generally self-chosen and are engaged in for affection, knowledge, or pleasure (Moss & Lawton, 1982). In terms of occupational therapy uniform terminology, the term discretionary activities is synonymous with play or leisure activities (AOTA, 1994). Although constraint characterizes obligatory activities and choice discretionary ones, the distinction is quite arbitrary. Any activity can fall into one or the other category depending on how it is carried out. For example, one can heat a frozen dinner to serve one's nutritional needs (obligatory) or one can try out new recipes for a dinner to be enjoyed with family and friends (discretionary). Similarly, an individual can chose to play bridge (discretionary), but by joining a bridge club with a fixed schedule, card playing takes on some constraints. On balance, however, obligatory activities have more constraint and fewer choice qualities than discretionary activities.

OBLIGATORY ACTIVITIES

Altergott (1988) examined day-to-day patterns of time use in American adults (18 to 88 years) and in the subset of older adults (75 years and older). This study is of particular value because by comparing the time use of older Americans and Americans in general, similarities and differences in their lifestyles can be elucidated. One measure of the involvement of an age group in an activity is the average time devoted to that activity by group members. From this viewpoint, Altergott found that adults 55 years and older spent about 14 to 15 hours per day doing obligatory activities. This includes an average of about 9

hours in sleeping, 2 1/4 hours in personal care, 2 1/2 hours in housework, 1 1/4 hours in paid work, less than 15 minutes in helping behaviors, and 5 minutes or less in child care. Women spent more time than men in housework and helping behaviors and less time in paid work. Overall, older Americans spent 1 to 2 hours less per day in obligatory activities than Americans in general, including an additional one-half hour sleeping.

A second measure of the involvement of an age group in an activity is the percentage of people who actually participate in the activity. This measure provides an indication of the intensity of involvement. From this viewpoint, all older adults participated in housework, personal care, and sleep. However, less than 40% participated in paid work, less than 30% in helping activities, and less than 20% in child care.

Lifestyle differences in obligatory activities were examined across three older age groups—55 to 64, 65 to 74, and 75 and older. About 1 hour more was occupied in obligatory activities by those in the 55 to 64 age group in comparison with the older age groups. Regardless of age group, married men and women also spent about 1 hour more doing these activities. These increases were largely accounted for by differences in paid work and sleep. For both men and women, work was concentrated in the youngest age group. Work for pay was also linked to being married. Sleep, including naps, increased with age. The time given to personal care was similar across gender and age groups. For women, there was a slight decrease in time for housework, whereas the time for men remained stable. Widows spent less time doing housework; widowers spent more time doing these tasks. For women, the time spent in helping activities decreased after age 75, but even then the time was more than triple that spent by men.

Time budget studies are difficult to compare because there is no uniform terminology for defining activities and no taxonomy for classifying such activities into categories. Keeping this in mind, the findings of Moss and Lawton (1982) have suggested that older adults spend approximately 1 to 3 hours less in obligatory activities compared with the results of Altergott (1988). Moss and Lawton's calculations indicate that approximately 2 1/3 hours is taken up by personal or sick care, about 2 hours in shopping, housework, and cooking, and about 7 1/2 hours sleeping. The figures for personal care are fairly comparable with those obtained by Altergott, whereas those for home management and sleeping are less.

DISCRETIONARY ACTIVITIES

The overall daily average of time spent by older adults in discretionary activities in Altergott's (1988) study was about 6 1/2 hours. This is about 1/2 hour longer than the average for American society in general. For men, the amount of leisure peaked at just over 8 hours each day in the 65 to 74 age range. For women, the peak was 7 1/2 hours and occurred after age 75. Moss and Lawton (1982) found that older adults spent considerably more time occupied in discretionary activities, with an average of 10 2/3 hours.

Altergott (1988) classified leisure activities into 10 categories:

1. Active leisure (golf, walking for pleasure, exercising)
2. Passive leisure (listening to music, reading, relaxing)
3. Television viewing
4. Social leisure
5. Religious practices (attending services, Bible study)
6. Voluntary organizations
7. Creative leisure (knitting, hobbies, artistic production)
8. Entertainment (going to a movie, museum, or fair)
9. Education (attending courses, working on homework for classes)
10. Travel to and from leisure.

Overall, men devoted about 50 more minutes per day to leisure activities than women. Men and women were similar in the time spent on social leisure, religious practices, voluntary organizations, entertainment, and education. The daily average for watching television was about 3 hours, and for participation in passive and social leisure it was about 1 1/3 to 1 1/2 hours, whereas daily averages for the other leisure categories were less than 20 minutes. Gender differences in participation levels were found in active leisure, passive leisure, television viewing, creative leisure, and traveling to and from leisure activities. Men spent more time than women in each activity, with the exception of creative leisure.

Almost all older adults participated in passive leisure, television viewing, social leisure, and travel for leisure. About 50% engaged in religious practices. One-fourth of the men and one-third of the women participated in voluntary organizations. About 16% participated in educational activities and about 10% participated in entertainment.

Lifestyle differences in leisure were examined across the three older age groups. As men age, they participate at a lower level in social and active leisure, whereas the participation of women remains fairly stable. For both men and women, passive leisure increases with age. For men, television viewing peaks in the 75 and older age range at about 3 1/2 hours per day. Throughout later maturity, men watch more television than women. Participation in religious practices increased for both genders across the age groups, more dramatically for women than for men. For men, participation in voluntary organizations remained low but stable over the age groups, while the participation of women over age 75 declined. Both men and women in the over 75 age group have higher levels of creative leisure than their younger counterparts. Entertainment, education, and travel for leisure remain fairly constant across the age groups.

From the viewpoint of social interaction, women spend about 6 1/2 hours alone each day; this is approximately 1 1/2 hours more than men. Compared with men, women also spend about 2 1/2 hours less with a spouse. These gender differences in solitude and marital interaction are likely indicative of the widowed status of a majority of older women. Women also spend less time than men with their children who share the same household, and less time with work colleagues, but more time with friends, relatives, and neighbors. In general, these older adults reflect the norms of American society in spending considerable time in solitude and having most of their social interaction within the family unit.

FACTORS INFLUENCING TIME ALLOCATION

The time budget study conducted by Moss and Lawton (1982) included dependent older adults and adds to the knowledge of temporal adaptation in late life. The four groups of elderly surveyed spanned the continuum from independent to dependent community living—community residents, age-segregated public housing residents, high-intensity in-home service users, and nursing home applicants. The effect of dependency was to reduce the time spent on obligatory activities. Compared with the service recipient groups, the independent groups spent more time away from the home, less time in personal and sick care or with social agency personnel, and more time shopping, doing housework, cooking and traveling. The only significant difference between the groups in discretionary activities is that independent groups spent less time resting and relaxing. The social context for activity, in terms of being alone or interacting with household family, family outside the household, friends, and others, was similar across the four groups. Most of the waking day was spent alone and inside the home.

Both age and gender influence time allocation. Other demographic characteristics, such as race, education, and income have also been shown to influence activity participation (Lawton, Moss, & Fulcomer, 1986–87). Beyond these basic demographic characteristics, however, health and the ability to carry out daily living tasks emerge as the strongest determinates of time allocation. Poor health and disability in personal self-care and home-management tasks have a substantial effect on time usage. Specifically, time spent in personal or sick care is increased, along with time spent with a social agency, listening to the radio, resting and relaxing, and time spent in the home.

Perhaps a more interesting question than how older adults spend their time, is whether they spend their time involved in activities that they enjoy. In this regard, time spent in obligatory activities does not seem to be based on liking; the same holds for interacting with family members (Lawton et al., 1986–87). For many discretionary activities, however, there is a clear relationship between time allocation and liking. More time is spent interacting with friends, reading, watching television, and recreating by those who enjoy these activities. Conversely, resting and relaxing is liked most by those who do it least. It is significant to note that it was the degree of liking for an activity, rather than the actual time spent in an activity, that contributed to personal adjustment (Lawton et al., 1986–87).

IMPLICATIONS FOR OCCUPATIONAL THERAPY

These studies indicate that older Americans spend more time in leisure activities than they do in activities of daily living or work and productive activities. Further, they suggest that as frailty develops, the time spent in obligatory activities declines, while the time spent in discretionary activities increases. The goal of occupational therapy in balancing performance areas is not to allocate equal time to each area, but rather to allocate sufficient time on a routine basis so that basic needs in each performance area are met (Reed & Sanderson, 1983). This contributes to a sense of control over a person's affairs and life. The diversity of time-use patterns identified, with some persons active in some areas and not in others, highlights the individualized nature of temporal adaptation. The balance of performance areas is then one that is appropriate for each individual.

This research also indicates that the ways in which older adults spend their time is consequential to their psychological well-being. The time spent in discretionary, but not obligatory activities, was related to the extent to which the activity was liked. Further, the liking for an activity, but not the time spent doing an activity, was related to personal adjustment. Occupational therapy practitioners concerned with the quality of life of disabled older adults will need to look beyond their capacities in personal care and home-management tasks. Not only do older adults spend more time in leisure activities than they do in other activities, it is their liking for these activities that enhances their psychological well-being. The activity balance that occupational therapy seeks to achieve in performance areas can relate more to the subjective connotation of activity participation than to the objective amount of time spent doing the activity (McKinnon, 1992).

PERFORMANCE AREAS IN LATE LIFE

The conceptual scheme underlying occupational therapy uniform terminology divides activities into three major performance areas—activities of daily living (ADL), work and productive activities, and leisure activities. Because ADL are expected of all humans, and an inability to perform any of these activities constitutes a disability, the most accurate estimates of disability are available for this performance area. Disability statistics for work and productive activities are more difficult to accumulate because these activities are not expected of all humans. Traditionally, for example, responsibility for activities such as cooking, laundry, and shopping have all been allocated to women. Therefore, the inability of men to perform these activities is not health-related, but is a result of their lack of experience. In addition, there is no consensus for the work and productive activities that should be included in disability surveys. Because of their individualized nature, it is more problematic to document disability in work and productive activities than in leisure activities.

In 1989, an estimated 14% of all noninstitutionalized persons in the United States had a disability. With age, the extent of disability increases. Whereas only 9% of adults ages 18 to 44 have a disability, the proportion increases to 22% in the 45 to 64 age group. The disability rate rises to 37% in the 65 to 69 age group, and further increases to 39% in those over 70 years of age (LaPlante, Rice, & Kraus, 1991).

ADL AND PRODUCTIVE ACTIVITIES: HOME MANAGEMENT

ADL refers to the ability to care for one's basic needs. Activities typically included under ADL are functional mobility, including walking, transferring, and moving in bed; feeding; bathing; performing hygiene, including caring for one's hair, teeth and mouth, fingernails and toenails; dressing; toileting, including bowel and bladder continence; and communicating one's basic needs. Synonymous terms for ADL are personal care, personal self-care, basic ADL, physical ADL, basic self-maintenance, physical self-maintenance, and personal self-maintenance (Fillenbaum, 1987; Lawton et al., 1986–1987; Lawton & Brody, 1969; Rogers & Holm, 1994).

Figure 4–1 displays disability statistics in regard to ADL for community dwelling persons 65 years of age and older. These data are based on the 1984 Supplement on Aging to the National Health Interview Survey (NHIS) (National Center for Health Statistics [NCHS], 1987b). Of the seven activities surveyed, older Americans are most likely to have difficulty walking. About 19% have this problem; this proportion is almost double that for any other ADL. In descending order, difficulty in walking is followed by difficulty in bathing and getting outside, performing transfers, dressing, and using the toilet. Eating was the least problematic activity.

Undoubtedly, difficulty in performing ADL indicates some loss in quality of life; task performance difficulty does not, however, necessarily represent a need for health or social services. A better measure of service need is the proportion of older adults who receive help with an ADL—a subset of those who have difficulty with the activity. Only one-fourth of those who experience difficulty with walking receive help for that activity (see figure 4–1). The proportion of those experiencing difficulty with a task and receiving help for it was more congruent for the other ADL. Four percent received help for one ADL, 2% received help for two activities, 1% received help with three activities, and 3% received help with four to seven ADL.

As illustrated in figure 4–2, as age increases, the proportion of older adults having difficulty with ADL also rises. At all ages, walking was the most difficult activity and eating the least. The order of difficulty for the remaining five activities varied slightly. Gender differences were seen in regard to bathing, transferring, walking, getting outside, and using the toilet, with women having more difficulty than men. These differences, however, can stem from the fact that, on the average, women in the age group 65 and over are older than men. Many of the gender differences were not significant when more narrowly restricted age groups were considered.

Home management involves the ability to carry out tasks inside and outside of the home that are required for independent living. Activities typically included under home management are

1. Advancing functional mobility, including entering and exiting the home, walking while carrying a weight, such as a purse or garbage, and moving around the community

Figure 4–1. Percentage of adults over 65 years of age who have task difficulty or receive help with ADL

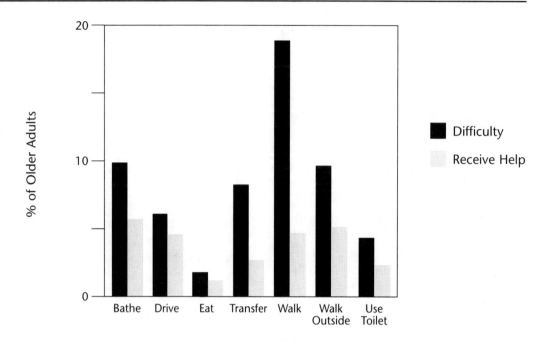

Source: National Health Interview Survey, National Center for Health Statistics, 1987b.

2. Managing medications
3. Managing finances
4. Managing more complex communication, including using the telephone and responding to mail
5. Shopping for food
6. Preparing meals and cleaning up after meals
7. Doing laundry
8. Doing light housework, including dusting furniture, cleaning floor surfaces, making beds, performing minor home repairs, raking the leaves, and watering the lawn
9. Doing heavy housework, including changing bed linens, washing floors, performing major home maintenance tasks such as putting up storm windows, painting the walls, shoveling snow, and weeding the garden.

Synonymous terms for home management are instrumental activities of daily living (IADL), independent living skills, and extended ADL, with IADL being the term used most frequently (Lawton & Brody, 1969; Nouri & Lincoln, 1987; Rogers & Holm, 1994).

Figure 4–3 displays disability statistics in regard to IADL. Almost 24% of older adults experience problems with heavy housework. This percentage is more than double that for any other home-management activity. In descending order, difficulty with heavy housework was followed by difficulty shopping, preparing meals, doing light housework, managing money, and using the telephone. At all ages, heavy housework was the hardest activity, whereas managing money and using the telephone vied for the easiest position.

Figure 4–2. Percentage of older adults who have ADL task difficulty, by age range

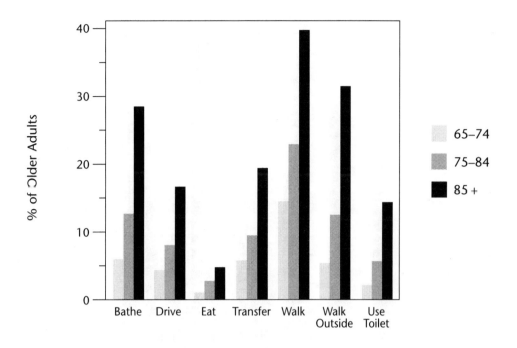

Source: National Health Interview Survey, National Center for Health Statistics, 1987b.

Figure 4–3. Percentage of adults over 65 years of age who have task difficulty or receive help with IADL

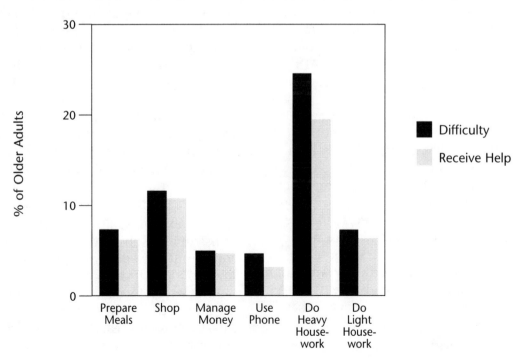

Source: National Health Interview Survey, National Center for Health Statistics, 1987b.

Figure 4–4. Percentage of older adults who have task difficulty by age range

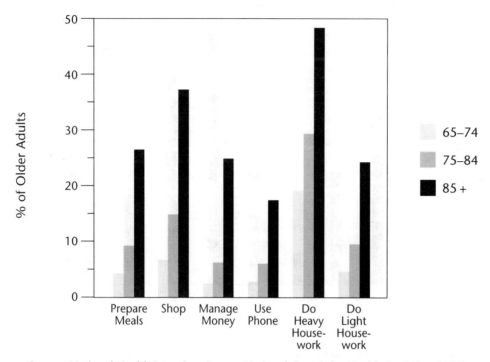

Source: National Health Interview Survey, National Center for Health Statistics, 1987b.

As found with ADL, the proportion of older adults experiencing difficulty with each IADL also increased with age (see figure 4–4), although more difficulty was experienced with these IADL than with ADL. Gender differences were seen in regard to four activities: preparing meals, shopping, doing heavy housework, and doing light housework, with men having less difficulty than women. However, these differences could have occurred because men were not as involved in home management as were women; therefore, men have less opportunity to experience such performance problems. The majority of older adults having difficulty with home management tasks receive help with those tasks, a trend dissimilar to that seen for personal care.

As is evident from these data of ADL and IADL disability, surveys ascer-taining the prevalence of disability in the American population have typically included only a small sample of the activities that could be included in each of these categories. As a result, these statistics probably underestimate the extent of disability in the older population. For example, if toenail care was among the activities surveyed, the prevalence estimates of disability would be higher, because this is a difficult task for older adults and one for which they often seek assistance.

The above disability statistics also translate into substantive ability in the community-dwelling older population. About 77% of those 65 years and over did not experience difficulty performing any of the seven ADL. Similarly, 51% of those 85 years and over had no performance difficulties at all. Further, 90% of all noninstitutionalized

Americans 65 years and over did not receive assistance for ADL. In regard to home management, 73% of those 65 years and over did not have difficulty performing any of the six IADL examined. In the age group over 85, 45% did not have difficulty in any IADL. No help was received for IADL by 78% of those 65 and older. Therefore, the detailing of the disabilities of the older population should not be allowed to obscure their remaining abilities.

These disability statistics are congruent with the classic portrait of decline and loss in biological, psychological, and social functions over late life. The increase in disability with age raises the question of the extent to which a disability should be viewed as a natural accompaniment of aging. Riley and Bond (1983) have argued that equating age with disability is a subtle form of age prejudice, and that it obscures the very real differences between the processes of normal aging and of disease. Separation of age and disease effects is supported by evidence from longitudinal studies of cognitive functions in which no declines were detected in the majority of older adults, except for the terminal decline frequently observed before death (Field, Schaie, & Leino, 1988; Riegel & Riegel, 1972). Further support is gleaned from the reversal of age effects on muscle tissue and the cardiovascular system through exercise. Such reversals led Gorman and Posner (1988) to hypothesize that about half of the functional decline observed between ages 30 and 70 is caused by a lack of exercise rather than age.

In view of the impact of disability in ADL and IADL on the need for health and social services, there is considerable interest in projecting future disability trends. Attention is currently focused on three theories linking age and disability—the Pandemic theory, the Compression of Morbidity thesis, and the Dynamic Equilibrium theory.

The Pandemic theory (Kramer, 1980; LaPlante, 1989) projects a substantial increase in the number of older adults with disabilities in the years to come. This projection is based on several factors. First, there is currently a high rate of disability in the older population. For example, when institutionalized and community-dwelling older adults are taken into account, 33% of those over age 65 have difficulty carrying out one or more basic daily living activities, such as feeding and dressing. Second, disability increases with age. Since the "oldest old" (those 85 years of age or older) is the fastest growing segment of the American population, it is logical to expect an increased proportion of disabled elderly. Third, advances in health and fitness are likely to lead to an increased life expectancy, with a proportional increase in the size of the older population itself. According to recent estimates, between the years 1990 and 2030, the number of elderly persons with disabilities will more than double from 6.2 million to 13.8 million (McBride, 1989).

A more optimistic outlook emerges from the Compression of Morbidity thesis. Fries (1980, 1984) used public health reports involving increased exercise, decreased smoking, and decreased saturated-fat intake to project an extension of health into advanced old age. Trends in actuarial data were used to project an average human life span of 85 years. Hence, although more people will live to be 85 years of age, the number beyond age 85 will not increase appreciably. Fries (1980, 1984) postulated that the time of health will be lengthened and the time of disability shortened (compressed), followed by death around age 85.

The position assumed by Manton (1982) in the Dynamic Equilibrium theory lies between the Pandemic theory and the Compression of Morbidity thesis. Accordingly, increases in life expectancy will be accompanied by delays in disability onset. Further, the rate of progression of disability will be slowed and the severity of disability will be decreased. Thus, people will be healthier and live longer, the onset of disability will be delayed, and when disability emerges, it will be less severe and progress at a slower rate. These theories await future disability surveys to confirm or dispute the projected trends.

PRODUCTIVE ACTIVITIES: WORK-RELATED

The ability of older adults to perform work-related activities can be viewed in reference to the following:

1. Those who continue to work
2. Those who retire for reasons other than health
3. Those who retire for health reasons.

Ten work-related activities common to many jobs were examined in the 1984 Supplement on Aging to the NHIS (NCHS, 1987a). The 10 activities tapped five motoric activity components—mobility, endurance, strength, range of motion, and fine motor skill. Mobility involved walking one-fourth mile and up 10 stairs without resting. Endurance for confined body movement involved standing for 2 hours and sitting for 2 hours. Lower- and upper-body strength took into account the ability to stoop, crouch, or kneel, and to lift 10 or 25 pounds. Range of motion involved reaching overhead and reaching out to shake hands. Fine motor skill consisted of grasp.

Fifty-eight percent of those 55 to 74 years of age, who had worked at some time since their 45th birthday, experienced no difficulty performing any of the 10 activities. Performance differ-

ences among employment groups were clearly evident. Among those who were still working, 73% had no difficulty with these activities. However, the percentage rates dropped to 60 for those who retired for reasons other than health and to 14 for those who retired because of health.

Figure 4–5 displays the percentage of people in the age ranges of 65 to 69 and 70 to 74 who had difficulty performing each of the 10 work-related activities. Stooping, crouching, and kneeling caused difficulty for the largest proportion of older adults, followed by lifting or carrying 25 pounds, standing for 2 hours, walking one-quarter mile, and walking up 10 stairs. Reaching out to shake hands caused the least difficulty in both age ranges. Only subtle age differences were evidenced for sitting, reaching up, and grasping. Activities emphasizing mobility, endurance, and strength were most affected by increased age, whereas those emphasizing range of motion and fine motor skill were the least affected.

In general, women had more difficulty performing these activities than men. The greatest discrepancies between older men and older women involved stooping, crouching, or kneeling, and carrying 25 pounds. The gender differences are more pronounced with increased age. For example, the percentage of older women having difficulty walking up 10 stairs without resting was 12% for those 55 to 59 years of age, 17% for those 60 to 64, 20% for those 65 to 69, and 25% for those 70 to 74. The corresponding percentages for men in these age ranges were 9%, 12%, 14%, and 18%. Of the women 70 to 74 years of age, 10% were unable to use the stairs, whereas 9% of the men in this age group were similarly disabled.

Figure 4–5. Percentage of older workers 65–74 years of age having difficulty with specific tasks

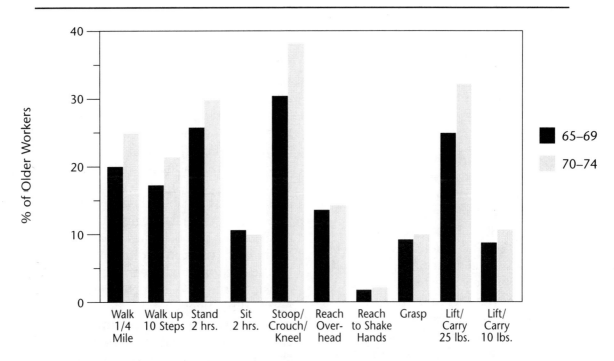

Source: National Health Interview Survey, National Center for Health Statistics, 1987b.

LEISURE

Changes in leisure activities because of aging or disease are difficult to track. Like work activities, leisure activities are also highly individualized. A defining characteristic of leisure is that it is discretionary. Hence, one can choose different activities at different points in one's life caused by changing interests, not capacity. A common set of leisure skills has not been identified for the compilation of disability statistics for leisure activities.

Data from the Duke Longitudinal Studies on Aging (Palmore, 1970, 1981)—one of the few longitudinal research projects to incorporate leisure variables—suggest that participation in social activities declines as people age. However, 17% of the subjects perceived no decline and 32% reported an increase in social activity. Considerably more change has been suggested by

cross-sectional studies. The classic study conducted by Gordon, Gaitz, and Scott (1976) is typical of the cross-sectional studies detecting change. Overall, as the age of the respondent increases, participation in leisure activity decreases. Decline was evident in eight categories of leisure activity:

1. Dancing and drinking
2. Movies
3. Sport and exercise
4. Guns
5. Outdoor activity
6. Travel
7. Reading
8. Cultural productive.

In seven other categories, no change was detected across the five groups spanning young adults (20 to 29), early maturity (30 to 44), full maturity (45 to 64), old age (65 to 74), and very old age

(74 to 94). These categories were

1. Television
2. Discussion
3. Spectator sports
4. Cultural consumption
5. Entertainment
6. Participation in clubs and organizations
7. Home embellishment.

Increased participation over the lifespan groups was observed in two categories, relaxation and solitude, and cooking, the latter for men only. Because cross-sectional studies are unable to separate the effects of aging from those of generation, these results are appropriately referred to as age differences rather than age changes. Overall, the results suggest a tendency to give up leisure activities that are strenuous or conducted outside of the home. Stability or increased participation is seen in activities that are of moderate or low intensity, centered in the home, or more sedentary.

Research then supports considerable continuity in leisure activities. Older adults continue to do what they previously did, except for a decline in activities requiring substantive energy. The leisure participation of men and women exhibits both similarities and differences. Gordon, Gaitz, and Scott (1976) found that throughout the life cycle, men were more involved than women in high intensity activities. No gender differences were ascertained in attending movies, reading, and entertaining friends, whereas participation in cultural consumption fluctuated over the life cycle. In all other activity categories, men were less active than women. Race differences have been found in religious participation, with Blacks being more active in church-related social activities (Arling, 1976). Declines in health have been consis-

tently related to changes in leisure participation (Covey, 1980; Gordon, Gaitz, & Scott, 1973).

IMPLICATIONS FOR OCCUPATIONAL THERAPY

Disability appraisal is a major focus of the occupational therapy evaluation. Activities that older clients are unable to perform or find increasingly difficult to perform become the targets of remedial and compensatory interventions. In the event that improved task performance is not feasible, the provision of care from informal caregivers or health or social services becomes a part of the overall care plan. In addition to disability, the occupational therapy evaluation considers the task competencies retained by older clients. These task competencies need to be enumerated as clearly as the disabilities so that task abilities can be enhanced and protected from overcare. *Overcare* refers to care that exceeds what is actually needed by the impairments of older clients. Eventually, overcare leads to excess disability—disability greater than that warranted by the accumulation of age-related and disease-associated impairments.

Occupational therapy intervention strategies can be directed at the level of occupational performance or the components of occupational performance. Occupational-performance-oriented strategies involve learning or relearning task skills, such as feeding, writing checks, and using the telephone. Because these interventions act directly on task performance skills, routine reassessments document progress or lack of progress attributable to the interventions. Occupational-performance, component-oriented strategies involve exercises in the enablers of task performance, such as range of motion, muscle strength, memory, or assertiveness. Because these interventions only act indirectly on task performance skills, occupational therapy practitioners must monitor the influence that they have on task competence carefully. For example, remedial interventions designed to increase muscle strength might need to be abandoned in favor of compensatory ones, if the increases in strength are insufficient to enable task performance or make it easier.

Activities in the areas of ADL, work and productive activities, and leisure activities constitute the domain of occupational therapy practice. These activities occur against a background of rest and relaxation, which influences the quality of participation in performance areas. Sleep disturbances are common in older adults. Biological aging alters stage duration and quality of sleep. The sleep sequence consists of non-rapid-eye-movement (NREM) and rapid-eye-movement (REM) sleep (Hock & Reynolds, 1986). Non-rapid-eye-movement sleep consists of four stages. As humans age, stages 1 (transition awake to sleep) and 2 (true sleep) increase in quantity, whereas stages 3 (deep sleep) and 4 (deepest NREM sleep) decrease. Rapid-eye-movement sleep occurs as frequently as it did at one's younger ages but the length of each episode decreases. REM sleep is considered important to learning, memory, and adaptation (Hauri, 1982). As a consequence of these biological changes, older adults take longer to fall asleep, awake more often, are sleepy during the day, need longer time to adjust to changes in a sleep-wake schedule, and spend more time in bed (Hock & Reynolds, 1986). Over adulthood and late life, total daily sleep time can decrease by about 1 hour. In addition to these biological changes, sleep can be aggravated by illnesses such as depression, Alzheimer's disease, and arthritis; psychological factors such as widowhood and retirement; and

medications such as hypnotics. In working with older clients, occupational therapy practitioners should be cognizant of the reciprocal relationship between the quality of sleep and the quality of activity. Sleep serves a restorative function. When sleep is inadequate, people are not protected against exhaustion, and the risk of injury could increase. Goals for temporal adaptation in older adults should incorporate sleep hygiene practices, including positioning, nutritional, activities, scheduling, and environmental interventions (Hock & Reynolds, 1986; Lerner, 1982).

ROLES

Activities are linked together by function in social roles. Social status and social roles are complementary concepts. Status refers to a position in a social structure, such as widow or widower. Role refers to the behavioral expectations associated with a role. In the case of widowhood, learning to cope alone again might be a behavioral expectation. Behavioral expectations such as these are normatively determined and can vary from one culture or subculture to another. All societies have age-based role structures.

People occupy many roles at the same time. An older adult can simultaneously be a spouse, parent, grandparent, friend, and a retiree. The configuration of roles shifts continually throughout the life cycle. During late life, role relinquishment is more common than role acquisition. Role transition is the gain or loss of a status. Widowhood and retirement fit this definition. In role change, status is maintained, but behavioral expectations change over time. Parenthood matches this description. Of the many roles occupied by older adults, this section highlights nine:

1. Worker-retiree
2. Leisure participant
3. Volunteer
4. Grandparent
5. Caregiver
6. Widowed person
7. Friend
8. Religious participant
9. Retired homemaker.

Worker-Retiree

Work is more than just a paycheck. Besides providing a means of earning a living, it is a source of personal identity, satisfaction, and social contacts; a focal point for organizing daily life; a means of contributing to society; and a vehicle for conferring social status (Roadburg, 1985). These functions then may be in jeopardy when work is terminated. Most older adults do not work for pay. The proportion of people over age 65 in the work force is estimated to be 12% (American Association of Retired Persons [AARP] & Administration On Aging [AOA], 1990). Maintenance of the worker role in late life is dependent on a host of factors, the most salient of which are job performance capability, desire to continue working, the opportunity to continue working, and work-related policies.

Changes in job performance capability might well be expected in older adults in view of age-related changes, such as decreased visual acuity, presbycusis, decreased reaction time, loss of muscle strength, and decreased speed of decision making. However, the extent to which these declines are evidenced in job performance depends to a considerable extent on the type of work. Most studies of clerical and sales workers have suggested that age has little to do with job performance. Interestingly, a study conducted by the U.S. Department of Labor (Sparrow, 1986) found that the performance of federal mail sorters started to decline at age 25, whereas the performance of older department store salespersons improved with age. In contrast, studies of semiskilled and skilled manual laborers have generally demonstrated improvement in performance until 30 to 40 years of age followed by declines (Clay, 1956; King, 1956). Despite those declines in performance, however, the performance of the older workers exceeded that of the youngest workers. Further examination of age-work performance relationships has suggested that the additional experience that accompanies job longevity can often account for presumed age effects (Schwab & Heneman, 1977). In a study of managerial workers, (Taylor, 1975) found that older managers sought more information before making a decision, thus extending the time needed to reach a decision. Further, because they were less confident about their decisions, they were more flexible about changing them. The link between age and work-performance capabilities of technical and professional workers has been difficult to study because of problems finding or devising adequate measures of job performance. Multiple studies of professionals in various fields have suggested that creativity as evidenced in publications, discoveries, and works of art, tends to peak during early to middle adulthood, depending on the specific field (Simonton, 1990). Strong achievement records can, however, extend into old age. In technical jobs in which pacing is a critical job function, the effects of age have been found. Studies conducted by the U.S. Civil Aeromedical Institute on air traffic controllers have repeatedly demonstrated that older applicants are at a disadvantage (Sparrow, 1986). Overall, the evidence does not support the belief that age influences performance, except in highly stressful jobs where the worker cannot control the pace of work. Generally, declines in job performance capability are more likely due to health declines than age (Roadburg, 1985).

Another critical factor influencing the maintenance of the worker role in late life is personal choice. Some older adults no longer have the desire to work. Retirement is attractive because it enables them to devote more time to their leisure pursuits. The number of older workers choosing to retire has been steadily increasing. Even though the Age Discrimination in Employment Act was amended in 1978 to safeguard work up to age 70 in most occupational groups, the number of older workers in the labor force has not increased. Older workers are opting for early retirement. The average age for taking such retirement options is 58.7 (Meier, 1988). Retirement has become more socially acceptable over the years and increased affluence has made it more feasible.

A desire to continue working in late life must be matched by market opportunities for work. Age discrimination and cutbacks in the labor force can make it difficult for older workers to find or continue employment. When older workers become unemployed, it generally takes them longer to become reemployed than younger workers. Older workers often become discouraged and give up the search for work. Some find the low wages offered in the available service jobs unattractive. Others find the part-time, flexible nature of many of these jobs appealing, because it provides an easy transition to full retirement. In comparison with younger workers, older workers tend to be more concerned about pay, working conditions, and company or agency policies; they are less concerned with advancement, recognition, approval,

and enjoying their work (Rosenfeld & Owens, 1965). Human resources management practices that are particularly useful in assisting older workers to remain on the job are evaluating job performance routinely and giving constructive help, training to update skills, and redesigning jobs to match older workers capabilities and interests. Even when these practices are a part of the management plan, they might not be made available to older workers (Schrank & Waring, 1989).

Company policies are a major factor in continuing employment. Private employers have been offering economic incentives to encourage early retirement. By hiring younger workers, paying them less, and giving them fewer benefits, employers can reduce labor costs. Although the private sector has been discouraging older workers from remaining in the work force, public policy is moving in the direction of encouragement. Mandatory retirement before the age of 70 for most occupations was outlawed in 1978. Beginning in the year 2000, the age for eligibility for full Social Security retirement benefits will gradually rise from 65 to 67 years. By advancing the age of Social Security retirement benefits, individuals contribute to the nation's production longer and draw fewer benefits. Given the declining worker to retiree ratio, it seems that our nation could benefit from workers remaining in the labor force longer.

When retirees were asked what they missed most about work, women indicated contact with supervisors and coworkers, whereas men indicated having something to do, and placed social contacts as a second priority (Roadburg, 1985). Loss of a daily routine and an income were less common responses. In another study, three-fourths of the respondents mentioned that they missed the money and the people at work. Other things missed about work were the work itself, the feeling of being useful, things happening around them, and respect from others (Harris & Associates, Inc., 1975).

Atchley (1976) described adjustment to retirement as taking place in four phases. In the initial or honeymoon phase, the retiree is intensely busy doing things largely precluded by employment, such as taking extended trips or remodeling the house. This phase is followed by a period of disenchantment, in which the retiree copes with the disparity between the expectations for and realities of retirement. Disenchantment is followed by a reorientation phase during which one's life situation is reevaluated, more realistic plans for time use are made, and a new daily routine is established. If adjustment does not occur, disenchantment persists, or the individual can seek to resolve it through reemployment. The termination phase of retirement is entered when the older adult becomes so disabled that independent functioning is no longer possible.

The satisfaction derived from retirement is in large part determined by pre-retirement factors in regard to finances, time use, and health (Schulz & Ewen, 1993). Having the financial means to satisfy one's retirement plans is critical. Retirees who were in higher paying jobs with sufficient retirement benefits will be likely to adjust well to their situation. Those who retired from low-level jobs with poor benefits are apt to encounter financial difficulties. Thus, most of the negative financial consequences commonly attributed to retirement are actually caused by preretirement financial status (Palmore, Fillenbaum, & George, 1984). The situation is similar in reference to time use and health. Those who have satisfying and meaningful leisure involvement before retirement will likely continue it

during the post-retirement years. Those who failed to develop strong leisure strengths over adulthood or in retirement are at risk for boredom and dissatisfaction. Similarly, retirement in and of itself does not negatively influence mental or physical health. Rather, poor health in pre-retirement most likely will continue into the retirement years, and will probably be compounded by further health problems as age advances.

Leisure Participant

Leisure is a highly individualized, discretionary activity (Gordon et al., 1976). People choose to participate in specific leisure activities for a variety of reasons. Functions commonly attributed to leisure are relaxation, diversion (recreation), knowledge, social participation, and creativity (Dumazedier, 1974; Riesman, 1952). Despite the high value attributed to leisure participation in gerontologic literature, there is a lack of research in the psychological benefits that older adults derive from their leisure experiences. In an early investigation, Donald and Havighurst (1959) had older adults identify the meaning of their favorite activities. Meanings that were frequently given included passing the time, an opportunity to achieve something, a chance to be creative, contact with friends, a change from work, and the newness of the experience. Nystrom (1974) found that most older adults defined leisure as pleasant anticipation or recollection. The most frequent uses of leisure were for social interaction or to be a spectator. Whereas workers emphasize leisure as freedom, retirees see it as a relaxing or pleasurable experience (Roadburg, 1985).

One barrier to research on the subjective meaning of leisure is the absence of a taxonomy of psychological benefits associated with leisure participation. A consensus appears to be developing among leisure researchers regarding the significance and comprehensiveness of eight factors for representing the psychological benefits of leisure (Tinsley, Teaff, Colbs, & Kaufman, 1985). These factors are

1. Self-expression
2. Companionship
3. Power
4. Compensation
5. Security (i.e., lack of a long-term commitment)
6. Service
7. Intellectual aestheticism
8. Solitude.

Tinsley and colleagues used these factors to characterize the motivation for 18 leisure activities in a sample of older men and women. Their results, although preliminary, not only provided some interesting perspectives of leisure motivation, but also hold potential for improving leisure programming. For example, older adults who played bingo or cards, or went bowling or dancing reported greater satisfaction of their need for companionship. Low scores on self-expression, companionship, power, security, service, and intellectual aestheticism attached to watching sports or television, were interpreted as forms of temporary escape from dealing with others and oneself. High scores on solitude and security suggested that older adults who raised houseplants, collected photographs or antiques, or read derived satisfaction in these activities from doing something alone without feeling threatened. Craft activities, such as knitting, crocheting, woodworking, and ceramics appeared to satisfy the need to use creative talents and to receive recognition for them. Participation in volunteer and professional service activities as well as attendance

at social and religious organization meetings satisfied the need of participants to be of service to others along with their needs to be in control of social situations and the pleasure of recognition. Picnicking was the only compensatory activity examined; it appeared to represent the need to escape from daily routines. Research such as this is necessary to foster a better understanding of the reasons why older adults engage in specific activities. By matching specific activities to specific psychological benefits a balanced program of leisure services can be developed for older adults, whether they are residing in the community or in institutional settings. As participation in some activities is precluded because of the development of impairments, it may be possible to substitute psychologically equivalent activities.

Although most retirees view leisure favorably, some do not. Roadburg (1985) found that older adults holding negative views of leisure had generally been socialized to see it as a waste of time and to have little meaning in their lives. They were often unable to find satisfactory activities to occupy their time or they preferred to be able to work.

Volunteer

The volunteer role provides a major means for older adults to serve others. Although only a small percentage of older adults perform volunteer work (roughly 22%), many more indicate a desire to do so (Crandall, 1980; Wan, Odell, & Lewis, 1982). This suggests a need for the availability of additional resources for meeting community needs. The major barriers to volunteering are poor health and lack of transportation. Volunteering has been associated with higher income and education, being employed, and being White (Harris & Associates, Inc., 1975).

Predominantly, volunteers are widowed women. Women and men tend to have divergent views of the volunteer role. Women focus on the expressive aspects, whereas men tend to view volunteering as a work substitute (Payne & Whittington, 1976).

Volunteer contributions can be made through a variety of formal and informal channels, including federally sponsored programs, religious groups, civic associations, and community organizations, as well as services and support given to family members and friends. Major services performed by older adults involve working in hospitals; driving the disabled; lobbying; registering voters; providing telephone reassurance for the homebound; and assisting in programs for family, youth, and children (National Council on the Aging, 1975).

Over the past few decades, several federally sponsored volunteer programs have been specifically developed for seniors. The Foster Grandparent Program (one of the oldest of such programs) enables older adults to work with children who have special needs, because of problems like drug and alcohol abuse, mental retardation, illiteracy, juvenile delinquency, and teenage pregnancy. In the similar Senior Companion Program, volunteers attend to adults with special needs, particularly the frail, homebound elderly, and those who reside in nursing homes. Both of these programs focus on the low-income elderly, and participants receive a stipend for their 20 hours of work per week. Volunteers in the Retired Senior Volunteer Program (RSVP) provide services in community centers, courts, schools, hospices, hospitals, and nursing homes. Participants can commit as much time as they wish to RSVP. The Service Corps of Retired Executives (SCORE), supported by the U.S. Small Business Administration,

provides a mechanism for retired executives to consult to small, public, and private sector organizations. In addition to these age-specific programs, seniors constitute about 20% of the Volunteers in Service to America (VISTA) Program, which requires a full-time commitment of 1 year. Seniors also account for about 10% of the Peace Corps. These federally sponsored programs are supplemented by private-sector ventures, including those by the American Association of Retired Persons, the National Council on Aging, and the National Executive Service Corps. Adequate training, careful placement, and meaningful task assignments enhance the effectiveness of volunteer service.

Volunteerism benefits both older adults and society in general. It affords individuals opportunities to use their lifetime experiences and skills to benefit others. In addition, volunteerism contributes to a sense of productivity and personal integrity, which can be particularly beneficial to those coping with losses related to retirement or widowhood (Crandall, 1980). The volunteer contributions of older adults over the past few decades have been instrumental in fostering attitudinal changes—leading younger persons to view older adults as physically and mentally able rather than disabled. Thus, older adults are perceived as service providers not just recipients (Ward, 1979).

Grandparent

Grandparenthood is a potentially important source of gratification for older adults. It affords the opportunity to interact with and enjoy one's grandchildren without the responsibilities of parenthood. The popular saying, "If I had known how much fun grandchildren were, I would have had them first," reflects the view of grandparents having warm, close, and enjoyable relationships with their grandchildren. Grandparenthood is rapidly becoming a role transition of middle age rather than late life, as it is increasingly common to have grandchildren in one's 40s and 50s (Kivnick, 1982). With adults becoming grandparents at a younger age and living longer, today's youth are likely to have some contact with one or more grandparents. About 75% of all older adults have living grandchildren (Peterson, 1989). The modern family often spans three and four generations.

In a classic study of grandparenthood, Neugarten and Weinstein (1964) examined the meaning of the role of the grandparent. The most common meaning attached to grandchildren was biological revitalization or continuity. Other grandparents emphasized that the grandparent-grandchild relationship provided emotional fulfillment. A small percentage stressed that being a grandparent enabled them to be a resource to their grandchildren and to experience vicarious achievement through their grandchildren's accomplishments. Interestingly, almost one-third of the respondents reported that grandparenthood had little effect on either their lifestyles or their personal identities. The respondents in Kivnick's (1982) survey stressed many of these same meanings. They detailed the rewards of indulging one's grandchildren without the burdens of parenthood, sensing immortality contingent to a family line of grandchildren as well as children, being viewed as a valued elder, and recalling pleasurable experiences shared with one's own grandparents.

Other researchers have focused on the reciprocal relationship between grandparents and grandchildren, that is, the ways in which they seek to influence each other. The legacy of grandparents tends to highlight values associated with areas such as religion, work, and social concerns (Cherlin & Furstenberg, 1986; Troll & Bengston, 1979). Grandchildren make their contributions in regard to new technologies (e.g., toys) and cultural styles (e.g., dress). Topics that are apt to lead to conflict are generally avoided by both sides (Hagestad, 1978).

Typically, grandparents do not live in the same household with their grandchildren, although they do have considerable contact with them. It is estimated that about 75% see their grandchildren at least twice a month and about 50% see them every few days (Harris & Associates, Inc., 1975). Interaction between grandparents and grandchildren generally takes place around special events, such as outings to the zoo or movies, telephone calls, or babysitting (Troll, 1980; Wood & Robertson, 1978).

Neugarten and Weinstein (1964) identified five patterns of grandparenting. In the formal style, contact between grandparent and grandchild was highly formal and limited. There was a clear distinction between parental and grandparental responsibilities. This was the most common style of grandparenting and was more frequently adopted by older grandparents (65 years or more). Conversely, the fun-seeking style was informal and focused on the sharing of leisure activities. In the surrogate style, the grandparent, who was usually the grandmother, assumed parental responsibilities in the absence of the mother, as a result of her working or otherwise being unavailable. This style was generally assumed out of necessity rather than by choice, and it was usually initiated by the parent.

In a fourth style, which might best be described as that of being the repository of family wisdom, grandparents viewed themselves as transmitters of information, advice, family traditions, and resources to their grandchildren. This style was the least common and was more characteristic of grandfathers than grandmothers. In the fifth style—the distant figure style—contact between grandparents and their grandchildren was generally limited to ritualistic events, such as birthdays and holidays. The fun-seeking and distant styles were more commonly adopted by younger grandparents below age 65. The variety of grandparenting styles reinforces the informal nature of this role. Because there are few normative guidelines, grandparents are free to develop a style that is congruent with their preferences. Overall, the styles portray grandparents as having relatively limited involvement in the lives of their grandchildren.

Caregiver

The majority of disabled elderly do not live in institutional settings, but rather in the community. Most of them are able to live in the community because they receive help, usually from family members—spouses, adult children, and siblings—who also might be elderly. The family plays a decisive role in warding off or delaying institutionalization (Day, 1985; Doty, 1986). Day (1985) estimated that in about one-third of the families providing care, the extent of care was so great that it was equivalent to a full-time work position. As the number of disabled elderly grows, so too will the number of family caregivers.

Aneshensel and colleagues (Aneshensel, Pearlin, Mullan, Zarit, & Whitlatch, 1995) applied the paradigm of career to the caregiver role. The increasing functional deterioration of the care recipient propels the caregiver through a series of transitions. The career sequence begins with the preparation for the caregiver role and the acquisition of the needed skills. Acceptance of the role is often subtle because initial demands can be very limited and readily incorporated into an individual's daily routines. This pattern is characteristic of caregivers for persons with dementia of the Alzheimer's type. When the need for care is sudden, which often happens with stroke, the caregiver role is assumed abruptly. In the second career stage, care is provided. The first site of care is usually at the home. As the need for care increases, or the caregiver fatigues, a decision to admit the care recipient to a nursing home might be made. Although some caregivers totally relinquish the caregiving role at this point, many others continue to provide care. This care can be in the form of direct hands-on assistance or in the more invisible types of aid, like washing and mending clothing. With the care recipient's death, the third, or postcare stage is entered. The caregiver disengages from the caregiving role and gradually restructures time and reorients activities. Both bereavement and social readjustment take place during this stage. The career analogy highlights the orderly progression from one stage to the next, and the responsibilities and stresses unique to each one.

Primary caregivers are more likely to be women who are also family members. When a married person becomes disabled, the spouse is almost always the caregiver (Aneshensel et al., 1995). The quality of the parent-child relationship influences who accepts the caregiving role. Although affect and obligation are strong motivating forces, they are not the only considerations. Adult children, having greater competing social obligations, such as being employed or being married, or living a distance from the care recipient, are less likely candidates for primary caregiving (Matthews & Rosner, 1988). Hasselkus (1988) identified five organizing themes of meaning regarding the caregiving experience:

1. Sense of self
2. Sense of managing
3. Sense of future
4. Sense of fear or risk
5. Sense of changes in role and responsibility.

The goals of caregiving were conceptualized as getting things done, and achieving a sense of health and well-being for the caregiver and the care recipient (Hasselkus, 1989).

Signs of caregiver stress are manifested in the health decline of the caregiver, a decision to institutionalize the care recipient, abuse or neglect of the care recipient, and conflicts within the caregivers family stemming from the energy given to caregiving. The effects of caregiving can have long-term consequences for caregivers. For example, those who leave the workforce to care for aging parents might not be able to resume the same job or reenter their work at the same level. These individuals will carry this disadvantage with them for the rest of their lives (Aneshensel et al., 1995).

Widowed Person

Widowhood is perceived as highly stressful and disruptive regardless of whether the marital relationship was harmonious or discordant, and regardless of whether death was sudden or preceded by a lengthy illness. Multiple losses, in addition to that of one's spouse, are intrinsic to widowhood. The most significant losses are the loss of an intimate companion, the loss of a partner for work and leisure activities, and the loss of a helper for structuring and organizing time (Glick, Weiss, & Parkes, 1974; Lopata, 1969). In late life, it can be difficult to develop relationships that satisfy these needs. The stress of widowhood is evidenced in the

increased risk of suicide during the first year of bereavement and of a life-threatening illness (Riley & Foner, 1968; Stroebe, Stroebe, Gergen, & Gergen, 1982).

The rate of widowhood is highest for those over 75 years of age. A disproportionate number of women are widowed. Nearly 70% of women over age 75 are widows, whereas only 23% of men in this age group are widowers (U.S. Bureau of the Census, 1975). Thus, widowhood is a predictable crisis for the majority of older women. The feminine characteristic of late-life widowhood reflects the longer longevity of women, as well as their tendency to marry men a little older than themselves. When men are widowed, they are more likely to remarry than women (George, 1980).

Widowhood is typically marked by an intense period of grief. This is followed by a period of adjustment during which the individual gradually develops a new lifestyle (Lopata, 1973). The primary adaptive challenges facing the remaining spouse involve learning to live independently and to successfully reengage with society (Lopata 1973). General coping strategies endorsed by widows are keeping busy and maintaining a sense that time heals all wounds (Glick et al., 1974). Pivotal to adjustment is the extent to which the spousal relationship was couple-oriented (Lopata 1973). More extensive lifestyle and personal identity changes are required by widows and widowers whose daily living activities were closely entwined with those of their spouses. Both genders are somewhat disadvantaged by traditional patterns of sex-role differentiation. For example, women can be unprepared for managing finances, while men might lack skills in housekeeping. Widowed persons receive task-oriented assistance as well as emotional support from others. Children, relatives, and close friends are the chief sources of this support (Glick et al., 1974; Lopata, 1973).

Feelings of loneliness can be especially problematic for widowed individuals. Lopata (1973) found that loneliness was particularly acute at dinnertime, when there was no one to cook for and individuals had to eat alone. Bereavement can be accompanied by feelings of relief, particularly if the marital relationship was stressful or death was preceded by a long illness (Lopata, 1973). If widowhood involves a loss of financial resources, adjustment can be more difficult. Atchley (1975) ascertained that adequate income was the strongest correlate of adjustment.

Most bereaved persons successfully adapt to widowhood. However, some develop serious health problems, such as severe depression, anxiety states, suicide, insomnia, and psychosomatic disorders (Schulz & Ewen, 1993; Stroebe & Stroebe, 1987). Pathological grief differs from normal grief in duration and intensity. Although an exact timetable does not exist, acute grief normally lasts for up to 2 months after death of the spouse, and healthy mourning can last up to 2 years. In pathological grief, acute grief is not resolved and readjustment to living without the loved one does not take place.

Friend

Friendship is based on a relationship that is voluntary, equal, reciprocal, flexible, and emotional (Brown, 1981). The number of friends an individual has appears to remain relatively stable throughout adulthood, with declines occurring in one's mid-70s and 80s (Riley & Foner, 1968). Interestingly, some studies suggest that for older adults, the frequency of contact with close friends, but not with family

members, is significantly related to general life satisfaction (Blau, 1981; Palmore, 1981).

Relatively little research has been conducted on the functions of friendship in late life. Responding to social and emotional needs seems to be particularly important. Support from relatives and friends strengthens an individual's mechanisms for coping with adverse life events, such as widowhood, residential relocation, and illness. However, the loss of long-lasting friends can be devastating. Friends and neighbors can also provide instrumental assistance by providing rides, shoveling snow, or helping in emergencies (Riley & Foner, 1968). Lee (1985) speculated that it can be more difficult for older adults to call on their adult children for help than it is for them to call on a close friend, because the former action might connote greater dependence. Friendships also serve as a vehicle for socialization. For example, a friend can serve as a model for using leisure time, adjusting to retirement, coping with widowhood, or obtaining senior services. The benefits of having friends and social contacts have been repeatedly demonstrated in lower mortality and better mental health (House, Robbins, & Metzner, 1982).

The quality of friendship can be more important than the number of friends. Lowenthal and Haven (1968) demonstrated that a confidant was invaluable for buffering social losses. They also found that such intimate friends were more common among women, married persons, and those of higher socioeconomic status. Whereas wives were the most likely candidates for men's confidants, women often selected their children, other relatives, or friends. Thus, women are less dependent on the marital relationship for emotional support.

Religious Participant

Two questions are of particular relevance in regard to religious participation in late life. The first relates to changes in religious involvement, the second to the association between religion and health. In exploring these questions, the distinction between organized and nonorganized religious activity must be kept in mind. The former considers attendance at formal church services that usually take place outside of the home, whereas the latter includes personal prayer as well as religious feelings.

Evidence from various cultural groups and religious denominations suggests that religious participation remains stable as people age, except for those with serious disabilities, whose attendance at organized religious events declines (Heisel & Faulkner, 1982; Markides, 1983; Ortega, Crutchfield, & Rushing, 1983). Ainlay and Smith (1984) ascertained that decreases in organizational religious activities were offset by increases in nonorganizational ones. Thus, it appears that the salience of religious involvement is maintained in late life.

The question of the relationship between religion and health as people age is more complex than that of age-related religious participation patterns, and the evidence also is somewhat mixed. The findings support positive associations between religious attendance and measures of health, personal adjustment, and life satisfaction in older people (Blazer & Palmore, 1976; Keith, 1979; Markides 1983; Usui, Keil, & Durig, 1985). In marked contrast, religious attitudes and self-rated religiosity are not related to these factors (Blazer & Palmore, 1976; Markides, 1983). More importantly, some evidence suggests that the relationship between nonorganizational involvement and health and well-being can be negative, that is, as nonorganizational religious involvement increases, health and well-being decline (Mindel & Vaughan, 1978). Alternatively, because nonorganizational involvement was greatest among those with the poorest health, it might be that health decline increases personal religious activities. From this viewpoint, recognition of increased frailty can draw an individual to religion in a very personal way.

Retired Homemaker

Housework is work without a paycheck or retirement benefits. Homemakers are often termed the forgotten workers, and this perspective carries into late life (Andre, 1981). As adults age, their work and leisure become more home-centered. As frailty develops, spouses provide in-home care for each other. Housecleaning and the ability to get out and around in the community become primary concerns (Warren, 1974). Adult children, other relatives, and friends gradually take over home-management responsibilities, sharing this perhaps with formal services, such as home-delivered meal services and chore services. The ability to complete home-management activities stands at the interface between community and institutional living. Home-management tasks play a pivotal role in the transition from independent to dependent living. Yet, little is known about the process of relinquishing these role responsibilities, and the meaning of this role transition to elderly homemakers.

IMPLICATIONS FOR OCCUPATIONAL THERAPY

The activities that older adults perform are linked together functionally in social roles. It is the role that provides the underlying and unifying theme for activity performance. The roles one occupies set dimensions for the activities that must be learned or relearned during intervention. Successful role performance involves the competence to perform the needed activities at the appropriate time. Hence, occupational therapy intervention incorporates training in task skills and time-use strategies.

By assessing role behavior, occupational therapy practitioners come to appreciate the diversity of roles enacted by an older client. The trajectory of an older adult's life is characterized by the stability and change that occurs in role responsibilities during late life. Roles might not be equally valued by an older client, and an assessment of roles enables the practitioner to determine the older client's priorities for treatment. As frailty emerges, successful role performance can switch from actually doing an activity to delegating and supervising its completion. By making older clients aware of their capacities, occupational therapy practitioners can assist them in making feasible choices in selecting the activities to retain and those to relinquish.

IMPAIRMENT, DISABILITY, AND TASK ABILITY

An *impairment* is a loss or abnormality of a biological or psychological structure or function (Granger, 1984). As documented in this chapter (see section by Linda Levy), older adults can experience multiple age-related and disease-associated impairments. An impairment may or may not result in a *disability,* that is, a restriction or inability to perform an activity in a normative manner (Granger, 1984). An impairment results in a disability if it becomes severe enough to warrant adaptive behavior, and the older adult fails to develop the necessary adaptive skill. Hence, a one-to-one correspon-

dence between impairments and disability does not occur. Typically, correlations between impairments and task performance are positive, but low to moderate, regardless of whether such impairments are neuropsychological (McCue, Rogers, & Goldstein, 1990) or physical (Badley, Wagstaff, & Wood, 1984). Thus, making inferences about older adults' task performance based on impairment (occupational performance components) measurements is hazardous.

Rather than focusing on declines in task performance, it might be more informative to explore the continuation of competence in late life. More specifically, one might respond to the question, in the presence of multiple impairments, how do older adults maintain their competence in routine tasks? Several skill maintenance strategies do come into play.

One of the strategies is, as the adage warns, "Use it or lose it." Accordingly, continued experience in performing an activity is hypothesized as enabling oneself to retain competence in it. Just as considerable practice is needed to develop competence, so too may be the case for retaining it. For example, if at the first sign of dysfunction in meal preparation skill, meals-on-wheels are provided, a cycle of decline can be triggered that cannot be stopped. Alternatively, by providing opportunities for older adults to develop skills for late-life roles, their adaptive capacity can be strengthened.

A second strategy for maintaining competence is through compensation. Compensation itself can take various forms. One of the first forms of compensation to be used is reducing the speed of task performance. In this way, older adults can still perform many tasks adequately, but they do so at a slower pace. Working slower reflects an increased investment of time in an activity, if not effort. Many older adults report that they continue to perform everyday activities, such as housework, shopping, and money management, but that they do so at a slower pace. A second form of compensation is work simplification. This process enables older adults to continue to be independent in an activity category, such as meal preparation, but the specific way in which the activity is carried out is simplified. The complexity of a five-course meal is replaced by a three-course one, a frozen entree, or a take-out meal. A third form of compensation is substitution. Substitution occurs when a performance component typically used to perform an activity becomes impaired, and a substitutable component replaces it. For example, as visual ability declines, tactile sensation might be substituted for vision so that meal preparation can still be carried out. Similarly, as hearing ability declines, many older adults substitute lip reading for hearing, so that they can continue to socialize. In a fourth form of compensation, referred to as selective optimization (Baltes, Dittmann-Kohli, & Dixon, 1984), older adults reduce the number of activity categories they engage in and target their energies on the remaining activity categories. In essence, they select certain activity categories to the exclusion of others, and compensate by optimizing their performance in the selected domains. The final compensatory form is the use of external aids. When memory begins to fail, it might be more functional to make lists and leave reminders in strategic locations than to try to improve memory skills. Similarly, when physical and mental energies fatigue, reliance on others for assistance becomes a viable alternative (Dixon, 1995).

Compensation provides a useful strategy for older adults to maintain a sense of control over their lives. It allows them to make decisions about how they invest their time and energies. Equally as important, compensation enables older adults to make arrangements for allocating control of some activities to others. They continue to make decisions even though someone else might implement them. In this way, they still have control over their activities. There is a plethora of research that supports the positive health effects of an enhanced sense of control for older adults. Occupational therapy interventions should be designed to foster and guide choice. To the extent possible, older adults with disabilities should be in charge of negotiating any needed support.

Activities

1. From the Case Studies, compare Mrs. G's time use, performance in activity areas, and role performance to the normative patterns suggested in this section.

2. Liking for an activity has been associated with personal adjustment. Mr. B, who retired from IBM 13 months ago, was admitted to an acute psychiatric unit for treatment of major depression. He was employed as a middle manager and indicates that the only thing that he likes to do is work. Suggest a strategy for getting Mr. B engaged in a meaningful role.

Case Studies

CASE STUDY 1

Mrs. G is 86 years old and married. On a typical day in June, she arises at 7:30 a.m. Mrs. G spends 20 minutes toileting, sponge bathing, and getting dressed. She fixes breakfast for herself and her husband while listening to the morning news on the radio. She joins her husband for breakfast and then spends about 45 minutes talking with him. Around 9:00 a.m., Mrs. G starts her housework—washing the breakfast dishes, tidying up the kitchen, making the beds, and paying the bills. She is interrupted by the mailperson, who hands her the mail and asks how she and her husband are doing. Around 10:45 a.m., Mrs. G prepares lunch and gets ready to go shopping with her daughter. She leaves the house at 11:15 a.m., shops for groceries for the next 2 hours, and returns home at about 2:00 p.m. After helping her husband with the groceries, she takes a nap around 2:30 p.m. Mrs. G arises at 3:30 p.m. and listens to an audiotape novel while she crochets. At 4:15 p.m., she prepares dinner and listens to music on tape. She spends 45 minutes fixing dinner; she and her husband eat as they watch the evening news. While her husband cleans up after the evening meal, she telephones her sister and daughter. At 6:30 p.m., Mrs. G joins her husband in the TV room for game shows. After these are over, she reads the newspaper. At 9:15 p.m., Mrs. G assists her husband in taking a bath, managing his medications, and getting ready for bed. After Mr. G retires at 10:00 p.m., she listens to the audiotape novel and sews a button on a coat. She gets sleepy at 10:30 p.m. and checks to make sure that the doors are locked and that the night lights are working. Mrs. G is in bed before 11:00 p.m.

CASE STUDY 2

Mrs. G, who was introduced earlier, is independent and safe and has adequate performance standards for all ADL. She goes to a beautician for hair care. Because of low vision caused by cataracts and macular degeneration and osteoarthritis, she exercises caution when walking. She is also independent in IADL, with the exception of community transportation and heavy housekeeping. Mrs. G has been unable to drive for 5 years and is dependent on relatives and friends for rides (her husband is also no longer able to drive). She routinely goes out at least three times a week to shop for food, get her hair washed, and attend church services. Financial management, shopping, watching television, and crocheting are the most difficult activities for Mrs. G. To aid her visual functioning, she uses a magnifier illuminated by a halogen bulb. Mrs. G also uses enlarged checks with raised lettering, enlarged dials or orange raised dots on equipment controls, and has a talking clock. She is retired from her position as an office manager. Mrs. G listens to books on tape, browses through the newspaper, crochets, and volunteers at the local hospital. She has an extensive social network and maintains frequent contact with her children, sisters, cousins, in-laws, and friends by telephone.

CASE STUDY 3

Mrs. G, introduced earlier in this section, retired from her position as an office manager 22 years ago at the age of 64. She had worked since the age of 14 until deciding that she wanted to spend more time at home. Mrs. G was in good health on retirement, and she and her husband had adequate savings to live comfortably.

Presently, Mrs. G's primary productive role is that of homemaker. Having worked outside the home throughout adulthood, she has always employed a housekeeper 1 day per week for major cleaning. She continues to supplement these services, but spreads heavier tasks out over the week. Some activities, like laundering clothes and running the dishwasher, are done less frequently now that her two children are on their own. Other activities, like check writing and managing the mail, are done at a slower pace because of her visual impairment. Mrs. G's move, 12 years ago, from an upstairs apartment to a ranch style house, has made tasks like carrying out the garbage and doing laundry easier for her. Her principal leisure activities are watching game shows on television (she sits within 12 inches of the screen); listening to audiotape books; reading the newspaper, giving particular attention to the headlines, obituaries, and food advertisements; clipping food coupons out of the paper; and visiting with her daughters, relatives, and friends over the telephone. Reading is extremely slow for Mrs. G because she must use a handheld magnifier. Hence, she no longer reads the newspaper from cover to cover, or reads books and magazines. The time spent watching television and crocheting has also declined as her visual impairment has increased. Mrs. G views her leisure activities as a means of keeping busy and helping others (e.g., making crocheted items for family members or the church bazaar). She has been a volunteer at the community hospital for over 40 years. During the majority of these years, Mrs. G has worked as a clerk in the gift shop. She has reduced her volunteer hours from 1 day per week to 1 day per month, because she is uncomfortable leaving her husband alone during the day and has difficulty getting to the hospital. Mrs. G views volunteering as a particularly important way of staying in contact with her friends. She attends church services every Sunday; she feels that one advantage of her relocation is that she can now walk to church, something that would have been impossible in her previous residence.

Mrs. G celebrated her 62nd wedding anniversary this year. She became a grandmother in her late 40s and has three adult grandchildren. They visit for birthdays and holidays and are also available to assist with chores. When her grandchildren were young, she babysat them frequently, taught them craft activities, and assisted with homework. Mrs. G became a caregiver for her own parents when they were in their late 70s; she was almost 60 years old. She now looks after her husband, who continues to undergo rehabilitation for a hip fracture. Mrs. G and her husband developed an extensive network of friends through their paid work, volunteer work, and organizational activities, including church and community service groups, parent groups, and Girl Scouts. Many of her close friends are now widows; she does not see them as often as she used to because they no longer attend dinners and other social events that are couples-oriented. However, they maintain weekly contact by telephone. Besides her husband, Mrs. G's closest friend is her sister, but she also feels that there are some things that are not to be discussed outside of one's home.

References

Ainlay, S. C., & Smith, D. R. (1984). Aging and religious participation. *Journal of Gerontology, 39,* 357–363.

Altergott, K. (1988). Social action and interaction in later life: Aging in the United States. In K. Altergott (Ed.), *Daily life in later life: Comparative perspectives* (pp. 117–146). Newbury Park, CA: Sage.

American Association of Retired Persons (AARP) & Administration on Aging (AOA). (1990). *A profile of older Americans.* Washington, DC: AARP.

American Occupational Therapy Association. (1994). Uniform terminology for occupational therapy (3rd ed.). *American Journal of Occupational Therapy, 48,* 1047–1054.

Andre, R. (1981). *Homemakers: The forgotten workers.* Chicago, IL: The University of Chicago Press.

Aneshensel, C. S., Pearlin, L. I., Mullan, J. T., Zarit, S. H., & Whitlatch, C. J. (1995). *Profiles in caregiving: The unexpected career.* San Diego, CA: Academic Press.

Arling, G. (1976). Resistance to isolation among elderly widows. *International Journal of Aging and Human Development, 7,* 67–86.

Atchley, R. C. (1975). Dimensions of widowhood in later life. *The Gerontologist, 15,* 175–178.

Atchley, R. C. (1976). *The sociology of retirement.* New York: Halsted.

Badley, E. M., Wagstaff, S., & Wood, P. H. N. (1984). Measures of functional ability (disability) in arthritis in relation to impairment of range of joint movement. *Annals of the Rheumatic Diseases, 43,* 563–569.

Baltes, P. B., Dittmann-Kohli, F., & Dixon, R. A. (1984). New perspectives on the development of intelligence in adulthood: Toward a dual-process conception and a model of selective optimization with compensation. In P. B. Baltes & O. G. Brim (Eds.), *Life-span development and behavior* (Vol. 6, pp. 33–76). San Diego, CA: Academic Press.

Blau, Z. S. (1981). *Aging in a changing society* (2nd ed.). New York: Franklin Watts.

Blazer, D., & Palmore, E. (1976). Religion and aging in a longitudinal panel. *Gerontologist, 16,* 82–85.

Brown, B. B. (1981). A life-span approach to friendship: Age-related dimensions of an ageless relationship. In H. Lopata & D. Maines (Eds.), *Research on the interweave of social roles:* (Vol. 2. pp. 23–50). Greenwich, CT: JAI Press.

Cherlin, A., & Furstenberg, F. F. (1986). *The new American grandparent: A place in the family apart.* New York: Basic Books.

Clay, H. M. (1956). Study of performance in relation to age at two printing works. *Journal of Gerontology, 11,* 417–424.

Covey, H. C. (1980). An exploratory study of the acquisition of a college student role by old people. *Gerontologist, 20,* 173–181.

Crandall, R. C. (1980). *Gerontology: A behavioral science approach.* Reading, MA: Addison-Wesley.

Day, A. T. (1985). Who cares? Demographic trends challenge family care for the elderly. *Population Trends and Public Policy, 9,* 1–17.

Dixon, R. A. (1995). Promoting competence through compensation. In L. A. Bond, S. J. Cutler, & A. Grams (Eds.), *Promoting successful and productive aging* (pp. 220–238). Thousand Oaks, CA: Sage.

Donald, M. N., & Havighurst, R. T. (1959). The meaning of leisure. *Social Forces, 37,* 355–360.

Doty, P. (1986). Family care of the elderly: The role of public policy. *Milbank Quarterly, 64,* 34–75.

Dumazedier, J. (1974). *Sociology of leisure.* New York: Elsevier.

Field, D., Schaie, K. W., & Leino, E. V. (1988). Continuity in intellectual functioning: The role of self-reported health. *Psychology and Aging, 3,* 385–392.

Fillenbaum, G. C. (1987). Development of a brief, internationally usable screening instrument. In G. L. Maddox & E. W. Busse (Eds.), *Aging: The universal human experience* (pp. 328–334). New York: Springer.

Fries, J. F. (1980). Aging, natural death, and the compression of morbidity. *New England Journal of Medicine, 303,* 130–135.

Fries, J. F. (1984). The compression of morbidity: Miscellaneous comments about a theme. *Gerontologist, 24,* 354–359.

George, L. K. (1980). *Role transitions in later life.* Monterey, CA: Brooks/ Cole.

Glick, I. O., Weiss, R. D., & Parkes, C. M. (1974). *The first year of bereavement.* New York: Wiley.

Gordon, C., Gaitz, C. M., & Scott, J. (1973). Value priorities and leisure activities among middle-aged and older Anglos. *Diseases of the Nervous System, 34,* 13–26.

Gordon, C., Gaitz, C. M., & Scott, J. (1976). Leisure and lives: Personal expressivity across the life span. In R. H. Binstock & E. Shanas (Eds.), *Handbook of aging and the social sciences* (pp. 310–341). New York: Van Nostrand Reinhold.

Gorman, K. M., & Posner, J. D. (1988). Benefits of exercise in old age. *Clinics in Geriatric Medicine, 4,* 181–192.

Granger, C. V. (1984). A conceptual model for functional assessment. In C. V. Granger & G. E. Gresham (Eds.), *Functional assessment in rehabilitation medicine* (pp. 14–25). Baltimore, MD: Williams and Wilkins.

Hagestad, G. (1978). Patterns of communication and influence between grandparents and grandchildren in a changing society. Paper presented at the World Congress of Sociology, Sweden.

Harris, L., & Associates, Inc. (1975). *The myth and reality of aging in America.* Washington, DC: National Council on Aging.

Hasselkus, B. R. (1988). Meaning in family caregiving: Perspectives on caregiver/professional relationships. *Gerontologist, 28,* 686–690).

Hasselkus, B. R. (1989). The meaning of daily activity in family caregiving for the elderly. *The American Journal of Occupational Therapy, 43,* 649–656.

Hauri, P. (1982). *Current concepts: The sleep disorders* (2nd ed.). Kalamazoo, MI: Upjohn.

Heisel, M. A., & Faulkner, A. O. (1982). Religiosity in an older black population. *Gerontologist, 22,* 354–358.

Hock, C., & Reynolds, C. (1986). Sleep disturbances and what to do about them. *Geriatric Nursing,* 24–27.

House, J. S., Robbins, C., & Metzner, H. L. (1982). The association of social relationships and activities with mortality: prospective evidence from the Tecumseh Community Health Study. *American Journal of Epidemiology, 116,* 123–140.

Keith, P. M. (1979). Life changes and perceptions of life and death among older men and women. *Journal of Gerontology, 34,* 870–878.

Kielhofner, G. (1977). Temporal adaptation: A conceptual framework for occupational therapy. *American Journal of Occupational Therapy, 31,* 235–242.

King, H. F. (1956). An attempt to use production data in the study of age and performance. *Journal of Gerontology, 11,* 410–416.

Kivnick, H. Q. (1982). Grandparenthood: An overview of meaning and mental health. *Gerontologist, 22,* 59–66.

Kramer, M. (1980). The rising pandemic of mental disorders and associated chronic diseases and disabilities. *Acta Psychiatrica Scandinavica, 62,* 382–397.

LaPlante, M. (1989). *Disability in basic life activities across the life span.* Disability Statistics Report, No. 1. San Francisco: Institute for Health and Aging, University of California.

LaPlante, M. P., Rice, D. P., & Kraus, L. E. (1991). *Disability statistics abstract. People with activity limitations in the United States.* San Francisco: Institute for Health and Aging, University of California.

Lawton, M. P., & Brody, E. M. (1969). Assessment of older people: Self-maintaining and instrumental activities of daily living. *The Gerontologist, 9,* 179–186.

Lawton, M. P., Moss, M., & Fulcomer, M. (1986–87). Objective and subjective uses of time by older people. *International Journal of Aging and Human Development, 24* (3), 171–187.

Lee, G. R. (1985). Kinship and social support of the elderly: The case of the United States. *Aging and Society, 5,* 19–38.

Lerner, R. (1982). Sleep loss in the aged: Implications for nursing practice. *Journal of Gerontological Nursing, 8,* 323–326.

Lopata, H. Z. (1969). Loneliness: Forms and composition. *Social Problems, 17,* 248–262.

Lopata, H. Z. (1973). *Widowhood in an American city.* Cambridge, MA: Schenkman Publishing.

Lowenthal, M., & Haven, C. (1968). Interaction and adaptation: Intimacy as a critical variable. *American Sociological Review, 33,* 20–30.

Manton, K. G. (1982). Changing concepts of morbidity and mortality in the elderly population. *Health and Society, 60,* 183–244.

Markides, K. S. (1983). Aging, religiosity, and adjustment: A longitudinal analysis. *Journal of Gerontology, 38,* 621–625.

Matthews, S. H., & Rosner, T. T. (1988). Shared filial responsibility: The family as the primary caregiver. *Journal of Marriage and Family, 50,* 185–195.

McBride, T. (1989). *Measuring the disability of the elderly: Empirical analysis and projections into the 21st century.* Washington, DC: The Urban Institute.

McCue, M., Rogers, J. C., & Goldstein, G. (1990). Relationships between neuropsychological and functional assessment in elderly neuropsychiatric patients. *Rehabilitation Psychology, 35,* 91–99.

McKinnon, A. L. (1992). Time use for self care, productivity, and leisure among elderly Canadians. *Canadian Journal of Occupational Therapy, 59,* 102–110.

Meier, E. L. (1988). Survey of retirees from early retirement incentive programs. (Issue Brief). Washington, DC: Public Policy Institute, American Association of Retired Persons.

Meyer, A. (1922). The philosophy of occupational therapy. *Archives of Occupational Therapy, 1,* 1–10.

Mindel, C. H., & Vaughan, C. E. (1978). A multidimensional approach to religiosity and disengagement. *Journal of Gerontology, 33,* 103–108.

Moss, M., & Lawton, M. P. (1982). The time budgets of older people: A window on four lifestyles. *Journal of Gerontology, 37,* 115–123.

National Center for Health Statistics (NCHS). (1987a). *Aging in the eighties: Abilities to perform work-related activities.* (Advance Data No. 136; DHHS No. [PHS] 87–1250). Hyattsville, MD: U.S. Public Health Service.

National Center for Health Statistics (NCHS). (1987b). *Aging in the eighties: Functional limitations of individuals 65 years and older* (Advance Data No. 133). Washington, DC: U.S. Government Printing Office.

National Council on the Aging. (1975). *The myth and reality of aging in America.* Washington, DC: Author.

Neugarten, B. L., & Weinstein, K. (1964). The changing American grandparent. *Journal of Marriage and the Family, 26,* 199–204.

Nouri, F. M., & Lincoln, N. B. (1987). An extended activities of daily living scale for stroke patients. *Clinical Rehabilitation, 1,* 301–305.

Nystrom, E. P. (1974). Activity patterns and leisure concepts among the elderly. *The American Journal of Occupational Therapy, 28,* 337–345.

Ortega, S. T., Crutchfield, R. D., & Rushing, W. A. (1983). Race differences in elderly personal well-being: Friendship, family, and church. *Research on Aging, 5,* 101–118.

Palmore, E. (1970). The effects of aging on activities and attitudes. In E. Palmore (Ed.), *Normal aging: Reports from the Duke longitudinal study, 1955–1969* (pp. 332–341). Durham, NC: Duke University Press.

Palmore, E. (1981). *Social patterns in normal aging: Findings from the Duke longitudinal study.* Durham, NC: Duke University Press.

Palmore, E., Fillenbaum, G. G., & George, L. K. (1984). Consequences of retirement. *Journal of Gerontology, 39,* 109–116.

Payne, B., & Whittington, F. (1976). Older women: An examination of popular stereotypes and research evidence. *Social Problems, 23,* 488–504.

Peterson, E. T. (1989). Grandparenting. In S. J. Bahr & E. T. Peterson (Eds.), *Aging and the family* (pp. 157–174). Lexington, MA: Lexington.

Reed, K., & Sanderson, S. (1983). *Concepts in occupational therapy* (2nd ed.). Baltimore, MD: Williams and Wilkins.

Riegel, K., & Riegel, R. M. (1972). Development, drop and death. *Developmental Psychology, 6,* 306–319.

Riesman, D. (1952). Some observations on changes in leisure activities. *The Antioch Review, 12,* 417–436.

Riley, M., & Foner, A. (1968). *Aging and society. Vol. 1: An inventory of research findings.* New York: Russell Sage Foundation.

Riley, M. W., & Bond, K. (1983). Beyond ageism: Postponing the onset of disability. In M. W. Riley, B. B. Hess, & K. Bond (Eds.), *Aging in society: Selected reviews of recent research* (pp. 243–252). Hillsdale, NJ: Erlbaum.

Roadburg, A. (1985). *Aging: Retirement, leisure and work in Canada.* Toronto: Methuen Publications.

Rogers, J. C., & Holm, M. B. (1994). Assessment of self-care. In B. R. Bonder & M. B. Wagner (Eds.), *Functional performance in older adults* (pp. 181–202). Philadelphia: F. A. Davis.

Rosenfeld, M., & Owens, W. A. (1965). *The intrinsic and extrinsic aspects of work and their demographic correlates.* Paper presented at the Midwestern Psychological Association, Chicago.

Schrank, H. T., & Waring, J. M. (1989). Older workers: Ambivalence and interventions. *Annals of the American Academy of Political and Social Science, 503,* 113–126.

Schulz, R., & Ewen, R. B. (1993). *Adult development and aging: Myths and emerging realties* (2nd ed.). New York: Macmillan.

Schwab, D. P., & Heneman, H. G. (1977). Effects of age and experience on productivity. *Industrial Gerontology, 4,* 113–117.

Simonton, D. K. (1990). Creativity and wisdom in aging. In J. E. Birren & K. W. Schaie (Eds.), *Handbook of the psychology of aging* (3rd ed., pp. 320–329). New York: Academic Press.

Slagle, E. C. (1922). Training aides for mental patients. *Archives of Occupational Therapy, 1,* 11–16.

Sparrow, P. R. (1986). Job performance among older workers. *Ageing International, 13,* 5–6, 22.

Stroebe, W., & Stroebe, M. S. (1987). *Bereavement and health.* Cambridge, England: Cambridge University Press.

Stroebe, W., Stroebe, M. S., Gergen, K. J., & Gergen, M. (1982). The effects of bereavement on mortality: A social psychological analysis. In J. R. Eiser (Ed.), *Social psychology and behavioral medicine* (pp. 527–560). New York: Wiley.

Taylor, R. N. (1975). Age and experience as determinants of managerial decision-making performance. *Academy of Management Journal, 18,* 74–81.

Tinsley, H. E. A., Teaff, J. D., Colbs, S. L., & Kaufman, N. (1985). A system of classifying leisure activities in terms of the psychological benefits of participation reported by older persons. *Journal of Gerontology, 40,* 172–178.

Troll, L. E. (1980). Grandparenting. In L. W. Poon (Ed.), *Aging in the 1980s: Psychological issues* (pp. 475–481). Washington, DC: American Psychological Association.

Troll, L. E., & Bengston, V. (1979). Generations in the family. In W. Burr, R. Hill, F. I. Nye, & I. Reiss (Eds.), *Contemporary theories about the family* (pp. 127–161). New York: Free Press.

Usui, W. M., Keil, T. J., & Durig, K. R. (1985). Socioeconomic comparisons and life satisfaction of elderly adults. *Journal of Gerontology, 40,* 110–114.

U.S. Bureau of the Census (1975). *Current population reports* (Series P–20, No. 287). Washington, DC: U.S. Government Printing Office.

Wan, T. T. H., Odell, B. G., & Lewis, D. T. (1982). *Promoting the well-being of the elderly: A community diagnosis.* New York: Haworth Press.

Ward, R. A. (1979). The meaning of voluntary association participation to older people. *Journal of Gerontology, 34,* 438–445.

Warren, H. H. (1974). Self-perceptions of independence among urban elderly. *American Journal of Occupational Therapy, 28,* 329–336.

Wood, V., & Robertson, J. F. (1978). Friendship and kinship interaction: Differential effects on the morale of the elderly. *Journal of Marriage and the Family, 40.*

Section 6.
Social Roles and Handicaps: The Performance Context

K. Oscar Larson, MA, OTR

Abstract

The authors introduce concepts about how aging adults continue social roles or experience handicaps in the performance contexts of the physical, cultural, and social environments.

Introduction

"Handicap Ramp," "Handicap Bus," and "Handicap Bathroom" are common labels in public places today. But, how do these objects differ—in design, use, and perception—from a ramp, bus, and bathroom? The World Health Organization defines a handicap as the disadvantages that someone who has a disability or impairment experiences in fulfilling a normal life role (WHO, 1980). These disadvantages occur on a systems level. In terms of occupational therapy, handicaps can be viewed in the physical, cultural, and social environments.

In many architectural designs, the first item above, the handicap ramp, appears to be an afterthought. The ramp can be set off to the side, concealed behind landscaping or walls, or blatantly tacked onto an existing set of stairs. An entryway is considered grand when steps rise from the street level to the portico. A rise from one level to another has grace when a curved staircase sweeps up and around. A front porch becomes quaint when steps creak as one walks up to sit on the porch swing. In contrast, a ramp is utilitarian. Ramps enable the masses to pass into train stations. Ramps move cargo into the storage rooms. Ramps are what one finds between levels of a parking garage.

How often have people using a ramp—whether because of using a wheelchair, cane, or baby stroller—found themselves separated from the rest of the people entering a building? They enter a side door, find themselves at the back of the building, or pass through the "Employees Only" area, which rarely has the same atmosphere as the rest of the building.

On the one hand, one could argue that at least they have access, which a decade ago they might not have had. Yet advocates of universal design and the independent-living movements would argue that we would all benefit from environments that encourage people of all levels of ability to function in their communities. (Reed, 1995). Changing the physical environment is only the beginning to changing the attitudes that lead to cultural and social handicaps. This section will briefly address some of the issues that older adults face each day as they go about their daily routines in the physical, cultural, and social environments.

Physical Environment

The most basic question a person should ask when contemplating the physical environment is what constitutes the older adult's physical environment. The answer will vary, of course, with each individual, but, for the most part, people age in the same environments in which they have lived most of their adult lives: home; work; church, synagogue, or mosque; stores and shopping malls; streets; freeways; parking lots; and places of recreation and entertainment (e.g., museums, theaters, beaches, casinos, mountains, golf courses, the porch). A few environments where older adults might spend more time than they did before revolve around their health and medical conditions: doctor's offices, hospitals, and nursing homes. Yet the majority of older people live and want to live in their own communities (Novack, 1995).

Environmental barriers in the home and community can lead to handicaps for the aging person by

1. Increasing social isolation

2. Fostering stereotypes and stigma against aging

3. Increasing the effort and risk to do tasks

4. Requiring that the aging perform tasks differently from others involved.

Conversely, environmental adaptations can reduce the experience of handicaps by

1. Increasing social contact

2. Reducing the preconceived ideas that others develop about aging adults

3. Reducing the effort and risk involved in doing tasks

4. Allowing all participants in a task to use the environment in a similar manner.

The following examples illustrate how the physical environment can contribute to or reduce handicaps. This is not a comprehensive list of either problems or solutions. Other chapters of this text will describe environmental barriers and adaptations in greater depth.

Isolation

A home can be either a refuge or a prison for an aging person. In either case, the older person is likely to spend more time at home and be more isolat-

ed from others. Those people in urban or suburban areas can find that the neighborhood has changed significantly, with familiar people moving away and community resources changing. They could be used to chatting with neighbors and running errands at certain stores. But, as those people and places are replaced, the older resident can have fewer social contacts and might lack a sense of security about going out. In rural areas, the distance between homes, the hazards of walking on uneven surfaces (e.g., stairs, unpaved driveways), and a limited number of places for people to congregate, could discourage older adults from venturing far from home. In urban, suburban, and rural settings, American society's sense of space has changed over several generations, with few homes having enough space for multigenerational households. People are less likely to move in with children or relatives as they age.

Technology and changing expectations about living environments offer opportunities for reducing the isolating effects of staying in the home environment. Telephones, television, radio, newspapers, and computers (see box on next page) allow those who spend more time at home to have access to family, friends, and information. Multiunit senior housing, assisted-living facilities, and shared homes allow aging people to congregate, having closer proximity to others who will use similar resources (Lord, 1995; Wechsler-Linden, 1994). Residents can have a greater sense of security by establishing relationships with neighbors, meeting for meals and social events in common dining and recreation areas.

Environmental and transportation barriers in the community can increase the older adult's sense of isolation. Stores with steps at the entryway, crowded merchandise aisles, and few

Cyberspace for Seniors!

Computers have become readily available during the later years of most older adult's careers. For those who have an interest in and access to computers, recent developments in on-line services give them access to other computer users in cyberspace. A study being conducted at Westchester University, in which nursing home residents have been provided with computer access to the on-line service Prodigy, has gathered preliminary data that indicate that the user's depression scores decreased and cognitive abilities increased (Noer, 1995). Below is a listing of some resources of interest to the senior cybernaut.

Elders Group
E-mail Patricia Davidson at patd@chatback.demon.co.uk

SeniorNet
http://www.seniornet.org
(800) 747-6848

Apple Computer's Worldwide Disability Solutions
(800) 776-2333

OutSpoken (text-to-speech software package)
http://access.becksys.com
(510) 883-6280

Senior Computer Information Project (funded by the Canadian Government)
http//www.crm.mb.ca/scip/

Senate Special Committee on Aging (United States Government)
http://policy.net/capweb/Senate/SenateCom/AGING.tml

Social Security Home Page
http://www.ssa.gov

Administration on Aging (United States Government)
gopher.os.dhhs.gov/DHHS-Resources by Organization/
Administration on Aging.

Source: Noer, 1995.

resting places can tax a person's endurance on a shopping trip. Workplaces that do not or cannot accommodate changes in the person's physical endurance can become inaccessible, encouraging the person who values his or her worker role to retire. Entertainment establishments and restaurants without parking facilities, or with parking lots that have narrowly spaced parking places, can prevent older patrons from parking close enough to warrant going out for recreation and meals. Narrow streets and small street signs make it difficult for older drivers to negotiate. Impatient drivers might intimidate older drivers. Some aging people will forego, or limit, their excursions away from home rather than try to overcome these hazards.

Responding to legislation and consumer demands, many public places are providing more accessible public environments. Many entrances now have automatic doors and sloped entrances. Shopping malls have started mall walker clubs, encouraging older adults to come out during morning hours, get some exercise, socialize with friends and, of course, shop a bit, when the malls are less crowded. Some transportation departments have made entrances more visible by using larger signs, traffic lights, and left-turn lanes.

Visual and auditory impairments are likely to interfere with older adults' ability to communicate as well as they have for most of their lives. The aging person could be less aware of sensory cues because of decreased acuity and difficulty distinguishing between important sights or sounds and glare or background noise. The person might perceive that he or she should be responding to someone, but respond in an irrelevant manner, such as answering a question incorrectly. In severe situations of sensory deprivation, the person can experience illusions or hallucinations in which misinterpretations or internal sensory stimuli substitute for actual stimuli. With visual or auditory sensory loss, the person can become more isolated and feel more vulnerable. The loss of familiar sensory cues can reduce the person's sense of security and competence to the point at which he or she becomes reluctant to go out into the community to run errands, carry out work and leisure tasks, or visit with family and friends.

Many charitable organizations exist in the community, some on the national level, such as Recordings for the Blind and Dyslexic (located at 20 Roszel Road, Princeton, NH 08540-9983), and some on the local level, such as civic or religious groups that provide eyeglasses and hearing aids to low-income citizens. More employers and physicians include basic vision and hearing screening as part of regular physical examinations. More books, magazines, and newspapers are offering text in large print or audiotape versions. Technology, ranging from low tech magnifying glasses or high tech computer-enlarged text and voice-

synthesized page scanners, are available on the market.

Stereotyping and Stigma

People can develop and hold prejudices against aging adults because of the appearance of their homes, their decreased ability to negotiate roads and buildings in the community, and their decreased ability to communicate because of sensory losses. Comments such as "they should be put out to pasture," "get the old biddy off the road," and "that crazy old woman down the street" express the younger person's assessment and attitude toward the aging person as someone who is obsolete, annoying, and odd.

Homes of older persons might stand out in the neighborhood. They might not be considered fashionable as the style in which they were built has changed. They might not be as well maintained because of the aging person's reduced physical stamina, decreased awareness of needed repairs, or lack of funds to hire someone to do yard and housework. Inside, the scents of years of living, as well as of collecting books, photographs, and clothes can mingle with the odors of cooking, bathing, and possibly defecating if the person has had difficulty with continence. Some older adults live in homes filled with evidence of years of living. Others live in disarray as short-term memories fade to confusion. And still others live in sparse, impoverished surroundings. Family, friends, health care professionals, apartment managers, and others who might come to an older person's home will have different degrees of comfort, acceptance, and prejudice toward the presentation of the older person's home.

Aging people often benefit from environmental adaptations and assistive technology that in the community carry a stigma of being different from others. As noted before, special ramp entrances physically separate people using the ramp from the rest of the people who move through the usual entrance. People using a handrail on stairs or a grab bar in a bathroom can be viewed as taking up more space and time than others. People using a lower counter height at a bank or office could be viewed as cumbersome (especially if they come in a wheelchair or request a chair to sit in during the transaction, thereby requiring more time from the employee, and lengthening the wait of other customers). People stepping up to the front of the line at an airplane or train to receive assistance for their "special needs" might be seen as slothful and freeloading (or at least slowing down everyone else who is in a hurry to get settled in).

Devices that help aging people communicate often mark them as different. Some people with whom the older person communicates might treat him or her with pity or disgust. How often does a younger person speak loudly, or even yell, at an older person who wears glasses, assuming that they cannot hear well, either? Or what about the puzzled looks young people have when they hear the whistling of a hearing aid turned up too loudly? What bionic images come to mind when a younger person talks with a person who uses a voice synthesizer after a laryngectomy (especially after the images of character Darth Vader's respirator and synthesized voice in the movie "Star Wars")?

Stereotyping and stigma never have been easy to overcome. If our general society's experiences offer hope, these prejudices should diminish with much education, personal exposure to people of various abilities, and many years of advocacy. With the graying of America, our fears about aging will come closer

to our lives (alas, we all are aging right now!). Yet, some popular images are offering new ways of conceptualizing older adults. Movies like "Cocoon," "Driving Miss Daisy," and "On Golden Pond"; television shows like "Golden Girls"; "Murder, She Wrote"; and "Matlock"; and magazines like *Modern Maturity* and *New Choices* offer different images of aging and relationships with older adults.

PHYSICAL EFFORT AND RISK

"When we get old, we'll move to a place without stairs" was the response a colleague recently gave me as we discussed her plans to buy a new home. She had her mind made up that she wanted a split-level home with the bedrooms and bathrooms upstairs, kitchen, living room, and dining room on the middle level, and recreation room and laundry area below. I tried to persuade her to seek a new home that had at least one bedroom and bathroom on the ground level. Working in an acute-care hospital, with many older adults who have difficulty managing in their own homes, I expected that I could educate her about the advantages of looking at a more accessible home now. She did not perceive a need to consider floor plans and doorways, beyond her sense of aesthetics. She did not see herself as aging. She is in her late 50s, has grown children and grandchildren, a husband who has retired early because of disability, and complains of being short of breath if she has to climb a flight of stairs.

Many aspects of the home environment are designed with the height, strength, and endurance of young people in mind. The aging person can experience a handicap when changing abilities no longer allow him or her to live at home with reasonable effort and safety. An apartment building with several steps in the lobby could discourage older people from going out to run errands, visit friends, or attend religious activities. Rooms without sufficient electrical outlets can become cluttered with extension cords that can cause trips or falls. Areas without adequate lighting can lead to confusion and a sense of vulnerability for someone with low vision or memory problems. Stoves and appliances with heating elements become a greater hazard when the knobs are difficult to turn or are attached behind the heating element. A person with balance problems could be at risk of accidentally touching the hot element. A person with memory problems might be at risk for not noticing that the appliance is still turned on. The combination of the environmental demands and physical decline can lead to a vicious cycle in which the person withdraws from prior routines, becomes more sedentary and isolated, and becomes weaker and less able to carry out daily tasks in the home environment.

As occupational therapy practitioners, we have been in the business of analyzing a person's ability to function in his or her environment. Often our client's ability to function has improved when relevant environmental adaptations and technology are matched with the person's current physical, cognitive, and psychological capacities. A few years ago, most of those recommendations would be based on products found in specialty catalogs and medical supplies outlets. With the aging of the consumer, the recognition of the commonsense practicality of environmental design and technology, and the independent-living movement, however, these products are beginning to move into the mainstream market.

Now, home improvement stores often carry raised toilet seats, bath benches, as well as grab bars. Retail chains and neighborhood drugstores may well stock reachers and long-handled sponges. Consumer-oriented mail order catalogs offer adaptive equipment (known commonly as gadgets, widgets, and gizmos) as fashionable ways of making one's life easier. Special niche catalogs exist for those interested in reading, with a host of book and magazine stands, page turners, and magnifying and lighting devices (see box on next page). Gardening associations are printing articles on adapted environments in their magazines (Staciokas, 1994). Recent issues of *Bird Watcher's Digest,* for example, included articles on low-vision bird watching and wheelchair-accessible bird trails (Maslowski, 1994; Smith, 1994). Trade publications are beginning to include articles (Clark, 1996; Wylde, Baron-Robbins, & Clark, 1994a) and publish texts (Peterson, 1995; Wylde, Baron-Robbins, & Clark, 1994b) on how to design accessible home environments.

SEPARATE WAYS TO ACCOMPLISH THE SAME TASK

When people must do a familiar task in a manner that is significantly different from their prior routine or is different from how other people do the same task, they experience a handicap. Many of the above examples demonstrate how aging people accommodate to environments that do not change with their changing abilities. There are other methods, too. They could select different hours of the day to run errands to avoid traffic. They might give up taking part in evening activities, such as movies, concerts, bingo, civic group meetings, or religious meetings because of difficulty seeing at night and a sense of vulnerability. They might limit housecleaning and cooking chores because of fatigue and difficulty in lifting vacuum cleaners, buckets of water, and laundry baskets. They could

Consumer Catalogs for Special Needs

AdaptAbility: Products for
    Independent Living
    S & S Worldwide
    P. O. Box 515
    Colchester, CT 06415-0151
    (800) 243-9232

AfterTherapy Catalog: Functional
    Solutions for Independent Living
    NCM Consumer Products
    Division
    P. O. Box 6070
    San Jose, CA 95150-6070
    (800) 235-7054

Brookstone: Hard-to-Find Tools
    17 Riverside Street
    Nashua, NH 03062
    (800) 926-7000

Enrichments: Products to Enhance
    Your Life
    Bissell Inc.
    P. O. Box 471
    Western Springs, IL 60558-0471
    (800) 323-5547

Levenger: Tools for Serious Readers
    420 Commerce Drive
    Delray Beach, FL 33445-4696
    (800) 544-0880

stop tending to the garden because of difficulty bending or enduring the heat of summer. As already mentioned, one of the social consequences of having to do tasks differently from others is that people might view older adults as being different, and begin to develop prejudices toward people who are aging.

Advocates of universal design and independent living argue most strongly against this handicap. By developing home and community environments that acknowledge that people come in a variety of sizes and have a variety of abilities, we design places for all to live.

For example, a short person might be a young child or an older adult with osteoporosis. Either benefits from aesthetic-appearing grab bars in the bathtub and a place to sit in the bathroom. Similarly, a person who needs to conserve energy could be a new mother who has recently come home after delivery or a grandmother who has chronic obstructive pulmonary disorder. Either benefits from lowered counters and an open area at the sink where she can sit while preparing a meal. A gently sloping ramp in a public park permits easier movement—whether for the businessperson, the parent with a stroller, an older adult with a cane, or the young lovers strolling arm-in-arm.

The reader might have noticed that in the discussion about handicaps, no reference was made either to literature in the occupational therapy profession or other academic literature. I have chosen, rather, to cite sources that are not part of our profession or related fields to demonstrate that this debate is occurring in the larger community. Also, we should be aware, as our society ages, that issues about the physical environment will become of greater concern. We offer much in our knowledge base about how people function and how to find solutions to the problems that lead to handicaps.

References

Clark, S. (1996, January). Opening kitchens to everyone. *Fine Homebuilding, 99*, 80–83.

Lord, M. (1995, June 12). Feathering a shared nest. *U.S. News and World Report*, pp. 86–88.

Maslowski, K. (1994). Caw Talk. *Bird watcher's digest. 16*(3), 67–69.

Noer, M. (1995). Senior cybernauts: Hint to retirees isolated by physical disabilities or suffering from depression: Get wired. *Forbes, 156*(7), 240–241.

Novack, J. (1995). Don't assume you will spend your declining years vegetating in a nursing home. *Forbes, 155*(2), 98.

Peterson, M. J. (1995). *Universal kitchen planning: Design that adapts to people*. Hackettstown, NJ: National Kitchen and Bath Association.

Reed, M. P. (1995). Designs for living and the frustrations of aging. *Generations, 19*(1), 13–14.

Smith, R. (1994). Wheelchair birding. *Bird watcher's digest, 16*(6) 67–69.

Staciokas, L. (1994). A "can-do" garden. *American Horticulturist, 73*(9), 23.

Wechsler-Linden, D. (1994). What's the best health care for the aged? Company: "Here, they don't have to compete." *Forbes, 153*(2), 102–103.

World Health Organization. (1980). *International classification of impairments, disabilities and handicaps: A manual of classification related to consequences of disease*. Geneva: Author.

Wylde, M., Baron-Robbins, A., & Clark, S. (1994a, May). Accessible bathrooms: Good design doesn't just accommodate wheelchair users; It makes a bathroom safer and easier to use for everyone. *Fine Homebuilding, 88*, 78–81.

Wylde, M., Baron-Robbins, A., & Clark, S. (1994b). *Building for a lifetime: The design and construction of fully accessible homes*. Newtown, CT: Taunton Press.

Section 7. Cultural Environment

Lela A. Llorens, PhD, OTR, FAOTA

The author acknowledges the assistance of Jill Chesley, Cindy Gracely, and Linda Matsumoto in the preparation of the section of this chapter on cultural environment.

Introduction

In Western culture, aging is viewed as negative, according to Papalia and Olds (1992). As a way to designate older persons with a less pejorative sound than *old*, Americans call older people by such names as senior citizens, golden-agers, elderly persons, persons in the harvest or twilight years, older Americans, or simply elders. The newest euphemism for old people is "chronologically gifted" (p. 472).

Ageism is defined as "prejudice or discrimination based on age, usually against older persons." (Papalia & Olds, p. 472) Feebleness, incompetence, frailty, and narrow-mindedness are the images associated with being old in America. In addition, many insensitive terms have been used to focus on negative factors of aging. Attitudes about older people are more negative than attitudes toward younger people. Kite and Johnson (cited in Papalia and Olds, 1992) reported a meta-analysis of 43 studies, in which older people were judged more negatively than their younger counterparts on all characteristics studied, particularly on competence and attractiveness.

To describe and define the older population more accurately and without negative stereotypes, gerontologists have suggested two categories: the young old—those who, regardless of chronological age, are "vital, vigorous, and active" (Papalia & Olds, 1992, p. 472); and the old old—those who are frail and infirm and who constitute the minority of older persons. Chronologically, the young old are generally between ages 65 and 75, the old old between 75 and 85, and the oldest-old, more than 85 years of age.

Some of the misconceptions about older people include that they have poor coordination, are lacking in energy, have poor health, are accident-prone, cannot learn new information or skills, have poor memory, sleep a great deal, and lack interest in sexual relationships. It is believed that elders live in institutions for older people, are isolated from friends and family, and generally are unpleasant in their demeanor. Other misconceptions, although somewhat positive, are just as erroneous. Such notions as old age being pictured as the "golden age" or as a time for "a carefree second childhood" are no more helpful to understanding aging than the negative ones (Papalia & Olds, 1992). Although both negative and positive stereotyping should be avoided, it is instructive to view the attitudes of other cultures about the aging population.

Aging and Culture

It is known that Asian cultures have shown great respect for their elders and the expectation is held that families will care for their older people. Asian American and Pacific Islander elders include those of Chinese, Japanese, Filipino, Southeast Asian, and Pacific Islander descent. Filial piety has traditionally been a value among Asian and Pacific Islander families. Filial piety refers to the children's care of their parents. While this value remains strong in many families, family mobility and working members can make it difficult for families to honor this responsibility in traditional forms (Morioka-Douglas & Yeo, 1990).

For Filipino elders, respect is an important value. This value is particularly important for health professionals to understand, as many Filipinos have reported that health providers' attitudes are as important, if not more important, to Filipino elders than the competence of the health professional. Specific prohibitions are expressed for health professionals who serve Southeast Asian elders. These should be studied in detail by health professionals who work with these populations. Sensitivity to handling, touching, and pointing behaviors should be observed.

Pacific Islanders include Tongans, Samoans, and the Charmarro culture on Guam. Respect is a very important factor among Pacific Islander elders (Morioka-Douglas & Yeo, 1990).

African cultures traditionally include extended families. The concepts of deep kinship are evident in African American families. There are, however, no typical Black elders. In America, Black elders might include those from the Caribbean Islands. Many Black elders bring attitudes to the health care setting that were developed in earlier times that were characterized by racial discrimination. These attitudes can manifest themselves as distrust of the health care "system." Extended family and informal support networks are important in the care provision of Black elders (Richardson, 1990). Reciprocity of shared goods and services is a characteristic of Black cultural values. According to Richardson (1990), "Black elders are believed to be entitled to reciprocity for the care they have provided their children and grandchildren when they were young and unable to care for themselves" (pp. 39–40). Socioeconomic factors such as limited financial resources can present problems in the care of Black elders. Research has shown that Black caregivers report less role conflict and generally indicated that they received more help from family and friends.

Hispanic and Latino cultures in America include U.S. Mexicans and Puerto Ricans, and U.S. Cubans and Central and South Americans. Strong family ties and the extended family are sources of support for older U.S. Hispanic and Latino elders. Many children of Hispanic and Latino elders also feel the bonds of filial piety and participate in the caregiving for their elder family member. This phenomenon is credited with the underutilization of extended care facilities such as nursing homes, residential care homes, and home care among Hispanic and Latino people (Villa, Cuellar, Gamel, & Yeo, 1993).

Native American health care cultural traditions include present orientation, variations in time consciousness with a propensity to task rather than time, generosity in helping, harmony with nature, respect for age, and roles for extended family as integral members of households. Specific practices can vary from one tribe to another, but some beliefs and values are held in common (Cuellar, 1990).

Cultural factors affect the interactions that health professionals will have with elders from any particular ethnic group. Ethnogeriatrics is the field of study specifically dedicated to the study of elders from different ethnic backgrounds. Readers are encouraged to study the work of the Stanford Geriatric Education Center, which has specialized in the development of resources that focus on the needs of ethnic elders for details of the personal and spiritual characteristics of the groups mentioned here and for further details on the health beliefs and practices of these groups (Yeo, 1988).

Elders in Western society include people with many different motivations, goals, experiences, and beliefs within the context of societal expectations for performance in the areas of work, play and leisure, and self-maintenance. The physical, social, and cultural factors can create an environment that can sustain and nurture or interfere with and disrupt the older person's ability to cope with and adapt to life roles as an aging person in the society (Christensen & Baum, 1991).

The cultural environment for the older person is cumulative. It originally was defined by the "sum total of socially inherited characteristics of a human group that comprises everything which one generation can tell, convey, or hand down to the next ..." (Fejos cited in Spector, 1991, p. 43).

Role Loss

Roles for older adults vary with socioeconomic status, choice or preference in activity orientation, presence or absence of illness or disability, and geographic location. Common occupational and social roles for older adults between 65 and 85 years of age, however, "may include parent, grandparent, son, daughter, grandson, granddaughter, friend, colleague, worker, volunteer, student, homemaker, and partner or spouse" (Llorens cited in Christensen & Baum, 1991, p. 60).

As an individual ages, adaptation to role acquisition and role loss involves adjustment to the following:

1. Changes in physical appearance
2. Decreasing physical strength and the possibility or reality of declining health

3. Possible retirement and reduction in income
4. The deaths of family members and friends, especially a mate
5. One's own impending death (Llorens cited in Christensen & Baum, 1991, p. 60).

Socioeconomic status, activity orientation, health status, and geographic location in a cultural context will influence the personal adjustment in roles for the older person.

In the old old age group, that is, those over age 85, some of the roles associated with the old adult age group continue but the succession of loss of roles becomes more prevalent. Decisions regarding continued growth through adaptation to the physical conditions, social, and cultural expectations increasingly are a part of the adaptation process.

Role transitions in old age are not demarcated well in Western society and often are viewed relative to middle age performance. Rosow (1985) described the phenomenon of role loss in which he indicates that "the loss of roles excludes the aged from significant social participation and devalues them" (p. 71). Some of the penalties of later life in Western society are rejection, intolerance, deprivation of vital functions that support a sense of self-worth and self-esteem, assignment to marginal status, and alienation from the mainstream of society. Old age is the first stage in the life cycle in which systematic loss of status is a factor to which an entire group is subject (Rosow, 1985).

Cultural competence in the health professional begins with respect for aging and for older people, respect for the diversity within the population, and respect for the aging process. Knowledge of the individual cultural preferences among elders and knowledge about elders' functional abilities and limitations is important for all health professionals to have.

As individuals age, culture, development, and maturity interact with occupation and adaptation. The complexity of living and the myriad factors to be considered in the aging process are challenges to adaptation.

In spite of their advancing age and role loss, the elders in the following case studies continue to occupy roles with which, for the most part, they find satisfaction. They have roles as worker, leisure person, mother, grandmother, friend, housekeeper, patient, retired person, daughter, son-in-law, and others. Each has experienced role loss. One has lost a spouse. All have relinquished roles—worker roles, leisure and special activity roles—some by choice and others because of the complications of aging such as arthritis, osteoporosis, or impaired vision. Adaptation to role and to role loss requires skill acquisition or use of skills acquired earlier in life. Continued involvement in activity in the context of occupation is embedded in role, which gives meaning to activity. Role is embedded in culture. Role can serve as extrinsic motivation and reinforcement for performance of occupation. Elders are exemplars of occupational beings. The cultural aspects of occupation and role can be learned from the stories of the lives of older persons. Learning to listen to those concerns that clients will share and to those that they might not yet be ready to share is particularly salient for occupational therapists who are becoming culturally competent.

Case Studies

Following are examples of adaptation in the context of aging, culture, and role loss.

CASE STUDY 1

Mr. C is 65 years of age. He retired as a biochemist and began work full-time as a courier for a bank at age 65. In addition to his work role, he actively engages in the roles of husband, provider, father, and grandfather. Mr. C has increased the time he spends in leisure activities on weekends since his retirement even though he works full time. His current job is less stressful than his previous one. His weekend activities include skiing, hiking, and yardwork. Mr. C is active with his family and his church, where he is director of the choir. In reflecting on his career, Mr. C reported that he regretted that he did not choose a better paying profession than biochemistry. He chose that career early as he has an interest in math and science, especially experiments and laboratory work.

Mr. C showed signs of aging such as wrinkles on his face and arms, graying hair, and decreased muscle tone. He wears glasses for visual correction. He reported that he tires more easily than in the past but he continues to engage in weekend activities of skiing, hiking, and yard work. At 65 years of age and given his lifestyle, Mr. C is classified as young old. He defies many of the stereotypes of aging such as lack of energy and inability to learn new activities. He admits to having less energy but has learned to adapt in both his work and leisure activities.

CASE STUDY 2

Mrs. B, a 66-year-old woman, is married and lives with her husband. She enjoys reasonably good health except for occasional episodes of acute rheumatoid arthritis and she is somewhat overweight. She is active in spite of these stated problems. Mrs. B retired from a full-time job as a packer in an industrial plant and is continuing her work as church secretary, a position that she has held for 40 years. She is a devout Catholic and would have become a cloistered nun if she had not chosen to marry. Mrs. B enjoys writing poetry and letters to family members and friends. She writes about her philosophy of life, about outings with family and friends and about unusual events in her life. Mrs. B participates in many community activities such as bake sales, rummage sales, carnivals, and events for charity. She enjoys shopping, especially browsing in mall shops and community stores.

Mrs. B is a good example of the role of relationships in adaptation to aging. Mrs. B has five adult children who live in different parts of the United States. The closest child lives about 4 hours away from Mrs. B. and her husband. Although Mrs. B admits and is observed as showing signs of aging, she nevertheless expresses great satisfaction with having created a good life.

CASE STUDY 3

Mrs. H is an 89-year-old widow. She lives with her daughter and son-in-law in a rural area. She has no responsibilities in the home and is driven by car by her daughter or son-in-law when she needs to visit family or has appointments. Her roles include grandparent, great grandparent, parent, sibling, and friend. Mrs. H came to the United States at age 17 with her parents. She was interned during World War II, for which she felt bitterness for many years; the bitterness, however, faded with the years. Before the war, her husband made all family decisions. After the war, she became more interested in their business.

Mrs. H has osteoporosis, a problem bladder, and arthritis; she walks with a walker, and carries out exercises prescribed by her physician. Mrs. H wears corrective lenses. She has lost most of her sense of smell and some of her sense of taste, but these losses have not affected her diet. Mrs. H's major concerns are stress, depression, and anxiety about the possibility of living a long life. She has been told that she could likely live 10 more years. As a result, she worries about the pain lasting for 10 years and worries about her finances not lasting as long.

Mrs. H gradually relinquished active participation in religious groups, a singing group, a flower arrangement group, and a crafts group. Most of her time is spent with family members. She expresses satisfaction with these relationships. She also listens to religious tapes, watches Japanese programs on television, and spends time in prayer. She would like to do more work with her hands but the pain from arthritis prevents this, as does as her impaired vision.

At 89 years of age, Mrs. H would be considered among the oldest old and demonstrates more of the effects of aging. She has changed in appearance, has decreasing physical strength, has some diagnosed chronic disease, has a reduction in her income, and has lived long enough to worry about whether her financial resources will last. Filial piety is operating in this family to support Mrs. H. She has lost her spouse and many of her friends and family members to death. She contemplates her own death as an impending reality.

References

Christensen, C., & Baum, C. (1991). *Occupational therapy: Overcoming human performance deficits.* Thorofare, NJ: SLACK.

Cuellar, J. (1990). *Aging and health: American Indian/Alaska native elders.* Stanford, CA: Stanford Geriatric Education Center.

Fejos, P. , (1959). Man, magic, and medicine. In I. Goldston (Ed.), *Medicine and Anthropology* (p. 43). New York: International University Press.

Morioka-Douglas, N., & Yeo, G. (1990). *Aging and health: Asian/Pacific Island American elders.* Stanford, CA: Stanford Geriatric Education Center.

Papalia, D. E., & Olds, S. W. (1992). *Human development.* New York: McGraw-Hill.

Richardson, J. (1990). *Aging and health: Black American elders.* Stanford, CA: Stanford Geriatric Education Center.

Rosow, I. (1985). Status and role change throughout the life cycle. In R. H. Binstock & E. Shinas (Eds.), *Handbook of aging and the social sciences* (pp. 62–91). New York: Van Nostrand Reinhold.

Spector, R., (1991). *Cultural diversity in health and illness.* Norwalk, CT: Appleton and Lange.

Villa, M. L., Cuellar, J., Gamel, N., & Yeo, G. (1993). *Aging and health: Hispanic American elders.* Stanford, CA: Stanford Geriatric Education Center.

Yeo, G. (1988). Introductory remarks. In L. A. Llorens (Ed.), *Health care for ethnic elders: The cultural context.* Stanford, CA: Stanford Geriatric Education Center.

Section 8.
The Social Environment

K. Oscar Larson, MA, OTR

Introduction

The August 16, 1995, edition of *The Washington Post* contained a stark contrast in articles about older adults. In the center of the front page, a photo of city workers burying a line of plain caskets precedes a headline, "For Chicago, a Tomb of the Urban Unmourned" (Walsh, 1995). On the first page of the next section of the newspaper, a photo of a smiling woman had a different headline, "Going Strong at 96, She's a Teacher for the Ages: Dyslexia Researcher Regarded a 'Grande Dame' for Her Contributions to the Field" (O'Hanlon, 1995). The former article chronicled the heat-related deaths of 591 people in the Chicago area, including 41 people for whom no family could be found to claim the body and prepare a burial. The mean age of those 41 people was 67 years, the median age was 70. The latter article described the gathering of teachers and researchers in the field of dyslexia to honor Margaret Rawson, who recently had published her third book about her studies on dyslexia. In one article, there is an account of social isolation; in the other article, an account of preserved social roles.

In regard to the social environment, one must consider what social roles aging people have performed throughout their lives; what social roles they continue to perform; and the consequence of losing, limiting, or discarding social roles. For many aging adults, the social environment will be support-ive and they will be able to maintain or adapt social roles. Handicaps, the disadvantages that others bestow on one related to impairments or disabilities, can occur in the social environment in the form of neglect, abuse, and abandonment. Handicaps also can occur in the context of bereavement and losses. Isolation, restrictions on sexual intimacy and expression, and financial insecurity are other forms of handicaps in the social environment.

For most aging adults, the changes in their social environments occur slowly. For those who have developed roles within the context of families, these relationships will most likely continue. Children will mature, leave home for college and work, marry, remain nearby, or move elsewhere. Sons- or daughters-in-law, with a host of other in-laws, might join the family. Grandchildren might be born. Business and civic roles can continue, though community or volunteer activities might replace paid work tasks after retirement. Religious organizations can take on greater importance, especially when the person no longer has the demands of a work schedule or turns to religion to define meaning over a lifetime and in the anticipation of death.

Periods of rapid change can punctuate one's continuity of relationships. Unplanned retirement or layoff without reemployment can leave the person without the daily contact with coworkers or substitute roles. Moving to a new area or retirement community can place the person in unfamiliar surroundings with few established friendships or roles. Unexpected or chronic illnesses can require the person to develop roles of caregiver or patient, and alter daily routines because of appointments, treatments, and exhaustion. The deaths of one's spouse, family, and friends can erode the foundation of one's social supports.

When learning about the life of an aging person, the occupational therapy practitioner should not assume that the person lives in a particular stereotyped manner. Rather, the practitioner should gather data that establish what constitutes the person's lifestyle. Some of this data can include information about past and present social roles, as well as changes that have occurred over the person's life and recent changes. Also important in developing an understanding of the person's social environment are the factors of the person's desires and expectations about relationships.

Neglect, Abuse, and Abandonment

Although most older adults are able to care for themselves as they age, some will need assistance from others for some period of time. They might need caretaking while recovering from an illness or injury, or returning to their prior living situations and relationships on recovery. Others could need caretaking over a longer period of time, such as when they can no longer manage their affairs, no longer demonstrate competency in making decisions, or become too frail or weak to care for themselves.

Caregivers primarily consist of family members, usually daughters, granddaughters, or even their older mothers. Other caregivers can include health care professionals, home health aides, live-in companions, housekeepers, guardians, financial managers, or lawyers who can assist with legal and financial matters. Although 96% of older adults live without the trauma of abuse or neglect, the 4% who do experience some form of abuse or neglect constitute about 1.1 million people in the United States (House Select Committee on Aging, 1985). Even if the percentage remains the same, as the number of aging adults increases, the total number of older adults experiencing some form of abuse or neglect will grow substantially in the coming decades.

Neglect occurs when the caregivers do not or cannot carry out the necessary services to maintain the older adult's safety, health, and comfort (see box on next page). This can include poor hygiene from lack of bathing and laundering of clothes; repeated falls or injuries when hazardous physical environmental conditions are not changed; malnutrition, dehydration, or electrolyte imbalances because proper food, fluids, and medications are not provided. The concept of neglect generally does not connote willful harm toward the dependent person.

The threshold between errors, ignorance, and neglect is not firmly defined because of the complex interaction of social values, lifestyles, and other demands on the caregivers. A caregiver can be very concerned about the well-being of the older person, but might lack the knowledge or skills necessary to provide adequate care; or the caregiver might have too many responsibilities, such as children, work, and other dependent family members that limit the amount of time and energy available for care for the older person. Professionals working with caregivers of older adults should not immediately assume neglect from the caregiver because of an accident or error. Rather, the practitioner should look for patterns of neglect over a period of time.

Abuse of older adults occurs when the caregiver acts willfully in a manner that harms or jeopardizes the safety, health, or comfort of the older person (see box on next page). Abuse can occur at home or within institutional settings. Physical signs of abuse can include multiple bruises, burns, or fractures, or similar injuries that cannot be

Definitions of Neglect and Abuse

Neglect—Failure of a caregiver to provide adequate care for the dependent person

Passive Neglect—Result of the caregiver's lack of knowledge about proper care and resources

Active Neglect—Result of the caregiver's lack of intervention to tend to a significant need, when the caregiver has adequate knowledge of proper care and resources

Abuse—A caregiver's acting in a manner that directly results in harm to the dependent person

Material or Financial Abuse—Result of the caregiver's misappropriation of funds or material resources

Physical Abuse—Result of the caregiver's handling of the dependent person, in which the person experiences physical pain, injury, or confinement

Sexual Abuse—Result of the caregiver's sexual activity with the dependent person without the consent of the person, or when the person cannot give adequate consent (e.g., the older adult with mental retardation or dementia)

Psychological or Emotional Abuse—Result of the caregiver's interactions (e.g., yelling, insulting, threatening, or silence) with the dependent person in which the person experiences mental anguish.

Source: Capezuti, 1989.

Questions That Could Elicit Information About Abuse or Neglect

1. Has anyone at home hurt you?
2. Has anyone scolded or threatened you?
3. Has anyone touched you without your consent?
4. Has anyone made you do things you didn't want to do?
5. Has anyone taken anything that was yours without asking?
6. Have you signed any papers that you did not understand?
7. Has anyone forced you to sign papers against your will?
8. Are you afraid of anyone at home? Are you afraid of anyone with whom you come in contact?
9. Has anyone failed to help you take care of yourself when you needed help?
10. Has anyone prevented you from seeing friends or other people whom you wish to see?

An answer of "yes" to any of these questions does not inherently indicate abuse or neglect, but should be followed up by the health care professional to determine more details about the situation. Also, the practitioner should gather corroborative evidence such as a physical examination, interviews with family, neighbors, or other involved people.

continued

continued from previous page

Conversely, an answer of "no" does not inherently indicate the lack of abuse. If the older adult has other objective signs of abuse or verbal accounts from people who know the person, the practitioner should inquire further. The older adult might have reasons to conceal or deny actual abuse (e.g., embarrassment, fear of retribution, guilt) or might have short-term memory deficits that limit her or his ability to give accurate answers.

Source: Morris, E. 1995, October 23. Internal memorandum, *Indicators of abuse, neglect, and/or exploitation.* Alexandria, VA: Alexandria Hospital.

accounted for by falls. Psychological signs of abuse can include fear of being touched, agitation, paranoia, or withdrawal.

Practitioners should be wary of accusing caregivers of abuse too quickly as this could result in an antagonistic relationship between the professionals and caregivers. Rather, the professional should attempt to develop an alliance with the caregiver to identify reasons for the abuse and resources that might resolve the situation.

Although some older adults might need to be removed from the abusive situation, others might be able to remain with the caregiver, after the precipitating factors have been identified and resolved. For instance, caring for an aging parent who has dementia and wanders frequently from the home can become draining for the adult child who has offered to take in the parent. The practitioner could work with the caregiver to identify visual cues and barriers that reduce the parent's wandering behavior, and alternative activities that the parent can do to become occupied in the task rather than wandering. The caregiver might need to have access to a support group in order to receive empathy and practical advice from other caretakers. She or he might need counseling to discuss

frustrations and fears of seeing one's parent lose the ability to live independently.

When a practitioner identifies signs of neglect or abuse of an older person (see boxes above), the practitioner should adhere to state laws regarding reporting of neglect or abuse. In addition to the ethical concerns about not reporting neglect or abuse, the practitioner could be obligated legally to report suspected neglect or abuse to the appropriate agencies.

Abandonment occurs when the caregivers forsake responsibility without securing consent from another caregiver to take on the dependent person. Recent sensational accounts have brought to the public's attention the issue of "granny dumping"—when family members have brought an older parent, aunt, or uncle to the emergency room of a hospital and then disappeared; or when an older man with dementia was left at a baseball stadium. Although we might be quick to conclude that these family members are cold, heartless people, some family members have later spoken out about their sense of desperation at the financial, emotional, and time demands of caring for their aging relatives. Some realized that their material resources would be quickly depleted to pay for long-term care. Others had made commitments to never let their family members be put away.

Beyond the immediate familial responsibilities are the issues of how larger communities have abandoned older adults. Advocates of people who are homeless, mentally ill, and aging would argue that the process of deinstitutionalizing long-term psychiatric hospital patients has resulted in a decline in health of some of these former residents (Bachrach, 1992; Bachrach, 1993; Cohen, Onserud, & Monaco, 1993; Saathoff, Cortina, Jacobson, & Aidrich, 1992). Some of these people had spent much of their adolescent and adult lives in institutional care, lacking many learning situations necessary to develop skills to live in the community. Other people have chronic mental illness, are resistant to treatment, and are growing older on streets that do not offer the freedom and comfort of younger days. Again, although these people might constitute a small percentage of the general population, they often develop illnesses or medical conditions for which they seek treatment at community clinics or hospitals.

Bereavement

Although "death and taxes" might be the two inevitable factors of living, most aging adults will grieve the loss of friends, spouses, and family members. The statistical numbers generated by epidemiological studies vary greatly depending on the inclusion criteria, yet Jacobs' (1993) analysis of research on bereavement has indicated that a notable number of people will experience some type of complication within a year of a major loss. Between 14% to 34% of the people experienced pathologic grief reactions; 4% to 31% experienced major depression; 13% experienced panic disorders; and 39% experienced generalized anxiety disorders.

Parkes (1965) identified three factors contributing to complication in grieving the death of a spouse: how suddenly or unexpectedly the death occurred; the intensity of emotions experienced after the loss, especially anger and guilt (e.g., anger toward the deceased person who has abandoned her or him); and the degree of ambivalence that the surviving spouse feels toward the relationship (e.g., unresolved issues about the relationship and remorse that one had not done more to make amends). The threshold between normal and pathological grief is a matter of degree, rather than radically different experiences (Jacobs, 1993). For most people, the grieving process would occur over several months, with periods of recurrent grief, such as during holidays and anniversaries.

The experience of bereavement appears to have several major processes (Parkes & Weiss, 1983). Although having major themes, the boundaries of each process are not rigid. The person can move from one process and back again during the course of grieving. In a normal grief reaction, the person would progressively experience an abating in the intensity of the emotions associated with the searching process, would begin to develop skills related to the different roles needed to perform daily tasks and social activities, and would develop a new sense of identity as a widow or individual. This person experiences the emotions, settles the estate, saves mementos, and establishes new routines.

In atypical or pathological grief, the person would not be able to tolerate the intensity of emotions associated with the searching process. In this situation, the person either becomes withdrawn and depressed or fights against anyone or anything that reiterates the loss. This person avoids confronting the emotions, leaves business unattended, does not clean the house or decide what possessions to keep, breaks off long-held relationships, and seeks to be reunited with the deceased person by maintaining vestiges of their life together.

Bereavement is not inherently an event in which the older adult will experience a handicap. Whether the person grieves normally or pathologically, however, other people might present obstacles to continuing prior social roles or establishing new ones because of their expectations about how widows or widowers should behave. This can occur in social situations where the person feels awkward around friends who are in couples, the fifth wheel syndrome. Or this can occur when others expect that the person should be sexually active or abstinent because of freedom from or loyalty to the deceased spouse. Or this can occur when the person loses financial security that was provided by the deceased spouse. Isolation, loss of sexual intimacy and expression, and financial hardship are three types of handicaps that people might experience in the context of bereavement.

Isolation and Loneliness

In addition to losses of partners, family members, and friends, many aspects of aging can result in isolation and loneliness. As pointed out in the section on the physical environment, changes in the aging person's physical mobility and sensory processing, in combination with home and community environments, can restrict the ability to go places where she or he could be involved with other people. Low vision and hearing, even if the person lives near other people, can result in isolation because the aging person has greater difficulty identifying when people want to interact or the content of the interaction.

Cognitive changes, especially short-term memory deficits, can lead to isolation as the person has greater difficulty seeking, finding, and remaining engaged in social activities.

The older adult's personality style also can be a factor in the development of social isolation and loneliness. Personality factors should be considered as extending along different continua, such as dependence to independence, histrionic to stoic, demanding to help rejecting, with either extreme potentially resulting in isolation. Most people will place somewhere along the midrange of the continuum, or could become more extreme in certain circumstances.

For instance, the demanding person is more likely to seek attention or assistance, whether this be calling 911, visiting the emergency room, or giving long testimonials about physical discomfort (known as organ recitals) at church or the senior center. People who routinely provide care and social contact with this person might begin to avoid meeting the person or treat her or him coldly, hoping to avoid initiating the long-winded, entangling conversations. The help-rejecting person might avoid assistance in any manner, remaining alone at home rather then taking taxi service, at a discount, to appointments and social events.

Sexual Intimacy and Expression

Aging adults can experience a restriction in participating or enjoying sexual intimacy or expressing themselves sexually because of la a partner, social attitudes, or m ceptions about physical limit Divorce and death can be tv tions in which the aging a becomes alone. The proba

Processes of Grieving

Process	Experience
1. Shock	Numbness, void of emotion, going through routines automatically (e.g., funeral, returning to home and work)
2. Disorganization	Depression, withdrawal, exhaustion, realization of the reality of the loss
3. Searching	Increase in the intensity of emotions (e.g., anger, guilt, remorse, hate); hostile toward people, places, or events that remind one of the loss; yearning or pining to have the deceased return; misinterpretations or hallucinations of the deceased being present; maintaining of familiar daily routines
4. Resolution	Begin to develop skills necessary to carry out daily tasks and social activities; clean house and save important keepsakes; settle estates and financial affairs; develop new or different relationships and traditions
5. Reintegration	Integrate new sense of identity, roles, and relationships.

Source: Parkes & Weiss, 1983.

Myths About Sexuality in Aging Adults

1. Aging adults have less interest in sex than younger people and cannot engage in sexual activity.
2. Intercourse, with mutual orgasm, should be the primary means of sexual expression. Other intimate behavior, such as cuddling, caressing, mutual stimulation, or oral sex, is foreplay and is not important sexual activity.
3. People who live in congregate residential situations (e.g., group homes, assisted-living facilities, nursing homes, etc.) should be segregated by gender and not have privacy.
4. As people age, they become physically unattractive and not desirable as sexual partners.

Source: Goldstein & Ruynan, 1993.

meeting another available partner for a heterosexual relationship is low in that, demographically, for every 100 older men, there are 149 older women, and for every widower, there are five widows (American Association of Retired Persons, 1991). Of course, this raises the question about whether sexual expression needs to be confined to heterosexual relations or could be directed to self-stimulation. For the current generation of older adults, social attitudes discouraging homosexual relationships and masturbation are likely to limit open pursuit of these means of sexual intimacy or gratification. In another decade or two, these attitudes might change as members of the sexual liberation and gay pride generations age.

Goldstein and Runyan (1993) have identified several myths about older adults and sexuality (see box on previous page). People who believe these myths can restrict the older adult from seeking sexual intimacy and expression. In addition to restricting the enjoyment of sexuality throughout the years, these attitudes can promote an acceleration in the normal age-related changes of sexual functioning. As Masters and Johnson (1966) noted, those people who remained sexually active as they aged tended to have fewer changes in sexual functioning.

In addition to believing these myths, aging adults who have experienced acute or chronic illnesses, and their partners, might have concerns about being sexually active. Some aging adults fear they will provoke a recurrence of the problem or exacerbate a problem, such as with heart attacks, angina attacks, hypertension, or strokes. Other older adults could have illnesses that require them to seek other means of sexual gratification, such as people who have arthritis, in which certain positions or touching

can be painful, or for someone after prostate surgery, in which a man is unable to have an erection. These situations can usually be overcome with some experimentation (e.g., different positions, lubricants, vibrators) and re-evaluation of attitudes that prohibit different sexual activity.

Economic Insecurity

People in the United States in the 20th century have seen the development of several economic safety nets. Public programs such as Social Security, Medicare, and Medicaid have been promoted as ways of preventing any citizen or worker from impoverishment. Private companies have offered employees pensions and tax-sheltered annuities. Individuals have had the opportunities, especially in the past 20 years, to pursue private investments through IRAs (individual retirement accounts), money market funds, and mutual funds, as well as traditional investments such as stocks and bonds. Home equity through home ownership offers a degree of security when the loan is paid off or when the person sells a home that has increased in value and moves to a smaller or less-expensive living situation.

Most families, however, experience a decline in income on retirement. A 1995 Rand Corporation analysis (Pasztor, 1995) indicated that the median household will replace only 69% of working income with retirement income (e.g., Social Security, pensions, savings). In essence, this is a 31% decrease in available income to pay for routine bills, as well as for retirement activities, such as traveling or activiti with the grandchildren, or for the potential increase in medical car tests, procedures, medications

Of great concern is the a son's available liquid assets

ments that could be readily sold, excluding real estate, which can consist of the home in which the aging adults live), especially across different ethnic groups. The median White household at age 60 had $15,000 in liquid assets, whereas Black and Hispanic households had less than $500 in liquid assets. Liquid assets are important in that these are the safety nets on which people can fall back in case of an emergency. In practical terms, a Black or Hispanic older adult paying his or her own heating bill during the cold winter of 1993–94, when much of the Midwest and Northeast remained well below seasonal freezing levels and had several more blizzards than usual, could easily have depleted much of the household's liquid assets to pay for the additional cost of keeping the home warm.

Financial insecurity can restrict someone from carrying out activities and social roles when the person has limited financial resources or fears using what is available. The person might not be able to afford the expense of joining a group, paying tuition for a class, buying supplies for a hobby, or paying for transportation to and from errands or activities. The person on a fixed or limited income might feel embarrassment about no longer having the previous standard of living or about not having the ability to pay his or her way as had been the habit earlier. The person could worry about whether finite savings will last as long as he or she does.

For the current generation of older adults, economic deprivation has been a real experience. Most 60-, 70-, and -year-old people lived through the t Depression of the 1930s and the ips of World War II. Whether young adults starting out in aising families, or adoles- ping a sense of identity,

they most likely saw the economic hardships of unemployment and war.

In addition, many adults of those generations had more strongly defined gender roles concerning money. Men were more likely to be the breadwinner and the person to manage the family finances. Given that women are more likely to survive their husbands, there is a good probability that a woman who has had a limited need to balance a checkbook, to buy and sell stocks or bonds, or to make financial decisions could find herself in charge of an estate. Often other family members will be able to assist, or a lawyer and accountant can be hired to manage financial affairs.

Summary

This chapter concludes an overview of the discipline of gerontology, the profession of occupational therapy, and the lives of the aging people we study and serve. The reader should recognize by now that all three of these entities are individual, complex, and constantly growing. The following three modules of this text will expand on these themes with details about service delivery, intervention techniques, and the interactions between the professional and the client.

Activities

1. Think about an older adult you know (grandparent, parent, relative, or neighbor). Write a brief essay that describes what his or her life is like. Consider the performance context, areas, and components that constitute his or her lifestyle. Does he or she have any impairments, disabilities, or handicaps?

2. Define the following terms (from AOTA Uniform Terminology):
   - Functional Performance Context
   - Functional Performance Areas
   - Functional Performance Components
     (From World Health Organization ICIDH)
   - Impairments
   - Disabilities
   - Handicaps.

   How are these definitions similar and different?

3. Compare your life to date with that of your grandparents. What technology did you grow up with that did not exist when your grandparents were children? What physical, cultural, or social environmental changes have occurred that have benefited your grandparents as they aged? When do you think you will consider yourself to be old? How do you believe you will live then? Write a brief essay about these questions.

4. Select an illness or medical condition that you would like to know more about (such as CVA, COPD, depression, hip fracture, or dementia). Using information from this chapter and additional texts (such as reference books, journals) available to you, write a brief description of the pathology, impairments, disabilities, and handicaps that could relate to that illness or medical condition.

Case Studies

While reading the following case studies, consider the person's functional performance context, areas, and components. How does the occupational therapist help the person respond to impairments, disabilities, and handicaps?

CASE STUDY 1—MR. A

(Contributed by Didi Olson, OTR)

Mr. A, a 73-year-old, retired Army sergeant, enjoyed an active lifestyle with his wife. They had a rich family life and a busy social schedule. When not in his garden growing prize-winning tomatoes, Mr. A was on the golf course. Although Mr. A had diabetes and high blood pressure, he appeared very physically fit and healthy. After suffering a right CVA, with left hemiplegia, he was hospitalized until his condition stabilized. Then he transferred to a skilled nursing facility for rehabilitation.

In an occupational therapy evaluation, Mr. A required moderate to maximum assistance with most activities of daily living (ADL) and functional mobility. His sitting balance was good, and standing balance fair. He could not ambulate. Although he had fair minus (3-/5) strength in his left upper extremity, profound sensory loss made it difficult to facilitate functional use of the extremity. His sensory loss included hemianopsia with left neglect, profound proprioceptive loss of both left upper and lower extremities, and impairment in light touch, pain, temperature, and stereognosis. Safety was a problem because of his left neglect. Although his cognitive and psychosocial statuses were intact, he needed assistance with impulse control.

Mr. A and his very supportive family thought that their goal was simple. They wanted Mr. A to return home to his previous lifestyle. This belief challenged the occupational therapist, who wanted to provide support, encouragement, and training to assist the patient in his functional recovery as well as to perform a realistic appraisal of his future capacities, limitations, and expectations. Therapy needed to include a treatment program that would focus on his ability to remain useful and productive. From the beginning, the family members attended therapy sessions to learn how to assist Mr. A. Their support was vital to the outcome.

The short-term occupational therapy goals were to ensure safety while teaching compensatory techniques, restoring and improving his abilities in performance components, and preventing further loss of functioning in performance areas. The occupational therapist accomplished these goals through various remedial and compensatory techniques, directed at his impairments that affected his ability to perform daily living tasks. Mr. A needed to coordinate and integrate those skills into effective living habits.

Mr. A's determination and Army training gave him the strength to pursue his goals. He persevered throughout the treatment program, always maintaining a terrific sense of humor. His left neglect interfered with his recovery and safety. He reached supervised goals with dressing through trial after trial. He began to have increased strength in his left arm and the necessary proprioceptive input to use the arm to help accomplish tasks. Occupational therapy included gross motor and weight-bearing exercises to improve the proprioception he would need to perform bilateral tasks.

After 6 weeks of therapy, Mr. A was ready for discharge. During a home evaluation, the occupational therapist made recommendations for safe environmental adaptations to compensate for his continued sensory loss. At discharge, he required supervision with cuing for safety, and could ambulate with a cane. He required setup for dressing, and minimal assistance for bathing. He had learned to compensate for his visual deficit to find his food on the table, and to look for obstacles on his left side while walking. His safety remained a concern, but again his personal strength and determination assured everyone that he could handle going home.

Three months later, Mr. A returned to the golf course. He reported that his game was awful and the ball hard to find, but he enjoyed the camaraderie of his friends and the exercise. His family continued to assist him as he need help. He expressed the opinion that his life, although different, was again full. Occupational therapy allowed Mr. A to recognize his disabilities while optimizing his independent functioning and intact decision-making skills. He continued to maintain a strong social involvement and his life remained useful and productive.

CASE STUDY 2—MRS. D

(Contributed by Anagha Deole, OTR, B.Sc.[OT])

Mrs. D is an 83-year-old woman with senile dementia, Alzheimer's type. She was admitted to the nursing home because she had been packing her clothes in a bag and running away from her home. At the nursing home, she continued to wander away. If a staff member attempted to stop her, she would slap that person. Physically, she was able to function, and her main impairments were her short-term memory deficits and a tendency to become agitated. The speech therapist worked with Mrs. D to evaluate and develop her cognitive skills.

Mrs. D was referred for occupational therapy after she fell in the bathroom and had a hip fracture. She returned from the hospital, where she had the hip fracture stabilized. She had become severely weak and was to be non-weight-bearing. She would not get out of bed and required moderate to maximal assistance for all ADL. The nursing staff, who were familiar with Mrs. D's periods of agitation and combative behavior, were hesitant to attempt transfers using non-weight-bearing precautions. Mrs. D's ability to comprehend instructions and learn techniques was limited by her dementia.

Occupational therapy first addressed her positioning in bed, following the standard precautions after a hip fracture (not crossing her legs, keeping the affected hip from ranging less than 90 degrees of flexion). The speech therapist helped Mrs. D become oriented to additional staff members and hip fracture treatment procedure, using a memory book. The occupational therapist posted instructions for proper positioning and transfer. One copy was placed near her bed and another at the nurses' station. For the first few days she remained in bed, with the subsequent risks of developing pulmonary problems and pressure sores.

To facilitate sitting and mobility for Mrs. D, a wheelchair was adapted with a wedge cushion slanting forward and a small roll cushion at the lumbar back level. These cushions accommodated for her kyphosis and improved her chest expansion during breathing. The seat level and leg rests were adjusted to her height. Occupational therapy and physical therapy personnel coordinated treatment to train unit staff to do transfers from the bed to wheelchair and from wheelchair to toilet.

The mutlidisciplinary team provided a variety of treatments. Physical therapy worked on pain management, applying hot packs to her lower back, where Mrs. D complained of pain. Occupational therapy increased her physical endurance, orientation, and cognition, and reduced her time in bed by provided activities that interested her, such as tossing a ball, playing cards, or crocheting. A respiratory therapist monitored her pulmonary status, and was pleased that she could spend more time sitting up rather than lying in bed. Mrs. D needed a posey vest during times that she was not eating a meal or involved in therapy because of her tendency to become agitated and wander. With her increased endurance to be involved in various therapies, she needed the vest restraint less often.

Within 3 weeks of initiating the treatment, Mrs. D had become much more involved in ADL, eating meals, and participating in therapy. She was able to move about the unit in her wheelchair, could feed herself, groom herself, and dress her upper body after setup and with standby assistance from staff. Mrs. D showed increased awareness of her non-weight-bearing precautions by keeping her effected leg slightly off the floor while doing functional transfers, with minimal verbal cues. She did not become agitated or combative with the therapists.

References

American Association of Retired Persons. (1991). *A profile of older Americans*. Washington, DC: Author.

Bachrach, L. L. (1992). What we know about homelessness among mentally ill persons: An analytical review and commentary. *Hospital and Community Psychiatry. 43*, 453–469.

Bachrach, L. L. (1993). The biopsychosocial legacy of deinstitutionalization. *Hospital and Community Psychiatry. 44*, 523–524, 546.

Capezuti, E. (1989). Preventing elder abuse and neglect. In R. Lavizzo-Mourey, S. C. Day, D. Diserens, & J. A. Grisso (Eds.), *Practicing prevention for the elderly* (pp. 167–181). Philadelphia: Hanley & Belfus.

Cohen, C., Onserud, H., & Monaco, C. (1993). Outcomes for the mentally ill in a program for older homeless persons. *Hospital and Community Psychiatry. 44*, 650–656.

Goldstein, H., & Runyan, C. (1993). An occupational therapy educational module to increase sensitivity about geriatric sexuality. *Physical and Occupational Therapy in Geriatrics. 11*(2), 57–76.

House Select Committee on Aging, Subcommittee for Health and Long-Term Care. (1985, May 10). *Elder abuse: A national disgrace* (Executive Summary). Washington, DC: United States House of Representatives.

Jacobs, S. (1993). *Pathologic grief: Maladaptation to loss*. Washington, DC: American Psychiatric Press.

Masters, W., & Johnson, V. (1966). *Human sexual response*. Boston: Little, Brown.

O'Hanlon, A. (1995). Going strong at 96, she's a teacher for the ages: Dyslexia researcher regarded as 'Grande Dame' for her contribution to the field. *The Washington Post*, pp. B1, B5.

Parkes, C. M. (1965). Bereavement and mental illness: Part 2. A classification of bereavement reactions. *British Journal of Medical Psychology. 38*(13), 13–26.

Parkes, C. M., & Weiss, R. W. (1983). *Recovery from bereavement*. New York: Basic Books.

Pasztor, A. (1995, July 25). Middle-aged, elderly have fewer assets than expected. *The Wall Street Journal*.

Saathoff, G. B., Cortina, J. A., Jacobson, R., & Aidrich, C. R. (1992). Mortality among elderly patients discharged from a state hospital. *Hospital and Community Psychiatry. 43*, 280–281.

Walsh, E. (August 26, 1995). For Chicago, a tomb of the urban unmourned. *The Washington Post*, pp. A1, A10.

Module II

Regena G. Stevens-Ratchford,
PhD, OTR, FAOTA
Editor

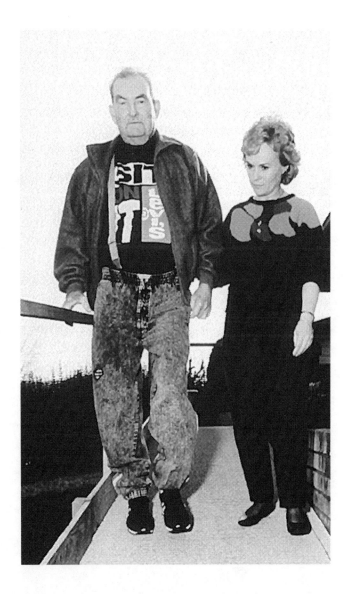

Author Biographies

Chris Cawley, OTR, received her bachelor's degree in occupational therapy from Texas Woman's University. Until recently, she was self-employed in Northern Virginia. In her more than 20 years as an occupational therapist, she has worked in a variety of traditional and nontraditional settings in both rural and metropolitan areas. As of this writing, she is in the process of moving to Atlanta, where she plans to continue her activities in promoting the use of assistive technology and environmental modifications as a strategy for enhancing function and safety of older adults.

Margaret A. Christenson, MPH, OTR, FAOTA, is president and founder of Lifease, Inc., the developer of a solution-generating, computerized evaluation (EASE2000) to facilitate home evaluations that health care professionals conduct. Located in New Brighton, Minnesota, she also consults with organizations, architects, interior designers, and administrators of senior housing, assisted living, and long-term care facilities concerning the environments used by elderly persons. She is a frequent lecturer and seminar leader on adaptations of the living environment to compensate for the changes of aging. She has written several articles on this topic as well as a book, Aging in the Designed Environment. In 1989, she was honored as the Minnesota Occupational Therapist of the Year. She is past chair of the Gerontology Special Interest Section of AOTA and was its delegate to the 1995 White House Conference on Aging.

Kathleen H. Conyers, MEd, OTR/L, is rehabilitation director for In-House Rehab at Twelve Oaks Health Care Center in Riverdale, Georgia. She earned her bachelor of science degree from Columbia University and her master's degree in education from Trenton State College. As a geriatric clinical specialist, she has had extensive experience in gerontology and rehabilitation of the older adult. She has worked in various settings, including skilled nursing facilities, rehabilitation centers, hospitals, and in home health and adult day services. In 1991, she received the Award of Merit for Geriatric Practice from the New Jersey Occupational Therapy Association. Ms. Conyers currently is on the editorial advisory board of AOTA's *O.T. Week*. She coauthored an article, "A Systems Approach to Eating Skills Programming in Long Term Care," published in Occupational Therapy Practice. She has been presenter at professional conferences at the local, state, and national levels. Ms. Conyers is a member of AOTA and other professional associations and president of the Georgia Black Occupational Therapy Caucus.

Phyllis Bauer Madachy, MHA, is the administrator of the Howard County, Maryland, Area Agency on Aging. She earned her bachelor of arts degree in political science from Wheeling Jesuit College and her master's degree in administrative science from Johns Hopkins University. She has a strong interest in programs that enable persons with disabilities to achieve maximum independence and has presented papers on these areas at local, state, and national conferences. Ms. Madachy's professional experiences include service as chairperson of the Howard County OPERATION INDEPENDENCE Steering Committee—a nationally recognized educational program on assistive technology, home modification, and occupational therapy intervention for persons with disabilities. She was president of the Maryland Association of Nutrition Programs and editor of Eating Together in Maryland, a survey of nutrition sites. Ms. Madachy was recipient of the Presidential Commendation Award from the Maryland Occupational Therapy Association in 1994.

Anne Long Morris, EdD, OTR, is the geriatric program manager for AOTA. She received her bachelor's degree in occupational therapy from New York University, her master's degree in public administration from the University of Oklahoma, and her doctorate in adult and continuing education at the Virginia Polytechnic Institute. She completed graduate work in gerontology at the University of Maryland. A national and international lecturer, seminar leader, and qualitative researcher, she focuses on improving the fit of older persons and their environments. Her doctoral study looked at the meaning, for older women, of learning to use assistive technology products at home. Grant projects with which Ms. Morris has been involved include Design for Aging; Strategies for Collaboration Between Architects and Occupational Therapists; A Part of Daily Life: Alzheimer's Disease Caregivers Simplify Activities and the Home; and Changing Needs, Changing Homes: Adapting Your Home to Fit You.

Steve Park, MS, OTR, is a research occupational therapist at the National Hospital for Neurology in London, England. He received his master's degree from the University of Illinois at Chicago and his bachelor's degree from the University of Puget Sound. He has taught occupational therapy courses in adulthood, aging, and rehabilitation at Pacific University in Oregon.

Jill Cohen Schie, MGA, OTR/L, is an acute care program manager at National Rehabilitation Hospital at Washington Hospital Center. She earned her bachelor's degree from Towson State University, Towson, Maryland, and her master's degree in general administration from the University of Maryland. For AOTA, she has been a reviewer for conferences and other types of projects. She has participated in a focus group with AOTA and the Commission on Aging and also contributed to the AOTA brochure regarding adapting to aging.

Regena G. Stevens-Ratchford, PhD, OTR/L, FAOTA, is an associate professor at Towson State University in Maryland. She received her doctorate in educational communications, with an emphasis on older adult development learning and programming, from the University of Maryland. She earned her bachelor's and master's degrees in occupational therapy from Ohio State University. She has 26 years of clinical experience and 21 years of college teaching experience in the areas of gerontology and physical disabilities. Her research has focused on qualitative and quantitative studies of reminiscence as a developmental task of old age, and she has given presentations and published in the area of gerontology.

Learning Outline

Chapter 7
Restoring Occupational Performance:
Rehabilitation Services for Older Adults 343

Steve Park, MS, OTR

Chapter 8
Environmental Design, Modification, and Adaptation 383
Margaret A. Christenson, MPH, OTR, FAOTA

Chapter 9
Consultation Amplifies the Impact of Occupational Therapy in the Community 417

Anne Long Morris, EdD, OTR; Phyllis Bauer Madachy, MHA; and Chris Cawley, OTR

Kathleen H. Conyers, MEd, OTR/L

Introduction to Module II

This module examines the roles and functions of occupational therapy in a variety of health care and community environments. The chapters in this module describe the delivery of occupational therapy services in both traditional and nontraditional settings. The client-centered delivery of gerontic occupational therapy services is stressed, and the clinical role and functions in hospitals and rehabilitation facilities is explained. Occupational therapy services in environmental adaptation and home modification for aging in place and continued independence are also explained. The therapist as a consultant is defined, and a description of consultation services is provided. The role of the occupational therapist in day care programming is also described. The role of the occupational therapist in the promotion of health and wellness is explained in relation to the adaptation and adjustment to the changes associated with normal aging and rehabilitation after serious illness.

This module emphasizes interventions in problems caused by normal aging and serious illness and describe the settings in which these interventions take place. The goal of gerontic occupational therapy is to help older adults to continue or resume their participation in everyday living at the highest quality of living (American Occupational Therapy Association, 1994; Christiansen, 1991) and the greatest sense of well-being. Occupational therapy provides the individual with opportunities to participate in occupations. Participation in occupations helps to develop the competence and self-esteem that are inherent in successful occupational performance and life role independence.

Chapter 5 examines the complexities of gerontic practice and the role and functions of occupational therapy geriatric health care. The well-being of the older adult as a primary goal of health care is emphasized. The clinician and consultant roles in gerontic occupational therapy are presented. The continuity of occupational therapy services follows the discussion of these practice considerations. Medical rehabilitation as a major focus and practice arena for gerontic occupational therapy is explained.

Chapters 6 and 7 examine the specific functions and delivery of services to older adults in acute care hospital and rehabilitation settings, respectively. The treatment process, including evaluation, intervention, and discharge planning functions, is described. Special considerations for occupational therapy services in acute care and skilled nursing facilities and home health care settings are detailed. Reimbursement and other issues and trends in gerontic occupational therapy practice are also discussed.

Chapter 8 emphasizes environmental design, modification, and adaptation practice functions and addresses both practice and ethical considerations in the use of assistive technology. Low- and high-technology devices are described in relation to continued aging in the home. Universal designs and barrier-free environments in relation to apartment, single home, and senior housing dwellings are explained.

Chapter 9 examines the role and functions of the occupational therapy consultant in promoting successful aging, health, wellness, and quality of life. The chapter explores the impact of change in health care delivery and the needs for services of the increasing older adult population. Several models for the delivery of consultation services and their application in a variety of community settings are examined.

Chapter 10 examines adult day care for the frail elderly. Continued community living for this population is emphasized. The chapter describes types of day care settings and performance levels in these day care settings. Evaluation for identifying remaining functional abilities and the need for personal care is explained. Recommendations for continued activity involve-

ment is stressed. Staff and caregiver consultation is detailed. Special program development to address the needs of the cognitively impaired and of other frail older adults is considered. Care issues and other practice considerations are also examined.

References

American Occupational Therapy Association. (1994). Uniform terminology for occupational therapy—Third edition. *American Journal of Occupational Therapy, 48,* 1047–1054.

Christiansen, C. (1991). Occupational therapy intervention for life performance. In C. Christiansen & C. Baum (Eds.), *Occupational therapy: Overcoming human performance deficits* (pp. 3–44). Thorofare, NJ: SLACK.

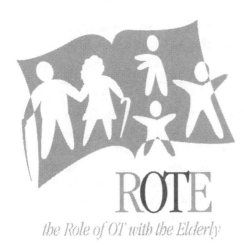

ROTE

the Role of OT with the Elderly

Occupational Therapy Services Within the Rehabilitation Health Care System

Regena G. Stevens-Ratchford, PhD, OTR/L, FAOTA

Abstract

Serious illness in later life often means hospitalization and loss of control over life situations, especially one's roles and routines. The older adult has had a lifetime of roles and experiences that reflect life autonomy. In this context, life autonomy is the ability to control and manage one's life situations with competence (Trombly, 1995a; Trombly, 1995c). This sense of life autonomy in turn contributes to one's physical, mental, and social well-being and overall health.

Well-being is a state of relative wellness—a positive state of being in mind, body, and spirit (Hales & Williams, 1986). In this state of wellness or well-being, the individual engages in "... an ever-expanding experience of purposeful, enjoyable living" (Hales & Williams, 1986, p. 4).

Serious illness or disability can disrupt this state of well-being and create a multidimensional set of health care problems (Gallo, Reichel, & Andersen, 1995). Serious illness may further complicate chronic conditions, such as arthritis, or disrupt family roles, such as caring for a disabled spouse or grandchildren. Such illnesses may also require changes in living arrangements and special care, such as rehabilitation or home health care, that are financial burdens to the individual and the family.

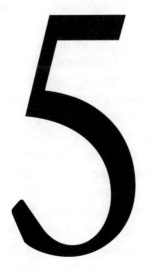

Caring for the older client is particularly challenging for the health care provider. A multidimensional approach that addresses the medical, psychosocial, and financial factors must be used to maximize the client's well-being. Maximization of the client's well-being is the primary focus of older adult health care (Bonder & Wagner, 1994).

Occupational therapy is a vital link to life autonomy and its accompanying independence because its emphasis is multidimensional. Occupational therapy addresses the physical, psychosocial, and occupational performance (Kielhofner, 1995b; Trombly, 1995b) problems that affect everyday function and living. Consideration of the individual's well-being is an inherent part of gerontic occupational practice.

This chapter examines the complexities of gerontic practice and the role of occupational therapy in geriatric health care. The well-being of the older adult is discussed as a primary goal of health care. The client-centered delivery of gerontic occupational therapy services is then examined. The clinician and consultant roles in gerontic occupational therapy are then presented and followed by a discussion of the special clinical and consultative considerations for the older adult. A discussion of the continuity of occupational therapy services follows, and medical rehabilitation as a major focus and practice area for gerontic occupational therapy is explained. The chapter concludes with an overview of all the practice settings in the medical rehabilitation sector of the health care system.

The Complexity of Gerontic Practice

The complexity of health care services for older adults is reflected in the roles and functions of the gerontic occupational therapist. Gerontic occupational therapy services for older adults involve the promotion of health and wellness (Reitz, 1992) as well as the prevention and rehabilitation of disabilities. Occupational therapy promotes health and well-being (Christiansen, 1991; Edwards, 1994) in physical, mental, and social realms of performance. This well-being is the foundation of occupational performance in home and community environments. The promotion of health and wellness is essential whether the individual is experiencing permanent or temporary impairments or disabilities (Christiansen, 1991).

The goal of gerontic occupational therapy is helping older adults to continue or resume their participation in everyday living at the highest quality of living (American Occupational Therapy Association [AOTA] 1994; Christiansen, 1991) and the greatest sense of well-being. Occupational therapy provides the individual with opportunities to participate in occupations, "the ordinary and familiar things that people do every day" (AOTA, 1995c, p. 1015). Participation in occupations helps to develop the competence and self-esteem (Trombly, 1995c) that are inherent in occupational performance and life role independence.

Particularly, participation in occupations promotes function (occupational performance) in life situations. In essence, "Occupational performance reflects the individual's dynamic experience of engaging in daily occupations within the environment" (Law & Baum, 1994, p. 12, as cited in AOTA, 1995c). This dynamic experience is closely related to what Hales and Williams (1986) refer to as wellness or well-being. In this instance, the "dynamic experience" (Law & Baum, 1994) may be equated with an ever-expanding experience of meaningful, enjoyable, purposeful living (Hales & Williams, 1986). Hence, a significant link can be inferred between the individual's experience of engaging in daily living (occupations) and the individual's well-being.

OLDER ADULT WELL-BEING

The importance of well-being (Hales & Williams, 1986) and quality of life (Bonder & Wagner, 1994; Kiernat, 1991) is fundamental for coping with and managing everyday life situations. The greater the older adult's physical, mental, and social well-being, the greater is his or her capacity to respond to and cope (Harke, 1991a, 1991b) with the physical or psychosocial problems that can occur in older adulthood, especially during serious illness. Serious illness creates a state of "non-well-being" that critically impacts occupational performance and the life autonomy that is experienced in later adulthood. When serious illness occurs, physical, psychosocial, or occupational performance problems may result. In short, life function is affected on a multidimensional level.

MULTIDIMENSIONAL HEALTH CARE PROBLEMS

The older adult who is admitted to the health care system (Levy, 1993) because of physical or mental illness experiences a loss of control over everyday management of life situations (life autonomy). The loss of autonomy that is associated with a health care admission affects mental and social well-being. When the older adult's well-being is threatened in this manner, the individual's response to treatment may be negatively influenced if the problems related to the individual's well-being are not addressed.

In addition to these well-being and life management concerns, the older adult who is admitted for health care services may present medical, psychological, social, and financial problems (Kelley, Kazamoto, & Rubenstein, 1991). The older adult's health care problems not only involve the medical diagnoses but may also include cognitive, psychological, and functional issues or limitations that further complicate the medical problems that instigated the need for health care services. These multidimensional problems can be further complicated by limited financial resources that can, in turn, restrict the individual from receiving the best and most comprehensive medical services.

Health care policies (Struthers & Schell, 1991) for older adults may also add to the complexities encountered during providing gerontic services. Cost containment policies, such as the perspective payment system (PPS) (DeJong & Sutton, 1995) and managed care (Repicky & Verynck, 1995), have limited hospital stays. Shorter acute hospital stays have resulted in the discharge of persons who still need medical care. This need for care can be especially problematic for the elderly. Older persons tend to have multiple diagnoses and chronic illnesses that affect their functioning. These individuals tend to need more care than the younger person; however, there are no differences in acute hospital stays for younger versus older adults. Moreover, there are increasing options for alternative postacute care that will be discussed later in this chapter.

Client-Centered Delivery of Services

THE EVOLUTION OF SERVICE DELIVERY

Provider-Driven Services

Historically, American health care has been provider driven (DeJong & Sutton, 1995). In this type of health care service presumed "experts" such as physicians and therapists know what are the most needed sets of services and how much of these services are needed by clients. The providers delivered an expert set of services and were paid on a fee-for-service basis. There was no attempt to contain health care costs, so third party payers instituted measures such as the perspective payment system and managed care (DeJong & Sutton, 1995). In response to the need for cost containment in the 1990s, health care has evolved from a provider- to a payer-driven system.

Payer-Driven and Consumer-Driven Health Care

In a payer-driven system of health care, the control of health care costs shifts from the provider to the payer. As a result of managed care, medical services are increasingly marketed and administered through health maintenance organizations. Such managed care plans attempt to maximize the market share of health care recipients by discounting services and maximizing financial gain by limiting services and marketing to low-risk populations (DeJong & Sutton, 1995).

A major criticism of such health care plans is the lack of proven quality as is indicated by published research data on the successful outcomes of services provided by managed care. Health care observers predict that health care will become increasingly consumer driven (DeJong & Sutton, 1995) as the demand for more services and coverage for high-risk populations, such as the elderly, increases. Additionally, as the demand for quality assurance (by demonstrating successful outcomes) increases, so will consumer-driven health care (DeJong & Sutton, 1995).

An understanding of who "drives" the health care system is essential if therapists and other health care providers are going to successfully market their services. In addition, successful marketing of services to payers and clients will require that service disciplines, like occupational therapy, develop treatment protocols that can be used to develop data for documentation of clinical outcomes (Bryant, 1995).

CLIENT-CENTERED SERVICE DELIVERY

It is important to note that AOTA (1995a) has officially identified occupational therapy as having a client-centered delivery approach. The client-centered approach to the delivery of occupational therapy services "considers systems, models, and contexts in making decisions that focus on the client's needs and ... engages the client as a participant" (AOTA, 1995a, p. 1029). The client is the person or organization for whom the occupational therapist provides service. A system here is an organized set of interdependent components that provide structure for function. Context refers to the temporal and environmental aspects of performance that can critically affect an individual's ability to engage occupations (AOTA, 1995a).

The occupational therapy client's values, needs, and priorities are central in this approach. As the health care system becomes more and more consumer oriented, the premises that underlie client-centered service delivery will place occupational therapists in a position to play a major and vital role in consumer-driven health care.

The Gerontic Occupational Therapy Role

Serious illness that results in the hospitalization and the loss of control over life situations makes the older adult particularly vulnerable to non-well-being and occupational dysfunction. The multidimensional nature of geriatric health care requires an approach that accommodates these complexities in treatment. The older adult who suffers impairments, disabilities, or handicaps (Trombly, 1995c) as a result of serious illness needs a practice approach that organizes the clinician's role and functions so that treatment always focuses on the older adult's well-being and return to some degree of competence and control over life situations.

The gerontic occupational therapist must not only be a clinician treating occupational and role dysfunction, but also be a consultant, providing advice, raising concerns, suggesting and weighing alternatives, and guiding the problem-solving process that will inevitably lead to the return of life roles that enable some degree of life autonomy. The clinical role addresses the more overt and immediate clinical manifestations of serious illness and disabilities, such as ADL dependence due to cognitive or sensorimotor impairments. On the other hand, the consultant role deals with the ongoing issues of well-being, life management, and life autonomy that accompany the role dysfunction and losses that result from disabling conditions. To ensure client-cen-

tered services that are truly comprehensive and holistic, the gerontic occupational therapist must develop strategies that accomplish short-term goals (Trombly, 1995b; Wells, 1986) that move the client inexorably toward productive living. These strategies need to encompass both clinical and consultative considerations.

Since the passage of the Older Americans Act in 1965 (Gelfand, 1993; Levy, 1993; Lewis, 1989) and the beginning of the era of health care reform, the array of older adult programs and services has continued to expand and create an even more complex service environment. In response to these factors, occupational therapy must develop methods for conceptualizing and implementing its services (Baum & Devereaux, 1983). Therapists need to create strategies that accommodate this expansion and complexity while at the same time capitalizing on occupational therapy's uniqueness of client-centered, holistic services.

One method of accommodating health care change and complexity is to better clarify the occupational therapist's roles and functions in geriatric care—especially in the areas of clinical and consultative services. Although occupational therapists often provide consultation in addition to clinical or direct services, these time-consuming functions are often viewed as part of the direct service process. When the therapist contracts to provide direct services, consultation may not be provided although some of the problems may require consultation during the problem-solving process.

Consultation is a valuable and needed service. It must be distinguished from direct services and recognized as an important part of the intervention process. Clinical services administered simultaneously with consultative services facilitate the organization of services so that the multidimensional problems of occupational performance, well-being, and life autonomy are continually considered as the individual proceeds through the recovery process.

These clinical and consultative roles are considered role components of the larger gerontic occupational therapy role. They are viewed as role components because both are essential in gerontic rehabilitation. The multidimensional health care problems of older adults; the fast-paced, short-stay nature of the health care system; and the complex environment of programs and services for older adults create rehabilitation circumstances that require both direct and consultative services. The occupational therapist must provide direct services that keep pace with short hospital stays and limited durations of service. The direct services allow practice and recovery of skills that return competence in self-care and other basic ADL functions. The delivery of these services demands treatment that incorporates organized and unhurried presentation of information and time to practice skills. Most clinical treatment sessions do not permit time to discuss the more complicated concerns of living arrangements, management of everyday living situations, and life autonomy in general.

However, occupational therapy can organize treatment protocols so that two to four 30-minute consultations are part of the overall treatment process. For example, if Ms. B, who has a residual left hemiparesis, is scheduled for 4 weeks of occupational therapy, the goal of therapy is maximum ADL independence. Ms. B's discharge plan is to return to her three-level townhome where she lives alone. She states,

"I think I'll be able to handle things if I can just get back to driving." She also states that she wants to reconnect with her social group activities and continue her volunteer work at the nursing home. Ms. B has physical, perceptual, and cognitive impairments as well as occupational performance problems that need to be treated during the clinical treatment sessions. The therapist plans to see her twice daily to treat these impairments and problems. The therapist also schedules four consultations to discuss and resolve problems that concern how she will manage her homemaker, social, and volunteer roles.

A similar need for consultation is seen in the case of a 70-year-old woman who has suffered a CVA and is admitted for acute care. In this instance, the gerontic therapist needs to be able to treat the client's immediate performance problems during a 1- to 2-week admission, as well as determine the client's needs for further occupational therapy. Additionally, the therapist must present alternative recommendations regarding living arrangements, activity involvement, or continued services. All of these service considerations must be geared toward restoring well-being and life autonomy. These multidimensional concerns are best addressed by organizing the gerontic occupational therapy role into two interrelating role components. The clinician component can deal with the immediate clinical issues, and the consultant role component can handle the broader, long-range issues of continued services and recovery of well-being and life autonomy. A role component in this view is a smaller role within the larger gerontic occupational therapy role. Each of the smaller roles has a particular set of practice considerations.

The Clinical Role: Older Adult Considerations

Occupational therapy's role in gerontic practice is helping older adults remain as active and independent as possible (Rogers, 1986) through both prevention (Edwards, 1994) and treatment strategies. As previously pointed out, the greatest threat to the older adult's well-being is serious illness that results in loss of autonomy and dependency. "Dependency is among the major fears of older adults" (Rogers, 1986, p. 117). Therefore, intervention focuses on developing ADL competence and self-efficacy (Trombly, 1995b) and recovering life role independence and autonomy—engagement in a dynamic, expanding experience of meaningful and purposeful activities (AOTA, 1995b, 1995c, 1995d; DeJong & Sutton, 1995; Hales & Williams, 1986; Kielhofner, 1995a; Trombly, 1995a).

EVALUATION CONSIDERATIONS

Evaluation is the process of obtaining and interpreting the data necessary for intervention. Assessment refers to specific tools or instruments that are used during the evaluation process (AOTA, 1994). The evaluation determines the client's functional level and is the first step in designing a treatment plan (Van Puymbrouck, 1993). The evaluation determines the individual's performance in self-care tasks and other higher-level ADLs. Because data from a comprehensive evaluation provides insight into the client's current and potential performance abilities, data must be gathered from a variety of sources. The occupational therapist gathers data on the following:

- Pre-morbid life roles and tasks
- The client's life story (Frank, 1996)
- Cognitive capacities
- Sensorimotor capacities
- Current impairments or disabilities
- Discharge plan
- Client's or family's goals (Van Puymbrouck, 1993)
- Present and alternative living arrangements
- Client's current well-being
- Potential well-being and life autonomy issues.

This comprehensive data set yields a picture of the balance of self-care, work, and leisure occupations that characterizes the person's lifestyle, the aging or medical conditions that have led to the person's current occupational status (Van Puymbrouck, 1993), and the client's well-being and potential for occupational independence and life autonomy. The older person's life history is of particular concern because it helps to explain who the individual is and where he or she has been. This knowledge of life history helps provide an understanding of the individual's well-being.

LIFE HISTORY, REMINISCENCE, AND THE CONTINUING LIFE STORY

The life history is the chronological or developmental story that is based on the important events in an individual's life (Frank, 1996). Persons 65 years of age or older have experienced more than 40 years of adult living. Their lives have included important events, role transitions, and coping with and adjusting to life's changes and challenges. These transitions and living strategies are often embodied in the stories that older adults share.

The older person's sharing of stories is an important part of the developmental process. As people age, they have an increasing tendency to engage in reminiscence or past-oriented thinking (Butler, 1963; Stevens-Ratchford,

1993). Reminiscence is not a therapy to help older persons experiencing psychological problems; it is a natural occurrence in old age (Butler, 1963). Reminiscence is manifested by nostalgia, recollection of past events and experiences, and storytelling (Stevens-Ratchford, 1990/1991). As in life history, stories and their telling are major characteristics of the reminiscence. Most older persons engage in life review reminiscence that involves an evaluative review of their lives that reflects on their satisfactions and accomplishments, as well as their disappointments and failures. The integration of these various past experiences into one's present life and living situation enables older persons to achieve a positive and acceptable view of their life's worth. Failure to accomplish this task can result in psychopathology (Butler, 1974). Reminiscence is also believed to promote successful adaptation in old age by maintaining self-esteem (Stevens-Ratchford, 1993). There continues to be a growing body of knowledge on the life story (Frank, 1996) and the use of life review reminiscence with older clients (Burnside, 1994; Stevens-Ratchford, 1993). As can be gleaned from the preceding case illustration, stories and reminiscence can have therapeutic benefits, especially in helping older adults who are depressed or need to integrate past experiences with present losses or challenges.

The gerontic occupational therapist can develop interview schedules that tap stories of the important events and transitions of the older person's life history. The therapist can also encourage reminiscing or the telling of stories about past events and experiences that indicated successful coping with challenges and adjusting to life changes. The sharing of such stories may promote the task of integrating the past with the present and achieving a positive acceptance of one's life as it has been (Butler, 1974; Erikson, 1959).

DEVELOPMENTAL TASKS CONSIDERATION

An understanding of later adult developmental tasks (Peterson, 1983) is important because it provides the therapist with a picture of the kinds of tasks and productive activities in which older adults should be involved. Several of these developmental tasks are related to adjustment to change and continued activity involvement (Peterson, 1983). These tasks include the following:

- Adjusting to age-related physical changes, such as decreasing vision or hearing
- Adjusting to the physical changes resulting from acute or chronic disabling conditions
- Adjusting to the changes that occur after the death of a spouse or a close friend
- Establishing satisfactory living arrangements in response to age-related physical changes, disabling conditions, or family changes
- Engaging in productive volunteer or leisure activities to replace work and family responsibilities
- Establishing explicit social relationships with other older persons.

A knowledge of these later adult developmental tasks provides a foundation for understanding the normal adjustment process in old age. This basic understanding can then be used to facilitate coping and adjusting to the acute situations that are a consequence of serious illness and disabling conditions.

Activity involvement and social relationships with peers are also important developmental tasks. Making referrals to senior centers and other older adult programs not only fosters well-being and life autonomy but also promotes continued older adult development.

THE OLDER ADULT LEARNER

One of the most important learning principles for older persons is that they benefit from self-pacing. In learning situations where information is presented quickly and in large chunks, learning is impeded. Information for the older adult learner needs to be presented in small units and delivered at a slower than normal pace. Presentation of units of information needs to be spaced. The elderly also need to be given time to respond to questions or performance commands. Highly organized presentations promote retention of information. In addition, learning conditions that oppose the older adult's values, habits, and preconceived notions impede learning (Stevens-Ratchford, 1990/1991).

These learning factors are important to consider and incorporate during treatment. The client-centered approach enables collaborative treatment planning that incorporates the client's priorities, opinions, and values. The client-centered approach facilitates learning and avoids situations that oppose the client's values.

The Consultant Role: Older Adult Considerations

CONSULTATION

In the context of this chapter, consultation is a process that involves raising concerns, identifying problems, counseling, giving advice or opinions, presenting and weighing alternatives, offering suggestions and recommendations, and providing help (Jaffe, 1992; Learner, 1992). The consultant is a professional who provides help through the sharing of expert knowledge in a variety of areas to help the client system resolve problems effectively and efficiently (Jaffe, 1992). The client system is the individual's treatment, family members, the social support system, or the residential support system. In short, the client system is all of the individuals or agencies involved in the problem that warrant occupational therapy consultation.

Consultation is different from the direct treatment services that are provided in the treatment of impairments, limitations, and disabilities (Trombly, 1995c). In the context of this chapter, consultation is the sharing of guidance and information that promotes the resolution of those problems that relate to advanced ADL tasks and life roles and that affect well-being, self-efficacy, productive living, and life autonomy.

In today's administration of direct services, there are time constraints that make it difficult to spend time with the client discussing adjustment, life role, and autonomy issues. Unless the gerontic therapist begins to develop strategies for delivering both direct and consultation services in gerontic settings, issues that relate to well-being and autonomy will receive cursory consideration. Cost containment and other service efficiency maneuvers have forced therapists to provide services in compressed time spheres. To make services cost-effective, treatment sessions are shortened, and the overall duration of occupational services is often limited by managed care policies.

The impetus to develop protocols that move the client quickly and efficiently through the treatment course (DeJong & Sutton, 1995) may present problems for the older adult recovering from a disabling condition. Older adults require more time than younger individuals to adjust and learn in new situations (Harke, 1991b). New service delivery methods and other responses to health care reform and cost containment may raise issues for older adults that will require the gerontic occupational therapist to play a consultant role. Occupational therapists will need to educate health care providers and payers regarding the characteristics and needs of older persons. They will also need to be advocates for the health care needs of older adults.

Additionally, as the gerontic occupational role continues to evolve in a changing health care environment, therapists will serve a growing number of older adults—especially those 85 years of age or older (Hasselkus, 1993). These individuals will need to understand and access the Aging Network (Gelfand, 1993). The Aging Network is an information resource that contains an array of medical, social, and community services for older adults. The network links individuals with clusters of people. The purpose of the Aging Network is to exchange information, share its resources, and facilitate self-help (Lewis, 1989).

Occupational therapists will need to be information specialists on the array of services of the Aging Network, especially those concerned with Medicare and Medicaid programs, medical care, in-home services, long-term-care residences and services, volunteer and educational programs, nutritional programs, adult day care, and multipurpose senior centers. The occupational therapist can provide consultation in the form of referrals, advice, alternatives regarding living arrangements, continued services, or involvement in productive pursuits in the community. This type of consultation not only contributes to the individual's well-being and life autonomy but also enhances the person's quality of life. Additionally, personnel working in the social

services component of the Aging Network, the area agencies on aging, senior centers, nutritional sites, chore services, and other agencies should be educated about occupational therapy clinical and consultative services (Rogers, 1986).

HANDICAPS AND THE LIFE STORY

Consultation is very necessary in developing the "post-disability" component of the individual's life story (Frank, 1996). The older adult, who must continue life with a handicap, often has to adjust to new living arrangements and living situations. The disabled older adult must continue to integrate his or her past with the present in order to continue to accomplish the final developmental task of accepting one's life as it has been (Stevens-Ratchford, 1990/1991, 1993). The individual needs to accomplish this acceptance of life with a validation of self-worth and self-esteem. The individual should be encouraged to reminisce and share positive experiences from the past (Stevens-Ratchford, 1993). This sharing of the past while living the present helps to integrate the two, continuing the life story with a new set of experiences that are positively connected to the past.

Medical Rehabilitation: A Major Focus for Gerontic Occupational Therapy

WHAT IS MEDICAL REHABILITATION?

Medical rehabilitation is an array of multidisciplinary evaluative, diagnostic, and therapeutic services that work to enhance the residual functional abilities of people who have suffered a disabling impairment as a result of congenital limitation, trauma, acute illness, chronic health condition, or other medical episode that has limited functional independence (DeJong & Sutton, 1995). The goal of medical rehabilitation is to enable the individual to live at his or her maximum level of independence in the least restrictive and most economical environment (DeJong & Sutton 1995; Rice & La Plante, 1992).

Sixty-four percent of the conditions treated in medical rehabilitation are stroke and orthopedic conditions, such as hip fracture (DeJong & Sutton, 1995; Rice & La Plante, 1992). During the 1980s, medical rehabilitation emerged as an essential component of the health care system. Medical rehabilitation purports to provide a full continuum of care for those individuals with physical or cognitive impairments. These impairments often afflict older adults who are major recipients of rehabilitation.

WHY IS MEDICAL REHABILITATION A MAJOR FOCUS?

There are several primary reasons for a therapeutic (especially occupational therapy) focus on medical rehabilitation. The following three reasons warrant focus on this area of care:

- The health care dollar. Services are reimbursable and a large proportion of health care dollars are in medical rehabilitation.

- Rehabilitation's rapid growth. The medical rehabilitation industry has experienced rapid growth during the 1980s and 1990s, and it is expected to continue to grow.

- The increasing older adult population. Medical rehabilitation provides services to a large population of older adults. This number of older adults is expected to continue to grow over the next 16 to 20 years as the "baby boom" generation reaches age 65.

Medical rehabilitation is estimated to be a $15 to $20 billion a year industry and is expected to exceed $45 billion by the year 2000 (DeJong & Sutton, 1995; Meili, 1993). Among the growing areas of medical rehabilitation are inpatient and outpatient services. Inpatient rehabilitation is provided in freestanding rehabilitation hospitals, in rehabilitation units within acute care hospitals, in long-term care facilities, and in subacute rehabilitation facilities, usually skilled nursing facilities (SNFs) (Haffey, Cayce, & Hallman, 1995; DeJong & Sutton, 1995). Some acute care hospitals are also developing subacute units in addition to their acute rehabilitation units.

Outpatient rehabilitation is provided in hospital-based outpatient facilities, non-hospital-based comprehensive outpatient rehabilitation facilities (CORFs), and through home-based rehabilitation (DeJong & Sutton, 1995).

Medical rehabilitation has grown rapidly during the 1980s and early 1990s and is viewed today as the most rapidly growing medical industry (DeJong & Sutton, 1995). This rapid growth is readily illustrated in the following data on the growth of the various areas of medical rehabilitation. Hospital-based rehabilitation includes the freestanding rehabilitation hospital or rehabilitation unit in acute care hospitals that have traditionally provided inpatient care. From 1985 to 1994, the number of rehabilitation hospitals has increased from 68 to 187 hospitals (275%). The number of rehabilitation units has increased from 386 to 804 units (208%) (DeJong & Sutton, 1995). Additionally, long-term care hospitals are another type of inpatient setting where medical rehab has grown. These facilities provide acute rehabilitation as well as care for individuals with chronic or terminal conditions. From 1985 to 1994, the number of long-term care hospitals has increased from 86 to 113 (18%). (DeJong & Sutton, 1995).

Another area of rapid growth is sub-acute care, including inpatient care in SNFs and in subacute rehabilitation units in hospitals. Subacute care is viewed as a less expensive alternative to inpatient medical rehabilitation. SNFs are thought to be the fastest growing part of rehabilitation. From 1985 to 1995, the number of SNFs has increased from 6,725 to 11,436 facilities (170%) (DeJong & Sutton, 1995). SNFs serve rehabilitation candidates who show little response to acute medical rehabilitation or who have chronic or acute conditions that render them unable to tolerate the intensity and pace of inpatient rehabilitation.

Comprehensive outpatient rehabilitation centers have also shown significant growth from 1985 to 1994. CORFs provide a comprehensive array of services, including vigorous day treatment programs for those individuals whose medical and nursing needs do not require 24-hour supervision and management. The number of CORFs has increased from 85 to 236 (278%).

Other outpatient rehabilitation centers, including hospital-based programs, hospital-based satellite centers, and freestanding outpatient centers, have also shown growth of 35% to 52% (DeJong & Sutton, 1995). These facilities serve clients who have only minor limitations in occupational performance or whose insurance does not cover inpatient rehabilitation.

Finally, home-based rehabilitation, a relatively new medical rehabilitation service, is another fast growing segment of the health care system. Home-based rehabilitation is usually provided through home health agencies in which occupational and physical thera-

py are well-established services (DeJong & Sutton, 1995).

OLDER ADULT NEEDS FOR MEDICAL REHABILITATION

In 1992, 64% of the medical rehabilitation discharges were people with stroke and orthopedically related conditions. Stroke is the largest impairment group served by medical rehabilitation. Stroke is one of the leading causes of disabilities in older people. Medicare is the largest payer for medical rehabilitation services.

As the 65-plus age population continues to grow, there will be an increasing demand for medical rehabilitation because disabling conditions increase with age (Rice & La Plante, 1992). The older adult population continues to be the fastest growing segment of population in the United States. From 1980 to 1991, the 65-plus age group increased by 24%, and the 85-plus age group increased by 41% (DeJong & Sutton, 1995).

The growing medical rehabilitation industry, the fact that these services are reimbursable, and the increasing older adult population are important reasons for occupational therapists to focus on providing gerontic services to older adults in this area of the health care system. As the medical rehabilitation industry continues to experience rapid growth and to serve an increasing number of older persons, the need for occupational therapists with special training in gerontology and geriatrics will grow. Gerontology is the study of aging theories, social and physical aspects of aging, and practice issues that address these age-related phenomena (Hasselkus, 1993). Geriatrics is the study of older adult health and medical care.

Gerontic occupational therapists not only need the knowledge and skills that will address the more simple problems of occupation and performance, but also need the clinical and consultative skills that will address the complex, multidimensional problems related to life roles, self-efficacy, and well-being.

Medical Rehabilitation in the 1990s

OUTCOME-ORIENTED REHABILITATION

Medical rehabilitation is an outcome-driven system. Outcome-oriented rehabilitation identifies outcomes (the results of rehabilitation intervention) for the client and measures the clinical outcomes to determine whether outcomes were achieved (Cope & Sundance, 1995). Cope and Sundance (1995) describe three kinds of outcomes for medical rehabilitation:

- Global outcome. The global outcome is the result of all clinical issues and treatment expressed in the most general form; it is the result of patient-specific outcomes, residual impairments, disabilities, and handicaps. It is also an expression of the objective recovery achieved and the subjective perceptions experienced that contribute to the person's quality of life.

- Outcome levels. Outcome levels are specific categories or groupings of patient problems and conditions that typically occur during the course of rehabilitation and recovery. Examples include achieving physiologic stability, being established in the residential environment, and returning to productive activity. There are six outcome levels ranging from 0 to V.

- Patient-specific outcomes. Patient-specific outcomes are the individual goals achieved through recovery and treatment of identified problems

specific to the patient and clinical condition. These may be medical, functional, psychological, social, or vocational in nature. "The collective result of achieving a group of patient-specific outcomes is typically the achievement of an outcome level" (Cope & Sundance, 1995, p. 44).

An outcome-oriented approach permits management of the complex problems involved in recovering from catastrophic losses.

Often there are two distinct age groups going through the course of rehabilitation: a young adult cohort that has received traumatic injuries and an older group coping with stroke and orthopedically related conditions. Each group needs a specialized approach that requires understanding of development and developmental tasks related to age-appropriate life roles and living situations. Dealing with catastrophic losses is a complex and difficult recovery and adjustment process at any age. However, this recovery and adjustment process is even more complicated and multidimensional for the older adult because of the interaction of age-related factors (Hasselkus, 1986, 1993). Again the multidimensional approach inherent in treating the individual's physical, psychological, and occupational performance needs is a unique approach that can readily be used in medical rehabilitation.

OUTCOME LEVELS

Level 0: Physiologic Instability

This is not truly an outcome level because the client has not yet been completely assessed, diagnosed, and managed. The category of physiologic instability is usually used to describe the client's appearance after the onset of the illness or injury (Cope &

Sundance, 1995). The individual generally has medical problems that require inpatient acute care.

Level I: Physiologic Stability

Physiologic stability is the first level of clinical outcome and is achieved when all major medical problems have been treated and managed. Some active medical and surgical problems may persist; however, they have been managed and the client no longer requires intensive physician or nursing supervision. The individual is discharged from the acute care hospital when outcome level I is achieved.

Level II: Physiologic Maintenance

The maintenance of the physiological system is the second clinical outcome. Although the outcome is usually achieved in acute care rehabilitation, it may also be reached in subacute rehabilitation, postacute residential, or outpatient or home settings. Limited mobility, self-care, communication, and cognitive and behavioral outcomes are part of this clinical outcome level and only to the degree that these functional abilities directly contribute to physiologic maintenance. This physiologic maintenance includes establishing adequate and safe systems of nutrition, prevention of aspiration, skin prevention, joint maintenance, and bowel and bladder management programs.

Level III: Primary Functional Goals (Home or Residential Integration)

Outcome level III is achieved when the client moves successfully through the necessary treatments to be able to function within the individual's selected long-term residence, home, nursing home, or other board and care facility (Cope & Sundance, 1995).

Level IV: Advanced Functional Goals (Community Reintegration)

Advanced rehabilitation outcomes are achieved at level IV. At this point in recovery, the client has developed those functional abilities that will enable appropriate function in the community with some degree of independence. This clinical outcome level is usually achieved by treatment delivered in home and community settings. The client's disability in relation to community reintegration depends on the client's disability and the community and environmental demands for functioning (Cope & Sundance, 1995). For example, a 75-year-old man with residual hemiparesis may be able to function fairly independently in a living arrangement where he lives with his son's family and walks to the neighborhood senior center to attend various activities. However, the demands of self-care and home and meal management would exceed his capabilities.

Level V: Productive Activity

Clinical outcome level V is the achievement of participation in productive activity within the individual's capacity (Cope & Sundance, 1995). Productive activities should be conducive to the client's interests and stage in life. These activities include work, education, recreation, and other leisure activities.

Levels III, IV, and V fall within the purview of occupational therapy because the outcomes are oriented to function in the occupational performance areas.

Summary

Medical rehabilitation and its array of services is the area of the health care system (Levy, 1993) that is servicing an ever-increasing number of older adults who have occupational performance problems. Medical rehabilitation and its continuum of services is an important focus of gerontic practice. Occupational therapists need to be aware of the trends and standards being established in rehabilitation services. Occupational therapy's emphasis on client-centered and holistic approaches to intervention provide valuable contributions toward achieving rehabilitation outcomes. In terms of the older adult, occupational therapists can play a salient role in helping older adults to achieve the more occupational-oriented outcomes with a sense of well-being, self-efficacy, and life autonomy. The occupational therapist can use life story and reminiscence strategies to help older adults recover their productive roles. Additionally, the multidimensional problems of the older adult can be more effectively addressed using both the clinician and consultant roles of the occupational therapist.

Case Study

The following case illustrates some of the complexities encountered in gerontic practice. The case illustration is presented in three parts:

1. Life story and role history
2. The serious illness and its effects on life roles
3. The treatment course and return to relative life autonomy.

The life story aspect of the case is presented because each older adult enters the health care process with a lifetime of well-established roles and routines and life management strategies. Life management strategies are the planning, organizing, functioning, coping, and adjusting tactics or maneuvers that enable productive activities, work, leisure, and other activities of daily living (ADLs). Knowing where the older adult has been helps the health care team to know how to help the patient return to productive participation in life.

The explanation of the serious illness and the circumstances contributing to the complexity of the case provide a background for understanding the client's multidimensional health care problems. The treatment course presents the issues and concerns encountered in the rehabilitation process.

LIFE STORY

Ms. J is an 80-year-old single woman. She was born in Durham, Connecticut. She was the youngest of six children. Ms. J has survived two brothers and three sisters. She has one living relative, a niece who lives in Pennsylvania and visits regularly. Ms. J attended Yale University and received a degree in biochemistry in 1921. She came to live in Baltimore in 1922. She worked as a biochemist and administrator for 45 years at Johns Hopkins Hospital. Ms. J participated in the development of pediatric antibiotics.

She was a patron of theater and arts. She enjoyed seeing plays that were comedies. Ms. J collected dolls, buttons, and depression glass. She was an avid reader of mysteries and historical novels. She has traveled all over the United States; her favorite place to visit was New England in the fall. She has always enjoyed doing things with friends.

In 1976 she moved from her long-time home in one of Baltimore's oldest neighborhoods to an apartment in a lifetime care community. Ms. J has been very active in community activities. She especially enjoyed going on community outings with her friends and playing bridge three times a week. She was a cashier at the center's Country Store. She attended an exercise group and took several daily walks around the community grounds.

SERIOUS ILLNESS

Ms. J survived a cardiovascular accident (CVA) 2 months ago. During the past 2 months, her medical condition has been very unstable. In addition to a severe residual left hemiplegia with upper and lower extremity contractures, the client has disphagia and hypertension and has experienced acute episodes of urinary tract infection and influenza. Currently she is experiencing depression. The patient has had two short hospitalizations since the 2-week hospital stay at the time of the stroke. The patient is now living in the skilled nursing facility of the lifetime care community. The physician's prognosis for recovery is poor. She was initially started on a rehabilitation program that included occupational, physical, and speech therapy beginning 2 weeks after the stroke. The therapies were discontinued after 1 week (4 weeks post stroke) because of influenza and other medical complications that necessitated hospitalization. The client has again been referred to occupational therapy for a program to improve her activities of daily living function.

Ms. J is currently very debilitated from both the stroke and the acute illnesses, dependent in self-care, and depressed. Ms. J is labile and appears listless and unmotivated during the occupational therapy screening. During the screening, a close friend and Ms. J's niece come into her room. They share with you that Ms. J does not like living in the nursing home and wants to return to her apartment. The niece asks, "Is there any way that my aunt will be able to return to living in her apartment?"

TREATMENT COURSE

Ms. J was seen in occupational therapy three times a week for a period of 2 months. The problems addressed during treatment were self-care dependence, cognitive impairment, and loss of productive roles. During the early phases of the treatment, Ms. J was tearful and uncommitted to treatment.

During the second week of therapy, the occupational therapist happened to witness a scene in which Ms. J yelled at the nursing assistant about giving her orange juice when she wanted cranberry juice. Ms. J explained to the therapist how having to wait to use the bathroom and for other care was really upsetting. She said the juice incident was "the last straw."

It was at this point in treatment that Ms. J began to tell stories of her premorbid life roles and activities. She told stories of being in charge of things, of bringing difficult workers "into line." During each succeeding treatment session, she would tell a story. As the therapist listened, the therapist began to develop a greater sense of who this woman was, where she had come from, and what she wanted. As these interactions increased, the depression lessened. Ms. J then became more involved in her treatment.

As Ms. J regained sitting balance, relearned to play bridge, and developed competence in some basic self-care skills, she became more and more assertive and idiosyncratic. She expressed her dislike of the nursing assistant's choosing her clothing and manner of dressing her hair. She once stated, "... and most of all, I hate waiting to go to the bathroom." Ms. J became a constant stream of complaints and a "problem" for nursing. The therapist spent a great deal of time talking with the niece, friends, the social worker, and the nursing staff in attempts to resolve some of the complaints. The outcome of these discussions was that Ms. J wanted to do what she wanted to do when she wanted. She wanted to "dictate" what and how things happened in the nursing facility. Of course this was not possible.

After 6 weeks of therapy with very minimal gains in ADL independence, Ms. J was transitioned from her apartment to a permanent residence within the nursing facility. Shortly after this time, Ms. J asked the therapist to help her hire an aide "so that I can dress the way I want to and have my hair as I like it." It was at this point that Ms. J began to regain control over her life.

She hired an aide for 10 hours a day for 7 days a week. Therapy was then directed at helping her to supervise and train the new aide. The aide became Ms. J's link to well-being and life autonomy; the aide was her mobility. With the aide's help, she was now able to go to the bathroom when she wanted to do so and to dress and groom herself in her own way. She could go on outings with friends, go for walks, be as mobile as she wanted. She continued her life story and participated in life, having overcome her handicaps and created a new version of independence.

CASE CONCERNS

Three areas of concern contribute to the complexity of this case: continuity of care, multiple medical diagnoses, and disruption of well-being.

CONTINUITY OF CARE

This client's primary diagnosis is one that warrants continued care in the form of both medical and rehabilitation services. The primary diagnosis here is RCVA because it presents the problems for primary consideration by the occupational therapist. The impairments underlying the occupational dysfunction that are experienced post cardiovascular accident require timely interventions of both pre-vention and remediation to ensure positive treatment outcomes in occupational performance. For example, range-of-motion problems might be lessened through a program of daily passive range-of-motion activities. Early participation in self-care activities helps facilitate tolerance for activities of daily living and prevents further debilitation.

Range-of-motion and endurance are essential factors in rehabilitation. The client's treatment experiences have focused on medical problems rather than the functional problems addressed in rehabilitation. The therapist in this case must treat occupational performance problems that resulted from the stroke, as well as treat the exaggerated performance component problems that have resulted because of the delay in initiating rehabilitation services.

MULTIPLE MEDICAL DIAGNOSES

In addition to the delay in initiating rehabilitation services for the cognitive and physical impairments that resulted from the stroke, the client is experiencing depression that may be a contributing factor to the listlessness and lack of motiva-tion. The recent acute illnesses and hospital readmission have not only added to the emotional stress experienced poststroke, they have further debilitated the client. Each condition has affected her occupational performance and participation in roles and routines and interrupted her autonomy in the general management of her life.

DISRUPTION OF WELL-BEING

Ms. J's participation in life was interrupted. She is now in a state of nonhealth and non-well-being. The security of independence and control over life situations has been replaced with uncertainty and dependence. Only with the return of a reasonable degree of self-efficacy can this client reestablish her well-being. In this instance, self-efficacy refers to the client's degree of competence and ability to be in charge of one's life (Trombly, 1995b).

Occupational Therapy Considerations

The preceding case presents not only a number of performance considerations (AOTA, 1994) but several medical and psychosocial problems for the occupational therapist's consideration. In the course of the initial screening, the occupational therapist is presented with both clinical and consultative problems. The patient's functional status and ADL dependence warrant the use of a number of clinical role functions; however, the niece's inquiry regarding the expected functional outcome (AOTA, 1994) necessitates the use of consultative role functions.

The gerontic occupational therapist must function as both a clinician and a consultant because of the complex nature of geriatric medicine. The older adult's medical and performance problems often necessitate changes in living arrangements that can seriously affect the client and his or her support system. If clinical outcomes are to be achieved, the occupational therapist must understand that the older adult must adjust to physical, environmental, and social changes. The client's well-being must be the central focus of the treatment.

During the treatment course, the therapist provided clinical services and consultation to resolve well-being issues and help the client reestablish self-efficacy and life autonomy. Life stories and reminiscing played a part in helping Ms. J reconnect with coping strategies that enabled adjustment to catastrophic losses and changes in living arrangements.

In summary, there are several complicating factors that contribute to the complexities of gerontic health care. Primary among these complicating factors is the well-being of the older adult. Well-being is central to self-efficacy and autonomy in life situations. The focus of health care is to maximize well-being. Serious illness in older adults often includes multiple medical conditions that disrupt one's control over life situations and one's sense of well-being. Serious illness in older persons present health care providers with a set of multidimensional care problems. The occupational therapist's unique emphasis on the treatment of physical, psychosocial, and occupational performance problems make occupational therapy a significant gerontic health care provider.

References

American Occupational Therapy Association. (1994). Uniform terminology for occupational therapy (3rd ed.). *American Journal of Occupational Therapy, 48,* 1047–1054.

American Occupational Therapy Association. (1995a). Concept paper: Service delivery in occupational therapy. *American Journal of Occupational Therapy, 49,* 1029–1031.

American Occupational Therapy Association. (1995b). Position paper: Broadening the construct of independence. *American Journal of Occupational Therapy, 49,* 1014.

American Occupational Therapy Association. (1995c). Position paper: Occupation. *American Journal of Occupational Therapy, 49,* 1015–1018.

American Occupational Therapy Association. (1995d). Position paper: Occupational performance: Occupational therapy's definition of function. *American Journal of Occupational Therapy, 49,* 1019–1020.

Baum, C., & Devereaux, E. B. (1983). Systems perspective—Conceptualizing occupational therapy in a complex environment. In H. Hopkins & H. D. Smith (Eds.), *Willard and Spackman's occupational therapy* (6th ed., pp. 799–814). Philadelphia: J. B. Lippincott.

Bonder, B. R., & Wagner, M. B. (1994). *Functional performance in older adults.* Philadelphia: F. A. Davis.

Bryant, E. T. (1995). Acute rehabilitation in an outcome-oriented model. In P. K. Landrum, N. D. Schmidt, & A. McClean (Eds.), *Outcome-oriented rehabilitation* (pp. 275–302). Gaithersburg, MD: Aspen.

Burnside, I. (1994). Reminiscence and life review: Therapeutic interventions for older people. *Nurse Practitioner,* 55–61.

Butler, R. N. (1963). The life review: An interpretation of reminiscence in the aged. *Psychiatry, 26,* 665–676.

Butler, R. N. (1974). Successful aging and the role of the life review. *Journal of the American Geriatrics Society, 22,* 529–535.

Christiansen, C. (1991). Occupational therapy intervention for life performance. In C. Christiansen & C. Baum (Eds.), *Occupational therapy: Overcoming human performance deficits* (pp. 3–44). Thorofare, NJ: SLACK.

Cope, D. N., & Sundance, P. (1995). Phsyiologic stability: Acute management. In P. K. Landrum, N. D. Schmidt, & A. McClean (Eds.), *Outcome-oriented rehabilitation* (pp. 57–67). Gaithersburg, MD: Aspen.

DeJong, G., & Sutton, J. P. (1995). Rehab 2000: The evaluation of medical rehabilitation in American health care. In P. K. Landrum, N. D. Schmidt, & A. McClean (Eds.), *Outcome-oriented rehabilitation* (pp. 3–42). Gaithersburg, MD: Aspen.

Edwards, D. F. (1994). Prevention of performance deficits. In B. R. Bonder & M. B. Wagner (Eds.), *Functional performance in older adults* (pp. 270–283). Philadelphia: F. A. Davis.

Erikson, E. H. (1959). Identity and the life cycle. *Psychological Issues, 1,* 87–98.

Frank, G. (1996). Life histories in occupational therapy clinical practice. *American Journal of Occupational Therapy, 50,* 251–264.

Gallo, J. J., Reichel, W., & Andersen, L. M. (1995). *Handbook of geriatric assessment.* Gaithersburg, MD: Aspen.

Gelfand, D. E. (1993). *The aging network: Programs and services* (4th ed.). New York: Springer.

Haffey, W. J., Cayce, L. E., & Hallman, L. E. (1995). Outcome-oriented subacute rehabilitation. In P. K. Landrum, N. D. Schmidt, & A. McClean (Eds.), *Outcome-oriented rehabilitation* (pp. 125–146). Gaithersburg, MD: Aspen.

Hales, D. R., & Williams, B. K. (1986). *An invitation to health* (3rd ed.). Menlo Park, CA: Benjamin/ Cummings.

Harke, R. J. (1991a). The aging process: Cognition, personality, and coping. In R. J. Harke (Ed.), *Psychological aspects of rehabilitation,* (pp. 45–72). Gaithersburg, MD: Aspen.

Harke, R. J. (1991b). The older adult's adjustment to the rehabilitation setting. In R. J. Harke (Ed.), *Psychological aspects of rehabilitation* (pp. 73–96). Gaithersburg, MD: Aspen.

Hasselkus, B. (1986). Assessment. In L. J. Davis & M. Kirkland (Eds.), *Role of occupational therapy with the elderly* (pp. 123–128). Rockville, MD: American Occupational Therapy Association.

Hasselkus, B. (1993). Aging and health. In H. Hopkins & H. D. Smith (Eds.), *Willard and Spackman's occupational therapy* (pp. 733–741). Philadelphia: J. B. Lippincott.

Jaffe, E. G. (1992). Theoretical concepts of consultation. In E. G. Jaffe & C. F. Epstein (Eds.), *Occupational therapy consultation: Theory principles and practice* (pp. 15–54). St. Louis: Mosby-Year Book.

Kelley, F. A., Kazamoto, T. T., & Rubenstein, L. Z. (1991). Assessment of the geriatric patient. In J. M. Kiernat (Ed.), *Occupational therapy and the older adult* (pp. 76–98). Gaithersburg, MD: Aspen.

Kielhofner, G. (1995a). The human system. In G. Kielhofner (Ed.), *A model of human occupation: Theory and application* (2nd ed.; pp. 9–26). Baltimore: Williams & Wilkins.

Kielhofner, G. (1995b). Introduction to the model of human occupation. In G. Kielhofner (Ed.), *A model of human occupation: Theory and application* (2nd ed.; pp. 1–8). Baltimore: Williams & Wilkins.

Kiernat, J. M. (Ed.), (1991). *Occupational therapy and the older adult.* Gaithersburg, MD: Aspen.

Law, M., & Baum, C. M. (1994). *Creating the future: A joint effort* (p.12). Washington University School of Medicine, St. Louis: Authors.

Learner, S. L. J. (1992). Hospital-based consultation. In E. G. Jaffe & C. F. Epstein (Eds.), *Occupational therapy consultation: Theory principles and practice* (pp. 311–324). St. Louis: Mosby-Year Book.

Levy, L. L. (1993). Occupational therapy's place in the health care system. In H. N. Hopkins & H. D. Smith (Eds.), *Willard and Spackman's occupational therapy* (pp. 357–367). Philadelphia: J. B. Lippincott.

Lewis, S. C. (1989). *Elder care in occupational therapy.* Thorofare, NJ: SLACK.

Meili, P. (April/May 1993). The rehabilitation market. *Rehabilitation Management,* 96–102.

Peterson, D. A. (1983). *Facilitating education for older learners.* San Francisco: Josey-Bass.

Reitz, S. M. (1992). A historical review of occupational therapies in preventive health and wellness. *American Journal of Occupational Therapy, 46*(1), 50–55.

Repicky, P. A., & Verynck, B. D. (1995). Outcome-based sales and marketing. In P. K. Landrum, N. D. Schmidt, & A. McClean (Eds.), *Outcome-oriented rehabilitation* (pp. 275–302). Gaithersburg, MD: Aspen.

Rice, D., & La Plante, M. (1992). Medical expenditures for disability and disabling conditions. *American Journal of Public Health, 82,* 739–741.

Rogers, J. C. (1986). Roles and functions of occupational therapy in gerontic practice. In L. J. Davis & M. Kirkland (Eds.), *Role of occupational therapy with the elderly* (pp. 117–121). Bethesda, MD: American Occupational Therapy Association.

Stevens-Ratchford, R. G. (1990/1991). The effectiveness of the reminiscence instructional systems design package in an educational program for older adults (doctoral dissertation, University of Maryland, 1990). *Dissertation Abstracts International, 49*, 5712.

Stevens-Ratchford, R. G. (1993). The effect of life review reminiscence activities on depression and self-esteem in older adults. *American Journal of Occupational Therapy, 47*, 413–419.

Struthers, M. S., & Schell, B. B. (1991). Public policy and its influence on performance. In C. Christiansen & C. Baum (Eds.), *Occupational therapy: Overcoming human performance deficits* (pp. 178–196). Thorofare, NJ: SLACK.

Trombly, C. A. (1995a). Purposefulness and meaningfulness as therapeutic mechanisms. *American Journal of Occupational Therapy, 49*, 960–972.

Trombly, C. A. (1995b). Planning, guiding, and documenting therapy. In C. A. Trombly (Ed.), *Occupational therapy for physical dysfunction* (pp. 29–40). Baltimore, MD: Williams & Wilkins.

Trombly, C. A. (1995c). Theoretical foundations for practice. In C. A. Trombly (Ed.), *Occupational therapy for physical dysfunction* (pp. 15–28). Baltimore, MD: Williams & Wilkins.

Van Puymbrouck, L. (1993). The occupational therapy evaluation of component skills. In J. Glickstein (Ed.), *Guide to functional assessment in geriatric rehabilitation* (pp. 25–30). Gaithersburg, MD: Aspen.

Wells, M. A. (1986). Treatment planning. In L. J. Davis & M. Kirkland (Eds.), *Role of occupational therapy with the elderly* (pp. 129–33). Bethesda, MD: American Occupational Therapy Association.

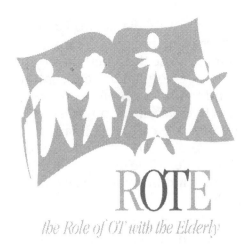

ROTE
the Role of OT with the Elderly

6

Primary Care

Jill Cohen Schie, MGA, OTR/L

Abstract

According to data from the National Center for Health Statistics (1989), senior citizens compose 12% of the United States population and consume more than 30% of all hospital resources. In 1995, 34 million Americans reached their 65th birthday, compared to 3 million in 1900. These increasing numbers are attributed to gains in life expectancy, especially in the age 85 and older category, one of the fastest growing segments of the elderly population. In 1900, the average life expectancy was 47.3 years. In 1993, the average life expectancy was 75.5 years, a gain of 28.2 years (Treas, 1995).

With a continuing increase in life expectancy, the elderly population represents a major consumer of rehabilitation services. In spite of this, the National Center for Health Statistics reported that rehabilitation services were available in only 44 to 56% of Medicare- and Medicaid-certified nursing facilities in 1989. According to Gill (1995), subacute care rehabilitation services have become a recognized entity along the continuum of care with the 1995 publication of standards for subacute care by the Joint Commission on Accreditation of Healthcare Organizations (JCAHO) and the Commission on Accreditation of Rehabilitation Facilities (CARF). Granger, Hamilton, and Gresham (1988) have shown positive outcomes of stroke rehabilitation following the completion of an acute rehabilitation program in the long-term care setting. The success was attributed to the need for a slower pace program and a longer period for the patient to achieve goals.

The decreased length of stay in the acute care hospital continues to produce more short-stay placement patients discharged to the subacute care setting (Brummel-Smith & Brody, 1995). This change has resulted in the workforce expanding into subacute care facilities and thus increased the recognition of the geriatric practitioner (Kiernat, 1991). Faust and Meaker (1991) found that as inpatient hospital stays shortened, the volume of occupational therapy services provided in the subacute care setting increased.

This chapter examines the changing service delivery model in the role of occupational therapy for the elderly population in both the acute care and the subacute care settings. First, acute care services are delineated from subacute care. The priorities for the occupational therapist during the evaluation, treatment, and discharge planning phases are presented for both settings. Second, other care issues and ethical considerations are discussed. These include issues related to culture, lifestyle, and assessment of outcomes. Finally, case studies are provided to illustrate the challenges that occupational therapy practitioners face in treating elderly patients.

Acute Care Versus Subacute Care

Acute care occupational therapy services are usually found in a general hospital. Occupational therapists in the acute care setting treat patients with a variety of medical and surgical diagnoses. The term *acute* refers to a condition that is "in crisis" and requires immediate medical attention. In contrast, subacute occupational therapy services are generally found in nursing homes, although there are subacute care rehabilitation units within the hospital setting. Subacute care rehabilitation can be defined in terms of the amount of therapy provided, the intensity of medical supervision necessary, or the complexity of the clinical profile (Salcido & Moore, 1995).

The increasing development of new subacute care programs in recent years can be attributed to two factors. First, there is intense pressure from payers to decrease the length of stay in the acute care hospital to help control costs, and to find an appropriate and cost-effective placement post discharge. Subacute care rehabilitation programs receive 80% of their revenue from Medicare, while exempt rehabilitation units and hospitals receive 70% (Gill, 1995).

Second, the patients who would traditionally have been transferred to an inpatient rehabilitation facility are leaving acute care facilities sicker and unable to tolerate a rigorous therapy regime. In addition, the increasing number of elderly patients who are discharged from the acute care setting do not meet the admission requirements of rehabilitation units and hospitals (Gill, 1995).

Subacute rehabilitation, unlike rehabilitation received in the acute hospital setting, is covered only under Medicare or other private insurance. Some of the elderly patients who enter a subacute rehabilitation program do not progress as expected and end up converting to long-term placement in a nursing facility. In this case, patients or their families must apply for Medicaid or other state assistance that covers long-term care. The option to pay privately is also available to those who can afford an extension beyond the days covered by Medicare.

Subacute rehabilitation programs have become more profitable due to the increased number of patients. Nursing facilities with subacute programs are able to provide a comparable product at a lower cost. The increased utilization of support personnel is one strategy used in subacute programs to provide the amount and intensity of therapy that is ordered. The stigma of the long-term care facility has changed with marketing efforts and a change in philosophy. Subacute programs now have a more interdisciplinary team of rehabilitation specialists that may include a consulting physiatrist. They are also improving their physical plant and equipment to entice practitioners as well as prospective patients and families.

Many subacute programs are looking toward contract agencies to fill the gap and provide the necessary staffing to meet the current demands of this growing specialty. Contract agencies will also provide marketing to build rehabilitation volumes which, in turn, may increase revenue. The contract agency and the rehabilitation professionals they employ work collaboratively with the facility on issues such as creating innovative programming, providing in-service training, and developing restorative programs.

In summary, the pressures of a decreased length of stay are helping to define the path the patient takes on the rehabilitation continuum beginning in the acute care setting.

Acute Care Evaluation

The elderly patient usually enters the acute care hospital with an acute medical condition. Quite often, it may be a significant event, such as a cerebrovascular accident (CVA) or the flare-up of a chronic condition, such as congestive heart failure (CHF), chronic obstructive pulmonary disease (COPD), or a change in mental status. The detail of the occupational therapy evaluation in the acute care phase depends on the severity and chronicity of the condition.

Standardized tests, performance checklists, and functional activities may be used to evaluate performance areas. The initial evaluation in acute care is usually general versus specific due to time limitations in the length of stay or the severity of the medical con-

dition. This allows the occupational therapist to proceed with the obvious treatment concerns quickly and follow up with more detailed standardized evaluations as needed (Kelley, Kawamoto, & Rubenstein, 1991).

An elderly patient admitted with a sudden onset of weakness or paralysis in the case of a CVA may be viewed differently than a patient with a fall resulting in a hip fracture or a patient in acute respiratory distress who is placed on a ventilator. Factors that need to be considered include how the patient was functioning before admission, what type of setting he or she came from, and what supports are available upon return to the previous living situation.

The occupational therapy evaluation of a patient who is admitted to the acute care setting with a more chronic condition or from a setting other than home, may have a completely different focus for evaluation and treatment. If there is no change in neurologic function, a change in mental status or decline in physical functioning may be the focus of the evaluation. When working with the elderly, involvement of family members is particularly important as they may be the primary caregivers. Caregiver training may include teaching family members how to assist the patient with basic activities of daily living (ADL), perform transfer techniques, or select the appropriate durable medical equipment (DME) and assistive devices. Caregiver training may also focus on teaching the family the best strategies to deal with cognitive impairment.

IDENTIFYING PERFORMANCE PROBLEMS

How is it that despite the decreasing length of stay in the acute care setting, an occupational therapist can identify the performance problems that are limiting independence and provide intervention in such a short time frame for a successful outcome? The key to identifying performance problems in the elderly patient is to obtain an accurate history and description of what the patient's status was before admission. For example, if the patient was bedridden and dependent in all ADLs except for feeding, it is probably unrealistic to set goals for independent dressing. It is essential to establish a baseline functional status. This can be obtained quickly by contacting a reliable family member.

Cognitive and motor deficits can be evaluated as the patient performs key functional tasks. Cognitive impairment is often a major limiting factor in an elderly patient's ability to achieve his or her prior level of function. Long, detailed standardized evaluations are being traded in for more functional tests that mean more to the patient. Medicare guidelines for occupational therapy have encouraged the use of functional-based evaluation and treatment. Repetitive and non-skilled interventions are not covered under Medicare (American Occupational Therapy Association [AOTA], 1987).

The role of the certified occupational therapy assistant (COTA) in evaluating ADL tasks in collaboration with the occupational therapist is common. Regulation of the COTA's ability to participate in the evaluation process is individual to each state practice act.

SETTING PRIORITIES AND GOALS

With the acute care hospital stay shrinking in number of days, priorities and goals for occupational therapy must be set quickly and carefully. The occupational therapist establishes priorities based on the evaluation findings and the patient's individual goals.

Goals must be relevant to a patient's lifestyle and current needs and may reflect a patient's prior level of functioning. The patient's input into the goal-setting process is critical. Discharge disposition, which is discussed later in this chapter, is also a factor that is considered when setting priorities and goals.

Priorities for a patient returning to an independent living situation are much different than those of a patient returning to an assisted living facility for a short stay or long-term placement. The priorities and goals for an elderly patient living in a senior citizen apartment which provides daily meals may be different than those for a patient who must prepare daily meals alone, or an elderly widow who has full-time help. The possibility exists that ADL may be a high priority for some patients and community skills or home management a priority for other patients, even if they have similar medical conditions.

ACCOMPLISHING GOALS WITHIN TIME CONSTRAINTS

Time constraints are a major factor to be considered when establishing a treatment plan and goals. There is little time to waste, and this may be complicated by unforeseeable changes in medical condition. In one urban teaching center in Washington, DC, the length of stay for an uncomplicated CVA has dropped from 11.8 days in 1993 to 6.3 days in 1995. If you count an average of 2 weekend days where occupational therapy may be unavailable, this leaves 4 days in which to plan priorities and accomplish occupational therapy goals.

A patient admitted for a total hip replacement is generally given 4 days in acute care (Blue Cross and Blue Shield of the National Capital Area,

1994). This may include admission on the day of surgery, beginning occupational therapy on postoperative day 1 or 2, and discharge on postoperative day 5. Short-term goals in the acute care setting that used to be set for every three to five sessions are now being set for every one to two sessions.

In summary, the occupational therapist seeing the patient through the acute care phase needs to quickly triage, evaluate, establish priorities, and set goals often all within the first occupational therapy session. Nursing personnel may be educated to carry out recommendations that have been made by the occupational therapist.

Subacute Care Evaluation

Evaluation for occupational therapy in the subacute care setting can be very different from that in the acute care setting. First, the patients may be more medically stable, although for patients being discharged from the primary care setting with more acute illness, this may not always be the case. The medical condition for which the patient was admitted to the primary setting is usually not as acute when the patient is admitted to the subacute care setting. The patient may have already begun to show signs of improvement or recovery. Second, referral for evaluation of occupational therapy may be more automatic for subacute patients than in the past. In the past, referral for occupational therapy or other rehabilitation services had to be solicited from physicians who were not always familiar with the reason or benefit from these type of services in the long-term care setting.

In the past, when a patient went into a long-term care setting, the plan did not include discharge to home as in the subacute care philosophy. If a discharge summary or evaluation is sent with the patient from the acute care setting, this can make the evaluation period more cost-effective by knowing what the patient's baseline on admission to acute care was and his or her progress thus far.

The occupational therapy evaluation of the geriatric patient in the subacute care setting should progress quickly and focus on the place where the treatment plan and goals in acute care ended. New problems may arise that were not previously evaluated in the acute care setting. These may include, but are not limited to, deficits with meal preparation, home management, access to public transportation, or return to driving. The need to obtain equipment to promote safety may require evaluation as well. This may include fitting and ordering of a wheelchair, bathroom equipment, or other adaptive aids.

Training caregivers or family members may also need to be addressed before discharge. The long-term goal for occupational therapy in the subacute care setting is to return the patient to the highest level of functioning and to enable the person to be discharged to return to his or her prior living arrangement as soon as physically able to do so.

IDENTIFYING PERFORMANCE PROBLEMS

The acute care evaluation or discharge summary is a good place to start in identifying performance problems for the geriatric patient in the subacute care setting. It is very important to understand and consider the patient's premorbid lifestyle, leisure interests, and functional status before he or she was admitted. If a patient had assistance with ADLs from a family member or other caretaker before being admitted, it may be unrealistic that goals are set to return to complete independence. It is important to talk to the patient and family members to learn what their priorities and goals are.

A common performance area that is addressed is the evaluation of the patient's ADL abilities. The presence of motor or sensory deficits can be observed during the evaluation. The degree to which the impairment will affect the patient's ability to achieve partial or full recovery can be estimated. With the general age in the United States increasing, more elderly patients are living longer and remaining far more active into their later years. Performance problems surrounding work and productive activities, such as driving or home management, may be an important part of a patient's lifestyle.

Cognitive deficits that may have been present to a lesser degree before admission to a subacute care setting may be more pronounced and prove to be the most difficult challenge facing the patient, the family, and the occupational therapy practitioner. Cognitive impairments, such as problems with short-term memory, safety or judgment, attention, or reasoning may limit the patient and his or her ability to return to independence more than the actual physical problems.

It is also important not to forget the psychosocial issues that accompany aging. These may include the loss of a spouse, close friends, or even a child. For many elderly patients, a senior center or housing provides the social interaction that families may be unable to provide. It is essential that elderly patients be able to make their own choices while still able, whether it be where to live or who is available to help them with their daily care.

SETTING PRIORITIES AND GOALS

Goals are very individual, and it is important that, when possible, the patient take part in setting them. It is also important that the goals be realistic and achievable in a reasonable time.

Goals for occupational therapy in the subacute care setting can focus on many different areas, including ADL, work and productive activities, or cognitive retraining.

Goals focusing on the area of ADL may include instruction in compensatory techniques during feeding, dressing, or bathing, and training in the use of adaptive equipment. Goals for work and productive activities may focus on simple meal preparation, transportation issues, or leisure issues. Goals for cognitive retraining may focus on the patient's ability to integrate the present level of cognitive function or safety issues within an individual ADL routine.

Discharge Planning and Follow-Up

Discharge planning may begin before the patient even enters the hospital. For preplanned surgeries and elective admissions, discharge often begins with a preadmission interview by a social worker or a more in-depth history taken by the physician during an office visit or preadmission testing. Preadmission evaluation by therapy professionals for planned admissions are also becoming more common practice.

Formulating a discharge plan for the elderly is often more complicated than for the average patient who enters for an elective procedure. The patient may have been living alone or in assisted living housing which is no longer possible. A patient may also have been living with family members who are now unable to care for their elderly parent due to heavy physical needs or the need for 24-hour supervision. In this case, long-term placement in a nursing facility may be indicated.

The social worker often acts as a liaison between the family and other team members, including the occupational therapist. The social worker often will relay information regarding progress, continued care needs, potential equipment needs, and family and caregiver training issues. Family conferences may be arranged for this purpose or when the family's expectations regarding progress or outcomes are unrealistic or unachievable from the rehabilitation professional's prospective.

In the case where the family decides it is unable to care for an elderly relative in the home, several options exist. Depending on the level of care the patient needs, there may be assisted living options or a senior citizens' apartment where meals are provided and home management services are offered. These environments may also provide safety features in the apartment, including pull cords to call for help, grab bars, or bath benches in the bathroom. Some of these housing arrangements will allow patients who are independent using a wheelchair; others may require a person to be ambulatory, with or without an assistive device.

A patient may receive post discharge follow-up at home or in a relative's home through a home care agency. Follow-up in the home can consist of any combination of nursing, occupational therapy, physical therapy, or speech therapy services. Home care has become more popular as many elderly individuals are unable to leave the house and families are unable to arrange transportation. A patient may require only an evaluation or several therapy sessions to continue working on goals initially established in the hospital. The advantage to follow-up in the home is the presence of real-life situations in which to practice and problem solve. Homemaker or nursing aide services may also be available to assist the patient and family in ADLs or work and productive activities.

Care Issues and Ethical Considerations

Culture plays a significant role in the patient evaluation, treatment planning, goal setting, and discharge planning in both the acute and subacute care settings. It is important to consider these factors and specific patient and family requests when formulating the occupational therapy plan.

Certain well-accepted occupational therapy evaluation or treatment approaches may be appropriate in one culture and not in another. Nonverbal communication, such as eye contact, personal space, or touch can be cultural barriers during treatment (McCormack, Llorens, & Glogoski, 1991). In addition, there may be particular customs associated with diet, dress, or other activities of daily living. It is important to identify any issues early on and ask permission, if necessary, so that the patient or family member is not insulted when asked to perform various tasks.

When it comes to discharge planning, some cultures would not consider placing a family member in a long-term care setting even for a short stay. They would rather care for the patient at home and will often go to great lengths to make sure the appropriate care is in place, such as a nursing aide to assist with ADLs or a homemaker to prepare meals.

Lifestyle and Habits

As previously mentioned, it is important to understand a patient's previous lifestyle and to plan accordingly. A patient who previously did not leave the house to grocery shop or socialize would probably not gain much benefit from this in his or her treatment plan. A homebound patient who prior to admission would have completed ADL and simple home management tasks could focus on these areas during treatment. If a patient has always had help with housecleaning then it is unlikely that he or she will need to focus on this skill.

In contrast, a very active and social elderly patient would want to resume as much of the previous active lifestyle as possible. Being able to play bridge or resume having meals in a community dining room may be very important and motivating for a patient. Some lifestyle habits can be modified to meet certain limitations and still provide a feeling of participation for the elderly patient.

Assessment of Outcomes

Assessment of functional outcomes is a popular topic in rehabilitation literature. There are many commonly known outcome measures, such as the Functional Independence Measure (Hamilton, Granger, Sherwin, Zielzny, & Tashman, 1987), the Rehabilitation Institute of Chicago Functional Assessment Scale (RICFAS) for acute medical rehabilitation (Heinemann, 1989), and the Minimum Data Set (MDS) (Health Care Financing Administration, 1990) for the long-term-care setting. Insurers are looking more closely at outcome measures throughout the continuum of care to determine the benefit of rehabilitation intervention.

There is more reported research on outcome measures in the acute inpatient rehabilitation setting than in the subacute care setting. As insurers begin to dictate where a patient goes following an acute hospitalization and cost is a factor in determining this placement, more research will be needed to determine whether the subacute care setting does provide positive outcomes along with a less costly price tag. There are limited research studies that specifically address the quality of outcomes received in the subacute care setting. Factors such as age and more aggressive rehabilitation have been cited as having a more positive outcome for decreasing impairment and allowing the patient to return home (Gill, Howells, & Hoffman, 1993).

In one study in the physical therapy literature, researchers concluded that only the intensity of therapy rather than baseline function in activities of daily living or cognitive function was associated with improvement in functional outcome. Furthermore, advanced age, dependence in ADL status, or cognitive impairment were not associated with poor outcomes (Chiodo, Gerety, Mulrow, Rhodes, & Tuley, 1992). It is clear that there is a need for more research on assessment of outcomes in the acute and subacute care settings.

Summary

This chapter focused on the changing role of occupational therapy in the acute and subacute care settings. As the length of stay continues to decrease in the acute care setting, occupational therapists will need to become more skilled in quickly assessing performance problems, setting attainable goals, and assisting with the discharge planning process. With the changes in the subacute care setting, the occupational therapist must now plan for patients who are more frequently discharged home rather than remaining in the subacute care setting.

Discharge planning is taking on a new role as well. Discharge planning may begin before the patient enters the hospital and can continue after the patient returns home. The challenge remains in finding a suitable placement for the elderly when the level of function has significantly changed and the patient cannot return to the previous living situation.

Ethical, cultural issues, and previous lifestyle are important to thoroughly understand, especially when dealing with the elderly patient. Elderly patients who suffer from chronic medical problems or an acute illness may require placement on life support. There is much debate on issues regarding medical futility in the elderly.

Cultural issues need to be understood to appropriately plan a meaningful treatment plan and gain maximal participation from the patient. An assessment of a patient's previous lifestyle and habits will assist in this process and allow the occupational therapist to plan accordingly.

With increasing competition in managed care, all types of healthcare facilities that provide rehabilitation are focusing on providing outcome data to third-party payers. Although there are data to support the benefit of rehabilitation in the acute inpatient setting, payers are more often choosing the subacute care setting due to a lower cost. Additional outcome studies are needed that show the benefits of subacute rehabilitation. A rehabilitation system that can market a product that provides services throughout the continuum of care may ultimately win the competition. In the end though, the insurance company makes the final decision, sometimes leaving the patient with a decision that does not lend much flexibility.

Two case studies have been provided, one for the acute care setting and one for the subacute care setting. Case studies provide an opportunity for clinical reasoning and help to illustrate how the evaluation, treatment planning, goal setting, and discharge planning processes actually occur. The case studies provided have been fabricated from the author's experience in acute care and subacute care settings and are meant to assist the occupational therapy practitioner in understanding the main concepts presented in this chapter.

Case Studies

CASE STUDY 1—ACUTE CARE

The patient is a 70-year-old, right-hand dominant man who sustained a left CVA with right hemiparesis and mild expressive aphasia. Other pertinent medical history included hypertension (HTN), a past history of myocardial infarction (MI), and diabetes mellitus (DM). The social history revealed that the patient lived with his wife in a one-story rambler. The patient had been retired from the federal government for 7 years. The patient and his wife enjoyed an active lifestyle taking day trips, going out to eat, and taking care of their grandchildren.

The patient was admitted to the acute care hospital after a 1- to 2-day onset of slurred speech and trouble holding onto objects, often dropping them. The patient status on evaluation revealed the following information.

ADL

The patient fed himself with minimal assistance after packages and cartons were opened using the left nondominant hand. The patient was unable to maintain a good grasp of the eating utensil with the right hand. Bathing tasks required moderate assistance to reach back and legs due to decreased endurance. Dressing required moderate assistance for upper extremities and maximum assistance for lower extremities.

Functional Mobility and Balance

The patient transferred from bed to wheelchair and from wheelchair to bed with minimum assistance. His static sitting balance was good; dynamic fair+. Standing balance was fair+ static and fair dynamic.

Upper Extremity Status

Within normal limits (WNL) in the left upper extremity; active isolated movement present at all joints in the right upper extremity, although quality of movement was decreased and the patient was noted to have a slight increase in tone which was greater proximal than distal. The right upper extremity tended to move in a flexor synergy pattern when the patient was asked to lift his arm. Gross grasp was present. Fine motor coordination was impaired. Patient had isolated finger movements throughout the right hand, but was unable to oppose thumb to the index finger. Patient could move the wrist against gravity. Sensation appeared WNL throughout the upper extremity. Patient had difficulty distinguishing movements of the right upper extremity as it was moved throughout space.

Cognition

The patient was alert and oriented to person, place, and time. He followed demonstrated instructions well. Visual memory was intact. Auditory memory and ability to follow verbal instructions were impaired. Judgment, reasoning and problem solving appeared to be intact.

Perception

The patient did not have any problem with body scheme or praxis; he showed evidence of homonymous hemianopsia.

Psychosocial

The patient had exhibited some signs of mild depression with his new disability and the inability to engage in his former active lifestyle.

Course of treatment

Six days after his discharge from the acute setting, the patient was able to perform ADL tasks with minimal assistance for his upper extremities and moderate assistance for his lower extremities. His feeding was independent, and his bathing required minimal assistance. Transfers required minimal assistance because of decreased standing balance. The patient was able to take several steps in the parallel bars with minimal assistance. The quality of active isolated movement had increased throughout the right upper extremity. The patient was transferred to an inpatient rehabilitation setting where he stayed for 3 weeks, followed by outpatient rehabilitation three times per week.

Outcome

The patient continued to show improvement and was able to ambulate with a quad cane, requiring supervision only for dressing and bathing, and using the right upper extremity as a gross assist. The outpatient treatment then focused on increasing the range of motion in his scapula and shoulder as well as fine motor coordination of the right hand to enable the patient to return to his hobby of gardening. The patient has learned to compensate for the residual effects of the hemianopsia.

The patient and his wife continued to enjoy an active lifestyle with modifications that are limited only by the patient's endurance and residual mild expressive aphasia. The patient and his wife appear to be coping with the changes in their lifestyle and receive continual support from their children and close friends.

CASE STUDY 2—SUBACUTE CARE

The patient is a 75-year-old woman who was admitted to the subacute care setting after an intertrochanteric fracture when she slipped and fell on the ice outside her apartment. In the acute setting, she had an open reduction and internal fixation (ORIF). She was transferred to the subacute care setting after 4 days. Her weight bearing status was as tolerated (WBAT). Social history revealed that the patient was otherwise healthy before this fall and lived in a senior citizen apartment building. She fixed a light breakfast and lunch in her apartment daily and went to the main dining room for dinner. She had previously walked without an assistive device. Patient was a widower and had several children in the area who drove her to the grocery store and doctor's appointments. There was a small grocery store in the building, so the patient was able to pick up a few groceries when she needed them. She was socially active in a book club and bridge group within the building. She received assistance with housecleaning every other week. When the patient was admitted to the subacute care setting, an occupational therapy evaluation revealed the following information.

ADL

The patient was independent with bathing using a long-handled sponge brush. She was independent with upper extremity dressing and required moderate assistance with lower extremity dressing using assistive devices.

Functional Mobility

The patient required supervision for transfers and was beginning to use a walker and moderate assistance for ambulation with cues to maintain WBAT status. Her pain and fear of falling were significant issues, although the patient remained motivated to return to her prior living situation. Bed mobility required minimal assistance for sit to and from supine.

Upper extremity status

WNL for range of motion, strength, and coordination.

Cognition

Alert and oriented to person, place, and time. No cognitive deficits noted that would impair functional abilities.

Course of treatment

The patient's treatment focused on basic ADL skills, including lower extremity dressing incorporating patient's use of walker into treatment to get into the bathroom and get clothes from the closet. She also practiced transfers on and off a shower bench and lifting legs into tub. She practiced preparing simple meals in the kitchen using the walker. Activities were limited by fatigue, with the patient requiring frequent rest breaks.

Outcome

The patient was discharged after 1 month, and she returned to her apartment. She had progressed to a cane at the time of discharge and was independent in all ADL using adaptive equipment and allowing increased time. There were already grab bars in her bathroom. A shower bench was ordered for the patient. Recommendations were made to remove loose rugs from the apartment and to build up the height of her favorite chair to make it easier to move from sit to stand. The patient used a wheelchair for long distances, including getting to the dining room for dinner and to social activities within the building. One month after discharge from the subacute care setting, she was able to walk to the dining room using the cane and with several rest breaks. The patient limits her walking outside in the community when her family comes to take her out, mainly due to fatigue.

References

American Occupational Therapy Association. (1987). *Occupational therapy Medicare handbook*. Rockville, MD: Author.

Blue Cross and Blue Shield of the National Capital Area. (1994). Length of stay guidelines for surgical procedures. Washington, DC: Author.

Brummel-Smith, K., & Brody, S. J. (1995). The nursing home population. In L. M. Gamroth, J. Semradck, & E. M. Tornquist (Eds.), *Enhancing autonomy in long-term care* (pp. 34–43). New York: Springer.

Chiodo, L. K., Gerety, M. B., Mulrow, C. D., Rhodes, M. C., & Tuley, M. R. (1992). The impact of physical therapy on nursing home patient outcomes. *Physical Therapy, 72*(3), 187–194.

Faust, L., & Meaker, M. K. (1991). Private practice occupational therapy in the skilled nursing facility: Creative alliance or mutual exploitation? *American Journal of Occupational Therapy, 45*(7), 621–627.

Gill, C., Howells, J. A., & Hoffman, E. H. (1993). Rehabilitation in the nursing facility. In L. Z. Rubenstein & D. Wieland (Eds.), *Improving care in the nursing home* (pp. 1–32). Newbury Park, CA: Sage.

Gill, H. S. (August/September, 1995). Subacute care in the inpatient setting. *Rehab Management,* pp.38–40.

Granger, C. V., Hamilton, B. B., & Gresham, G. E. (1988). The stroke rehabilitation outcome study—Part I: General description. *Archives of Physical Medicine & Rehabilitation, 69,* 506–509.

Hamilton, B. B., Granger, C. V., Sherwin, F. S., Zielzny, M., & Tashman, J. S. (1987). A uniform national data system for medical rehabilitation. In M. J. Fuhrer (Ed.), *Rehabilitation outcomes: analysis and measurement* (pp. 137–150). Baltimore: Paul H. Brookes Publishing.

Health Care Financing Administration. (1990). *Resident assessment for long term care facilities*. Washington, DC: Author.

Heinemann, A. W. (1989). *Rehabilitation Institute of Chicago functional assessment scale (revised)*. Chicago: Rehabilitation Institute of Chicago.

Kelley, F. A., Kawamoto, T. T., & Rubenstein, L. Z. (1991). Assessment of the geriatric patient. In J. M. Kiernat (Ed.), *Occupational therapy and the older adult.* (pp. 76–98). Gaithersburg, MD: Aspen.

Kiernat, J. M. (Ed.). (1991). *Occupational therapy and the older adult.* Gaithersburg, MD: Aspen.

McCormack, G. L., Llorens, L. A., & Glogoski, C. (1991). Culturally diverse elders. In J. M. Kiernat (Ed.), *Occupational therapy and the older adult* (pp. 11–25). Gaithersburg, MD: Aspen.

National Center for Health Statistics. (1989). *Vital and health statistics* (DHHS Publication No. PHS 89–1758). Washington, DC: U.S. Government Printing Office.

Salcido, R., & Moore, R. W. (August/September, 1995). Cost-effectiveness of Subacute Rehab. *Rehab Management,* pp. 33–40.

Treas, J. (1995). Older Americans in the 1990s and beyond. *Population Bulletin, 50*(2), 2–41.

Related Readings

Bohannon, R. W. (1994). Acute care occupational therapy, functional performance and discharge disposition. *International Journal of Rehabilitation Research, 17*(1), 61–63.

Brodie, J., Holm, M. B., & Tomlin, G. S. (1994). Cerebrovascular accident: relationship of demographic, diagnostic, and occupational therapy antecedents to rehabilitation outcomes. *American Journal of Occupational Therapy, 48*(10), 906–913.

Bruhn, J. G. (1991). Occupational therapy in the 21st century: An outsider's view. *American Journal of Occupational Therapy, 45*(9), 775–780.

Crabtree, J. L. (1991). Occupational therapy's new mandate: Providing services to the elderly. *American Journal of Occupational Therapy, 45*(7), 583–584.

Deitch, C. J. , Gutman, S. A., & Factor, S. (1994). Medical residents' education about occupational therapy: Implications for referral. *American Journal of Occupational Therapy, 48*(11), 1014–1021.

Feiner, C. F. (1993). Another model for delivering primary medical care to the elderly. *Mount Sinai Journal of Medicine, 61*(2), 492–494.

Garfield, R., Broe, D., & Albano, B. (1995). The role of academic medical centers in delivery of primary care: An urban study. *Academic Medicine, 70*(5), 405–409.

Melin, A. L., & Bygren, L. O. (1992). Efficacy of the rehabilitation of elderly primary health care patients after short-stay hospital treatment. *Medical Care, 30*(11), 1004–1015.

Narzarko, L. (1991). Improving care for elderly people. *Nursing the Elderly, 3*(2), 6.

Reuben, D. B., Zwanziger, J., Bradley, T. B., & Beck, J. C. (1994). Is geriatrics a primary care or subspecialty discipline? *Journal of the American Geriatrics Society, 42*(4), 363–367.

Rodriguez, G. S., & Goldberg, B. (1993). Rehabilitation in the outpatient setting. *Clinics in Geriatric Medicine, 9*(4), 873–881.

Rogers, J. C., & Holm, M. B. (1994). Accepting the challenge of outcome research: Examining the effectiveness of occupational therapy practice. *American Journal of Occupational Therapy, 48*(10), 871–876.

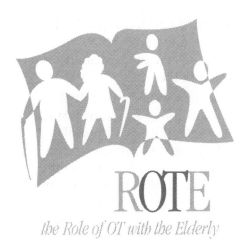

ROTE

the Role of OT with the Elderly

Restoring Occupational Performance: Rehabilitation Services for Older Adults

Steve Park, MS, OTR

Abstract

For occupational therapy practitioners who work with older adults, the general objectives when providing services are:

1. Restore function

2. Maintain function

3. Develop function

4. Prevent dysfunction (Canadian Association of Occupational Therapists [CAOT], 1991).

For those occupational therapy practitioners who work with older adults in rehabilitation settings, such as inpatient rehabilitation units, skilled nursing facilities, and home health agencies, the primary objective is to restore an older adult's ability to *function* so that he or she can return to or continue to live in the community. However, other rehabilitation professionals (e.g., nurses, physical therapists, and psychologists) also are concerned with function. To delineate the role of an occupational therapy practitioner from other professionals who work in rehabilitation settings, function must be defined from the unique perspective of an occupational therapy practitioner.

From the perspective of an occupational therapy practitioner, function is framed in an older adult's daily *occupation*—that is, an older adult's engagement in and performance of daily life tasks that are meaningful and purposeful, such as self-care, instrumental activities of daily living (ADL), work, education, play and leisure, and rest and relaxation

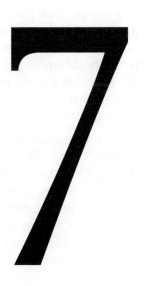

activities (American Occupational Therapy Association [AOTA], 1994b; Christiansen & Baum, 1991; Fisher, 1992a). The engagement in and performance of daily life tasks, from an occupational therapy practitioner's viewpoint, is termed an older adult's *occupational performance.*

For an older adult, engaging in and performing daily life tasks may become difficult due to the onset of various *impairments* (e.g., vision loss, major depression, or limited short-term memory) resulting from medical or psychiatric conditions, age-related physiological changes, or both (Rogers, 1990). Further, an older adult's ability to successfully engage in and perform desired life tasks may be restricted due to factors within the physical, social, and cultural *environment* (e.g., multistory buildings with no elevators, a limited social support network, ageist beliefs that older adults are unproductive workers). If the degree of the impairment(s) or the environmental factor(s) becomes of sufficient magnitude to interfere with an older adult's performance of a daily life task, a *disability* may result—that is, a restriction in or an inability to perform daily life tasks (World Health Organization, 1980). The resultant disability is the primary concern for occupational therapy practitioners. Within rehabilitation settings, such as geriatric inpatient rehabilitation units, skilled nursing facilities, and home health agencies, occupational therapy practitioners work with their patients to restore their occupational performance. This does not imply that maintaining function, developing function, or preventing dysfunction is not a component when providing rehabilitation services. Rather, it implies that the primary reason why older adults receive services within these rehabilitation settings is because they have become disabled (i.e., a restriction in or

an inability to perform daily life tasks) and they demonstrate the potential to become more *able* in their ability to perform daily life tasks.

In contrast, other rehabilitation professionals frame function from a different viewpoint. For example, physical therapists and physical therapist assistants frame function within a physical capacity framework, nurses within a health framework, and psychologists within a cognitive and emotional framework (Fisher, 1994). The primary focus from which physical therapists and physical therapist assistants provide intervention is framed within an older adult's physical function (e.g., mobility, strength). In contrast, the primary framework for nursing intervention is an older adult's health function (e.g., physiological or psychological signs and symptoms). Psychologists use a framework that examines an older adult's cognitive and emotional functioning. This is not to say that each rehabilitation professional's framework is exclusive and does not overlap with another professional's (Fisher, 1994). Rehabilitation professionals do share some common knowledge and skills, and all rehabilitation professionals are concerned with an older adult's function. However, each rehabilitation professional brings a unique perspective to the rehabilitation setting. As a result, the role of occupational therapy practitioners is distinctly different from other professionals during the evaluation and intervention process of an older adult's rehabilitation.

One challenge that occupational therapy practitioners may face when providing services in geriatric inpatient rehabilitation units, skilled nursing facilities, and home health agencies (the settings in which restoring occupational performance is the primary objective) is that current rehabilitation evaluation and intervention approaches for older adults continue to be framed predominately within a medical model framework (Levine & Gitlin, 1993). This presents a unique challenge as occupational therapy practitioners are working with other professionals who tend to follow a more traditional medical model framework that focuses more on an older adult's underlying functional impairments. The framework from which occupational therapy practitioners view an older adult is not a medical model framework, and the evaluation and intervention process for occupational therapy practitioners is directed at the more global issue of performing daily life tasks.

This distinction does not imply that occupational therapy services are not warranted within systems that follow a more traditional medical model. Occupational therapy practitioners do have an interest in bridging medical systems and everyday life (CAOT, 1991). Older adults who receive services from geriatric inpatient rehabilitation units, skilled nursing facilities, and home health agencies have experienced some degree of limitation in their ability to perform daily life tasks. For example, older adults may be experiencing difficulties with toileting, preparing meals, shopping for groceries, visiting with friends, or volunteering at the local food bank. When older adults are experiencing these types of difficulties, they receive occupational therapy services to restore their ability to participate in valued daily life tasks. On the basis of their expertise in occupational function, occupational therapy practitioners focus the evaluation and intervention process on an older adult's ability to resume the performance of daily life tasks in the environments in which he or she lives, works, and plays. As occupational therapy practitioners understand how the environment influences an older adult's occupational performance, their expertise is needed in both institutional and community settings (CAOT, 1991). Thus, occupational therapy services are a vital link from the more traditional medical model systems to the older adult's home in the community.

Another challenge presented to occupational therapy practitioners working in systems with a more traditional medical model focus is a tendency for those systems to operate from a practitioner-centered perspective rather than a client-centered one (Levine & Gitlin, 1993). Occupational therapy practitioners are committed to client-centered practice—that is, the client's knowledge and experience of his or her daily life are of central concern during client-practitioner collaboration. When providing occupational therapy services, practitioners are guided by an ethical commitment to listen and respond to a client's goals and priorities regarding meaningful and purposeful occupations in his or her daily life (AOTA, 1994a; CAOT, 1991). Levine & Gitlin (1993) advocated that all healthcare practitioners need to develop a perspective that extends beyond the current medical model that emphasizes intervention that is symptom-based and practitioner-driven to a client-centered model that incorporates the specific goals and issues of older adults.

Central to the issue of client-centered practice is the consideration of culture in an older adult's daily life. Culture is defined as the customs, beliefs, activity patterns, behavior standards, and expectations accepted by a group of individuals (AOTA, 1994b). Persons receiving occupational therapy services judge the quality of those services through a filter that is based on three beliefs:

1. The meaning of one's life and activities

2. The meaning of illness and health

3. The perception of the therapy process (Levine, 1987; Ramsden, 1993).

Occupational therapy services will be perceived as meaningful and purposeful only if the process and outcome is relevant to a client's and caregiver's daily life and their perceptions of how illness should be treated and how health should be maintained and promoted. (The term *caregiver* refers to those individuals [e.g., spouses, partners, family members, friends, or paid assistants] who are involved in the primary care of an older adult.)

Particularly for those practitioners working on geriatric inpatient rehabilitation units and skilled nursing facilities, the "medical" culture of the facility should be examined with respect to the client's values and beliefs regarding traditional medical intervention. For example, older adults from minority ethnic groups may have different health beliefs and practices than those of the rehabilitation staff (McCormack, Llorens, & Glogoski, 1991; Wells, 1992). Thus, older adults' expectations regarding the type of care and intervention that they should receive may be different from the care and intervention the rehabilitation staff will provide. Older adults admitted to an inpatient rehabilitation unit or skilled nursing facility may believe that a "sick" role is appropriate within these settings, and they may expect the staff to take care of them. This may conflict with the rehabilitation staff's beliefs and expectations that older adult clients should be more participatory and independent in their own care.

Accounting for an older adult's cultural background requires occupational therapy practitioners to be attentive to their own values and beliefs about one's quality of life. Practitioners cannot impose their own values and beliefs on their clients and clients' caregivers (Ramsden, 1993). For example, values and beliefs regarding daily life and health practices may influence an older adult's caregivers when they are deciding who should take care of the older adult, how much care should be provided, and how the care should be performed. Independence may not be valued by all older adults, and one's cultural background may contribute to a belief that older adults should be taken care of when they have an illness or a disability. A practitioner's suggestion that an older adult should be independent when dressing may be perceived as insensitive and inappropriate by some older adults and their caregiver(s) if they do not value independence for an older adult (Ramsden, 1993). Thus, setting goals and planning intervention for older adults requires that clients and their caregivers be actively involved in the planning and that cultural beliefs and practices be taken into account (McCormack et al., 1991).

Framed with a focus on occupational function and guided by a value for client-centered practice, the remainder of the chapter delineates the role of occupational therapy practitioners within the three healthcare settings in which the primary objective is to restore occupational performance: geriatric inpatient rehabilitation units, skilled nursing facilities, and home health agencies. Each section provides an overview of the unique role of occupational therapy practitioners within each setting, the occupational therapy process, and the parameters that occupational therapy practitioners must consider when working within each health care setting. The primary role of an occupational therapy practitioner—restoring an older adult's occupational performance—does not change significantly among settings. The main difference among the three settings is how that objective is pursued and achieved given the unique characteristics of each setting. Thus, much of the information on geriatric inpatient rehabilitation (presented in the first section) is applicable to both skilled nursing facilities and home health agencies and therefore will not be repeated.

Geriatric Inpatient Rehabilitation

Geriatric inpatient rehabilitation units, either hospital based or freestanding, provide a comprehensive array of rehabilitation services by professionals who specialize in services for older adults. Admission to a geriatric inpatient rehabilitation unit requires that the patient be medically stable, capable of benefiting from rehabilitation services, and able to participate in 3 hours of therapy services a day (i.e., physical and occupational therapy, although speech and language pathology services may qualify in unique situations) (Bachelder, 1994; Miller & Kirchman, 1991). (The term *patient* refers to an older adult who is receiving services at an inpatient rehabilitation unit.) Further, admission to the rehabilitation unit is predicated on the requirements that a client must be discharged to a living situation in the community (a nursing facility does not qualify) and that he or she must make regular progress toward the established goals and discharge plan. The length of stay may vary from as short as 7 days to as long as 3 weeks, depending on the patient's diagnosis and the magnitude of the functional impairments.

The evaluation and intervention process focuses on the patient's func-

tional limitations and problems that interfere with his or her ability to live in the community (Bachelder, 1994). However, as previously described, function is framed from the perspective of each rehabilitation team member, and each brings a unique viewpoint to the rehabilitation process. The core team members of a geriatric inpatient rehabilitation team and their primary functional concerns (Clark, 1994; Fisher, 1994; Kelly, Kawamoto, & Rubenstein, 1991; Steinberg, 1994; U.S. Department of Health and Human Services, 1995) are as follows:

- Physician—Leads the team and coordinates the medical and rehabilitation services. Primary area of expertise is the patient's health function.

- Nurse—Educates patient and caregiver(s) about physical and psychological issues, such as medication management, bowel and bladder function, skin care, and health and caregiving issues. Reinforces the skills learned during rehabilitation therapies. Primary area of expertise is the patient's health function.

- Social worker—Educates and counsels patient and caregiver(s) about the consequence of the patient's condition from a system perspective (e.g., family, social, community, economic). Evaluates community and family resources and facilitates discharge planning. Primary area of expertise is the emotional and social functions of the patient and the social support system.

- Physical therapist and physical therapy assistant—Focus on the patient's physical function, such as motor control, mobility, strength, endurance, balance, coordination, range of motion, motor control, and pain. Primary area of expertise is the patient's physical function.

- Speech and language pathologist—Facilitates the patient's communication and language functions, and often focuses on patient's swallowing ability. Primary area of expertise is the patient's communicative function.

- Neuropsychologist—Assesses the patient's mental, cognitive, and emotional status and provides patient and caregiver counseling. Primary area of expertise is the patient's mental, cognitive, and emotional function.

- Therapeutic recreation specialist—Facilitates the patient's participation in leisure and community activities. Primary area of expertise is patient's recreational and leisure function.

Other professionals, such as dietitians, pharmacists, audiologists, dentists, optometrists, clergy, prosthetists, orthotists, respiratory therapists, and consulting physicians also may work with the core rehabilitation team members (Clark, 1994; Kelly, Kawamoto, & Rubenstein, 1991).

The unique focus of occupational therapy practitioners, when compared to other inpatient rehabilitation professionals, is the client's and caregiver's occupational function—that is, the client's and caregiver's performance of daily living tasks. To be an effective rehabilitation team member, occupational therapy practitioners must be confident in their own role and the unique focus associated with that role (CAOT, 1991). Occupational therapy practitioners working on geriatric inpatient rehabilitation units bring their expertise in occupational function—that is, working with patients and their caregiver(s) to enhance their performance of basic self-care tasks, such as eating, grooming and hygiene, toileting, dressing, and bathing, as well as other daily living tasks, that the patients and their caregivers deem important. Thus, occupational therapy practitioners are concerned with how patients and their caregivers are able to safely and efficiently carry out the tasks that are valued and needed for living in the community. Examples of such tasks include the following:

- A patient is able to eat safely and independently with minimal risk of aspiration.

- A patient, with the assistance of the caregiver, is able to safely transfer in and out of a standard bathtub.

- A patient requires only minimal verbal prompts to play a favorite card game with a friend.

- A patient and caregiver are able to safely work together in a kitchen to prepare a grandchild's favorite cookies.

Finally, although each rehabilitation team member brings his or her own expertise, a blending of roles also may occur to achieve a patient's rehabilitation goals (Miller & Kirchman, 1991). For example, physicians, nurses, physical therapists, and occupational therapy practitioners all bring some knowledge regarding techniques to manage edema for a patient's hand. While some techniques may be specific to a discipline (e.g., the use of medications would be specific to a physician), other techniques may not be discipline-specific (e.g., the use of Coban wrap is not specific to any one discipline). In this case, there is an overlap among the team members' responses on how to manage edema. Thus, although occupational therapy practitioners' primary expertise is not the management of hand edema, practitioners would contribute their expertise in how patients could carry out their daily living tasks while also managing the edema. The primary reason why occupational therapy practitioners are members of a rehabilitation team is their unique knowledge and skills regarding how best to enhance a patient's and caregiver's performance in daily living tasks despite the patient's current functional limitations and impairments.

OCCUPATIONAL THERAPY EVALUATION PROCESS

The rehabilitation team members conduct a comprehensive evaluation of the patient to discover the patient's medical, physical, cognitive, and psychological problems; problems within the patient's physical, social, and cultural environments; and how the identified problems may affect the patient's quality of life and ability to live in the community (Bachelder, 1994). With this in mind, each rehabilitation professional brings a perspective of function to the evaluation process, as does the occupational therapy practitioner.

From an occupational therapy practitioner's perspective, the expected outcome of occupational therapy intervention is the patient's and caregiver's enhanced performance of daily life tasks. Thus, the occupational therapy evaluation process should begin with a focus on the daily life tasks of concern to the patient and the caregiver (Fisher, 1992a). Trombly (1993) advocated that occupational therapy practitioners adopt a top-down approach when gathering information during the evaluation process. (When referring to the evaluation process, it is implied that an occupational therapist and occupational therapy assistant are working together and that they are following AOTA guidelines regarding those evaluation procedures that an occupational therapy assistant can complete independently and those evaluation procedures that are completed in collaboration

with an occupational therapist.) The occupational therapy practitioner should begin at the "top" with an appraisal of the patient's occupational function—that is, the patient's self-care, instrumental ADL, work, play, and leisure performance. This contrasts with the practice of beginning the process with an evaluation of the patient's occupational performance components (e.g., level of depression, muscle strength, or mental status). The occupational therapy practitioner should begin the evaluation process with a predominant focus on the patient's and caregiver's roles, routines, interests, values, and perceptions with regard to their daily life tasks and the environments in which they perform those tasks, including observations of the patient's performance of daily life tasks (Park, 1995). Thus, for an occupational therapy practitioner, the evaluation process should consist of an interview that focuses on daily tasks and observations of the patient's performance of those daily life tasks.

Finally, when conducting an initial evaluation, occupational therapy practitioners should examine the practice of using the same assessment tools and evaluation procedures that other rehabilitation professionals (e.g., physical therapists, nurses, or psychologists) use to evaluate a patient's functional status (Fisher, 1992a). The use of such assessment tools and evaluation procedures implies that the primary focus of occupational therapy is the patient's underlying functional impairments (e.g., memory loss, depression, weakness) rather than the patient's ability to carry out daily life tasks. Research has not demonstrated a firm, reliable relationship between a patient's medical diagnosis or degree of impairment and the performance of daily life tasks (Fisher, 1992b; Steinberg, 1994). Thus, using evaluation procedures that focus on the patient's impairments to begin the occupational therapy evaluation process is inappropriate for occupational therapy intervention because such an assessment does not focus on the patient's and caregiver's ability to safely and efficiently perform daily life tasks. However, Trombly (1993) advocated that once information about the patient's and caregiver's concerns with daily life tasks was gathered and the occupational therapy practitioner had observed the patient performing daily life tasks, then the practitioner could "drop down" and perform additional evaluations, as appropriate, to further clarify why the patient may be experiencing difficulty with the performance of daily living tasks. For example, it may be appropriate, at times, to evaluate a patient's mental status. However, such an evaluation should only be performed in the following instances:

1. The occupational therapy practitioner has observed that the patient's diminished cognitive status interferes with his or her ability to perform a daily life task.

2. No other rehabilitation professional has conducted a similar assessment of cognitive function.

Thus, the use of evaluation procedures that focus exclusively on the patient's sensorimotor, psychosocial, and cognitive-perceptual performance components outside the context of the performance of daily life tasks should be used sparingly.

Gathering Information During an Initial Interview

As a client-centered approach to intervention requires that an occupational therapy practitioner actively seek information of concern to the patient and the caregivers (CAOT, 1991), the evaluation process should begin with an interview of the patient and, if possible, the patient's caregiver(s). Beginning the evaluation process with an interview also establishes rapport with the patient and the important individuals in the patient's life (Kelley, Kawamoto, & Rubenstein, 1991). The focus of the interview is on the patient's roles, interests, motivations, and values with regard to his or her daily living tasks, as well as the patient's and caregiver's perceptions and concerns about the patient's ability to live in the community (Park, 1995).

The occupational therapy practitioner is particularly concerned with identifying those daily life tasks in which the patient and caregiver(s) are experiencing problems or that they anticipate will be a problem after discharge to the community. The Canadian Occupational Performance Measure (Law, Baptiste, Carswell, McColl, Polatajko, & Pollock, 1995), which was developed from a client-centered perspective, is one formal assessment tool that can be used to identify problems with daily living tasks from either the patient's or caregiver's perspective. Many other interview formats are also available. For example, interviews developed from the model of human occupation (Kielhofner, Mallinson, & de las Heras, 1995) can be useful to structure the interview process. Regardless of which interview procedure—formal or informal—is used, it is imperative that the occupational therapy practitioner quickly identify those areas of immediate concern to the patient and caregiver(s) so that the practitioner can complete the evaluation process with observations of the patient's performance of those daily life tasks that are of particular concern.

Finally, during the initial interview, the occupational therapy practitioner should begin to gather information regarding the home environment to which the patient is to be discharged. Typically, this approach will involve soliciting the assistance of the patient and caregiver(s) to report information regarding the home environment. The use of brochures or booklets, such as *A Consumer's Guide to Home Adaptation* (Adaptive Environments Center, 1993), that focus on the home evaluation process from a patient's and caregiver's perspective, can be very helpful to the patient and caregiver(s).

Identifying Problems by Observing Patient Performance

One of the most objective targets for rehabilitative intervention is the performance of daily life tasks, particularly self-care tasks (Stineman & Granger, 1994). Small gains in the ability of an older adult to perform daily life tasks can be of enormous benefit to personal health, can result in less care required by the patient's caregivers, and may decrease the amount of community resources required to maintain living in the community. One of the valuable contributions that occupational therapy practitioners provide to the rehabilitation team is an evaluation of the patient's and caregiver's ability to safely perform those tasks that are required so that the patient can return to and live in the community.

Following the initial interview, the occupational therapy practitioner should observe the patient performing those daily life tasks that are of concern to the patient and caregiver. If possible, this also could entail observing how the patient's caregiver assists the patient with self-care or other daily life tasks. However, because evaluations on inpatient geriatric rehabilitation units are usually completed within 3 days, an observation of the caregiver's performance may be infeasible. Nonetheless, following the initial inter-

view, the occupational therapy practitioner should focus the evaluation process on observing the patient's performance while eating, grooming, toileting, dressing, and bathing, as well as other occupational performance tasks that the patient and caregiver(s) identified as problems.

Self-care tasks are an important component of the occupational therapy evaluation process. Typically, one of the primary reasons why older adults are admitted to geriatric inpatient rehabilitation units is the adult's inability or limitation in performing these tasks. Older adults who have difficulties with self-care performance are more likely to require services (including financial) when living in the community (Bonder & Goodman, 1995). Further, older adults who are not motivated to perform self-care tasks or are severely limited in their ability to perform those tasks will need a caregiver to assist them when they return to the community. Thus, caregiver training with regard to self-care tasks is an important component of rehabilitation intervention and should be addressed whenever possible during the evaluation process.

The use of standardized assessment tools to measure self-care independence, such as the Functional Independence Measure (State University of New York at Buffalo, 1990), is common on geriatric inpatient rehabilitation units. Rehabilitation professionals use such tools to determine the level of independence (or conversely, the level of care) that a patient demonstrates while performing self-care tasks. The patient's level of care is established by observing the patient performing self-care tasks and determining the amount of assistance required. However, some people are concerned with relying on standardized assessments to structure the occupational therapy evaluation process. To the extent that the independent performance of self-care tasks is relevant to a patient's daily life, the results will be useful for the occupational therapy practitioner (Rogers & Holm, 1994). However, other daily living tasks may be of more importance to a patient. If the occupational therapy practitioner relies solely on standardized assessment tools to observe the patient's performance, the practitioner has a tendency to be concerned only with the tasks contained in the assessment. This practice does not reflect a client-centered approach and does not respect the importance of the patient's and caregiver's viewpoint.

It is imperative that the occupational therapy practitioner not begin the evaluation process with a direct evaluation of a patient's functional limitations or impairment, such as muscle strength, mental status, or level of depression (Park, 1995). Older patients typically present with a multitude of various limitations and impairments. It is the interplay of those limitations and impairments during the performance of daily life tasks and the environments in which the patient performs those tasks that is the primary focus of the occupational therapy practitioner's evaluation process. Thus, the patient's impairments are best observed and evaluated in the context of the patient's task performance (Park, 1995; Rogers & Holm, 1994). To this end, it is essential that an occupational therapy practitioner use evaluation procedures that capture the full range of a patient's occupational function and that do not address a patient's cognitive, sensorimotor, and psychosocial functions outside the context of a patient's engagement in and performance of daily life tasks. For example, handing a patient a shirt and slacks to don would identify limitations in the patient's physical ability to don the clothes but would fail to identify the patient's potential

cognitive limitations to decide which clothes to wear or potential psychosocial limitations to initiate getting dressed for the day (Rogers, 1990).

If occupational therapy practitioners believe that a person's cultural background is an important consideration when focusing on a person's occupational function, then practitioners must account for a person's cultural background when considering the use of standardized assessments (Dickerson, 1994). Occupational therapy assessment tools need to consider cultural differences, and practitioners must be certain that the assessment tools they use are free of cultural bias. One example of an occupational therapy assessment that accounts for a person's cultural background is the Assessment of Motor and Process Skills (AMPS) (Fisher, 1995). For the assessment, the person is allowed to choose and perform instrumental ADL tasks (e.g., meal preparation or simple household chores) that are culturally relevant and that the person is motivated to perform. Patients are encouraged to perform tasks in their usual manner. Depending on their cultural background, patients may perform tasks that are typical of Hispanic, Swedish, British, or Canadian cultures, as well as tasks that are typical of American culture. Although the AMPS focuses the occupational therapy practitioner's observation on the performance of instrumental ADL, the assessment is very useful to use on inpatient rehabilitation units for those patients who have at least assisted mobility within their environment and are able to engage in simple daily living tasks (Park & Fisher, 1995).

One concern that may emerge during the evaluation process on geriatric inpatient rehabilitation units is the influence of the environment on older adults' performance of instrumental

ADL. Environmental influences on older adults' performance have been demonstrated (Nygård, Bernspång, Fisher, & Winblad, 1994; Park, Fisher, & Velozo, 1994), and occupational therapy practitioners must consider that their patients' performance in the rehabilitation setting may be different than their performance in the home environment. As the long-term goal of rehabilitation is to return the patient to community living with the highest quality of life, the occupational therapist must consider the patient's discharge environment when evaluating the patient's performance of daily life tasks, and the practitioner should attempt to evaluate the patient's performance under conditions that are similar to the patient's anticipated discharge environment.

Finally, it has been noted that few assessment tools are designed specifically for occupational therapy practitioners and are based on occupational therapy frames of reference (Kelley, Kawamoto, & Rubenstein, 1991). Many standardized assessments that were developed from other rehabilitation professionals' perspective and framework on function are available. Occupational therapy practitioners should be cautious of using these assessments and should rely more on their expertise in evaluating a patient's performance of daily life tasks based on their observations of the patient's performance of those tasks.

SETTING GOALS THROUGH PATIENT-PRACTITIONER COLLABORATION

One current concern in rehabilitation settings is that professionals may not be taking a patient's wishes and personal goals fully into account when planning intervention (Neistadt, 1995;

Northern, Rust, Nelson, & Watts, 1995; Steinberg, 1994). By focusing on goals that are important to the patient and beginning intervention with those goals, the occupational therapy practitioner can provide a purposeful experience that is immediately relevant to the patient's life (Levine & Gitlin, 1993). If an occupational therapy practitioner has followed a patient-centered practice, gathered information from the patient's and caregiver's perspectives, and observed the patient and caregiver(s) perform tasks that are of concern to them when they return home, then setting goals from the patient's perspective should be an easier process.

Before the actual goals can be determined, though, the occupational therapy practitioner must be certain that the patient's and caregiver's baseline performance of daily tasks has been observed and documented (Park, 1995). That is, the occupational therapy practitioner must determine the patient's and caregiver's current level of ability to perform daily life tasks. This typically has been defined as the patient's level of independence, delineated by a rating scale that describes the amount of assistance associated with each level of performance (dependent through independent). However, the level of safety, efficiency, or difficulty of the patient's and caregiver's performance also could be used to describe baseline performance (Park, 1995). For example, an occupational therapy practitioner, through an observation of a caregiver assisting a patient to bathe in the morning, may determine that the caregiver is not performing the task safely. The occupational therapy practitioner observed that the caregiver did not give clear verbal directives to the patient and the caregiver experienced moderate difficulty assisting the patient from the wheelchair to the bath bench, putting the patient at risk for a fall. If both the patient and caregiver agree that bathing is a priority when they return home, a goal could be established that states, "Caregiver will safely assist the patient during bathing." Thus, through a collaborative process, the practitioner, patient, and caregiver agree to important goals. Further, as the occupational therapist documented the caregiver's original baseline performance and the goal, the therapist can observe the caregiver assisting the patient at a later date and determine if the caregiver is capable of assisting the patient safely and, thus, if the goal has been achieved.

All occupational therapy goals should reflect the quality of the performance of daily life tasks that the patient or caregiver is expected to achieve. A good rule of thumb to follow is that if the patient or caregiver does not understand the goal, it is probably inappropriate to use. Of particular note, goals should not reflect the functional perspective of other professionals nor should they describe the type of intervention the occupational therapy practitioner intends to use (Park, 1995). For example, goals such as "Patient will be able to lift right arm to 130 degrees" or "Patient will perform 10 repetitions of shoulder flexion with a 5-lb. weight" are inappropriate. Goals should reflect the daily life tasks that the patient will perform when he or she is discharged to home. Goals such as "Patient will safely transfer into bathtub with standby assistance of caregiver" or "Patient will require only minimal verbal cues to dress in the morning" would be considered appropriate. Finally, the expected outcome of occupational therapy is a change in occupational performance, either the patient's or the caregiver's. Thus, to evaluate the effectiveness of occupa-

tional therapy services, goals must reflect the client's and caregiver's expected change in their performance of daily living tasks.

ACHIEVING GOALS THROUGH OCCUPATIONAL THERAPY INTERVENTION

To achieve the primary goal of geriatric inpatient rehabilitation (restore the patient's ability to perform daily life tasks) occupational therapy, intervention is focused on the practice of those tasks that the patient and caregiver have identified as important and will need to perform at home when discharged. Further, the establishment of a self-care routine on the ward, such as eating, grooming, toileting, dressing, undressing, bathing, or managing medications, will allow the patient to practice those important daily life tasks in preparation for discharge. Thus, the occupational therapy practitioner should work closely with the nursing staff to establish self-care routines that reinforce the goals agreed upon with the patient and caregiver(s).

As patients may be discharged in as few as 7 days, the occupational therapy practitioner should begin to plan caregiver training as soon as possible. Again, close collaboration with the nursing staff is important when providing caregiver training as it can be confusing for the patient's caregiver(s) to receive conflicting information regarding, for example, how to best assist a patient with dressing or toileting. Therefore, although it can be difficult, occupational therapy should be scheduled at those times that are appropriate for daily life tasks to occur. Thus, if eating, dressing, or bathing, for example, are important to the patient, then occupational therapy should be scheduled at times that these tasks normally take place. Typically, patients on rehabilitation units are scheduled for a morning self-care session and one or two other sessions throughout the day. To meet their patients' goals, occupational therapy practitioners should examine the practice of scheduling additional sessions when, in fact, the patient may need more time during the morning routine to practice those tasks of importance. Finally, occupational therapy intervention should occur in as realistic a context as possible. For example, it does not benefit a patient on a rehabilitation unit to practice transfers with clothes on, including shoes, onto a bath bench in a wheelchair-accessible bathroom when this is not the routine that will be followed at home nor the type of environment in which the routine will take place.

DISCHARGE PLANNING UPON ADMISSION

Occupational therapy practitioners bridge the gap between the geriatric inpatient rehabilitation unit and the patient's home in the community (Maloney & Kasper, 1991). From the beginning of a patient's admission, occupational therapy practitioners are constantly thinking about what the patient requires to return to and live in the community. However, as lengths of stay become shorter, there is less time to achieve goals on geriatric inpatient rehabilitation units. Therefore, discharge planning begins when the patient is admitted to the unit.

If feasible, the occupational therapy practitioner should conduct a home evaluation as soon as possible during the patient's rehabilitation stay. Information from the home evaluation is invaluable to all the rehabilitation team professionals and is extremely useful to plan intervention before discharge. Further, if the occupational therapy practitioner can arrange for the patient to be at home

when the evaluation is conducted, the information gained is even more valuable. However, this arrangement may not be possible for all patients because of contraindications, such as limited cardiovascular endurance or poor medical stability. Nonetheless, the occupational therapy practitioner can gain important information from an observation of the home environment and the patient's caregivers during a home evaluation.

Of particular concern to occupational therapy practitioners is the adaptive equipment that may be required to perform daily life tasks when the patient returns home. Discharge planning is often hampered by a lack of options (Trace & Howell, 1991), and the availability and financing of adaptive equipment is no exception. Most of the adaptive equipment for rehabilitation patients is not reimbursable, so the occupational therapy practitioner must work with the patient, the caregiver(s), and the social worker to find some creative options to procure the needed adaptive equipment. To complicate the matter, it may be difficult to determine a patient's exact adaptive equipment needs during a patient's stay in the rehabilitation unit (Maloney & Kasper, 1991). For example, it may be difficult to determine the exact type of bath bench that a patient will require without accurate information regarding the home environment. The occupational therapy practitioner may be unable to conduct a home evaluation and the information from the caregivers may be insufficient with which to make a reasonable decision. In these instances, the occupational therapy practitioner should arrange that home health services begin immediately upon discharge from the rehabilitation unit and specify that a first priority for the home health practitioner is to evaluate the need for a bath bench and assist the patient and caregiver to procure an appropriate one.

In addition to providing recommendations to the patient and caregiver(s) about adaptive equipment for the home environment, the occupational therapy practitioner should know what resources are available in the community to support a patient's engagement in desired daily life tasks and provide clear information to the patient and caregiver as to how to access those resources (Maloney & Kasper, 1991). For example, a patient may want to continue to attend a local church, but the caregiver is unable to transport the patient in that person's car. The occupational therapy practitioner can work with the patient and caregiver to identify options for community transportation that are within the capability of the patient and caregiver. Social workers typically are the most knowledgeable regarding community resources. However, occupational therapy practitioners can facilitate the referral to community resources, particularly if the patient is motivated to engage in desired activities in the community.

EVALUATION OF OUTCOMES IN OCCUPATIONAL THERAPY

From an occupational therapy practitioner's perspective, the outcome of occupational therapy services could be measured by a change in the patient's or caregiver's occupational function. Typically, this is measured using standardized assessments that tend to focus on the independent performance of self-care tasks, such as the Functional Independence Measure (State University of New York at Buffalo, 1990). If a patient is admitted to an inpatient geriatric rehabilitation unit and requires moderate assistance with most self-care tasks and if the patient is then discharged 2 weeks later and requires over-

all supervision for self-care tasks, it can be stated that the rehabilitation outcome was beneficial to the patient. Further, if the patient's caregiver also demonstrates a change in performance and is now capable of assisting the patient safely and with minimal risk of injury to the patient and himself or herself, the rehabilitation outcome can also be considered successful.

However, if self-care tasks are unimportant to the patient, and it is agreed that a caregiver will assist the patient with those tasks, the use of standardized self-care assessments to evaluate rehabilitation outcomes will not necessarily indicate that rehabilitative intervention was beneficial. For example, a patient, who initially requires overall moderate assistance with self-care tasks, may be admitted to an inpatient rehabilitation unit. Although the occupational therapy practitioner will instruct and teach the caregiver to safely assist the patient during the morning routine, the results of the standardized assessment at discharge may indicate that the patient still requires moderate assistance. In other words, the patient requires the same level of assistance but the caregiver's ability to provide assistance has greatly improved.

The evaluation of rehabilitation outcomes should encompass not only the degree of change in a patient's functional status but also the relevance of rehabilitation services from the patient's, caregiver's, and society's perspective (Stineman & Granger, 1994). From the patient's perspective, an occupational therapy practitioner might ask, "How does the patient perceive that personal life satisfaction has changed as a result of intervention directed at self-care skills?" A similar question also could be asked from the caregiver's perspective, such as, "How does the caregiver perceive that his or her life has changed as a result of caregiver training?" From a societal perspective, the occupational therapy practitioner could pose the question, "How has the patient's improved performance reduced the financial burden on the family and the community, lessened the need for institutionalization, and enhanced the role that the patient occupies in the community?" (Stineman & Granger, 1994).

Assessing the benefits of rehabilitation from these perspectives is a relatively new proposition. Currently, occupational therapy practitioners do not possess all the evaluation procedures to comprehensively evaluate the outcomes of occupational therapy intervention. However, occupational therapy practitioners should remember that it is the patient's and caregiver's quality of life that is of ultimate concern, and in some cases, this quality of life may bear little relationship to the patient's level of independence in self-care tasks. Ultimately, the patient's goals should guide occupational therapy intervention, and the patient's achievement of those goals is the benchmark by which to evaluate the outcomes of occupational therapy intervention (Park, 1995).

DOCUMENTATION OF OCCUPATIONAL THERAPY SERVICES

Documenting rehabilitation services constitutes a significant amount of a rehabilitation professional's time; in many cases, the process takes away time that could be spent in direct patient care (Wilson, 1992). However, documentation is a very important process because the medical record is a legal document and it is the "measure" by which reimbursement for services is determined by third-party payers (Scott & Somers, 1992). Wilson (1992), a former manager of a large occupational

therapy department, stated that despite the amount of time spent documenting occupational therapy services, the written documentation typically failed to produce a coherent picture of the occupational therapy services that were provided or the outcomes of those services. If this is the case, then documentation fails to serve as an effective communication mode for both the rehabilitation team and third-party payers.

Wilson (1992) also provided some recommendations to improve the documentation process. Those recommendations were as follows:

1. To develop a training program to improve the occupational therapy practitioner's interview skills to focus on identifying practical, realistic, and achievable functional goals from the patient's and caregiver's perspective

2. To develop and refine the occupational therapy practitioner's observation skills of the patient's task performance to focus on identifying the underlying factors that limit the patient's performance

3. To reduce the direct evaluation of underlying limitations and impairments.

To paraphrase Wilson, if an occupational therapy practitioner adopts a client-centered approach and focuses on the occupational function of the patient and caregiver(s), then the written documentation should consume less time and accurately reflect the outcomes of occupational therapy.

One of the first considerations when documenting occupational therapy services is to ensure that the description of the occupational therapy services provided does not resemble the other services that the patient is receiving (Scott & Somers, 1992). If the occupational therapy practitioner is aware of the functional perspective of the other professionals and if the practitioner focuses on the patient's occupational function, this should not be an issue. The second consideration is that, while it is important to document the occupational status of the patient and caregiver, it is also important to document why occupational therapy services are needed. This typically reflects the underlying functional limitations (i.e., performance components) that affect the patient's ability to perform daily living tasks. However, those functional limitations should always be documented in the context of the patient's performance. For example, if a patient has limited cognitive skills, such as a poor short-term memory, it should be documented how the short-term memory limitation affects the patient's ability to perform daily living tasks. Further, only those functional limitations that affect performance need to be documented by an occupational therapy practitioner. It is important to document the patient's abilities that support performance of daily living tasks. Occupational therapy practitioners must justify that a particular patient will benefit from rehabilitation; thus, documenting the strengths of a patient that will enable him or her to learn and demonstrate progress is very important.

The final consideration is that all occupational therapy practitioners should be aware of the needs and requirements of third-party payers with regard to documentation (Robertson, 1992). They should work with the business department of the inpatient geriatric rehabilitation unit and learn the specific requirements of the various third-party payers. However, this does not mean that the occupational therapy documents only what the third-party payers want to see in the written notes. Occupational therapy practitioners have an ethical responsibility to accurately document the services that are provided without distorting the description of those services to meet third-party payer requirements for reimbursement.

REIMBURSEMENT FOR OCCUPATIONAL THERAPY SERVICES

Unfortunately, some occupational therapy practitioners tend to distance themselves from issues of reimbursement for occupational therapy services (Faust & Meaker, 1991). It is imperative that all occupational therapy practitioners understand the parameters of reimbursement that may vary depending on the source of the reimbursement. Payment for geriatric inpatient rehabilitation services is derived from the following sources:

1. The federal government, of which the primary reimbursement source is Medicare, Part A

2. State governments, of which the primary source is Medicaid (MediCal in California), a joint venture between the federal and state governments to provide services to the poor and medically indigent

3. Private and commercial insurers, which may either be a fee-for-service or health maintenance organization plan (Scott & Somers, 1992).

For most older adults, the primary source of reimbursement for geriatric inpatient rehabilitation is from the federal government in the form of Medicare, Part A (Scott & Somers, 1992). To qualify for Medicare, Part A, reimbursement, patients who are admitted to an inpatient rehabilitation unit must meet the following criteria (Phillippi, 1996):

• The patient must have one of six functional limitations (self-care, mobility, safety dependence, communication deficits, swallowing disorders, or cognitive dysfunction).

- The patient must be medically stable.

- The patient must be capable of benefiting from therapy services and able to participate in 3 hours of therapy a day (a combination of occupational therapy and physical therapy).

- The patient must demonstrate a level of consciousness that allows for a response to a command.

- The patient must not have previously participated in an intensive rehabilitation program for the same functional limitation unless a significant change in status warrants further rehabilitation services (Phillippi, 1996).

After admission to the rehabilitation unit, Medicare, Part A, guidelines for reimbursement further stipulate that:

1. The patient's functional condition will improve significantly within a reasonable and predictable length of time.

2. The patient requires the provision of rehabilitation services by skilled and qualified rehabilitation personnel and not lay persons.

3. Intervention services must be specific and effective for patient's functional limitations.

4. Services must reflect the standards of practice for individual rehabilitation disciplines (Phillippi, 1996).

When reviewing the documentation to determine if rehabilitation services should be reimbursed, representatives of third-party payers may note any of the following issues or concerns (Phillippi, 1996):

- The documentation fails to reflect intervention that must be provided by skilled personnel.

- The documentation fails to show functional goals and outcomes.

- The documentation fails to include comparative data by which to judge if functional progress was made (i.e., the documentation of the patient's baseline performance).

- The data documented (e.g., range of motion, mental status) does not show a correlation to functional performance (e.g., daily life tasks).

- The information included is subjective in nature and overgeneralized.

- The intervention plan is inappropriate for the patient's medical diagnosis and original care plan.

For any of these reasons, a third-party payer may deny payment for rehabilitation services. Thus, occupational therapy practitioners should be aware of the documentation requirements and work closely with the hospital's business department and third-party payers to ensure that all documentation requirements are met.

Of particular concern from an occupational therapy practitioner's perspective is the issue of reimbursement for durable medical equipment. Durable equipment is that which can withstand repeated use, is primarily and customarily used to serve a medical purpose, and is generally not useful to a patient who does not have a functional limitation (Scott & Somers, 1992). On the one hand, a bedside commode will be considered durable medical equipment if it is documented that the commode is medically necessary to maintain or improve the patient's bowel and bladder function (e.g., to prevent incontinence or infections) and that the patient is unable to walk or wheel into a bathroom without great difficulty. On the other hand, a raised toilet seat is not considered a piece of durable medical equipment because it is not considered medically necessary for a patient to use. In these cases, as with most adaptive equipment that is recommended by occupational therapy practitioners, the practitioner should consult with a social worker to identify options to procure and fund necessary adaptive equipment.

Skilled Nursing Facilities

Geriatric rehabilitation programs within skilled nursing facilities follow an interdisciplinary team approach, and the rehabilitation process is similar to hospital-based inpatient rehabilitation programs (Clark, 1994). (Among the various long-term-care facilities, only skilled nursing facilities provide comprehensive rehabilitation services where the primary objective is to restore daily living skills.) Typically, a percentage of beds within a nursing care facility will be designated for skilled rehabilitation services, and these beds will be collectively referred to as the skilled rehabilitation unit. The long-term goal for residents admitted for rehabilitation services is that the resident will be discharged to live in the community, requiring less assistance with his or her daily life tasks. (The term *resident* refers to an older adult receiving services within a skilled nursing facility.) Thus, it is not considered a permanent living situation, and the resident is expected to be discharged to a home environment (e.g., his or her own home or an adult foster care home).

The main difference between inpatient rehabilitation and skilled nursing facility rehabilitation is the intensity of the services provided. While a patient on a geriatric inpatient rehabilitation unit receives intensive rehabilitation services (3 or more hours a day) for a short period of time (e.g., 1 to 3 weeks), a resident within a skilled nursing facility rehabilitation program receives less intensive services over a longer period of time, typically 1 to 2 hours a day over the course of 1 to 3 months or

longer. Unlike hospital-based inpatient rehabilitation programs, no minimum requirement exists for the number of therapy hours a resident must receive each day. Residents admitted for skilled nursing facility rehabilitation typically are unable to participate in the rigorous demands of inpatient rehabilitation due to their medical status (e.g., limited cardiovascular endurance or limited cognitive ability to learn new skills). However, these older adults still demonstrate a potential to regain skills to allow them to return to and live in the community, although it may take a longer period of time in which to do so.

As most older adults are covered by Medicare insurance when they are admitted to a skilled nursing facility, the facility must be Medicare-certified, the resident must be assigned to a Medicare-certified bed, and the resident must require some form of daily skilled service (Phillippi, 1996). The daily skilled service can be one of the following:

1. Skilled nursing care 7 days a week
2. Skilled occupational therapy, physical therapy, and/or speech and language pathology 5 times a week
3. A combination of nursing and rehabilitation services.

Further, the resident must have had a qualifying acute hospital stay of at least 3 consecutive days, the resident must have been transferred to the skilled nursing facility within 30 days of the hospital discharge, and the care provided in the skilled nursing facility must be related to the condition that was treated in the hospital (Phillippi, 1996).

The emphasis of rehabilitation within a skilled nursing facility continues to focus on the resident's functional problems that interfere with his or her ability to live in the community. However, the core team members of the skilled nursing rehabilitation team tend to be slightly different from those of a hospital-based inpatient rehabilitation program (Glantz & Richman, 1991; Kaufmann, 1994). The physician assumes a less predominant role on the interdisciplinary care team as nursing home regulations require that a physician only see the resident at least once every 30 days for the first 90 days after admission (Kaufmann, 1994). Nursing staff members continue to be involved, and a nurse often will serve as the care plan coordinator (Glantz & Richman, 1991). Social workers continue to play a key role in skilled nursing facilities, educating and counseling the resident and family members about the resident's condition and assisting with discharge planning. The dietitian also assumes a prominent role, monitoring and maintaining a resident's nutritional status (Glantz & Richman, 1991).

If a resident does require rehabilitation therapy services, speech and language pathologists, physical therapists and physical therapist assistants, and occupational therapy practitioners are part of the team as well. Another key team member in skilled nursing facilities is the activities director, a professional not found within inpatient rehabilitation settings. The activities director is responsible for planning an activities program for all nursing home residents regardless of whether they receive rehabilitation therapy services. Finally, as with geriatric inpatient rehabilitation programs, a variety of professionals, such as psychologists, dentists, pharmacists, audiologists, optometrists, and podiatrists, among others, may provide additional services as needed (Glantz & Richman, 1991; Kaufmann, 1994).

The primary role of the occupational therapy practitioner working at a skilled nursing facility does not differ from an occupational therapy practitioner working at a geriatric inpatient rehabilitation unit. The occupational therapy practitioner continues to focus on a resident's occupational function, that is, a resident's ability to safely and efficiently perform those daily living tasks of value and that are needed to return to and live in the community. As with patients at inpatient rehabilitation units, the ability of residents at skilled nursing facilities to perform self-care tasks are compromised, as well their abilities to engage in valued instrumental ADL, leisure, and work activities. Thus, the occupational therapy practitioner works with residents and their caregivers to identify those daily living tasks that are required to live in the community and to provide intervention that will enable the resident to return to and live in the community.

The Ombudsman Budget Reconciliation Act (OBRA) is a federal regulation that was implemented in 1990 to monitor and improve the quality of life for residents living in long-term-care nursing facilities (Glantz & Richman, 1991). (As of November 1995, it is unclear if the House of Representatives and the Senate will dismantle the federal regulations regarding the monitoring of long-term-care facilities and turn over this responsibility to the state governments.) This legislation guarantees that residents have basic rights, such as respect, dignity, choice, a comfortable home-like environment, and an opportunity to interact with the community outside the nursing facility (Kaufmann, 1994). The OBRA also guarantees that long-term-care residents have the right to choose how they want to live their lives and receive care (Glantz & Richman, 1991). This federal legislation mandates that residents should be able to function as independently as possible and that residents should have a choice in determining the activities of daily living in which they want to participate, including community activities.

The predominant role that occupational therapy practitioners (both occupational therapists and occupational therapy assistants) assume within skilled nursing facilities is that of a direct service provider of occupational therapy services to enhance a resident's ability to perform daily life tasks. However, rather than provide direct services, occupational therapy practitioners may choose the role of a consultant to a long-term-care nursing facility. Typically, an occupational therapist will assume this role, but occupational therapy assistants can assume the role of a consultant, provided they seek, if required, an appropriate level of occupational therapist supervision to meet regulatory and professional standards (AOTA, 1993). As a consultant, occupational therapy practitioners can assist the long-term-care nursing facility by evaluating how OBRA's guidelines are implemented. They can also make recommendations regarding the facility's practices to enhance the residents' quality of life (Glantz & Richman, 1991). This may mean providing consultation regarding the physical environment of the facility, the administration policies and procedures, the activities program (as well as other programs), and the specific issues with resident care plans.

The third role that occupational therapy practitioners may choose within a long-term-care nursing facility is that of an activities director. As the OBRA mandates that an activities program be available to all residents, opportunities for residents to participate in activities that are based on the resident's background and needs and that are of interest to individual residents must be provided (Glantz & Richman, 1991). Federal legislation mandates that the activities program

must be directed by one of the following:

1. A recreational therapist
2. An occupational therapist or occupational therapy assistant
3. An individual with 2 years of experience in an activities program in a health care setting
4. An individual who has completed a trained course approved by the state (Peckham & Peckham, as cited in Kaufmann, 1994).

Thus, either an occupational therapist or an occupational therapy assistant can assume the role of an activities director, drawing upon his or her expertise in human occupation and activities to provide a wide array of meaningful activities that are tailored to an individual resident's interests and that make use of each resident's strengths and capabilities (Glantz & Richman, 1991). It should be noted that restoring a resident's occupational function is not the primary objective of the consultant and activities director. However, key concerns of people in these roles include maintaining a resident's occupational function and preventing occupational dysfunction. However, as Medicare reimbursement limits reimbursement with respect to rehabilitation services for these objectives, these roles are not the primary ones that occupational therapy practitioners assume within long-term care nursing facilities. Since Medicare will reimburse to restore occupational function, most occupational therapy practitioners work as direct service providers at rehabilitation programs within skilled nursing facilities.

OCCUPATIONAL THERAPY EVALUATION PROCESS

When a physician prescribes occupational therapy services, the occupational therapy practitioner will begin the evaluation process within the skilled nursing facility. The OBRA also has provided evaluation guidelines to ensure that the quality-of-life objectives are achieved for each resident, and the occupational therapy practitioner can assist the skilled nursing facility staff in gathering this information. Although the OBRA does not mandate that specific care approaches must be utilized, it does mandate that the facility use a structured approach to assessment. This approach is referred to as the Resident Assessment Instrument (RAI) (Glantz & Richman, 1991).

The RAI provides a consistent and comprehensive format for evaluating each resident living within a facility that receives Medicare or Medicaid reimbursement, ensuring that the staff members focus on the resident's strengths as well as needs with regard to his or her current functional ability and potential for improvement (Glantz & Richman, 1991). To begin this process, the OBRA mandates that the admission of a resident to a skilled nursing facility, requires physician orders, and that an evaluation (the RAI) must be completed within 14 days of admission and a care plan completed within 7 days of the RAI's completion. A component of the RAI is the Minimum Data Set (MDS), a form on which to record the evaluation results for each resident. The categories of the MDS include the following:

1. Identification and background information
2. Customary routine
3. Cognitive patterns
4. Communication and hearing patterns
5. Vision patterns
6. Physical functioning and structural problems
7. Continence

8. Psychosocial well-being
9. Mood and behavior patterns
10. Activity pursuit patterns
11. Disease diagnoses
12. Health conditions
13. Oral and nutritional status
14. Skin condition
15. Medication use
16. Special treatments and procedures (Glantz & Richman, 1991).

The structured format of the MDS assists the long-term care nursing facility staff to identify the functional problems that a resident may have, as well as the resident's strengths and potential for improvement.

Of particular concern to occupational therapy practitioners is the section on physical functioning and structural problems. This section focuses on the resident's abilities in the areas of bed mobility, transfer, locomotion, dressing, eating, toilet use, personal hygiene, bathing, body control problems, mobility appliances and devices, task segmentation, and ADL functional rehabilitation potential. Although occupational therapy practitioners are skilled in observing human behavior and can assist the long-term-care staff to gather this information, the expertise of the occupational therapy practitioner is understanding and observing the performance of daily activities, such as those found in the physical functioning and structural problems section of the MDS. If occupational therapy has been ordered upon admission to the skilled nursing facility, the occupational therapy practitioner can share the results of the occupational therapy evaluation and integrate this information into the MDS.

Conducting an Interview, Observing Resident Performance, and Setting Goals Through Patient-Practitioner Collaboration

The rehabilitation process for skilled nursing facilities is very similar to that on inpatient rehabilitation units. Thus, to gather information during an initial interview, to identify occupational performance problems by observing performance, and to set goals through resident-practitioner collaboration, the occupational therapy practitioner should follow the occupational therapy evaluation process guidelines outlined in the previous section on geriatric inpatient rehabilitation.

The information gathered for the MDS is from the long-term-care nursing facility staff's perspective; however, it is important to gather information from the residents' perspectives (Lawson, 1994). From a study conducted in a long-term-care nursing facility, residents tended to perceive themselves as more capable when performing the self-care tasks delineated in the MDS (the exception being the task of bathing) than did the staff members (Atwood, Holm, & James, 1994). Residents also tended to report higher capability in those self-care tasks that the resident valued the most. The conclusion from this study was that a resident's perceptions of his or her self-care capability is important information to gather. This perception reinforces the value that conducting an occupational therapy evaluation from a client-centered perspective is equally important to implement within a skilled nursing facility.

The MDS was designed to gather information for the nursing facility staff in order to develop a resident's nursing care plan. This by no means restricts the occupational therapy practitioner from gathering information that is important to the resident regarding personal concerns about daily life tasks, as well as information about roles, values, interests, routine, and occupational history. Further, goals that are decided upon among the occupational therapy practitioner, resident, and caregiver(s) are not restricted to the content of the MDS. This is only the minimum amount of information required by federal regulation. The occupational therapy practitioner, guided by a respect for client-centered practice, will interview residents and caregivers to identify their concerns of daily life tasks, observe their performance of daily life tasks, and set goals that reflect an improvement in the ability to perform daily life tasks.

ACHIEVING GOALS THROUGH OCCUPATIONAL THERAPY INTERVENTION

If the occupational therapy practitioner has interviewed the resident and caregiver, observed the resident's performance in as many daily living tasks as possible, and collaborated with the resident and caregiver(s) to prioritize goals, then the occupational therapy practitioner can structure a routine by which to meet those goals. One of the primary reasons that residents are admitted to skilled nursing facilities for rehabilitation is that they have difficulty with performing self-care tasks. To prepare for discharge to a less-structured environment within the community (e.g., home or adult foster care), one of the strategies that can be adopted is to establish a consistent daily self-care routine, which is based on each resident's unique values, needs, capabilities, limitations, and the resources available within the skilled nursing facility (Glantz & Richman, 1991). Older adults benefit from consistent practice in those tasks that they will need to perform when they return home and those tasks that they want to engage. Thus, establishing a consistent morning routine with the nursing staff becomes very important to facilitate a resident's and caregiver's ability to perform self-care tasks. Although a resident may not value independence in self-care skills, it is important that he or she learn to work with the caregiver(s) and to make the process as easy as possible for both of them when the resident returns home.

DISCHARGE PLANNING UPON ADMISSION

The process for discharge planning is not that different from the process on inpatient rehabilitation units. That is, the occupational therapy practitioner, upon the admission of the resident, must consider the resident's and caregiver's requirements for when they return to live in the community. However, one advantage in skilled nursing facilities may be the greater length of time in which to prepare the resident and caregivers for discharge and develop home programs for daily living tasks. The occupational therapy practitioner works with the resident's caregivers, as well as the social worker, to secure needed adaptive equipment and information regarding resources in the community.

EVALUATION OF OUTCOMES IN OCCUPATIONAL THERAPY

As with inpatient geriatric rehabilitation units, a resident's success with regard to occupational therapy intervention is the degree of change in the resident's and the caregiver's occupational performance. That is, their ability to return to and live in the community and engage in those daily life tasks that are important and necessary to maintain their quality of life. Thus, the success of occupational therapy intervention within skilled nursing facilities

should be measured by the achievement of the patient's and caregiver's goals that were established upon admission to the facility.

DOCUMENTATION OF OCCUPATIONAL THERAPY SERVICES

The documentation requirements for skilled nursing facilities are essentially the same as those required for inpatient rehabilitation services. A representative for third-party payers will examine the documentation for evidence that skilled nursing care was required and that rehabilitation services were warranted. As in all rehabilitation settings, the occupational therapy practitioner should document the resident's level of ability to perform daily life tasks, the reasons why the resident is having difficulty, the resident's potential to benefit from occupational therapy intervention, goals that reflect the resident's or caregiver's expected level of performance with daily life tasks, and an intervention plan that supports the stated goals.

REIMBURSEMENT FOR OCCUPATIONAL THERAPY SERVICES

As with geriatric inpatient rehabilitation, the primary source of reimbursement for occupational therapy services provided in skilled nursing facilities is Medicare, Part A (Scott & Somers, 1992). The qualifications for reimbursement are similar to those for inpatient rehabilitation in that it must be documented that the resident requires and receives skilled care by a qualified practitioner or under his or her supervision, that the resident could benefit from an extended rehabilitation program, and that discharge to a lower level of care is anticipated. Further, to be admitted and reimbursed for rehabilitation services, the resident must have had a qualifying acute hospital stay of at least 3 consecutive days, must have been transferred to a skilled nursing facility within 30 days of discharge from the hospital, and must receive care in the skilled nursing facility that is related to the condition that was treated in the qualifying hospital stay (Phillippi, 1996). If any one of these requirements is not met, the representative for the third-party payer may deny payment for the services (Crabtree, 1995).

One unique feature regarding reimbursement for Medicare rehabilitation services in skilled nursing facilities is related to the direct cost to provide the services (Faust & Meaker, 1991). Medicare reimburses rehabilitation service providers for a portion of the fixed overhead costs that are allocated to the rehabilitation services within the facility. This means that if more rehabilitation services are provided within the facility, the rehabilitation service provider will receive a larger payment for services relative to the actual cost to provide those services. This method of reimbursement has the potential for abuse—that is, rehabilitation service providers may ask occupational therapy practitioners to meet a quota of units per day in order to generate more revenue. In such instances, practitioners may be providing more services to residents who may not need the services. Under these circumstances, occupational therapy practitioners are referred to the Occupational Therapy Code of Ethics (AOTA, 1994a), which states that "Occupational therapy personnel shall provide services in an equitable manner for all individuals" (p. 1037) and that "Occupational therapy personnel shall refrain from using or participating in the use of any form of communication that contains false, fraudulent, decep-

tive, or unfair statements or claims" (p. 1038). When occupational therapy practitioners are providing services that may be unwarranted, they may be in violation of the AOTA Code of Ethics and subject to sanctions imposed by AOTA and state regulatory bodies, as well the potential for legal action, from both state and federal agencies (Kornblau, 1995).

A related reimbursement issue is billing the provision of a nonoccupational therapy service as occupational therapy (Kornblau, 1995; Reitz, 1992). For example, it is a fraudulent practice to bill as occupational therapy the time that a certified nursing assistant spends dressing a skilled nursing facility resident in the morning. In these cases, not only is it an ethical issue for the occupational therapy practitioner, but also it is a legal issue. Billing for occupational therapy services that are not provided by occupational therapy practitioners is illegal and is a phenomenon within the long-term care nursing facility industry that is of growing concern.

Home Health Agencies

Providing rehabilitation services in home settings differs from the more traditional settings of inpatient rehabilitation and skilled nursing facilities (Paulson, 1991). The rehabilitation practitioner is a guest in a client's home, and the practitioner must be acutely aware that the client and caregiver(s) are the individuals in charge within the home environment and that the client's cultural background is a very important consideration when entering the home. (The term *client* refers to an older adult who is receiving rehabilitation services from a home health agency.) For example, it may be customary for visitors (whether they be friends or healthcare professionals) to remove their shoes at the front door, or it may be expected that visitors accept an offer of food or drink (Chin, 1994). Thus, it is very important that the rehabilitation practitioner follow a client-centered approach, accounting for a client's beliefs and preferences when interacting with clients and caregivers within the clients' homes.

Providing rehabilitation services in a home setting offers a rehabilitation professional a unique perspective as he or she can observe the client's and caregiver's ability to function in their living environment and ability to learn new adaptive skills (Bachelder, 1994; Paulson, 1991). Further, a major advantage of providing services in the home is that rehabilitation professionals can accurately evaluate the need for specific home environmental adaptations and monitor the effectiveness of those adaptations (Frank & Miller, 1994). Receiving services in the home affords those clients with cognitive or affective impairments an optimal opportunity to learn and practice new skills within a familiar environment (Bachelder, 1994; Keenan, 1990). Finally, receiving rehabilitation services at home is a viable alternative for those patients who are discharged from a hospital before they have sufficiently recovered and who lack the ability to participate in an inpatient rehabilitation program (Bachelder, 1994) and for those patients who may benefit from rehabilitation services but do not require the full services of an inpatient or skilled nursing facility rehabilitation program.

As with inpatient rehabilitation and skilled nursing facilities, certain criteria must be met for a client to receive rehabilitation services in the home. Most important, the client must be considered homebound—that is, the client requires a device to assist with mobility and experiences difficulty when leaving the home (e.g., the client uses a wheelchair and there is

no accessible ramp in and out of the home) or the client has been advised by a physician not to leave the home because of the effort required (e.g., a compromised cardiovascular system limits the client's physical endurance) (Jackson & Kavalar, 1993). Clients with a psychiatric disorder may qualify for homebound status if the client requires supervision outside the home or refuses to leave the home because of psychiatric symptoms (Menosky, 1995; Reichenbach, 1992). However, this is not to say that clients can never leave the home. A client may leave the home if the absences are infrequent and of a relatively short duration (Jackson & Kavalar, 1993). For example, a client would be able to leave the home for a physician's appointment without compromising his or her homebound status.

Many of the same professionals found on inpatient rehabilitation and skilled nursing facility teams are core members of the home care rehabilitation team. For home health agencies, nurses typically serve as the team coordinator, and they are the primary liaison with the physician. A physician must authorize all home health services, and then will receive reports of all the services provided. However, the physician's role is less prominent within a home health agency as he or she is typically not on site, similar to the physician's role within a skilled nursing facility. Further, the nurse is often the one who will initiate a referral for rehabilitation therapy services (physical therapy, occupational therapy, speech and language pathology) and secure a physician's prescription for these services (Jackson, 1993). If the home health care team specializes in psychiatric disorders, a nurse with appropriate psychiatric accreditation will serve as the team coordinator (Hunt, 1994). Home health aides, another member of the home health care team, assist with the personal care of a client, such as hygiene, grooming, dressing, and bathing, and with the monitoring of a client's health indicators, such as vital signs, skin integrity, and medication side effects. Home health aides must be supervised and monitored by a rehabilitation professional who is typically a nurse, but physical therapists, occupational therapists, or speech and language pathologists may serve as a supervisor of home health aides (Jackson, 1993; Young & Youngstrom, 1995). Home health aides are assigned a specific number of hours a week to assist a client, the most common responsibility being that of assisting with bathing. Homemaker aides may be members of the team, assisting with such home chores as meals, cleaning, and shopping (Jackson, 1993). However, although Medicare insurance will reimburse for the services provided by home health aides, it will not reimburse for homemaker aide services; consequently, funding for these services must come from other community agencies or private funds (Hunt, 1994; Young & Youngstrom, 1995). As with other rehabilitation settings, social workers, physical therapists, physical therapist assistants, and speech and language pathologists compose the remaining core members of the rehabilitation team, as well as occupational therapists and occupational therapy assistants (Hunt, 1994).

Although many of the same professionals are present on the home health care team, how the team operates is very different from how rehabilitation teams operate at inpatient and skilled nursing facility settings. While the team approach is important in the home health agency, a major difference from other rehabilitation settings is the limited time for the rehabilitation team members to meet together

formally (Paulson, 1991). Regularly scheduled team meetings are held, but given the larger client caseload for each professional, each client is not discussed at each meeting. When informal teaming takes place, it typically occurs in the morning when most of the home health staff members are in the agency. However, for the remainder of the day, the telephone typically serves as the primary means of communication between team members. Some home health team members who begin their day in the field may conduct regularly scheduled team meetings by telephone. Thus, it can become more difficult to plan and implement a coordinated team effort as there is much less time spent working alongside other team members. Consequently, rehabilitation professionals in home health agencies may be more autonomous when planning intervention (Clark, 1994) as they typically spend a great portion of their workday by themselves.

The role of the occupational therapy practitioner does not change when providing services in clients' homes. The main objective of occupational therapy intervention continues to focus on the performance of daily living tasks that are most important to the client and caregiver(s) (Friedman, 1986; Jackson, 1993). If anything, providing services in a client's home compliments an occupational therapy practitioner's expertise—a focus on an older adult's occupational function within the environment in which he or she performs daily life tasks. Within the home setting, the occupational therapy practitioner can observe the client and caregiver(s) engaging in those tasks that are of concern. If bathing is an issue, the practitioner can observe the process and provide recommendations and additional intervention to enhance safety and efficiency. If lack of social interaction is an issue, the practitioner can collaborate with the client and caregiver(s) to identify social activities of interest to the client and develop a plan to solicit community volunteers who might visit the home. If wandering behavior is an issue, the practitioner can recommend environmental modifications to reduce the possibility of the client wandering from the home. As Friedman (1986) wrote, "Occupational therapists are wizards at finding the most efficient way for a disabled patient to accomplish the activities of daily living" (p. 73).

Although the role of the occupational therapy practitioner remains the same within a home health agency, how the role is enacted is quite different. The major difference between home health services and inpatient rehabilitation or skilled nursing facility services is the amount of time spent with the client. Typically, home health visits are 45 to 50 minutes, with 10 to 15 minutes set aside for documentation (Steinhauer, 1995). Further, clients are typically seen anywhere from one to three times per week, depending on the need for services or the number of visits that are authorized by the funding agency. In addition to the reduced number of sessions per week, another major difference for occupational therapy practitioners working for home health agencies is that typically no other team members are in the home at the same time, and often no other practitioners are immediately available to answer questions and help solve problems (Paulson, 1991). Occupational therapy practitioners who work in home health settings require a greater level of independent problem solving than practitioners who work in more structured rehabilitation settings. Another difference in home health care is the scheduling of visits to the client's home. Scheduling and coordinating

visits with other home health care personnel and around the routines of the client and caregiver(s) can be complicated (Steinhauer, 1995). Further complications can result when attempting to schedule visits that focus on daily life tasks that are more time sensitive, such as dressing or bathing, which typically are done in the morning or in the evening during the hours that an occupational therapy practitioner may be unavailable. Occupational therapy practitioners are guests in the client's home and must respect the client's wishes as to when a practitioner may visit. For some clients, the time of the visit may be very important or not important at all (Ramsden, 1993). Also, it is always the client's prerogative to refuse a visit from a home care team professional (Keenan, 1990).

OCCUPATIONAL THERAPY EVALUATION PROCESS

As in other rehabilitation settings, various professionals from the home health team conduct evaluations. However, one major difference in home health care is that not all team members will evaluate the client. Only those professionals whose services are requested per a physician's prescription will conduct an evaluation. Typically, a nurse will be the first team member to visit a client and conduct an initial intake evaluation. If occupational therapy services are needed and were not initially ordered by a physician, the nurse may request occupational therapy services by soliciting a physician's prescription.

One unusual aspect of home health care is that although a nurse, physical therapist, or speech and language pathologist may be the first team member to visit a client, under Medicare, Part A, guidelines, an occupational therapy practitioner may not be the first one. (The same is true for social workers and home health aides.) If occupational therapy services are required, either nursing, physical therapy, or speech and language pathology services must be required. In other words, a home health client could receive only occupational therapy services if he or she was receiving nursing, physical therapy, or speech and language pathology services. However, once occupational therapy services are initiated in conjunction with another professional service, occupational therapy services may continue even if the other services are discontinued. Thus, it becomes important for occupational therapy practitioners to educate other professionals regarding the need to appropriately screen for occupational performance difficulties that would warrant the intervention of an occupational therapy practitioner.

Occupational therapists and occupational therapy assistants both practice in home health settings. Because of the relatively brief visits and the limited number of visits per week, the occupational therapist will conduct the initial evaluation, establish the goals, and develop the intervention plan (Jackson, 1993; Young & Youngstrom, 1995). In some cases, when service competency has been established, the occupational therapy assistant may conduct further evaluation procedures as warranted. For example, it may not be possible to observe a client bathing during the first visit. However, once the intervention plan has been established, an occupational therapy assistant could conduct an evaluation of bathing at a later date.

The primary focus of the evaluation for an occupational therapist does not change significantly from an inpatient or skilled nursing facility setting. That is, the therapist is still concerned with the client's and caregiver's abilities to perform the tasks that are of impor-

tance to them in the home. However, it becomes very important that the occupational therapist not evaluate the client on the basis of the therapist's values and beliefs, particularly when observing the client in the context of his or her social system (May & Dennis, 1993). Occupational therapy practitioners bring their own values and beliefs regarding how families should function and how families should interact with each other. In the course of evaluating the client's daily living skills, the occupational therapist should account for those values and beliefs when interpreting the family's behavior and be very cognizant that his or her initial perspective may be biased.

Gathering Information During an Initial Interview

Because of the time constraint of a short home visit, the occupational therapist is unable to conduct a comprehensive evaluation. Following a client-centered approach, the practitioner must quickly get to the areas of concern identified by the client and caregiver(s). This approach does not negate the importance of understanding the roles, interests, and values of the client with respect to his or her daily life tasks. However, the occupational therapist may not have the opportunity to explore these issues in depth on the first visit. Essentially, the occupational therapist should structure the interview to solicit the client's perspective of the difficulties experienced when performing daily life tasks and what tasks the client is unable to do but would like to be able to do. The evaluation process should not evolve solely from the client's medical diagnosis or the client's level of independence with daily living tasks (Levine & Gitlin, 1993). If an occupational therapy practitioner approaches the client in the home with this perspective, the practitioner may ignore the multiple concerns and needs that confront clients in their homes.

It is very important that the occupational therapist address the concerns of the client's caregivers during the initial interview. Thus, the occupational therapist must quickly identify the members of the client's social system who are primarily responsible for the client's care (May & Dennis, 1993). It is highly unusual for a client's caregiver(s) not to be present in the home when home health professionals are present; therefore, the occupational therapist should take advantage of the opportunity to interview the caregiver(s) to gather information regarding the caregiver's need for assistance, additional information, and any fears and concerns (May & Dennis, 1993). It may be helpful, at times, to talk with the caregiver separately. However, this conversation is not a general rule, and the occupational therapy practitioner should be cautious when attempting this talk, as it may not be viewed favorably by the client.

Identifying Problems by Observing Client Performance

The therapist not only should accept the verbal report of the client or caregiver but also should attempt to observe the performance of daily living tasks (Paulson, 1991). A client may report that he or she does not require any assistance when toileting, but this may not be the case when the occupational therapist or the caregiver assists the client to the toilet. If an occupational therapist is unable to observe the performance, the therapist should always designate the information on the evaluation form as "per patient report" or "per caregiver report."

As a result of the time constraints, it is not possible to observe the client in all daily living tasks that may be of concern. The occupational therapist conducting the initial evaluation may choose to select a few tasks for observation following the interview. The observations of the client's performance of daily life tasks should be based on the client's primary concerns, but the occupational therapist may have a good idea from a previous discharge summary, if one is available. For those tasks that are not observed, the occupational therapist may choose to document that further evaluation for those specific tasks is warranted. For example, during an initial interview, a caregiver reported experiencing great difficulty in assisting the client with bathing. Further clarification with the caregiver led the occupational therapist to document that, per the caregiver's report, the client requires moderate assistance to bathe and that an occupational therapy evaluation of bathing is warranted. In this case, either an occupational therapist or an occupational therapy assistant could return the following week to observe and assist the client and caregiver during bathing, make an evaluation, and document the results in a progress note.

One of the requirements for continued home health services is the documentation of the need for services based on the functional status of the client (Spector, 1993). It becomes critical that the occupational therapist evaluate what the client is able and unable to do in order to justify continued occupational therapy services. The client's safety during performance of daily life tasks is a primary area of concern, and observing the client's and caregiver's performance is the most accurate method to assess safety in the home environment. Further, the occupational therapist can observe any potential risks and hazards within the home, such as slippery bathtub surfaces, lack of grab bars, and poor lighting.

Finally, if the client's third-party payer is Medicare, it is required that all home health professionals provide some teaching on the first visit (Paulson, 1991). Thus, although the occupational therapist is gathering information from which to complete the occupational therapy evaluation, he or she is also expected to begin intervention on the first visit. To satisfy this requirement, an occupational therapist will often give a client and caregiver a brochure or handout that describes potential risks and hazards in the home environment for individuals with disabilities and that also provides suggestions to reduce those risks and hazards. The occupational therapist can review the handout with the client and caregiver, answer any initial questions, and, in doing so, satisfy the Medicare teaching requirement.

SETTING GOALS THROUGH PATIENT-PRACTITIONER COLLABORATION

Because of the time constraints imposed on the length and number of visits, it becomes necessary for the occupational therapist, client, and caregiver(s) to prioritize potential goals (Hunt, 1994). The occupational therapist needs to balance the immediate concerns of the client with those identified problems that have the best potential for resolution within a limited time frame (Austill-Clausen, 1995). The practitioner can collaborate with the client and caregiver, offer a professional opinion as to which concerns and problems are more amenable to intervention, and arrive at an agreement as to which concerns and problems should be a priority. For example, a client and caregiver may identify five

potential areas of concern:

1. Difficulty with toileting
2. Inability to prepare dinner
3. Lack of socialization with friends
4. Difficulty getting a snack in the afternoon
5. Inability to easily exit from the house in case of a fire.

Through a collaborative process, the occupational therapist may offer, based on professional judgment of the situation, that with regard to safety, exiting from the house should be a priority; that toileting, when compared to preparing a snack or dinner, may be more amenable to intervention; and that the lack of socialization is important to address because the client is experiencing some minor depression. Thus, the client and occupational therapist initially can agree on those three goals, particularly as the goals were among the client's five original concerns.

It is very important for the occupational therapist to identify the underlying cause of the occupational performance problem. A client who is experiencing a loss of self-confidence and self-esteem as a result of a disability is often at risk for further disability because of a lack of motivation to engage in daily life tasks (Hunt, 1994). Therefore, although independence in feeding may be a very appropriate goal, the occupational therapist should identify and document the underlying reason why the client does not eat independently, particularly if the underlying cause is a psychosocial issue. From one study that examined the documentation of home health occupational therapy practitioners, although practitioners said that they addressed psychosocial issues during intervention, no evidence of psychosocial issues appeared in any documented notes (Kunstaetter, 1988). Occupational therapists need to establish goals that reflect the daily life tasks that are important to the client and document why the client is experiencing difficulty with those tasks, including any psychosocial issues affecting the client's performance of those daily life tasks.

ACHIEVING GOALS THROUGH OCCUPATIONAL THERAPY INTERVENTION

Occupational therapy practitioners must identify the key members of the client's social system (e.g., family members, caregivers, friends, or neighbors) and develop insight into the important relationships with the social system (May & Dennis, 1993). Such insight will help occupational therapy practitioners, as these key members of the client's social system will most likely be the people interacting with the client when the client is not receiving occupational therapy services. It is important that the client and the key members of his or her social system understand the intervention plan to achieve the goals.

An additional consideration that occupational therapy practitioners should address is coordinating their services with those provided by home health aides (Jackson, 1993). If safety and independence are valued by a client and a home health aide is providing bathing services, the occupational therapy practitioner needs to coordinate the intervention plan with the home health aide (Young & Youngstrom, 1995). If such coordination does not occur, the home health aide and the occupational therapy practitioner may be working at cross purposes, and diminishing the likelihood of achieving the goal, for example, greater independence when bathing.

DISCHARGE PLANNING

One issue of concern is that when home health services are discontinued, the client and caregiver(s) may feel abandoned (Hunt, 1994). In many cases, clients and their caregivers accept the practitioner as a valued confidant and receive great emotional support from the practitioner's visits. It is not unusual for a home health client to invite a practitioner to sit down for something to drink or eat and visit for awhile before beginning the actual intervention for daily life skills. Thus, the practitioner may be a valuable support, and it may be difficult for the client and caregiver(s) to accept that the support may no longer be available. Thus, occupational therapy practitioners must prepare clients and caregivers in advance that occupational therapy services will eventually be discontinued. When discharge is imminent, it is very important that the client and caregiver(s) understand what community resources are available to them in the absence of an occupational therapy practitioner's services (Hunt, 1994).

EVALUATION OF OUTCOMES IN OCCUPATIONAL THERAPY

As with other rehabilitation settings, the evaluation of outcomes in home health settings depends on the accuracy of the practitioner's documentation of the client's and caregiver's baseline performance. For example, at the end of 3 weeks of occupational therapy intervention, it is readily apparent to the practitioner that the caregiver is able to safely assist the client with all home care tasks, that grab bars are installed in the bathtub and around the toilet, that the client requires supervision in bathing and toileting, and, per the client's report, that the client enjoys playing cards with the volunteers from the local hospital.

However, unless the occupational therapy practitioner had documented, either during the initial visit or on subsequent progress notes, that the client's caregiver was not safely assisting the client, that the client required moderate assistance with toileting and bathing, and that the client was not engaging in social activities, then an accurate evaluation of occupational therapy intervention outcomes would not be possible. Further, achievement of the client's and caregiver's goals determines the ultimate effectiveness of occupational therapy intervention.

DOCUMENTATION OF OCCUPATIONAL THERAPY SERVICES

Documentation for home health agencies remains just as important as in other rehabilitation settings. As with the other settings, the documentation must be easily understood by other professionals and representatives from funding sources (Spector, 1993). The occupational therapy practitioner should document that a client is benefiting from occupational therapy intervention and that the results can result in reduced health care costs (Reichenbach, 1992). For example, if, as a result of occupational therapy intervention, a client and his or her caregiver(s) demonstrate the ability to safely and independently bathe at home, the services of a home health aide may no longer be required. Thus, an additional expense would be saved by the third-party payer. Further, the occupational therapy practitioner should establish a correlation between the client's improvement with daily life tasks and the reduced possibility of admission to a nursing home, a potentially greater expense for a third-party payer. For these reasons, it is critical that occupational therapy practitioners document intervention to enhance a

client's and caregiver's safety and independence during the performance of daily living tasks.

The documentation of occupational therapy intervention should reflect the client's and caregiver's progress with carrying out daily living tasks and the unique focus of occupational therapy (Paulson, 1991), not the focus of other professionals. In many instances payment for home health occupational therapy intervention was denied by third-party payers because the insurers declared that the occupational therapy goals and intervention plans were very similar to the physical therapy goals and intervention plans. Consequently, the insurer would not pay for duplicate services. Thus, occupational therapy notes should not resemble physical therapy notes (Paulson, 1991), as Medicare will not pay for duplicate services (Reichenbach, 1992). (Occupational therapy intervention should not resemble physical therapy intervention!) Another potential issue is when the occupational therapy practitioner documents that a client is experiencing problems with instrumental activities of daily living and does not document that the client also is experiencing difficulty with basic self-care tasks. In these cases, the occupational therapy services will most likely be ineligible for reimbursement under Medicare, Part A, guidelines (Spector, 1993).

Another important consideration is that the documentation should reflect a requirement for skilled intervention (Jackson & Kavalar, 1993). That is, the occupational therapy services provided could not be provided by a lay person. Thus, occupational therapy practitioners should document the underlying limitations and the rationale for the intervention, which reflect solid clinical reasoning that is based on professional standards of practice. When occupational therapy practitioners document the limitations and problems that clients are experiencing with basic self-care tasks and instrumental activities of daily living, they are supporting the eligibility for reimbursement by third-party payers (Spector, 1993). Further, establishing a maintenance program and teaching the client's caregivers how to carry out the program is considered a skilled service and is eligible for reimbursement by Medicare (Jackson & Kavalar, 1993). However, if the documentation reflects that the occupational therapy intervention is merely maintaining the client's current level of performance and progress is not being made, then payment for the services will more than likely be denied.

Another important aspect of documentation in home health care is that all practitioners must document that caregiver teaching and training has occurred over the course of intervention. Thus, occupational therapy practitioners should document when home program instructions are provided (Jackson & Kavalar, 1993; Reichenbach, 1992) as well as the response of the caregivers when providing caregiver training. Finally, under Medicare guidelines, the discharge visit must be conducted and documented by an occupational therapist, not an occupational therapy assistant (Young & Youngstrom, 1995).

REIMBURSEMENT FOR HOME HEALTH OCCUPATIONAL THERAPY INTERVENTION

Medicare, Part A, is the major reimbursement source for older adults who receive home health services, and Medicare will reimburse for skilled nursing, rehabilitation therapies, and home health aides (Frank & Miller, 1994). Medicare, Part A, will reimburse for occupational therapy services provided that the following criteria are met (Jackson & Kavalar, 1993; Phillippi, 1996; Reichenbach, 1992; Spector, 1993):

- A physician must certify the need for occupational therapy services.
- The client must be considered homebound.
- The services could be provided effectively and safely only by a qualified practitioner.
- The client must demonstrate potential for reasonable progress.
- The client must make significant progress in practical daily living tasks.
- The progress must occur within a reasonable amount of time considering the client's diagnosis and prognosis.
- The services cannot be for the maintenance of functional skills.
- The intervention services must be provided through a certified home health agency.

As in other settings, Medicare, Part A, will reimburse only for adaptive equipment that is considered durable medical equipment (Phillippi, 1996), such as bedside commodes, hospital beds, or wheelchairs. Finally, occupational therapy practitioners should be aware that while Medicare will reimburse for services provided by occupational therapists and occupational therapy assistants (with the exception of evaluations and discharge visits), some private insurance companies and state Medicaid programs may not allow occupational therapy assistants to provide occupational therapy services (Young & Youngstrom, 1995). (Occupational therapy practitioners need to work with reimbursement agencies to educate them regarding the valuable services that occupational therapy assistants provide.)

Future Trends in Rehabilitation Services for Older Adults

Occupational therapy practitioners are now at a crossroads with the provision of healthcare services in the United States (Baum, 1991). Health care reform is a major issue in the United States, particularly the issue of funding health care so that the services are available and equitable for all individuals. Occupational therapy practitioners are grappling with the rapid changes in health care and the effects those changes are having on the delivery of occupational therapy services (Devereaux & Walker, 1995). Of current concern to occupational therapy practitioners who work with older adults in rehabilitation settings is the rapid change in the funding of rehabilitation services from fee-for-service plans to managed care plans (Joe, 1995a). In all rehabilitation settings, occupational therapy practitioners, who traditionally have valued the benefit of therapeutic relationships with clients, are now being asked to move their clients quickly through the health care system, keeping occupational therapy intervention to a minimum and within a specified time frame, while at the same time not compromising the quality of their services (Joe, 1995b). Occupational therapy practitioners are now faced with the fact that they must promote the continued existence of the system where they work—if health care costs are not contained, the financial stability of their place of employment may be at stake (Joe, 1995b). This promotion may create an ethical conflict between wanting to provide quality services for occupational therapy recipients and maintaining the financial viability of one's place of employment. In some cases, occupational therapy practitioners have been asked by their employers to provide rehabilitation services to clients who did not need them in order to generate more revenue for the facility (c.f., Joe, 1995a; Sophia, 1995). The rising cost of health care and the subsequent changes in how health care is provided are spurring some occupational therapy practitioners to rethink how they provide rehabilitation services and, in some cases, whether they can even work within those systems that do not appear to hold the same values for quality client care.

Many other changes are occurring within rehabilitation health care systems. Discipline-specific departments are no longer the norm in hospital-based practice (Joe, 1995b). Rehabilitation professionals are increasingly being required to receive advance authorization from third-party payers for their services, particularly from managed care plans (Joe, 1995a). It is expected that in the future a greater proportion of direct client care will be provided by rehabilitation aides that are supervised by rehabilitation practitioners. Those practitioners will provide more indirect intervention with more emphasis on evaluation, program development, and supervision and less hands-on, direct intervention (Joe, 1995b). The demand for home health services is increasing as a result of the rising cost of providing rehabilitation services within inpatient rehabilitation units and skilled nursing facilities (Menosky, 1995), and changes in Medicare's reimbursement system are starting to shift the responsibility for rehabilitation services away from hospital-based systems, such as inpatient rehabilitation, and toward alternative settings, most notably home care (Spector, 1993). An increased demand exists for mental health services for older adults who are homebound and require rehabilitation services (Menosky, 1995).

Such changes in the provision of rehabilitation services mean that occupational therapy practitioners must refine how their role within each rehabilitation system is enacted. Traditionally, occupational therapy practitioners have focused the provision of occupational therapy services on restoring an individual's occupational function (Devereaux & Walker, 1995). However, the current changes in how health care is provided do not mean that the objective of restoring an individual's occupational function will go by the wayside and no longer be important. Occupational therapy practitioners must continue to show that their rehabilitation services will produce outcomes that are functionally relevant and meaningful to older adults and their caregivers in their natural living environments and that those outcomes are sustainable over time (Foto, 1995). In doing so, practitioners will be promoting the health of the recipients of their services, while also holding down the cost of those services (Foto, 1995).

A major thrust of the current health care reform debate is an attempt to redefine health care delivery in terms of maintaining and restoring health and preventing illness, rather than solely emphasizing the cure of an illness (Devereaux & Walker, 1995). Occupational therapy practitioners are poised to become a major service provider in health care because of their focus on how people engage in occupation and how that engagement influences the state of their health and wellness (Baum, 1991). Occupational therapy practitioners can maintain their important role in rehabilitation settings by maintaining a commitment to the provision of services that promote independent living in the community and to their expertise in evaluating and providing intervention for occupational performance dysfunction (Baum, 1991). In doing so, occupational therapy practitioners will serve their clients well by promoting and enhancing not only their ability to perform daily life tasks, but also their health, wellness, and quality of life.

Review Questions

1. What expertise does an occupational therapy practitioner possess compared to other rehabilitation professionals? Explain the differences among the specialties.

2. Why should an occupational therapy practitioner follow a client-centered approach in rehabilitation settings?

3. Describe the process that occupational therapy practitioners should follow during the evaluation process in each of the three rehabilitation settings. Why should they follow this process?

4. What are the major requirements of Medicare insurance when deciding to reimburse for rehabilitation services? What are the different requirements among the three settings?

5. Compared to inpatient rehabilitation units and skilled nursing facility settings, what factors are unique within home health care settings with regard to providing rehabilitation services?

References

Adaptive Environments Center. (1993). *A consumer's guide to home adaptation.* Boston, MA: Author.

American Occupational Therapy Association. (1993). Occupational therapy roles. *American Journal of Occupational Therapy, 47,* 1087–1099.

American Occupational Therapy Association. (1994a). Occupational therapy code of ethics. *American Journal of Occupational Therapy, 48,* 1037–1038.

American Occupational Therapy Association. (1994b). Uniform terminology for occupational therapy (3rd ed.). *American Journal of Occupational Therapy, 48,* 1047–1054.

Atwood, S. M., Holm, M. B., & James, A. (1994). Activities of daily living capabilities and values of long-term-care facility residents. *American Journal of Occupational Therapy, 48,* 710–716.

Austill-Clausen, R. (1995). Clinical considerations for the treatment of patients with physical disabilities in home health. In *Guidelines for occupational therapy practice in home health* (pp. 29–42). Bethesda, MD: American Occupational Therapy Association.

Bachelder, J. (1994). In B. R. Bonder & M. B. Wagner (Eds.), *Functional performance in older adults* (pp. 296–305). Philadelphia: F. A. Davis.

Baum, C. (1991). The environment: Providing opportunities for the future. *American Journal of Occupational Therapy, 45,* 487–490.

Bonder, B. R., & Goodman, G. (1995). Preventing occupational dysfunction secondary to aging. In C. Trombly (Ed.), *Occupational therapy for physical dysfunction* (pp. 391–404). Baltimore: Williams & Wilkins.

Canadian Association of Occupational Therapists. (1991). *Occupational therapy guidelines for client-centered practice.* Toronto: Author.

Chin, M. (1994, April 14). Treating a culturally diverse clientele at home. *OT Week,* 36–37.

Christiansen, C., & Baum, C. (1991). Occupational therapy: *Overcoming human performance deficits.* Thorofare, NJ: SLACK.

Clark, G. S. (1994). Rehabilitation team: Process and roles. In G. Felsenthal, S. J. Garrison, & F. U. Steinberg (Eds.), *Rehabilitation of the aging and elderly patient* (pp. 439–448). Baltimore: Williams & Wilkins.

Crabtree (1995). To prevent fraud, try going by the book [Letter to the editor]. *Advance for Occupational Therapists, 11*(43), 3.

Devereaux, E. B., & Walker, R. B. (1995). The role of occupational therapy in primary health care. *American Journal of Occupational Therapy, 49,* 391–396.

Dickerson, A. (1994). Considering culture in the assessment of elderly persons. *Gerontology Special Interest Section Newsletter, 17*(3), 1–2.

Faust, L., & Meaker, M. K. (1991). Private practice occupational therapy in the skilled nursing facility: Creative alliance or mutual exploitation? *American Journal of Occupational Therapy, 45,* 621–627.

Fisher, A. G. (1992a). Functional measures, part 1: What is function, what should we measure, and how should we measure it? *American Journal of Occupational Therapy, 46,* 183–185.

Fisher, A. G. (1992b). Functional measures, part 2: Selecting the right test, minimizing the limitation. *American Journal of Occupational Therapy, 46,* 278–281.

Fisher, A. G. (1994). Functional assessment and occupation: Critical issues for occupational therapy. *New Zealand Journal of Occupational Therapy, 45*, 13–19.

Fisher, A. G. (1995). *Assessment of motor and process skills.* Ft. Collins, CO: Third Star Press.

Foto, M. (1995). New president's address: The future—Challenges, choices, and changes. *American Journal of Occupational Therapy, 49*, 955–959.

Frank, J. C., & Miller, L. S. (1994). Community-based rehabilitation for the elderly. In G. Felsenthal, S. J. Garrison, & F. U. Steinberg (Eds.), *Rehabilitation of the aging and elderly patient* (pp. 477–485). Baltimore: Williams & Wilkins.

Friedman, J. (1986). *Home health care.* New York: W. W. Norton.

Glantz, C. H., & Richman, N. (1991). *Occupational therapy: A vital link to the implementation of OBRA.* Rockville, MD: American Occupational Therapy Association.

Hunt, L. A. (1994). Home health care. In B. R. Bonder, & M. B. Wagner (Eds.), *Functional performance in older adults* (pp. 284–295). Philadelphia: F. A. Davis.

Jackson, B. N. (1993). Health care providers: Functions and issues. In B. J. May (Ed.), *Home health and rehabilitation* (pp. 25–53). Philadelphia: F. A. Davis.

Jackson, D. E., & Kavalar, M. K. (1993). Reimbursement and documentation. In B. J. May (Ed.), *Home health and rehabilitation* (pp. 311–327). Philadelphia: F. A. Davis.

Joe, B. (1995a, October 26). Bracing for change: NARA's Zigenfus tells it like it is. *OT Week*, 14–15.

Joe, B. (1995b, October 12). Case managers confront managed care. *OT Week*, 14–15.

Kaufmann, M. M. (1994). Activity-based intervention in nursing home settings. In B. R. Bonder, & M. B. Wagner (Eds.), *Functional performance in older adults* (pp. 306–321). Philadelphia: F. A. Davis.

Keenan, J. M. (1990). In-home geriatric rehabilitation. In B. Kemp, K. Brummel-Smith, & J. W. Ramsdell (Eds.), *Geriatric rehabilitation* (pp. 357–369). Boston: College-Hill.

Kelly, F. A., Kawamoto, T. T., & Rubenstein, L. Z. (1991). Assessment of the geriatric patient. In J. M. Kiernat (Ed.), *Occupational therapy and the older adult: A clinician manual* (pp. 76–98). Gaithersburg, MD: Aspen.

Kielhofner, G., Mallinson, T., & de las Heras, C. G. (1995). Methods of data gathering. In G. Kielhofner (Ed.), *A model of human occupation: Theory and application* (pp. 205–250). Baltimore: Williams & Wilkins.

Kornblau, B. (1995). Can we stop the values shift? [Letter to the editor]. *Advance for Occupational Therapists, 11*(43), 4.

Kunstaetter, D. (1988). Occupational therapy treatment in home health care. *American Journal of Occupational Therapy, 42*, 513–519.

Law, M., Baptiste, S., Carswell, A., McColl, M. A., Polatajko, H., & Pollock, N. (1995). *Canadian occupational performance measure* (2nd ed.). Toronto: Canadian Association of Occupational Therapists.

Lawson, S. R. (1994). Maximizing independence in activities of daily living. *Gerontology Special Interest Section Newsletter, 17*(1), 4–5.

Levine, R. E. (1987). Culture: A factor influencing the outcomes of occupational therapy. *Occupational Therapy in Health Care, 4*, 3–16.

Levine, R. E., & Gitlin, L. N. (1993). A model to promote activity competence in elders. *American Journal of Occupational Therapy, 47*, 147–153.

Maloney, C. C., & Kasper, P. K. (1991). Discharge planning for the geriatric patient. In J. M. Kiernat (Ed.), *Occupational therapy and the older adult: A clinician manual* (pp. 137–154). Gaithersburg, MD: Aspen.

May, G. J., & Dennis, J. K. (1993). Caregivers. In B. J. May (Ed.), *Home health and rehabilitation* (pp. 269–288). Philadelphia: F. A. Davis.

McCormack, G. L., Llorens, L. A., & Glogoski, C. (1991). Culturally diverse elders. In J. M. Kiernat (Ed.), *Occupational therapy and the older adult: A clinician manual* (pp. 11–25). Gaithersburg, MD: Aspen.

Menosky, J. A. (1995). Mental health services in the home health setting: Special considerations. In *Guidelines for occupational therapy practice in home health* (pp. 43–54). Bethesda, MD: American Occupational Therapy Association.

Miller, M. A., & Kirchman, M. M. (1991). Geriatric rehabilitation programs. In J. M. Kiernat (Ed.), *Occupational therapy and the older adult: A clinician manual* (pp. 99–122). Gaithersburg, MD: Aspen.

Neistadt, M. E. (1995). Methods of assessing clients' priorities: A survey of adult physical dysfunction settings. *American Journal of Occupational Therapy, 49*, 428–436.

Northern, J. G., Rust, D. M., Nelson, C. E., & Watts, J. H. (1995). Involvement of adult rehabilitation patients in setting occupational therapy goals. *American Journal of Occupational Therapy, 49*, 214–220.

Nygård, L., Bernspång, B., Fisher, A. G., & Winblad, B. (1994). Comparing motor and process ability of persons with suspected dementia in home and clinic settings. *American Journal of Occupational Therapy, 48*, 689–696.

Park, S. (1995). Treatment planning. In A. Fisher (Ed.), *Assessment of motor and process skills* (pp. 61–72). Ft. Collins, CO: Third Star Press.

Park, S., & Fisher, A. G. (1995). Case studies: Evaluation and treatment planning—Roberta: The use of the AMPS in treatment planning for an older adult who had a stroke. In A. Fisher (Ed.), *Assessment of motor and process skills,* (pp. 81–98). Ft. Collins, CO: Third Star Press.

Park, S., Fisher, A. G., & Velozo, C. A. (1994). Using the Assessment of Motor and Process Skills to compare occupational performance between clinic and home settings. *American Journal of Occupational Therapy, 48*, 697–709.

Paulson, C. P. (1991). Home care programs. In J. M. Kiernat (Ed.), *Occupational therapy and the older adult: A clinician manual* (pp. 220–240). Gaithersburg, MD: Aspen.

Phillippi, L. M. (1996). Medicare documentation: The paperwork challenge. In C. B. Lewis (Ed.), *Aging: The health care challenge* (3rd ed., pp. 425–447). Philadelphia: F. A. Davis.

Ramsden E. L. (1993). Cultural considerations. In B. J. May (Ed.), *Home health and rehabilitation* (pp. 243–254). Philadelphia: F. A. Davis.

Reichenbach, V. (1992). Special considerations II: Home health. In J. Acquaviva (Ed.), *Effective documentation for occupational therapy* (pp. 105–112). Rockville, MD: American Occupational Therapy Association.

Reitz, S. (1992). Ethical issues in documentation. In J. Acquaviva (Ed.), *Effective documentation for occupational therapy* (pp. 219–229). Rockville, MD: American Occupational Therapy Association.

Robertson, S. C. (1992). Why we document. In J. Acquaviva (Ed.), *Effective documentation for occupational therapy* (pp. 23–33). Rockville, MD: American Occupational Therapy Association.

Rogers, J. C. (1990). Improving the ability to perform daily tasks. In B. Kemp, K. Brummel-Smith, & J. W. Ramsdell (Eds.), *Geriatric rehabilitation* (pp. 137–155). Boston: College-Hill.

Rogers, J. C., & Holm, M. B. (1994). Assessment of self-care. In B. R. Bonder & M. B. Wagner (Eds.), *Functional performance in older adults* (pp. 181–202). Philadelphia: F. A. Davis.

Scott, S. J., & Somers, F. P. (1992). Orientation to payment. In J. Acquaviva (Ed.), *Effective documentation for occupational therapy* (pp. 5–21). Rockville, MD: American Occupational Therapy Association.

Sophia, S. (1995). How do we work in an unethical system? [Letter to the editor]. *Advance for Occupational Therapists, 11*(43), 3.

Spector, M. (1993). Assessing status and function. In B. J. May (Ed.), *Home health and rehabilitation* (pp. 75–102). Philadelphia: F. A. Davis.

State University of New York at Buffalo (1990). *Guide for the use of the uniform data set for medical rehabilitation including the Functional Independence Measure (FIM)*. Buffalo, NY: Author.

Steinberg, F. U. (1994). Medical evaluation, assessment of function and potential, and rehabilitation plan. In G. Felsenthal, S. J. Garrison, & F. U. Steinberg (Eds.), *Rehabilitation of the aging and elderly patient* (pp. 81–96). Baltimore: Williams & Wilkins.

Steinhauer, M. J. (1995). Home health practice: Considerations for the practitioner. In *Guidelines for occupational therapy practice in home health* (pp. 9–14). Bethesda, MD: American Occupational Therapy Association.

Stineman, M. G., & Granger, C. V. (1994). Outcome studies and analysis: Principles of rehabilitation that influence outcome analysis. In G. Felsenthal, S. J. Garrison, & F. U. Steinberg (Eds.), *Rehabilitation of the aging and elderly patient* (pp. 511–522). Baltimore: Williams & Wilkins.

Trace, S., & Howell, T. (1991). Occupational therapy in geriatric mental health. *American Journal of Occupational Therapy, 45*, 833–838.

Trombly, C. (1993). The Issue Is—Anticipating the future: Assessment of occupational function. *American Journal of Occupational Therapy, 47*, 253–257.

U.S. Department of Health and Human Services (1995). *Post-stroke rehabilitation* (AHCPR Publication No. 95–0662). Rockville, MD: Author.

Wells, S. A. (1992, December 3). Issues in minority affairs: Aging among minority populations. *OT Week, 7*.

Wilson, D. (1992). "If I had known then what I know now...." In J. Acquaviva (Ed.), *Effective documentation for occupational therapy* (pp. 1–3). Rockville, MD: American Occupational Therapy Association.

World Health Organization (1980). *International classification of impairments, disabilities, and handicaps (ICIDH)*. Geneva, Switzerland: Author.

Young, J. A., & Youngstrom, M. J. (1995). Teamwork, personnel, and supervision in the home health setting. In *Guidelines for occupational therapy practice in home health* (pp. 15–20). Bethesda, MD: American Occupational Therapy Association.

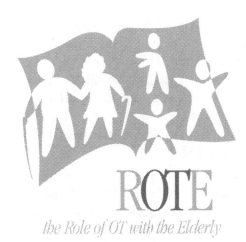

the Role of OT with the Elderly

Environmental Design, Modification, and Adaptation

Margaret A. Christenson, MPH, OTR, FAOTA

Abstract

"We are accustomed to adapting ourselves to the built environment rather than adapting the built environment to meet our needs" (Wylde, Baron-Robbins, & Clark, 1994). Because environment has the greatest effect on persons with the least capabilities, as people age, they become more dependent on their environments. "Design that adapts for the changes that occur with aging is crucial in providing an environment in which the older person can function to the maximum of his/her competence." Kiernat (1982) describes the environment as the "hidden modality."

This chapter discusses ways to improve these environments. Various housing types are described, followed by general principles that should be considered for all types of housing for older people. The chapter concludes with a discussion on assistive technology.

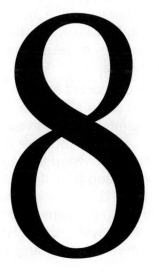

Housing Options

The decision to live in an independent, semi-independent, or dependent setting is usually determined by need, cost, and available choices. However, the level of dependency may not be closely defined because of supports and services provided.

When older people's needs increase, the family often is unable to provide assistance because, in part, older people today do not live as near their children as they did when society was less mobile. Home care services are often the only intervention considered. Before such services begin, the home needs to be analyzed for possible modifications that can increase the independence of the person living there.

If older people are purchasing a home, they prefer one that is on one level; however, two-story condominiums and townhouses are still the norm. Most older people are willing to have less square footage in exchange for having the main living areas on one floor. Because this type of housing usually requires more land, the trend is still to build two-story dwellings. The growing number of older people, compared to the growth of our Western population, calls for changes in the housing industry. When developers realize the preference for one-story homes, the industry will, it is hoped, focus more on that type of dwelling.

As older persons develop more problems and become less independent, they may desire some type of support. They might consider senior housing or assisted living, or they might desire to remain in their single-family dwelling and use 24-hour care service. However, this kind of service is not only expensive, but it also requires space for a live-in attendant.

When both physical and cognitive needs increase, a long-term-care facility is not only the logical but the best housing option. If dementia is present, the supports incorporated in special care units can maximize the quality of life for those who reside there.

Single-Family Dwelling or Apartment

The preference of 85% of older people (American Association of Retired Persons [AARP], 1990) is to continue to live in their own home as long as possible. Being older does not lessen the desire for home ownership, including freedom, privacy, and comfort. Many

people are willing to pay extra for the adaptations that will make a home more accessible. The phrase "aging in place" is often used to designate an older person's ongoing ability to live in their chosen type of housing. This may range from a single-family dwelling to assisted living.

Adaptable housing refers to houses and apartments that are consciously designed by adding or adjusting certain elements to eliminate barriers for those who have physical limitations (Branson, 1991). These designs not only meet the needs of a person with a disability but also make the home more efficient for persons in the household who are not disabled. Local building codes and zoning regulations should be checked before beginning any construction (Johnson, 1993).

Because 60% of the accidents that occur to older people happen in the home (Phillips & Roman, 1984), injuries can be prevented with appropriate design schemes. "More people can potentially benefit from accessible design than from conventional design. We estimate that at one time or another, 90% of us will be disabled by conventional building design" (Wylde et al., 1994).

Designing housing for persons with severe physical or cognitive problems requires in-depth evaluation. These assessments are best performed by an occupational therapist.

In a study conducted in Canada, it was found that about 80% of the people with Alzheimer's disease live at home with a caregiver, usually a husband or wife (Canada Mortgage and Housing Corporation [CMHC], 1990). Practical physical changes were made to the dwellings to accommodate the behavior of people with Alzheimer's disease and the needs of their caregivers.

Designed Housing

In this chapter, the term *designed housing* refers to buildings planned for older residents. The requirements of the physical, sensory, and cognitive changes of aging should be incorporated into all areas of the design of this type of housing.

GENERAL CONSIDERATIONS

Three types of housing based on the increased dependence needs of the residents are discussed: senior and congregate housing, assisted living, and long-term-care facilities. (Special care or dementia units within long-term-care facilities is also discussed.) A variety of other housing types exist, but they are generally a subcategory of one of these three. When all three types of housing exist on the same campus, it is referred to as a continuing care retirement center (CCRC).

Each design team, directed by the developer, determines what areas to incorporate into a particular building. In the discussion of each housing type, the descriptions of the areas and spaces are not all inclusive. Spaces that are significantly different or have components addressed differently from those of the other types have been addressed. Inclusive environmental checklists for various building types are available (American Institute of Architects [AIA], 1985).

Spaces within designed housing should range from the most public to the most private of places. This sequence parallels the traditional home and community environment (Regnier, Hamilton, & Yatabe, 1991). This transition is illustrated as follows:

- The main entry, main lounge, and corridors leading to the elevator are public spaces.
- The dining room, meeting room, craft rooms, and any outpatient areas are semi-public.
- The corridors to resident rooms or apartments, lounges, and laundry are semiprivate.
- The resident's unit is private.

Wayfinding through these spaces must be a priority in planning the design (Christenson & Raschko, 1989). Interaction with the resident should convey and complement the public-to-private concept.

CODE RESTRICTIONS

In some types of designed housing, building codes favor low-maintenance materials. The codes do not yet reflect changes in technology, such as updated fire-retardant products. These outdated constraints result in facilities that have negative side effects, creating dehumanizing environments (Regnier et al., 1991).

DESIGN COLLABORATION

"... [I]t is increasingly clear that the information needs of design for older users go beyond the expertise of any one profession" (Ware, 1993). Occupational therapy practitioners with specialized knowledge about aging can work effectively with the non-health care team of architects, interior designers, contractors, and suppliers to provide quality environments for the elderly.

The occupational therapy practitioner can provide insights for the members of the team on the functional needs of older people. "Growth in the aging population points to an increased demand for occupational therapists' skills in new construction as well as retrofitting" (Ware, 1993).

SENIOR AND CONGREGATE HOUSING

Senior housing is marketed to active older people who are generally able to care for themselves without supervision or extensive medical attention (AIA, 1985). Today, the average age of the first occupants in a new complex is 78. Most are still driving their own cars. Few are thinking about their future accessibility needs (D. Lindh, personal conversation, September 15, 1995).

When senior housing was first introduced, developers gave little thought to the needs of these people as they became more frail. Today, senior housing is still marketed to active older people, but plans to accommodate later aging changes are incorporated. These modifications usually begin 5 to 7 years after the first people take occupancy. Some of these strategies include additional lighting, roll-in showers or planned ways to adapt current showers, and wall reinforcements to accommodate handrails. In one facility, the current card room is wired to allow for a future home care office. Plans to add a new chapel will allow the current chapel space, which is adjacent to the dining room, to become an additional dining area when wheelchair users increase (D. Lindh, personal conversation, September 15, 1995). When design decisions have not been based on compensating for aging changes, problems arise and often the building must undergo major expensive remodeling.

The design team should consider the following when planning a facility:

- Garages and parking spaces should be major concerns, because of the active and mobile nature of senior housing residents. Increased quality lighting, enlarged parking spaces, and large signs are crucial.

- Outdoor spaces should be as extensive as site and budget will allow. Active sports areas, including swimming pools, horseshoe, boccie or lawn bowling, shuffleboard, and putting greens may be considered. Places for residents to garden, socialize, and entertain visitors should also be included.

- Exercise rooms and equipment should foster wellness. A lot of health fitness equipment is appropriate for senior housing.

- Reception areas should be near entries and include a place where residents can sit and wait comfortably. Direct visibility of drive-up areas will facilitate pickups and dropoffs.

- Resident mail and package facilities with boxes at the residents' eye level, quality lighting, and large numbers should be included.

- Dining rooms should be designed not only for efficient food service but also to respond to socialization needs.

- Meeting rooms should provide enough room for all the residents as well as space for visitors.

- Libraries and craft or activity areas should provide places to share interests.

Generally, people with dementia are not initially admitted in senior housing. However, aging in place occurs, and cognitive problems may develop. Often senior housing is occupied by couples, and one person may have cognitive needs while the spouse does not. Thus, senior housing must be designed to accommodate people with cognitive as well as physical and sensory changes. The latter part of this chapter discusses ways these changes can and should be incorporated into the design.

ASSISTED LIVING

Assisted living is designed for persons with more limitations and needing more supports. It is a residential environment equipped with professionally delivered personal care services in a way that avoids institutionalization and keeps older, frail individuals independent for as long as possible (Regnier et al., 1991). Theoretically, housing and medical care are separate and may be provided by different organizations.

Some buildings are specifically designed and marketed as assisted living. Size may vary, but smaller dwellings have a more home-like quality. However, it is economically infeasible to have the building too small and still provide adequate services.

Other buildings have been converted from housing originally designed as senior housing. Assisted living may also be a package of services brought into senior housing. Regardless of the setting, four basic concepts underlie the philosophy of assisted living:

- Create a place of one's own in a private housing unit.
- Serve the unique individual through services that respond to a range of competencies.
- Share responsibilities among caregivers, family members, and residents, including family input in decisionmaking and care plans.
- Allow residents choice and control that reinforces self-esteem, self-reliance, and self-respect (Regnier et al., 1991).

The typical resident in assisted living is a frail woman in her mid-eighties. She most likely fits one of two profiles: an older cognitively alert, physically frail individual who needs assistance with some activities of daily living, or a physically able but mentally frail individual who exhibits early signs of dementia.

Common spaces are similar to senior housing, except handrails should always be included in the corridors because these residents are quite frail.

Some assisted living buildings have "unit clusters." These are semiprivate spaces around which several apartments may be grouped. This arrangement provides the apartment residents a common space in which to develop a sense of "family."

The living units in most assisted living facilities are apartments. These units may be smaller than those in senior housing, and they should provide features to support the more frail, older person. In bathrooms, walk-in/roll-in showers are less dangerous than tubs or showers with curbs. If the person needs a bath chair, it's easier to place in space. Also, a roll-in chair can be used.

The health care office should be easily accessible to the residents. Rehabilitation services are often not included because of the separation of medical and residential components. Occupational therapy practitioners need to market services to assisted living residents because of the need for training in ADLs and programming that will maximize the cognitive levels of the people with dementia. Space for therapy should be available because the need for occupational and physical therapy services in assisted living is growing as the needs of the residents increase.

LONG-TERM-CARE FACILITIES

The long-term-care facility generally has three types of residents, each of whom has different needs:

- Frail elderly persons who require a wide range of medical services.
- Subacute residents who have had an acute episode of some type and are in the facility for a short period of time, primarily for rehabilitation.
- People who have dementia.

When we consider the long-term-care facility, one of the most overlooked areas is the physical environment and how its design can promote the well-being of its residents. Too often, plans for the long-term-care facility have been for the convenience of the administration, focusing on upkeep and the needs of the staff. Sometimes the design accommodates the desires of the resident's children or the corporate owners (Andreasen, 1985; Aranyi & Goldman, 1980). The possibility of motivating the resident through thoughtful design may not even be explored. It is essential for occupational therapy practitioners to share their knowledge with the decisionmakers so that new products, materials, and application of the theories of aging can be incorporated into the nursing home environment.

Because age-related sensory changes do occur gradually, and most people continue to function in familiar surroundings, it often isn't until persons are admitted to the nursing home that the impact of the need caused by the person's sensory changes becomes most obvious. When major sensory losses are present, the person's functioning in a new environment is difficult at best. Wolanin and Phillips (1981) state, "Sensory alteration as a possible cause of confusion among the elderly cannot be ignored." Their reduced sensory acuity and a nursing home environment with little variety can often lead to sensory deprivation.

When an older person does not respond to "normal" amounts of stimulation, increased stimulus is required. However, too many changes result in sensory distortion. For example, with impaired hearing, usually the higher ranges of tones are affected. When the volume is increased to hear these higher tones, even fuzzily, the volume may be too loud in the low ranges where hearing is relatively normal. Thus deprivation, distortion, and overload may exist simultaneous-

ly for the older person (Wolanin & Phillips, 1981).

The subacute setting in the nursing home may be designed like a rehabilitation hospital. The occupational therapy clinic in the subacute setting should have an ADL apartment that will provide space for the occupational therapy practitioner to review the capability of the residents according to the discharge setting demands. Ideally, a home evaluation needs to be conducted shortly after the person's admission to determine those demands.

Many of the longer-term-stay residents are in wheelchairs. Residents use handrails to pull themselves down the hall. The *Uniform Federal Accessibility Standards* (Architectural and Transportation Barriers Compliance Board, 1984) recommends that handrails be placed 33 to 36 inches from the floor

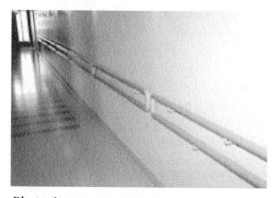

Photo 1.

on both sides of the corridor. Koncelik (1976) suggested a second handrail be placed on the same wall at approximately 26 inches (see photo 1). It has been observed that many ambulatory, frail elderly persons actually lean on the handrail with their lower arm rather than their hand. If this is true, the current height may be too low, but no research has been published to justify this change.

For the new residents, finding their way easily through the corridors can be challenging. Design to promote wayfinding should be included (Christenson & Raschko, 1989). Landmarks or prominent features marking a particular locality can help older persons find their way in a space. Just as certain buildings, monuments, and such, serve as focal points in a city, picture groupings or special textured objects or surfaces can be used as landmarks in an older person's immediate environment. These landmarks give cues concerning where to sit, turn, or stop.

Human recognition of pictures is superior to recognition of words. When actual architectural landmarks are not present, murals and pictures representing different scenes should be used as landmarks (Christenson & Raschko, 1989). Staff members can help residents orient themselves by explaining the landmarks and using them when giving directions to the resident, for example, "This is your room, Mrs. Jones; it is by this large picture of red flowers."

For a new resident in the long-term-care facility, personal possessions can contribute to adjustment. Familiar pieces of furniture, bedspreads, quilts, pillows, pictures, and other memorabilia are only some of the items to consider. Because objects often provide older persons with crucial links to their past, a space to store and display personal things that can be easily reached and touched is crucial. When older persons have personal belongings, they are perceived in a more positive light by others than when these artifacts are missing (Millard & Smith, 1981). Studies indicate that including easily attainable items can decrease offensive behavior (Windley & Scheidt, 1980).

Resident rooms, including the bathroom, should be designed for the resident and meet their needs, not those of the staff, should the two conflict.

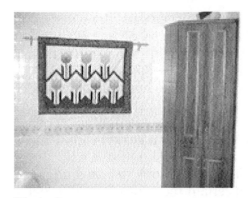

Photo 2.

For instance, equipment used by staff, particularly that of a less residential look, such as bedpans, urinals, and wound care equipment, should be stored elsewhere.

Tub rooms or central bathing areas are usually included in long-term care facilities because many of the residents require complete assistance in bathing. These rooms have traditionally been very cold and clinical and designed for staff efficiency only. Design that responds to the residents can promote privacy and create a more aesthetically pleasing space (see photo 2).

Because of its height, the nurses station counter may create a communication barrier for the residents. To increase communications with staff, nurses stations have been designed with at least one area lowered to desktop height. A place for nurses to document is placed away from residents.

Special Care or Dementia Units

The impact of the environment on the person with cognitive impairment is crucial. In fact, "a therapeutic environment can slow the decline expected over time in the functional abilities of people with dementia" (Cohen & Weisman, 1991).

As a resident becomes more confused, often fewer personal belongings are around. Sometimes these items are mislaid or taken by other residents. Family and friends may remove them because those people assume that if the resident does not talk about the item or the loss of these objects, he or she is unaware of them. Keeping personal items near a person with dementia enhances links with the past. Because specific objects may bring back certain memories, it may be helpful to provide a kit of familiar items to stimulate reminiscing. Hellen (1992) has suggestions for reminiscing kits.

Because movement may reduce agitation in the resident with dementia, areas where the resident can pace should be incorporated into the unit. If practitioners want to increase the understandability of the layout for the residents, hidden areas and corners should be avoided when possible (Calkins, 1988). Self-contained outdoor spaces should be included, even in climates where year-round use is not possible.

Techniques to reduce incontinence may preserve an individual's autonomy and dignity. Placing toilets so they are more visible, arranging the bed so it is nearer the bathroom, and painting toilet seats so they contrast with the floor are strategies to increase continence (Cohen & Day, 1993).

Sometimes the confused resident can be deterred from opening a door or entering an elevator by camouflaging the door handles or call buttons. However, because a confused resident will often follow the behavior of others, care should be taken by staff and visitors how they enter and leave the unit (Schafer, 1985). Because the staff members do not routinely use emergency exits, these exits can successfully be camouflaged with barriers or room dividers.

In a study by Steffens and Thralow (1987), the visual field of advanced Alzheimer's patients was investigated. The study showed a significantly reduced visual field in the patients with Alzheimer's disease in comparison to the findings with the other demented patients. This reduction gives additional credence to the appropriate placement of signs and pictorial landmarks as well as the necessity of the staff using these landmarks when attempting to orient the resident. (Sign placement is discussed in the next section of this chapter.)

In another study exploring the use of lighting with residents diagnosed with Alzheimer's disease, subjects were videotaped at mealtime under bright fluorescent lighting and indirect lamp lighting. "Findings demonstrated a decreased frequency of agitated behaviors during the indirect light periods and a return to increased frequency and intensity when fluorescent lights were used" (Kolonowski, 1992).

Inappropriate behavior in the resident with dementia may be traced to faulty perception of the environment (Wolanin & Phillips, 1981). It has been suggested that the increased agitation, referred to as Sundown Syndrome, which often occurs at dusk, can be reduced by clearly illuminating the environment (Kolonowski, 1992). This can be done quite effectively by using timed dimmer switches.

The recent increase in the development of Alzheimer's or special care units designed for residents with dementia requires that those designing these environments attempt to perceive them "through the senses" of these residents. Neither an overall highly sensory-stimulating nor a markedly subdued environment should be the goal. Rather the environment should have controlled stimulation with visual, tactile, and auditory cues designed into it that will have meaning for the resident. Because persons with dementia will be experiencing the normal age-related changes, adapting the physical environment to meet the needs of persons with dementia must begin with creating an environment that compensates for age-related changes. These adaptations will be discussed later in this chapter.

Legislative Influences

The Americans With Disabilities Act (ADA) has created many positive changes for persons with disabilities. The law's intent was to extend civil rights protection to persons with disabilities and to prohibit discrimination against this group in employment, state and local government services, public transportation, telecommunications, and public accommodations (Perry, Jawer, Murdoch, & Dinegar, 1991).

Some of these guidelines affect senior housing, assisted living, and nursing homes. Areas such as lobbies, dining rooms, restrooms, and admitting offices are considered public. The residents' apartments are not.

ADA has also had a negative impact on design guidelines for older people. If those involved in housing design look to ADA standards as absolutes, they may discover their designs impede rather than enhance independence of older people. One example is thresholds. The American Disability Accessibility Account Guidelines (ADAAG) Sections 4.13.8 and 4.1.63)(d)(ii) read as follows:

> Maximum threshold height: 1/2" (3/4" at exterior sliding doors). Raised thresholds and floor level changes shall be beveled with a slope no greater than 1:2. Alterations/Existing Conditions: If existing thresholds are 3/4" high maximum, and have (or are modified to have) a beveled edge on each side, they may remain (Perry et al., 1991).

If manufacturers and installers believe they have met the needs of all older people by adhering to these guidelines, they are wrong. Thresholds that pass ADAAG may be too high for both wheelchair users and persons who can walk. The wheelchair users will have difficulty getting over the projection; the frail elderly person, whose balance and proprioception is poor, may trip on such raised thresholds.

In a Swedish study conducted on causes of injury to the elderly in the home environment, it was noted that "fall injuries induced by the door threshold (doorsill), ladder and step chair, and throw rugs resulted in more severe injuries than did snow or ice, water, and stairs" (Sjorgen & Bjornstig, 1991). No threshold should be the goal. Level surfaces are possible but require innovative designers, contractors, and installers.

Another law that affects older people is the Fair Housing Amendment Act (FHAA) of 1988. This amendment "requires landlords to make reasonable accommodations in rules and procedures and to allow reasonable modifications to the premises to meet the needs of tenants with disabilities" (Edelstein, 1994). These modifications are usually made at the tenant's own expense and may require that the premises be restored to the original condition when the tenant moves out. The landlord must pay for the costs of modifications to common areas of the building.

Aging Changes as a Foundation for Design Decisions

Thousands of possible modifications, adaptations, and devices exist to compensate for aging changes. These solutions must in no way compromise personal safety. Ideally, the solutions should enhance a person's security.

COMPENSATING FOR PHYSICAL LIMITATIONS

The following solutions to compensate for physical changes are grouped by functional category. Many of these solutions have more than one use. For example, grab bars not only assist someone sitting and rising, but they also provide support for a person with stability problems. In addition, lamps that respond to touch are helpful for persons with limited pinch ability as well as a limited range of motion.

Mobility

When it is impossible to eliminate the threshold, gently sloped reducer strips may be incorporated. These strips will allow the person's foot or walker or wheelchair to slide over the space.

When elevation changes make a ramp necessary, the ramps used should have a pitch no greater than 1:20; that is, for every foot of elevation, the ramp must extend horizontally 20 feet. If the pitch is greater than 1:20, the individual will probably be unable to manage the distance independently, and a steeper pitch may be unsafe.

Stairs are a significant problem for many older people. Handrails are needed on both sides of the stairs. To eliminate the need for stairs, planners may need to rearrange the living setting. A dining room or part of a living room may be converted into a bedroom. If need, desire, and resources warrant it, a bathroom can be built on the main level. A glider with a seat may be placed to run up and down along the stairs, or a single-passenger elevator may be installed. Less expensive modifications include a commode placed near the bed in the converted sleeping space.

Stability

Handrails on each side of the stair will give the person added stability. Through hallways or any other open area with no support, handrails may be installed on the wall, or stable furniture may be placed to provide support (see photo 3).

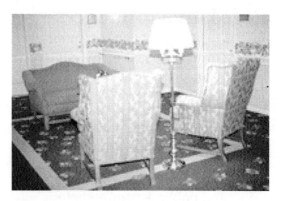

Photo 3.

Strategically placed grab bars in the bathroom are crucial for persons with poor balance. Often a horizontal bar is placed on the long wall above the tub. This bar is helpful while showering, but a vertical bar is needed to assist the person entering or exiting the tub or show-

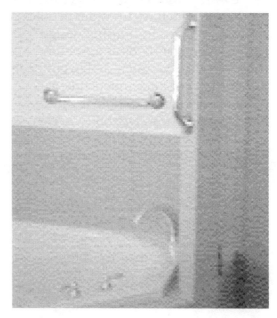

Photo 4.

er (see photo 4). Other compensations for stability are listed under solutions for changes in the kinesthetic sense.

Endurance

For the person with little endurance, a place to sit to prepare food or fold laundry can be very helpful. Strategic places to sit may increase the person's endurance because knowing there is a place to sit often gives the person the incentive to walk more.

Sitting and Rising

Chairs for older persons should have arms extended to aid in sitting and rising. The seat should be at a height, depth, and density that gives firm but comfortable support, is easy to rise from, and allows the feet to be placed securely on the floor (Christenson, 1990).

Bending

Adjustable closet shelves placed in the person's easy-reaching range while either standing or sitting make retrieving clothing and other items much easier. For the greatest comfort, the best location for these shelves, closet rods, outlets, door hardware, etc., is between 45.5 inches and 27.3 inches from the floor (Raschko, 1982). Roll-out trays on shelves in cupboards or closets reduce the need to bend down and reach under cabinets.

Arm Movement

Jar openers help compensate for weakened grasp. Persons who have difficulty with tremors (regardless of the cause) can be helped with products such as Dycem®, plate guards, and weighted eating utensils. If the person has difficulty reaching his or her feet, a sock aid or long-handled shoe horn is helpful. A reacher can compensate for a limited range of motion.

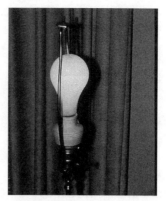

Photo 5.

Grasp and Pinch

Lever door handles can help the person with limited grasp. Sink faucets are available that can be operated with a closed fist. The shape of the handrail should provide a comfortable grip. The best handrail design is cylindrical and 1 1/4 to 1 1/2 inches in diameter.

Rocker light switches, Velcro®, touch-operated lamps or lamp converter, and button hooks are only a few of the assistive devices that can help a person who has problems with pinch (see photo 5).

One-Handed Activities

Many products are designed for people using one hand whether caused by a stroke, an amputation, or a broken arm. Most of these products stabilize an item while it is being worked on, such as an embroidery hoop with a clamp, a wall-mounted bag closure, or a cutting board with spikes and a corner guard.

ADAPTATIONS THAT COMPENSATE FOR PERSONS WITH SENSORY CHANGES

Sensory changes are common among elderly people, but these problems vary in severity and usually occur gradually. Care must be taken when recommending adaptations for groups of individuals. Solutions for one person may complicate functioning for another, for example, increased light that is needed for one person may be too intense for another (Christenson, 1990).

Vision Adaptations

When a person holds reading material farther away because it is difficult to read, it is a normal age-related difficulty of accommodation known as

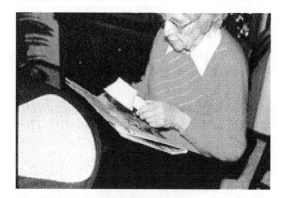

Photo 6.

presbyopia. In the early stages, corrective lenses will rectify the difficulty of reading fine print. Correction for this type of low vision is more difficult in later stages. A magnifier, preferably lighted, may be helpful (see photo 6).

Books and periodicals with larger print and good color contrast benefit people with low vision. Adapted watches and clocks are available. Other solutions include a cutting board, dark on one side but light on the other, which provides contrast with the items with which the person is working; a slicing knife with an adjustable, detachable guide that allows a person to select a slice width of from 1/16 to 1/2 inch; and a liquid level indicator that alerts the user with an audible signal to different levels of liquid in a glass, cup, or pan.

Glare. Glare is an overload problem caused by too much illumination. Direct glare occurs when light reaches the eye directly from its source. Direct glare from the sun can be reduced by mini-blinds, pleated polyester window shades, tinted windows, glare-reducing film directly applied to a window, or roller-type Mylar shades. Outdoor seating areas need sun screens, such as gazebos, wood trellises, and fences. Roof overhangs, awnings, or building recesses help protect from direct sunlight. Trees can shade courtyards and major glass areas.

Glare distracts older people, especially those who have difficulty concentrating. They can recognize faces better when there is less glare. Being able to recognize people often improves communications.

Indirect glare arises when the light rebounds off another surface and reflects into the eye. Indirect glare results from bright structures or surfaces outside a window, water from a pond or lake, sunlight reflecting off a highly polished floor, or light reflecting off stainless steel appliances such as walkers, plastic-covered furniture, and waxed floors. Even dishes and silverware can reflect an uncomfortable level of light. To reduce glare, avoid anything

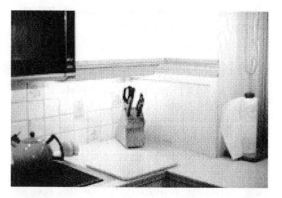

Photo 7.

highly polished, such as glossy paint, shiny laminated plastic table tops, or highly polished floors. Glass-covered surfaces should have nonglare glass.

Wall-mounted valances, light bars, or cove lighting that conceal the source of light also reduce glare. In a kitchen, task lighting under cabinet should be installed with a decorative board to eliminate direct glare (see photo 7). Fluorescent bulbs may be used in fixtures, but they must be selected carefully, and the ballasts must be checked regularly to ensure flickering is minimized. Fluorescent lighting should be combined with incandescent lighting in reading areas or where extensive lighting is needed, such as bathrooms. Whenever fluorescent light sources are used, warm-white deluxe or prime color tubes should be chosen. Paraboloid-patterned fixture covers on fluorescent lights provide better light distribution and eliminate glare (Christenson, 1990).

Lighting guidelines. Increased lighting permits more independence in home living. A 60-year-old needs three times the light that a 20-year-old needs to accomplish the same visual task. Because the lens of the eye becomes more opaque as one gets older, more light is needed to penetrate the lens.

Reading and close work can be aided by increased task lighting from floor or table lamps with three-way bulbs. However, bulbs should not be exposed or installed directly in the older person's line of vision because this lighting creates direct glare.

The eyes of an older person adjust more slowly when moving from light to dark or dark to light areas. Because of this delayed adaptation, furniture or other objects should not be placed directly inside an entry door where an older person might fall over them. Night lights should be used exten-

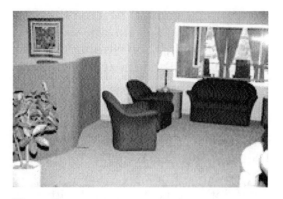

Photo 8.

sively, especially in and on the way to the bathroom.

Color perception. With increasing age, the lens of the eye takes on a yellowish color, which alters the quality of light entering the pupil. This impairs the perception of certain colors, particularly greens, blues, and purples. Dark shades of navy, brown, and black are discernible only under the most intense lighting conditions. Differences among pastel colors, such as blues, beiges, yellows, and pinks, are often hard to detect. In the nursing home, color takes on additional significance for the elderly. Color should be used not only for aesthetics but also to contrast different areas and distinguish objects from their backgrounds (see photo 8). For instance, adjacent corridors should not be painted pastel shades of green and blue or peach and gold.

Cuing by color alone should not be used to give directions to older people. Uniquely shaped objects, unusual architecture, distinctive furniture, large plants, a window with a view, etc., as well as smells, air currents, and tactile cues all provide spatial orientation.

Using definite color contrast in many activities of daily living is helpful. For instance, dressing is easier if buttons contrast in color with a shirt or sweater. Other tasks can be made easier by creating a contrast between the toothbrush and the sink, the slippers and the floor, the cookies and the plate, or the handrail and the wall.

Eating is easier when light-colored dinnerware and a dark tablecloth are used when serving dark foods; dark dinnerware and a light-colored tablecloth are used when serving light-colored foods. Dishes, place mats, and tablecloth should all contrast with each other.

The absence of color can assist persons with cognitive deficits. In long-term-care facilities or assisted living facilities, doorways that have no functional meaning for the residents, e.g., storage, linen room, locker rooms, etc., can be painted the background color of the walls. When visual information is reduced, the resident has fewer decisions to make (Christenson, 1990).

Depth perception. Depth perception is the ability to recognize relative distances to different objects. Increasing contrast or using nonglare lighting influences depth perception. This can be done by highlighting the edges of steps with light or a contrasting color; increasing nonglare lighting in dining areas so that the position of dishes is easier to discern; or adding a contrasting colored tape to the edge of the shower stall.

Depth perception may be hindered for persons wearing bifocals or trifocals. Older persons wearing glasses should be reminded that these glasses are designed to facilitate reading, and they may hinder walking because they blur the feet and ground. Older persons should be more cautious when relying on vision when walking or climbing stairs.

Figure-ground discrimination. Figure-ground illusions occur when an object or figure is perceived as background and the background as a figure. It is more difficult to recognize an object when it is placed on a highly patterned carpet. Patterns (including stripes, checks, and designs) on a floor surface, particularly in hallways, living rooms, or dining rooms, should be avoided.

Upward gaze. For many older people, upward gaze becomes problematic. This difficulty may be due to several reasons: the presence of bone spurs in the neck may prevent the person from looking upward; the older person is usually shorter than the population as a whole; often the eyelid itself does not open as wide. A combination of these difficulties makes it mandatory that signs and other instruction material be placed from 32 to 48 inches above or within the visual field of most older people.

Hearing Adaptations

"Poorly managed and designed acoustical settings can be as great a barrier to older people as steps are to a wheel-chair user" (Hiatt, 1985). Reducing background noise through acoustical treatment, replacing products with too little volume or too high a frequency, and using devices that compensate for hearing loss will help compensate for hearing changes.

Background noise and acoustics. Many elderly people with impaired hearing feel isolated. They may be reluctant to eat in restaurants or attend large social gatherings because they cannot enjoy the conversation of people around them. Noise from conversations, fans, dishes, television, traffic, music, etc., interferes with hearing. Furnishings and materials should absorb sound, reduce echoes, and muffle irrelevant noise.

Acoustical ceiling tile is usually the most economical way to lower sound levels, but carpeting, draperies, textured wall covering, and other upholstery fabrics also help reduce noise levels.

Decorative ceiling baffles, wall hangings, and wall panels reduce background noise and add aesthetic appeal. Panels should be placed on at least two adjacent walls between 2 feet 6 inches and 6 feet 8 inches from the floor (Leibrock, 1993). Insulation should be used around noisy areas, such as kitchens and laundry rooms.

In rooms where interaction is desired, noise reduction should be a priority. In the dining room, persons with a hearing loss should not be seated at the end of the table. Other potentially disturbing sounds, such as the television, radio, and air conditioners, should be eliminated. People with hearing loss should not be placed near the kitchen or other noisy areas.

In a nursing home, intercoms produce additional background interference, and the inability to identify a sound or to determine the source of a sound can create confusion.

Snyder (1978) demonstrated that wandering and confusion increased in nursing homes during shift changes and other periods of high noise level. Hall, Kirschling, & Todd (1986) reported that patients on an Alzheimer's unit that had minimum traffic, no television sets, no intercom or public address system, and no ringing phones showed less anxiety. No medications were passed at mealtime, and residents ate in small groups, thus reducing noises related to the traditional dining room.

In an area where incontinence may be a problem, such as an Alzheimer's unit, furniture upholstered with polyester fabric furnishes the texture and sound absorbency of traditional fabric while simplifying maintenance problems. This upholstery is installed with Velcro, has a vapor barrier, and can be laundered in a clothes washer and line dried.

Adaptive devices for hearing loss. Hearing aids should be encouraged. Many older people who tried a hearing aid more than 5 years ago may have been told nothing could help them. Hearing aid technology has made enormous improvements, and newer products should be examined.

Telephones, door bells, and appliances should be analyzed for their decibel and frequency levels. Many electronic-toned products have high frequencies that cannot be heard by the hearing impaired. Buzzers, bells, and ringers can be replaced with lower frequency mechanical tones. People with hearing loss may require a fire and smoke alarm (which usually have high frequency sounds) with a visual cue, such as a flashing light.

Radio, television, and music in a nursing home need to be assessed carefully. Generally, it is helpful for older people if the bass is turned up and the treble is turned down (Hiatt, 1979).

Sense of Smell Adaptations

The sense of smell provides both protection and pleasure. Literature on olfactory (smell) sensitivity is contradictory, but sensitivity appears to decrease with age. Older people have not only a reduction of pleasant smells but also a reduced sensitivity to body odors and smoke or gas fumes. In a study in England (Chalke & Dewhurst, 1957) of 892 deaths caused by domestic gas poisoning, over 75% of the people who died were over 60 years of age. Because many of these people are living alone, the inability to sense the presence of gas fumes or smoke is a safety issue. Smoke detectors are crucial, and when gas appliances are present, gas detectors should be added.

Tactile and Touch Interventions

Carpeting, velour, textured upholstery, and wood not only cut down on glare but also add warmth and tactile input. Wall hangings made from burlap, carpet, heavy yarn, or rope add texture. Varied floor coverings likewise increase the degree of texture in an area. Outdoors, a distinctive surface treatment such as brick or stone can lead the older person to a particular seating area. However, when using varied floor or ground treatments, close attention must be paid to their levels, in light of mobility and kinesthetic problems (see photo 9).

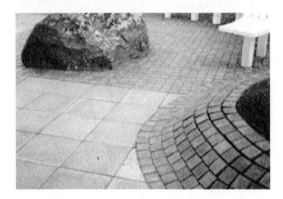

Photo 9.

Tactile information can be used for other cues. Variations on the surface of handrails, such as knurling or grooves, can give cues to turns or the approaching end of a wall. Fire and exterior doorknobs must have some type of textured surface for safety purposes.

Kinesthetic Input

Many aids can compensate for kinesthetic loss. Handrails add support for the person with balance problems. Ramps are often seen as helpful for all older people. Indeed, they are necessary for the wheelchair user and for the person who has difficulty with foot position sense. However, because of lowered gaze and increased forward tilt due to osteoporosis, stairs rather than ramps may be safer and easier for some older people to negotiate (Hiatt, 1979). Handrails along both sides of the ramp are absolutely essential.

Ramps should be as gradual as possible both for the frail ambulatory person and the older wheelchair users who have less upper extremity strength. ADA has been helpful in reducing the recommended ramp pitch from 1 foot up for every 10 or 12 feet of length (1:12) (Architectural and Transportation Barriers Compliance Board, 1984) to 1 foot up for every 20 feet of length (1:20) (Perry et al., 1991).

Because elderly people fall more easily (Hasselkus, 1974) and have less balance because of a reduced righting reflex, the floor covering is important. The following factors regarding floor treatment should be considered:

- Carpet has approximately the same installation price as sheet vinyl.
- Carpet maintenance is usually cheaper than vinyl composition tile if immediate attention is taken for cleaning of spills.
- Carpet produces a feeling of warmth and comfort.
- Carpet is quiet, but it traps bacteria and dust.
- Carpet has a wide color and texture range.
- Residents appear to feel more secure on carpet. Gait speed and step length have been demonstrated to be significantly greater on carpet than on a vinyl surface (Wilmott, 1986).
- Vinyl composition tile (VCT) is relatively inexpensive to install and has adequate color choices.
- VCT has high maintenance requirements, is noisy, produces glare, and has an institutional appearance.

- Sheet vinyl does not require high gloss maintenance.
- Installation costs for VCT are the least expensive; however, a user-cost comparison shows that carpet, over the lifetime of the product, is less expensive (Reznikoff, 1979).
- Wheelchair users are affected by the floor surface.
- Carpet produces more drag on wheels, which causes difficulties for some wheelchair users.
- Carpet will have less drag if it has no padding and it is glued down directly to the subfloor.
- Either sheet vinyl or VCT is easier for wheelchair users to roll on.

Basis for Decisions for Aids and Supports for Persons with Dementia

Assistive devices have traditionally been designed for persons with physical disabilities. Products for persons with dementia and increasing memory loss need to be developed. Such persons, especially those with probable Alzheimer's disease or an Alzheimer's related disorder (ARD), are trying to make some sense out of what has become a very confusing existence. Some devices can help these people who no longer have accurate decision-making abilities. These products include timers, monitors, organizers, etc.

The needs of the caregiver must be considered. Their needs include more than assistance with lifting and physical care. Interventions that compensate for memory loss reduce some of the psychological problems of caregiving. A timer that, after a predetermined period of time, automatically turns off the stove eliminates the concern that the stove might be left on and unattended.

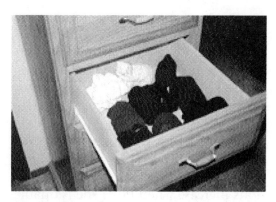

Photo 10.

Surroundings for people with dementia must be as calm and consistent as possible, including the reduction of objectionable noises.

Items should be placed so the client can see them easily. For instance, open shelving should be provided for toothpaste, toothbrush, soap, washcloth, electric razor, etc., and should act as a visual reminder of good grooming.

To simplify dressing, caregivers should (1) visually sequence the task by putting an outfit such as a pair of pants and shirt on the same hanger; (2) position an adjustable closet rod and hangers at eye level; (3) place cupboards and drawers at appropriate heights for the person; and (4) place one type of item, such as socks, in a drawer (see photo 10). Coated wire baskets will permit contents to be seen more easily.

When a person with dementia is faced with a situation he or she does not understand, "catastrophic reactions" (Hellen, 1992) often occur that are out of proportion to the magnitude of the incident that triggered the reactions. Thus it is important to avoid situations that might create conflicts or confrontation.

If the individual should not be using appliances, caregivers should turn off the stove with a hidden lock switch rather than removing the knobs. If the person is still capable of using a stove for a short period of time and the concern is more with leaving the stove on or a pan burning dry, the range timer described previously can be used in addition to a heat-sensitive safety device called a heatguard.

Dementia clients are often upset by locked cupboards or closets, as well as childproof latches. The person thinks that something is stuck, and frustrations increase when he or she is unable to open a drawer or door. Inconspicuous magnetic closures are better. This magnetic lock is mounted on the

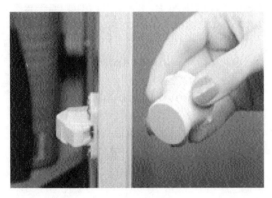

Photo 11.

inside of the cabinet so no locking hardware appears on the exterior of the door. To open the door, the magnetic "key" is placed on the outside cabinet area that corresponds to the locking mechanism. This releases the magnetic-closure hold so cabinets and doors will open (see photo 11).

Items not commonly used by the person should be stored out of sight. Things that may appear to be something else should be removed. These items might include wastebaskets or other objects that are mistaken for a toilet.

Pacing is often a characteristic of persons who have dementia and should not be thwarted. A secure enclosed area in the garden can allow the individual a place to pace and release excess energy

and tension. Appropriate indoor walking space is also important.

Rocking behavior is commonly seen in disoriented elderly. Is this self-induced movement an attempt to increase vestibular stimulation? If so, the need for self-determined vestibular input can be encouraged by including rocking chairs. Outdoor porches are a good investment for resident well-being, particularly if porch swings and rocking chairs are included in this area. Ideally, the arms of the swing should be part of the support system of the swing and not movable.

When there are security concerns about the person leaving the house, monitoring schemes can be tried. A simple alarm, such as a bell, can be installed to indicate that the door has been opened. Some security systems can be programmed to alarm when there is movement in only certain areas. If this is a temporary setting, a security bar that emits a loud noise when disturbed can be placed on the door.

Preventing the person from getting lost can be helped by monitoring devices. These are often used in long-term-care facilities, but some are available for home use. A local nursing home might be able to provide suggestions.

Many existing products are available at hardware stores, lumber yards, pharmacies, mail order catalogs, etc., that are not marketed specifically for persons with dementia.

Persons with dementia have a tremendous need for research and development of new products. For people to live as independently as possible in their homes, additional products are needed to compensate for memory loss. As designers and manufacturers discover the demand, these products will be developed.

Environmental Attributes

The competence of older people is affected by less tangible social and psychological attributes. These following attributes must be addressed in all housing for older people (Christenson, 1990; Regnier et al., 1991).

COMFORT

Many comfort features are addressed by meeting age-related sensory and physical changes, that is, adequate light, reduced background noise, comfortable temperature, and chairs that provide for long-duration sitting.

ACCESSIBILITY

Accessibility is the ease in getting from point A to point B and the ability to meet the physical challenges of aging, bending, reaching, manipulating objects, etc.

SECURITY

A person needs to feel secure in his or her setting. This sense of security may be protection from forced entry or the ability to reach help in time of an emergency.

LEGIBILITY

Legibility is defined as how clearly information is portrayed and displayed and is affected by a person's ability to receive and process the information (Windley & Scheidt, 1980). Therefore, adapting for age-related sensory changes is crucial. Orientation in designed housing must foster a sense of orientation that reduces confusion and facilitates wayfinding.

FAMILIARITY AND MEANING

Historical references and solutions influenced by tradition can provide a sense of familiarity and continuity by evoking memories. Objects help us develop and maintain our concept of self.

PRIVACY

Privacy is the ability to decide what information and under what circumstances a person wishes to communicate. It is the opportunity for seclusion where one can be free of intrusion.

PERSONALIZATION

This ability allows an individual to convey ownership of a space. In resident units—regardless of the level of care—adequate display and space must be provided.

SOCIALIZATION

Spaces should be planned to foster social connectedness. Seating that not only meets design criteria but also encourages eye contact should be planned.

Assistive Technology, Adaptative Equipment, and Assistive Devices

DEFINITION

The American Occupational Therapy Association recognizes the definition of assistive technology, which was established by the enactment of Technology-Related Assistance of Individuals with Disabilities Act in 1988:

> Assistive technology is any item, piece of equipment, or product system, whether acquired commercially off the shelf, modified, or customized, that is used to increase, maintain, or improve functional capabilities of individuals with disabilities.

In this discussion, assistive devices and assistive technology are used interchangeably.

HISTORICAL PERSPECTIVE

In the context of this definition, assistive technology has been a part of occupational therapy since its beginning. Many assistive devices still recommended today may have been developed through early problem-solving techniques of the reconstruction aides during the early 1900s. Perhaps when a person needed something to hang onto when rising from a seated position, a pipe was placed at a convenient height. Thus the grab bar was born. When a client was unable to move from a chair to the toilet, a piece of scrap lumber was sanded. Thus the transfer board became a reality. When a patient could not button a shirt, a button hook used to button shoes was adapted to meet dressing needs.

Today thousands of products can be considered assistive devices. McCuaig and Frank (1991) identify those items that are commercially available and could be considered adaptive because of specific characteristics and application as "transparent" equipment. Examples include lightweight kettles, typewriters with well-spaced keys, felt-tip pens, and slip-on shoes.

An assistive device is any product that makes performing daily tasks or leisure activities easier. A vegetable peeler is easier for most people to use than a knife—thus the peeler could be considered an assistive device. When that peeler has a large, easy-to-grip handle, we may consider it a device for a person with a disability. However, when that large grip handle is designed and marketed as "easy for everyone to hold onto and easy for everyone to use," (Good Grips, 1993) the design takes on a universal appeal.

UNIVERSAL AND TRANSGENERATIONAL DESIGN

Both terms focus on suitability with aesthetic appeal, service, and accommodation. Universal design means providing good design for all people by incorporating knowledge about the ranges of abilities of all people into the design (Universal Design Initiative, 1993). It does not mean every product should accommodate every person regardless of age or physical capability. "Transgenerational design is the practice of making products and environments compatible with those physical and sensory impairments associated with human aging, which limit major life activities" (Pirkl, 1994). "Transgenerational design extends the traditional boundaries of 'barrier-free accessibility' to embrace the various functional limitations we may acquire as we grow older" (Pirkl, 1994).

CONSUMERS' PERSPECTIVES

Whether assistive technology is used is ultimately the consumer's decision. A determiner will be the consumer's understanding of the extent of the disability, including the prognosis for the particular problem. Solutions will be quite different if the problem is a rapidly deteriorating neurological condition, a temporary difficulty such as a hip fracture, or more permanent disability where an individual has reached a plateau.

A study of 86 older people with impairments revealed that the activities they most missed doing were not the traditional self-care but rather leisure activities (Mann & Lane, 1995). We must look at consumers' needs from their perspectives.

Understanding the Options

Does the person understand the wide variety of options available? If devices are not being used by older people with disabilities, it is often because they are unaware that devices exist to compensate for a problem.

A study conducted in Minnesota concerning older people's familiarity with technology showed a high level of awareness and positive attitudes toward technology. Throughout the state, 101 older people participated in focus groups. The guided discussions centered on the older person's awareness, attitudes, and needs for technological interventions. Among older Minnesotans, technological innovation was both welcome and needed (Minnesota Gerontology Society, 1989).

In another study, it was found that, when a group of older people were asked about devices that would be helpful and that they would like to have manufactured, all of the suggested products already existed (Mann & Lane, 1995). The University of Buffalo has established Project Link to help people learn about assistive devices. Project Link can be reached at 1-800-628-2281.

Cost as an Issue

Often the professional assumes no resources exist to purchase the needed items, so none are recommended. This lack may not be the case. Clients need variously priced options so that they can decide what they wish to purchase.

A National Health Interview Survey performed in 1990 revealed that about one-half of the assistive devices and more than three-fourths of the accessible modifications to homes had been paid for by clients or their families without contributions from third-party payers (Enders, 1995).

Some states have loan programs that may provide needed funds (Wilner, 1995). Some simple low- or no-cost solutions can be tried first. The simpler solution may solve the problem, or the individual may see that investing in a device of a more permanent nature

would allow him or her to do the task even more easily.

FINDING SOLUTIONS

Home Environment Checklists

Numerous home environment checklists have been developed to determine client needs. Some are designed to be self-administered. The occupational therapy practitioner can gain insight from these self-administered reports but will no doubt be more interested in those that are designed to be administered by the professional. (A listing of some of these checklists is provided at the end of this chapter.)

HyperHome Resource

HyperHome Resource is a computerized management tool that helps home modification service providers handle diverse technical information on environmental design ideas and products. HyperHome Resource can provide clients with illustrations of home modifications (Mann & Lane, 1995).

EASE2000

It is virtually impossible for occupational therapy practitioners to be aware of all the assistive devices that are available (Christenson, 1995). EASE2000 Software was developed by Lifease, Inc., to provide ready access to the wide array of devices and ideas that are possible to compensate for problems of people and to help them live at home more safely and independently. EASE2000 is a computerized assessment that guides the evaluation of the functional demands of the environment for a specific client and identifies appropriate solutions where needed.

In EASE2000, the functional abilities of the person are compared with the functional requirements of the home. For each defined problem, the software retrieves optional solutions: products, adaptation recommendations, and services. Together, the therapist and client choose product solutions. EASE2000 then documents the selections, including information such as price, supplier's order phone, and catalog number. Ideas that are already in the database may be retrieved, or the practitioner may add his or her own ideas. Local services and individual therapist's ideas may be entered. If additional products or ideas are desired, these may be found by using the search function. The selected recommendation paragraphs are printed and may be edited by the user.

A Taxonomy of Generic Names

Manufacturers often describe a product with their own "catchy" titles. Little thought may be given as to whether the name actually describes the product. Many products may be designed to serve the same basic purposes, for example, reachers, grab bars, and magnifiers, but these may be called by different names. Lifease, Inc., has developed a taxonomy or nomenclature of generic names that will guide practitioners to identify more quickly the product(s) desired. The generic names provide a cascading selection system. The first term is the most general, and then two or three subsequent terms are more specific about the product.

Because some items may still be difficult to understand from just reading a description, 400 of the generic names have been illustrated. The illustrations as well as the complete taxonomy of names have been developed into *The Pictorial Dictionary of Assistive Technology*. AOTA is scheduled to publish this book in 1997.

Local Sources

An occupational therapy practitioner may use a variety of methods to find the right product for a client. The practitioner may order products from specific durable medical goods companies. Additional solutions may be available in local optometry, hardware, or specialty stores.

Catalogs

Catalogs of assistive technology distributors offer products for a variety of deficits. Certain companies concentrate on one area of concern, such as vision or hearing.

Computer Databases

For a specific product, the practitioner might go to a database such as ABLEDATA, which describes products and sources for the items. This database is available on RELIABLE SOURCE. Specific products can be identified using EASE2000 as well. Products are beginning to appear on the Internet and CD-ROM.

Summary

Occupational therapy training and practice provides knowledge to understand interactions between a user's daily activities and environments that may create barriers. This insight places the occupational therapy practitioner in the unique position of being able to work with other professionals to recommend environmental adaptations for older people regardless of the client's problem(s). The occupational therapy practitioner can and must become involved in helping create environmental quality for older persons.

Activities

1. Follow the instructions on the Environmental Checklist in the Appendix.

2. At a local hardware store, find at least twenty products that fit the description of "transparent" equipment as it has been described in this text.

3. In homes, apartments, senior housing, assisted living, or long-term-care facilities, find twenty examples of good and bad adaptations for age-related sensory and physical changes. Document these situations with photos or drawings and explain why you selected this situation. Only five of the examples should be outdoors.

Case Studies

CASE STUDY 1

Mrs. D is a 90-year-old woman who lives in an assisted living facility (ALF). She has been living in this facility for 2 years. Because of an increase in her rent, she moved from a previous ALF where she had been for 3 years. She took the initiative to find the second ALF. Before living in the ALFs, she had shared a townhouse with her daughter, who has a professional occupation. Mrs. D was a clerk in a retail store but retired 25 years ago. She enjoyed gardening on the deck of the townhouse and entertaining friends, particularly for afternoon coffee.

Her change in living settings occurred after a hospitalization due to coronary heart disease. She and her family decided it would be better for her to have more supervision during the day, so she moved into the ALF. She also has osteoarthritis, which affects her mobility.

Her daughter lives nearby and gives her showers and sets up her medications. Other family members share with caregiving.

An aide helps her get up and get dressed each morning. She uses a wheelchair to move about the facility. When necessary, she is wheeled to the dining room for meals.

The apartment consists of a living room, bedroom, kitchen, and bathroom. The bathroom has a roll-in shower. The living room and bedroom have windows facing south.

Physical adaptations were made to her apartment to make it easier for her and her daughter to perform tasks. A bath chair and hand-held shower were put in the bathroom. Additional strip task lighting was placed in the kitchen. Lamps were converted to touch lamps, and a vertical pole was placed by the chair in the living room to aid in her sitting and rising. A large button control for her television replaced one with small numbers.

She continues with some of her previous roles. She has plants by both her bedroom and living room windows. She has friends in for coffee on a regular basis.

CASE STUDY 2

Mrs. V is an 82-year-old woman who lives alone in the home she has lived in for 55 years. Her husband died 10 years ago after a stroke. She cared for him at home for 2 years before his death. She has osteoarthritis and has difficulty hearing.

Three years ago, following a flair-up of her arthritis, she began verbalizing concerns about her ability to continue to live independently in her home. Her family requested an EASE home assessment be performed.

Using the EASE report, the family made the necessary changes, including the following: touch lamps in the living room and bedroom, a light-activated doorbell at the front and back doors, grab bars and a hand-held shower in the bathroom, a bath chair in the tub, marking of the chair legs so they contrast with the carpet in the dining room, new lighting in the bathroom, installation of a cupboard organizer in the kitchen, placement of handrails on both sides of the stairs between the attic and the main level and on both sides of the front steps, and placement of a handrail on the wall from the garage to the backdoor.

After these modifications were made, Mrs. V was encouraged to see her physician, who placed her on anti-inflammatory medication for her arthritis. Mrs. V realized she did not need supportive housing at this time and now states that she wishes to remain active in her home as long as possible.

Appendix A.
Environmental Checklist Exercise

In the following locations, observe the various elements in that space and consider whether the environment compensates for age-related changes.

HALLWAY

Floor Surface
- Floor treatment has a resistant surface of high pile.
- Floor treatment has a surface of low pile.
- Floor treatment is similar to a throw rug on a waxed surface.
- Floor treatment is a nonslip unwaxed surface.
- The floor surface has no reflected glare.

Wall Surface
- Wall treatment has no reflected glare.
- Cove base is the same color as wall.
- Handrails are available.
- Handrails contrast in color with the wall.
- A window is at the end of the corridor.

Lighting
- No direct glare from the sun is created through a window at the end of the corridor.
- Ceiling light does not create a direct glare.
- Fluorescent bulbs have a warm white, rather than a cool white, tone.
- Fluorescent lighting does not hum.
- No burned-out light bulbs are present.

Doors
- Door handles are lever type.
- Width of door permits passage of wheelchair or walker.

Acoustical Treatment
- Ceiling has acoustical tile.

LOUNGE

Floor Surface
- Floor treatment has a resistant surface of high pile.
- Floor treatment has a surface of low pile.

- Floor treatment is similar to a throw rug on a waxed surface.
- The floor surface has no reflected glare.

Lighting
- Ceiling light does not create a direct glare.
- Fluorescent bulbs have a warm white, rather than a cool white, tone.
- Fluorescent lighting does not hum.
- No burned-out light bulbs are present.
- There are light sources other than in the ceiling to prevent corners and furnishings from falling into shadows.
- Lights can be switched on from two or more places.
- Localized light exists for special tasks.
- A lamp near a chair encourages reading and hand work.
- Reading lamps have incandescent bulbs that do not create direct glare.

Windows
- Windows have been designed to eliminate glare (e.g., wide eaves, elongated roof, slope of windows).
- Window treatment that eliminates glare has been installed (e.g., vertical blinds, mini-blinds, glare-reducing film, shades, sheers, draperies).
- Window sills are at a height that permits looking outside while seated, approximately 2'6" from the floor.

Door
- Door handles are lever type.
- No objects are on floor by door that could cause someone to trip and fall.
- Width of door permits the passage of a wheelchair or walker.

Furniture
- Furniture is arranged to provide a clear traffic path.
- Furniture has no sharp edges.
- Coffee table edge contrasts in color with floor covering.
- Lock-casters are on heavy, hard-to-move furniture.
- Chairs provide good support to the neck and back.
- Chairs provide a handhold to allow ease in sitting and rising.
- Chairs, tables, and storage units (e.g., bookcases, desks) are sturdy enough to function as a support when a person is walking.

Acoustical Treatment
- Ceiling has acoustical tile.

BATHROOM

Lighting
- Light over mirror is approximately 150 watts.
- Direct glare from lighting is reduced with the use of globe or lenses over bulbs.
- Fluorescent bulbs have a warm white, rather than a cool white, tone.
- Fluorescent lighting does not hum.
- No burned-out light bulbs are present.
- Electrical switches are from 3' to 4'8" above the floor.
- Bathroom light switch is located directly inside the door.
- Switches are rocker type.

Floor Surface
- Floor surface provides stability when wet.
- The floor surface has no reflected glare.
- Carpet or vinyl floor material does not curl at the edges.
- Resilient flooring is waxed with a low shine, slip-resistant wax.

Wall Surface
- Wall treatment has no reflected glare.
- Cove base is the same color as the wall.

Door
- Pressure to open the door is approximately 5 pounds.
- Bathroom door opens outward.
- Door handles are lever type.
- No objects are on the floor by the door that could cause someone to trip and fall.
- Width of door permits the passage of a wheelchair or walker.

Acoustical Treatment
- Ceiling has acoustical tile.

Toilet
- Stool is at height that allows ease in sitting and rising.
- Grab bars are located in a position to facilitate sitting and rising.

Mirror
- A full-length or large counter mirror is located so that glare does not reflect.

Sink
- Red markings are on hot water faucets.
- A liquid soap dispenser is present.

- Towel dispenser or hand dryer is easily accessible by a person in a wheelchair.
- Sink can be reached by a person in wheelchair.
- Sink controls are easy to manipulate by someone having difficulty with grasp.

ENTRY

Door
- Pressure to open the door is approximately 5 pounds.
- Door opens outward.
- Door handles are lever or bar type.
- No objects are on the floor just inside the door that could cause someone to trip and fall.
- Width of door permits passage of wheelchair or walker.
- Glass doors have decals or other indication that this is not an open space.

Sidewalk
- The sidewalk has surface that would provide stability when icy or wet.
- Area is well-lighted.

Curb
- Curb edges are marked.
- Curb cuts are of different material or well-marked.

Ramp
- Ramp is at a scale of at least 1:20.

Steps
- Step edges are well-marked.
- Stable railings are along both sides of steps.

DINING ROOM OR RESTAURANT

Floor Surface
- Floor treatment has a resistant surface of high pile.
- Floor treatment has a surface of low pile.
- Floor treatment is a nonslip unwaxed surface.
- The floor surface has no reflected glare.

Lighting
- Ceiling light does not create a direct glare.
- Fluorescent bulbs have a warm white, rather than a cool white, tone.
- Fluorescent lighting does not hum.

- No burned out light bulbs are present.
- A light source is directly over table or booth.

Windows
- Windows have been designed to eliminate glare (e.g., wide eaves, elongated roof, slope of windows).
- Window treatment has been installed that eliminates glare (e.g., vertical blinds, mini-blinds, glare reducing film, shades, sheers, drapery).
- Window sills are at a height that permits looking outside while seated, approximately 2'6" from the floor.

Door
- Door handles are lever type.
- No objects are on floor by door that could cause someone to trip and fall.
- Width of door permits the passage of a wheelchair or walker.

Tables
- Tables are arranged to provide a clear traffic path.
- Tables have no sharp edges.
- Tables are sturdy enough to function as a support when a person is sitting or rising.

Chairs
- Chairs provide good support to the back.
- Chairs provide a handhold to allow ease in sitting and rising.
- Chairs are sturdy enough to function as a support when a person is walking.

Booths
- Booths provide good support to the back.
- Seat surfaces of booths have a finish upon which it is easy to slide.

Acoustical Treatment
- Ceiling has acoustical tile.

References

American Association of Retired Persons. (1990). *Understanding senior housing: For the 1990s*. Washington, DC: Author.

American Institute of Architects. (1985). *Design for aging: An architect's guide*. Washington, DC: AIA Press.

Architectural and Transportation Barriers Compliance Board. (1984). *Uniform federal accessibility standards*. Washington, DC: Author.

Aranyi, L., & Goldman, L. (1980). *Design of long-term care facilities*. New York: Van Nostrand Rheinhold.

Branson, G. D. (1991). *The complete guide to barrier-free housing: Convenient living for the elderly and the physically handicapped*. White Hall, VA: Betterway Publications.

Calkins, M. P. (1988). *Design for dementia: Planning environments for the elderly and the confused*. Owings Mills, MD: National Health Publishing.

Canada Mortgage and Housing Corporation. (1990). *At home with Alzheimer's disease: Useful adaptations to the home environment*. Ottawa: Author.

Chalke, H., & Dewhurst, J. (1957). Coal gas poisoning: Loss of sense of smell as a possible contributing factor with old people. *British Medical Journal, 2,* 1915–1917.

Christenson, M. A. (1995). Assessing an elder's need for assistance: One technological tool. *Generations, 19*(1), 54–55.

Christenson, M. A. (1990). *Aging in the designed environment*. Binghamton, NY: The Haworth Press.

Christenson, M. A., & Raschko, B. B. (1989). Environmental cognition and age-related sensory change. *Occupational Therapy Practice, 1*(1), 28–35.

Cohen, U., & Day, K. (1993). *Contemporary environments for people with dementia*. Baltimore: The Johns Hopkins University Press.

Cohen, U., & Weisman, G. D. (1991). *Holding on to home: Designing environments for people with dementia*. Baltimore: The Johns Hopkins University Press.

Edelstein, S. (1994). *Fair housing laws and frail older tenants*. Los Angeles: National Eldercare Institute on Housing and Supportive Services.

Enders, A. (1995). The role of technology in the lives of older people. *Generations, 19*(1), 7–12.

Good Grips. (1993). *Kitchen utensil packaging*. Terre Haute, IN: OXO International.

Hall, G., Kirschling, M., & Todd, S. (1986). Sheltered freedom: An Alzheimer's unit in ICF. *Geriatric Nursing,* 132–137.

Hasselkus, B. (1974). Aging and the human nervous system. *American Journal of Occupational Therapy, 28*(1), 16–21.

Hellen, C. R. (1992). *Alzheimer's disease: Activity-focused care*. Boston: Andover Medical Publishers.

Hiatt, L. G. (1985). Understanding the physical environment. *Pride Institute Journal of Long Term Care, 4*(2), 12–22.

Hiatt, L. G. (1979, November/December). Architecture for the aged: Design for living. *Inland Architect,* 6–18, 41–42.

Johnson, P. M. (1993). *Creation of the barrier-free interior*. Millville, NJ: A Positive Approach.

Kiernat, J. (1982). Environment: The hidden modality. *Physical and Occupational Therapy in Geriatrics, 2*(1), 3–12.

Kolonowski, A. M. (1992). The clinical importance of environmental lighting in the elderly. *Journal of Gerontology Nursing, 18*(1), 10–14.

Koncelik, J. A. (1976). *Designing the open nursing home.* Stroudsburg, PA: Dowden, Hutchinson, and Ross.

Leibrock, C. (1993). *Beautiful barrier-free: A visual guide to accessibility.* New York: Van Nostrand Reinhold.

Mann, W. C., & Lane, J. P. (1995). *Assistive technology for persons with disabilities.* Bethesda, MD: American Occupational Therapy Association.

McCuaig, M., & Frank, G. (1991). The able self: Adaptive patterns and choices in independent living for a person with cerebral palsy. *American Journal of Occupational Therapy, 45*(3), 224–234.

Millard, P. H., & Smith, C. S. (1981). Personal belongings—A positive effect? *Gerontologist, 21*(1), 85–90.

Minnesota Gerontology Society. (1989). *Technology and aging in Minnesota.* St. Paul, MN: Author.

Perry, L. G., Jawer, M. A., Murdoch, J. R., & Dinegar, J. C. (1991). *BOMA International's ADA compliance guidebook: A checklist for your building.* Washington, DC: Building Owners and Managers Association International.

Phillips, A. H., & Roman, C. K. (1984). *A practical guide to independent living for older people.* Seattle, WA: Pacific Search Press.

Pirkl, J. J. (1994). *Transgenerational design: Products for an aging population.* New York: Van Nostrand Reinhold.

Raschko, B. B. (1982). *Housing interiors for the disabled and elderly.* New York: Van Nostrand Reinhold.

Regnier, V., Hamilton, J., & Yatabe, S. (1991). *Best practices in assisted living: Innovations in design, management and financing.* Los Angeles: Long Term Care National Resource Center at the University of California at Los Angeles and the University of Southern California.

Reznikoff, S. C. (1979). *Specifications for commercial interiors.* New York: Whitney Library of Design, Watson-Guptill Publications.

Schafer, S. C. (1985) Modifying the environment. *Geriatric Nursing, 6*(3), 157–159.

Sjorgen, H., & Bjornstig, U. (1991). Injuries among the elderly in the environment. *Journal of Aging and Health, 3*(1), 107–125.

Snyder, L. H. (1978). Environmental changes for socialization. *Journal of Nursing Administration, 8*(1), 44–50.

Technology-Related Assistance of Individuals with Disabilities Act, Pub. No. 100–407. (1988).

Universal Design Initiative. (1993). *Toward universal design* (videotape). Washington, DC: Author.

Ware, C. (1993). *Design for aging: Strategies for collaboration between architects and occupational therapists.* Washington, DC: AIA Press.

Wilmott, M. (1986). The effect of vinyl floor surface and carpeted floor surface upon walking in elderly hospital in-patients. *Age and Aging, 15,* 119–120.

Wilner, M. A. (1995). *Fix it!: A report from the First National Conference on Home Modifications Policy.* Raleigh, NC: Center for Accessible Housing.

Windley, P., & Scheidt, R. (1980). Person-environment dialectics: Implications for competent functioning in old age. In L. Poon (Ed.), *Aging in the 1980's.* Washington, DC: American Psychological Association.

Wylde, M., Baron-Robbins, A., & Clark, S. (1994). *Building for a lifetime: The design and construction of fully accessible homes.* Newton, CT: The Taunton Press.

Home Environment Checklist References

American Association of Retired Persons, Consumer Affairs Section. (1992). *The perfect fit: Creative ideas for a safe and livable home.* Washington, DC: Author.

American Association of Retired Persons, Consumer Affairs Section. (1991). *The doable renewable home.* Washington, DC: Author.

American Occupational Therapy Association. (1995). *Growing older in your home: Bathroom modifications for your changing needs.* Bethesda, MD: Author.

American Occupational Therapy Association. (1995). *Growing older in your home: Bedroom modifications for your changing needs.* Bethesda, MD: Author.

American Occupational Therapy Association. (1995). *Growing older in your home: Kitchen modifications for your changing needs.* Bethesda, MD: Author.

Canada Mortgage and Housing Corporation. (1989). *Maintaining seniors' independence: A guide to home adaptions.* Ottawa: Author.

Consumer Care Products/Consulting, Inc. (1985). *Independent living appraisal.* Sheboygan, WI: Author.

Information and Advisory Services Section of the City of Toronto Housing Department. (1991). *Your safe-home checklist: Your guide to safety in your home.* Toronto: City of Toronto Housing Department.

National Association of Home Builders Research Center. (1994). *Retrofitting homes for a lifetime.* Upper Marlboro, MD: Author.

Pynoos, J., Cohen, E., Lucas, C., & Davis, L. (1985). *Home evaluation checklist for the elderly.* Los Angeles: Long Term Care Gerontology Center and the University of California at Los Angeles and the University of Southern California.

Rabizadeh, M. (1982). *Housing for the elderly: A self-help guide.* Eugene, OR: University of Oregon Books.

U.S. Consumer Product Safety Commission. (1985). *Home safety checklist for older consumers.* Washington, DC: U.S. Government Printing Office.

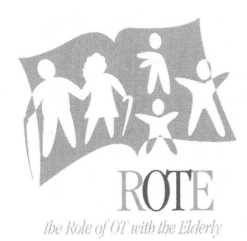

Consultation Amplifies the Impact of Occupational Therapy in the Community

Author block
Anne Long Morris, EdD, OTR
Phyllis Bauer Madachy, MHA
Chris Cawley, OTR

Impact of Change

HEALTH CARE DELIVERY

Dramatic changes are under way in the health care delivery system in the United States regarding the depth and duration of interventions available for older persons. Occupational therapy (OT) practitioners describe their concern regarding the impact of cost-cutting efforts on the quality of services delivery as they struggle to find the most ethical solution to implementing a managed care approach. Practitioners indicate feelings of stress as they strive to provide appropriate services for increased numbers of clients in less time. Concomitantly, reimbursement mechanisms have been modified, and the locus of service delivery has shifted from the institutional facility to diverse community settings (AOTA, 1995a).

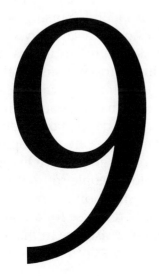

DEMOGRAPHIC SHIFTS

Demographic changes in the age 60-plus population are having a profound impact on the interaction of occupational therapy practitioners and supportive services in the community. America is growing grayer. The fastest growing age segment in America is in the population over age 75. The significance for OT practitioners and community-based aging specialists is that this age group is more likely to have functional impairments caused by disease or chronic age-related conditions. These functional deficits create difficulties in both physical and instrumental activities of daily living (ADL), affecting the independent living ability of many older people.

ACTIVITY LIMITATIONS

According to data from the National Medical Expenditure Survey of the Department of Health and Human Services, "… approximately 21% of older persons (age 65 and above) in the population had at least some Activity of Daily Living, Instrumental Activity of Daily Living, or walking difficulty" (Leon & Lair, 1990).

Elders living in the community are frequently identified as being dependent on family caregivers. In the U.S. Health Care Financing Administration's 1982 Long-Term-Care Survey, informal (nonpaid) caregivers represented 84% of all caregivers for older disabled men, and 79% for older women (U.S. Senate Special Committee on Aging, American Association of Retired Persons, Federal Council on the Aging, & U.S. Administration on Aging, 1991).

Older people consume health services at a higher rate than the younger population. "On the average, people 65+ visit a physician eight times a year, compared with five visits by the general population. They are hospitalized over three times as often as the younger population, stay 50 percent longer, and use twice as many prescription drugs" (U.S. Senate Special Committee on Aging et al., 1991).

Although older people consume health services at a higher rate than other segments of the population (U.S. Senate Special Committee on Aging et al., 1991), only 5% of the population over 60 years of age is receiving institutional services at any one time. The remaining 95% of older people are living in the community, with the level of functional impairment noted above. For older people in the community receiving services through a home health agency, from an outpatient department of a hospital, or from a freestanding outpatient rehabilitation facility, OT practitioners are a valuable resource. They help people with functional impairments compensate for functional deficits through direct treatment, task analysis, provision of and training about assistive technology, recommendations about environmental modification, and other activities.

However, many more people are not touched by the medical model or may continue to have difficulties in independent living after the standard reimbursement for OT services has ended. Even for older people receiving services in an institutional setting, the length of time for OT intervention following the implementation of prospective payment systems is limited. Hospitals are under increasing pressure to discharge patients quickly, limiting the time available for intervention in the facility. Nursing homes are being pressured to carefully screen incoming residents to ensure that the need for skilled care (not simply the need for supervision or personal care assistance) is the basis for admission for residents who depend on public funding. Many states are developing community-based alternative living options for older people so that medical model nursing homes are no longer the only recourse for an older person needing assistance in maintaining routine tasks of daily living.

CAREGIVER EDUCATION INCREASINGLY IMPORTANT

Elders living in the community are frequently identified as being dependent on family caregivers. In the U.S. Health Care Financing Administration's 1982 Long-Term Care Survey, informal (nonpaid) caregivers represented 84% of all caregivers for older disabled men and 79% for older women (U.S. Senate Special Committee on Aging et al., 1991).

Cynthia Epstein, MS, OTR, Director, OT Consultants, Inc., New Jersey, emphasized in her chapter "Long-term care," in the text *Willard and Spackman's Occupational Therapy,* that long-term care affects family ties and caregiving; places demands on personal and family resources; requires expanded medical, therapeutic, and social service interventions; and mandates options that help people live in the least restrictive home environment (Epstein, 1993).

Occupational therapy practitioners involved with community services delivery increasingly recognize the need to identify new client, caregiver, and family education strategies that will continue to facilitate the ease of caregiving, yet enable the caretaker to maintain his or her own well-being. When this is achieved, the burdens of caregiving can be minimized, and the staff or the family member can sustain the responsibilities more successfully and for longer periods of time (Levine, Corcoran, & Gitlin, 1993).

HEIGHTEN AWARENESS OF SUCCESSFUL AGING STRATEGIES

Although a proliferation of new technologies have increased a person's average life span, similar advances in the management of chronic health conditions that elders typically experience have not been made. Occupational therapy practitioners engaged in community geriatric rehabilitation through home health services delivery regularly use the environment to promote optimal function in those with chronic disabilities. These practitioners regularly use consultative techniques when working with clients, family members, and other community aging services providers. Practitioners typically facilitate appropriate assistive device selection for clients, instruct them in how to use these devices, and reinforce their continued use. This clinical reasoning process of issuing assistive devices relies on a "… complex series of decisions and skilled clinical judgements" (Levine, Corcoran, & Gitlin, 1993).

Clearly, practitioners must become ever more mindful of the increased potential that new developments in assistive technology product design could hold for older adults and persons with disabilities. It is important to note that among the 18,000 products described in the HYPERABLE computerized database, few were originally designed with the complex needs of older persons in mind. In a recent qualitative research study, a phenomenological inquiry drew co-researchers from a purposefully selected sample at a local senior center. These older women identified specific improvements needed in the basic design of some assistive technology products. Practitioners recognize the need for improved occupational therapy technology assessment tools that can better discern performance improvement as individuals learn to use assistive technology or modify their home and community work environments (Morris, 1995). Longitudinal outcomes research studies in these areas can aid in determining which component of a technology system or feature of an assistive technology device better improves task performance.

Occupational therapy interventions regularly incorporate environmental interventions, such as recommendations to older adults about home modification, as a strategy to facilitate ease of task performance. This information can be critically significant to people aging with disabilities, as well as for the increasing numbers of older adults who are experiencing sensory loss and concomitant activity limitations but who strongly prefer to remain in their current living arrangement. Practitioners can identify new avenues and new audiences with whom to share proven rehabilitation strategies that have been shown to facilitate continued activity by the older adult. A successful proposal led to a funding award from the Retirement Research Foundation to the American Occupational Therapy Foundation. The writer, in collaboration with architects at the Center for Universal Design, has developed a consumer education video and printed materials intended to heighten the awareness of home modification as a strategy for aging more successfully (Morris, Connell, Sanford, & Kolm, 1996). Occupational therapy practitioners can better provide community education that facilitates increased independence at home for older adults. This same information can assist those who provide informal support to their aging parents, thereby reducing caregiver burden as well.

AGING AS A GLOBAL PHENOMENON

The graying phenomenon will continue to pervade the global scene as the numbers in aging populations escalate dramatically. Critically needed are occupational therapy interventions that enable older people to live pro-

ductively and meaningfully in the community as long as possible. Ethnically and culturally diverse elder populations, significantly represented in the changing demography, create challenges in the need for developing culturally sensitive screening and assessment tools (Price & Fitz, 1990). Practitioners need to facilitate delivery of services that maximize an aging person's autonomy and minimize family and social burden (Morris, 1995).

Canadian and American OT practitioners explored challenges in the changing economic climate for their health care delivery systems in joint sessions at the 1993 Canadian-American (CANAM) Conference held in Boston, Massachusetts. Stanton wrote that historically, practitioners may have limited their scope by relying on funding that led to services delivery within the medical setting (Stanton, 1995). Stanton proposed that therapists view this pervasive challenge as an opportunity: One must search for expanding funding opportunities despite shrinking budgets. The international rehabilitation literature further supports positive outcomes as seen through the application of OT practitioners' skills in environmental interventions. The issue of growing concern appears to be, "How can the occupational therapy practitioner identify new settings where these same skills will be sought after to facilitate more successful aging in place within the rapidly escalating numbers of elderly persons?"

Fortunately, occupational therapists are now providing valued consultation for a diverse array of community-based programs, the growing number of aging services' providers, and the rapidly escalating numbers of older adult consumers. The publication *Design for Aging: Strategies for Collaboration Between Architects and Occupa-*

tional Therapists (Aging Design Research Program, 1993) described consultation by therapists for architects in the United States and Canada. Individual case studies demonstrated occupational therapists' roles in the design of an assisted living facility (Roseville, Minnesota), in the interior design for renovation of the psychiatric ward of a geriatric teaching hospital (Ontario, Canada), and in the retrofitting of an urban row house for elderly residents (Baltimore, Maryland).

In the article, "Occupational Therapy in the 21st Century: An Outsider's View," Bruhn (1991), a medical sociologist, commented that, "… professions are initiators of change as well as products of its effects." He believes that OT practitioners may not endure the impact of societal change; instead, they may prefer to seize the opportunity to shape the future by directing social change. Issues of significance that he noted as needing change included ongoing OT personnel shortages; methods of coping with the changing boundaries of the profession; and an in-depth clarification of practitioner roles, such as evaluator, supervisor, researcher, and consultant.

In another article, "New Landscape, New Models, New Roles," (Hettinger, 1995) a clinical psychologist and faculty member at the Texas Women's University's OT program, encouraged practitioners to adopt a proactive stance and to broaden their role perspectives. Opportunities beckon in multiple settings where a consultative model (i.e., a social services model) is used instead of a medical model. Hettinger's consultant's role addresses issues related to the Americans with Disabilities Act (ADA). Recognizing that OT interventions strive to improve accessibility, Hettinger suggests that the OT practitioner should consult more with architects and builders. She believes that it is important that practitioners increase their knowledge base about business aspects of health care. Hettinger stresses the critical need for education of the managed care entities, or third-party payers, and consumers about the dramatic benefits of OT services.

NEED TO EXPAND OCCUPATIONAL THERAPY SERVICES

The challenge is that the settings in which OT services are currently delivered need to be expanded beyond the traditional medical model and integrated into the community network of supportive services. In the same way that OT practitioners are currently an integral part of a health team with other medical support personnel, they must now begin to see themselves as part of the community team in settings such as social service agencies, housing organizations, senior centers, home repair programs, and other community-based efforts. Meeting this challenge will require innovation, creativity, and the willingness to identify and form consulting relationships with community-based organizations and specialists in aging.

Understanding the Network of Community Aging Services

Occupational therapy consultation with community-based programs is full of promise and challenge. The promise is created by the fact that increasing numbers of older adults are living longer, and options are expanding for these adults to remain in their communities. Therefore, OT practitioners face increased employment and consultation opportunities to the extent that they can learn about the community-based long-term-care networks that exist outside the medical model. It is the latter task—that of learning about the community-based long-term care network—that constitutes the challenge.

The older adult interacts with as many diverse organizations in the community as does any adult, depending on the needs of the individual. With that as a premise, the breadth of the aging service community can be more readily understood. Just as health services can be found in a variety of settings provided by a range of professionals, aging services also come in a wide array of programs, forming a network in the community.

Because the structure of aging services is national to some extent, and adults with disabilities often require the same services regardless of where they live, similar services can be found in many communities. However, the OT practitioner should be aware that the titles of services may vary, urban and rural service delivery systems vary, and the way in which programs interact with each other in the network may differ. It also cannot be assumed that specific services in one community (or state) will exist in another, or that similar services will exist to the same extent.

KEY PLAYERS IN THE AGING SERVICES NETWORK

Where in the community would an OT practitioner start to explore consultation or employment opportunities outside the traditional medical facility or beyond home health agencies? Aging services can be provided by both formal sources (agencies, organizations, or individuals providing services for payment) and informal sources (spouses and other family members, church groups, neighbors, friends). Although it is important to recognize the formal sources within a community, it is equally important to note that approximately 80% of the care provided to older disabled adults is provided by the informal network of family and friends (U.S. Senate Special Committee on Aging et al., 1991). This involvement of informal providers (also called caregivers) means that OT practitioners should view the caregiver community as an equally appropriate recipient of OT education as the older adult. Sometimes the older disabled adult is also a caregiver, so the two audiences overlap.

The best starting point is with the public aging network. Although it is only one of the players in the formal community-based service network, the aging network can identify other key organizations in the community for interested occupational therapists.

OLDER AMERICANS ACT (P.L. 102–375)

In aging services, a federally authorized network was established in 1965 by Congress as part of the Older Americans Act (OAA). This act is up for reauthorization at the end of 1995. By creating a national network of federal, state, and local agencies, OAA ensures that organized planning and services will exist to meet the needs of persons age 60 and above. The Declaration of Objectives for Older Americans includes the pledge to provide "Full restorative services for those who require institutional care, and a comprehensive array of community-based, long-term-care services adequate to appropriately sustain older people in their communities and in their homes, including support to family members and other persons providing voluntary care to older individuals needing long-term care services" (Compilation of the Older Americans Act of 1965 and the Native American Programs Act of 1974, 1993).

ADMINISTRATION ON AGING (AOA)

The Department of Health and Human Services directs the AOA. Funds from the Older Americans Act are allocated to state units on aging (SUAs) or territories; these units exist as identifiable parts of state governments or as subunits of other state departments. Older Americans Act funds are also channeled to more than 190 Native American tribal organizations for special aging programs. State units add specific state policy to the federal mandates, coordinate activity with related state agencies and institutions, and develop individual state initiatives in areas such as community-based long-term care. Federal and state grants pass through the state units to the local Area Agency on Aging (AAA), which may be part of public government or organized as a private, nonprofit agency. Over 670 AAAs (titled commissions, departments, offices, or similar designations) cover geographic areas that may be a single political jurisdiction or multi-county in scope. Reporting requirements and common goals link all three of these networks.

The AAA is responsible at the community level for carrying out the mandates of the Older Americans Act and administering specific state programs. Most important, an AAA is required to assess the needs of older adults in its service area and to establish plans to develop comprehensive, community-based services to ensure meeting those needs. The AAA can provide services directly if no other vendor exists or can contract with other organizations. AAAs also play a role in local communities to advocate for the needs of older adults, and the organization may be a player with other health and human service agencies to encourage and coordinate services from other parts of the community.

Recent trends promoted by the Administration on Aging should be of particular interest to OT practitioners. Because the aging network is dealing with larger numbers of disabled older adults within the community, some communities are seeking stronger linkages with the community of younger people with disabilities to address the similar issues faced by both groups. In addition, as more people with lifelong disabilities experience longer life spans, they are encountering age-related conditions and are beginning to use community-based aging services in greater numbers. Both networks are reaching out toward each other to explore common areas of interest, advocacy, and need. This is a rich area for OT practitioners who wish to move into community practice. Occupational therapists can provide environmental assessment and modification, education about assistive technology, and training of personal assistants and other support staff in the community. OT practitioners can help both age groups focus on independence.

Because Congress decides the level of funding under the Older Americans Act, there can be changes in federal mandates establishing specific services and funding levels for individual programs. Congressional reauthorization of the Act is how these changes occur. That decision is affected by the same political and fiscal debates that shape the discussion of all publicly funded programs. It is likely that the extent of services publicly funded in the past will be decreased in the future because of the reduction in federal and state funding levels or elimination of selected services. However, at the local level, funding streams often include a variety of sources, and communities may continue at least some level of service in various categories. In addition, the AAA is not the only provider of services for older adults in the community; other organizations involved in aging services will also affect assistance available in any single community.

In addition to the public aging network funded through the Older Americans Act, other federal agencies fund programs targeted to older adults. For instance, the Assistive Technology Related Assistance to Individuals with Disabilities Act (Tech Act) of 1988 and its reauthorization, Tech Act Amendments of 1994, has funded 50 state technical assistance programs (TAPs) for disseminating assistive technology information to the community. Older adults are one of the target populations identified in the amendments to the Tech Act, and in some locales, there are active partnerships among the state units on aging, AAAs, and the state TAPs. In Iowa, for example, the TAP, entitled "small changes, BIG DIFFERENCES," developed outreach efforts by training older adults for peer education about selected low-technology assistive products and environmental modification (Gay, 1995).

The federal and state departments of Housing and Urban Development (HUD) have funded housing in many local communities for older adults with limited income. Because of the length of time this type of housing has been available, many residents have "aged in place" and have acquired age-related disabilities, affecting their ability to live independently. Many communities with senior housing (whether originally funded by HUD or not) provide services like environmental assessment and modification, information on assistive technology, and other efforts to provide a level of supportive housing to residents.

Like federal agencies, state and local governments also have agencies outside of SUAs and AAAs that provide services to older adults. For instance, county governments often have a Department of Recreation and Park Services that may have an active role in providing recreational and leisure activities for the older adult, including persons with disabilities.

State and local health departments in some states provide publicly funded in-home, multidisciplinary evaluations for people who have difficulty maintaining an independent life in the community, especially if they are considering applying to a nursing home. Such services are invaluable for families trying to determine what the community has to offer older disabled adults.

Private, nonprofit organizations play a well-known part in community-based, long-term-care services. Home health agencies are the primary vehicle for skilled care provided in the home: nursing services, physical therapy, occupational therapy, and social work services combine as a team for persons who need medical assistance at home. Nonprofit groups also represent a much broader role in the community as a support to community residents, often filling in the gaps between public services and private resources. Church groups, civic organizations, neighborhood committees, urban foundations, and many more offer a wide range of assistance.

Finally, the community-based aging network has a growing number of providers who operate as private, for-profit entities. Case management, for example, can be purchased from professionals who offer to "manage" the mix of services often needed by older adults in the community. For family members who may be concerned about relatives several states away, private case managers provide useful contact between the client, the service network, and the family. Many services, including a wide range of housing alternatives, are available for purchase in communities. In light of the increasing number of older adults who are looking for ways to remain in the community, private providers will play an important role in ensuring that options are available for persons with the resources to purchase services.

TYPES OF SERVICES IN THE COMMUNITY LONG-TERM-CARE NETWORK

The types of services generally found in the community may be publicly or privately funded (nonprofit and for-profit) and may represent a partnership of agencies. The most useful way of recognizing the types of services that constitute the community-based long-term-care system is to think of the network as a continuum of care. Theoretically, a complete network will range from wellness and prevention activities for the mobile older adult to services delivered to adults who are totally dependent on others for their care. The network also provides assistance to caregivers of the older person as well as to the older client.

The organization of a continuum reflects the fact that some older people may literally move from one type of setting to another to receive needed services (from their own home, to assisted or supportive housing, to a nursing home) or that increasingly intensive services are introduced into the setting itself (services delivered in the home or on site). The continuum also has access services available throughout the span; these services help clients identify and use what they need.

PRACTITIONER USE OF THE NETWORK

The public aging network of services is broad and typically incorporates some of the following services:

- Access services information and referral case management
  —Transportation (may be fixed route or paratransit)
  —Elder abuse prevention or protective services
  —Preadmission services (required by many states before public funding is authorized for nursing home placement)
  —Public or private guardianship
  —Health insurance counseling and advocacy legal counseling
- Community facility services
  —Senior centers and congregate meal sites
  —Wellness promotion
  —Exercise programs
  —Recreational and leisure activities
  —Educational lectures
  —Volunteer opportunities
  —Nutrition education
  —Trips
  —Employment counseling and placement volunteer opportunities
- Adult day care (for persons who need special support to participate in a group program)
  —Medication administration
  —Specialized programming
  —Social work services
  —Family counseling
  —Access to prescribed therapy
- Services delivered in-home
  —Home-delivered meals
  —Home health services
  —Skilled care—personal, chore, and respite (may be publicly

subsidized in communities with specific long-term-care programs)

—Friendly visitor telephone reassurance

—Assistance with or weatherization of homes

—Minor home repair

—Emergency response systems

—Low-income loans for housing renovation

- Services delivered in nursing home facilities

—Skilled health care

—Ombudsman services—protection of residents' rights, advocacy, and complaint resolution between resident or family and nursing home administration; investigation of abuse or neglect; Pets on Wheels; and friendly visiting recreational programs.

Many different agencies and organizations will offer these services, often with different service criteria, costs, and capabilities. Consumers who need services often find the network fragmented and difficult to access. Services providers need to be well grounded in how to use the network so they can advise on and advocate services for the older adult consumer or the family caregivers.

UNTAPPED OPPORTUNITIES IN ELDER HOUSING CONTINUUM

Many communities are beginning to develop residential housing alternatives for older adults who want or need additional support services up to or including skilled medical services traditionally found in a nursing home. These residential options may have different titles from state to state, but they are viable alternatives to older adults who wish to minimize the changes in their lives created by the reduction in self-care capacity. Some

housing options receive public funding to keep them affordable for low-income persons. Other types of housing are paid for by the residents, requiring substantial income and assets.

It is important to become familiar with the licensing requirements imposed by states and local jurisdictions regarding specialized housing. Information and referral services offered by the local AAA are a good place to start to learn what an individual community has to offer. The licensing and monitoring requirements are helpful to understand because they shape the kinds of clients served by the facilities and govern the types of services that can be offered within the residential setting. State and local laws also help protect the community from unlicensed housing providers who may place vulnerable residents at risk of neglect.

Some examples of specialized housing include the following:

- Alternative senior housing—apartment-style facilities that may offer personal care, light chores, congregate meals, and some degree of case management for selected apartment units. Requires moderate degree of independence and often lacks 24-hour supervision.

- Assisted housing—small to large group setting, with 24-hour non-medical supervision, personal care, meals, and medication management. Licensing requirements determine staffing requirements, but generally the staff does not provide skilled medical care as a regular service.

- Foster homes—small, family-style homes.

- Individual assisted units within larger facilities.

- Retirement communities—designed for apartment-style independent living with varying levels of assistance (meals, personal care, chore service) provided on site as needed by the resident. Basic services may be part of the monthly fee, with additional charges for more intensive care.

- Continuing care facilities—designed for independent living with varying levels of assistance, including traditional nursing home care and supervision provided within the facility although not in the individual apartment. Basic services may be part of the monthly fee, with additional charges for more intensive care.

In summary, organizations such as senior centers, area agencies on aging, home repair programs, nutrition sites, day care centers, respite services, retirement communities, and human services departments provide a wide range of support services, including monitoring, consultation, referral, education, and health promotion activities as part of their efforts to support and maintain older adults in their communities. These types of activities offer the OT practitioner multiple opportunities for consultation and direct service.

Working in the Community: New Clients, New Roles, New Strategies

The scope of current occupational therapy activities in community-based social service settings is very broad, and sometimes difficult for new or clinically oriented practitioners to grasp. Additionally, the nature of the client-practitioner relationship, the expectations and outcomes of this relationship, and the cluster of skills required to function effectively in community systems can be very different from that of the traditional medical model.

The nonmedical, advisory nature of the relationship between a human service provider and his or her client has parallel implications for the relationships and roles assumed by the OT practitioner working within a social or human service setting. In a nonmedical, social, or human service system, the client maintains control of and responsibility for the actions and decisions that affect his or her life or work. The OT practitioner functions as a problem identifier, adviser, educator, linker to resources, strategizer, and collaborative problem solver rather than as the expert providing "treatment." This relationship reflects the "consultative" mode of practice common to social service settings.

The term *consultation* can and should be intimidating to those unfamiliar with its dynamics or requirements. In the text *Occupational Therapy Consultation: Theory, Principles, and Practice,* co-authors Evelyn Jaffe, MPH, OTR, FAOTA, and Cynthia Epstein, MA, OTR, FAOTA (1992), offer a comprehensive look at the field of OT consultation. They provide an in-depth presentation of the preparations, processes, pitfalls, and challenges inherent in consultation. In their text, consultation is described as an interactive process designed to help someone solve problems and develop skills needed to work effectively. Jaffe stated:

> ... Study of various theoretical consultation models and levels will help you assess given situations and determine the appropriate approaches you need.... Keys to successful consultation include the ability to diagnose situations accurately and develop, organize and help implement the most appropriate strategies for change (Jaffe, 1992, p. 52).

An understanding of the different models and levels of consultation can provide practitioners with a framework for organizing and defining their activities in the community.

Levels and Models of Consultation

Jaffe and Epstein (1992, pp. 20–43) discussed and outlined nine models for consultation and three levels for consultation (pp. 49–51). It may be easier to understand the relationship between models and levels if the levels are discussed first.

LEVELS OF CONSULTATION

Consultation can occur at three levels: case centered, educational, and program or administrative.

Case-Centered Consultation

OT practitioners have the potential to be employed or hired by an agency or organization to act as a consultant to the agency's or organization's clients, to the client's caregiver, or to the professional working with the client. The primary goal of case-centered consultation is to produce appropriate behavior, physical change, or psychological well-being in the individual (Jaffe, 1992, p. 49).

Educational Consultation

Educational consultation is targeted at the community caregiver, staff, professional, etc. The focus is still client centered, with the goal of improving the functioning, efficiency, and ability of the individual by increasing knowledge, skills, and expertise (Jaffe, 1992, p. 49).

Program or Administrative Consultation

Intervention at this level is targeted to the system or organization that wishes to change. Activities may include program planning, development, reorganization, training, etc. (Jaffe, 1992, p. 51).

MODELS OF CONSULTATION

Jaffe and Epstein (1992, pp. 20–43) describe nine models of consultation:

- Clinical or treatment model
- Collegial or professional model
- Behavioral model: modification of learned behavior
- Educational model: informational approach through seminars, in-service training, and workshops
- Organizational development model: management-focused approach based on organizational structure
- Process management model: focus on the dynamics and processes of the organization
- Program development model: focus on the modifications and development of service models
- Social action model: focus on changing social values and policies to effect change
- Systems model: focus on development of mission, goals, values, and culture of a given system.

The authors, from personal experience, identified three of these models as most likely to be used by new or inexperienced practitioners just entering community-based practice: the clinical or treatment model, the collegial or professional model, and the educational model.

Clinical or Treatment Model

The clinical or treatment model is derived from the traditional medical model for consultation. In this model, the consultant or OT practitioner is considered the expert. The consultee is another professional or person capable of making appropriate decisions.

The consultant may be asked to assist in identifying the problems experienced by the individual receiving services and to recommend a solution or set of strategies to ameliorate those problems. For example, many OT practitioners are called upon to help identify factors contributing to an individual's difficulty in performing a specific daily living task. The consultee, whether it be the individual, the caregiver, or the professional providing services, is to be provided with recommendations for modifications, products, alternative task performance processes, and services that can ameliorate the problem and support the individual's continued safe function and residence in the community. A limiting factor in this type of relationship is the inherent assumption that the consultant possesses specialized technical skills or knowledge that enable only him or her to solve the problem. Additionally the relatively passive and limited nature of the client's participation in this process may bode poorly for the active follow-up with the recommendations made.

Collegial or Professional Model of Consultation

Jaffe (1992, pp. 22–23) defines the collegial or professional model as a peer-centered, joint problem-solving process with the primary goals of brainstorming options and discussing alternative courses of action to assist the consultee in identifying the approach to take to remediate or address the problem. In this model, the problems are identified mutually, and the consultant assists the consultee in identifying and exploring the pros and cons of different alternative courses of action. Jaffe states that professionals respond positively to this type of consultation when seeking to broaden their base of knowledge and skills to solve particular problems, obtain another opinion, and develop, modify, or expand programs.

Personal experience has shown this model can be effective when working with individuals and caregivers. For caregivers and clients, as well as professionals, using this method of consultation enhances the likelihood of positive reactions and follow-through on the options discussed. The use of this method also provides consultees with invaluable practice and experience in using the problem-solving process.

Educational Model

Jaffe (1992, p. 26) describes the educational model as information centered. Integral to this model is the process of analyzing and assessing client needs, conceptualizing issues in terms of deficits in knowledge and skills, and facilitating the provision of information in ways that will broaden the knowledge base of the organization and enhance the ability of its employees to address the issues. The consultee participates in this process as an equal, again enhancing the likelihood of a positive outcome and reaction to the educational effort.

SELECTING A STRATEGY

Many factors should be considered in selecting the strategies that will best meet the client's needs and the practitioner's objectives. In general, practitioners select different models for consultation based on the following:

- The target of their consultation, whether individual, caregiver, professional, team, or organization
- The objectives for the target
- The level at which they are intervening.

Likewise, practitioners select the level at which to intervene based on

- Their target
- The objectives
- The consultation model that they think will best help the target meet its goals.

The two are related. Certain models of consultation fit more appropriately at different levels of consultation and vice versa.

For example, if a consultation was targeted to an individual or to a case, a practitioner would most likely use strategies congruent with the clinical or collegial model. Whereas if the target was a group of employees of an agency providing services to older adults, the collegial or educational models might more likely be used. If the client was the administration of an agency, the educational or program development model of consultation might be used.

When working with community organizations, it is not unusual for a practitioner to be involved in a number of interventions at different levels simultaneously. For example, a practitioner may find him or herself involved in providing direct care to some clients, consulting with the caregivers of others, consulting with individuals or teams of professionals, assessing the need for and guiding the development of staff education, participating in program development activities with the administration, and representing the agency in working as part of a community team in developing communitywide education programs for the public, all at the same time. No matter the client or the level at which a practitioner is working, he or she is always aware of the importance of selecting the strategy that has the greatest positive long-term impact on that particular client's ability to perform desired tasks.

Some examples that illustrate the variety of roles a practitioner might assume when working with community agencies are presented as case studies at the end of this chapter.

Survey of Community-Based OT Practitioners

In November 1995, the authors conducted an informal telephone survey with a number of practitioners working for and with community-based agencies. Their activities further illustrate the wide range of roles assumed by practitioners both in consulting and direct service.

Joyce Deily, OTR

While employed as the director of Meals on Wheels for the Charlottesville, Virginia, Area Agency on Aging during the 1980s, Deily was familiar with the parameters of the extensive rural aging network. Identifying some gaps in service, she advocated for the development of a program similar to Independent Living of Madison, Wisconsin. Independent Living provided home safety assessments and long-term loans of assistive technology products that facilitated home safety. With the support of the agency director, Deily submitted a grant proposal for 1 year of funding. In subsequent years, community support for the program secured funding from city and county governments. In Virginia, Deily's program focused on safety and access and provided OT consultation to over 1,100 clients, including aging services providers, housing departments, and a variety of city and county agencies. Additionally, Deily developed and sold two manuals with a videotape for use with family caregiver education programs. These products introduced coping strategies and instructed caregivers in how to use assistive technology to compensate for sensory as well as cognitive losses.

Valerie Lee, OTR
Arthritis Foundation of
Columbus, Ohio

Lee provides case-centered occupational therapy consultation service, education, and referral to residents with arthritis. Lee screens calls from the community, identifying those residents who will be able to benefit from her services. During a home visit, Lee has the client take her on a room-by-room tour of the home, soliciting client input on particular problems he or she may have with features, tools, and task performance in that room.

Lee also observes the client during this tour. She recommends products and practices that could make daily living safer and easier, instructs in appropriate energy conservation and work simplification techniques, and provides guidance in the appropriate use of joints. Lee also provides individual educational intervention on what she describes as common topics of interest with her older adult clients: medication, communication with their physicians, benefits of exercise and staying active, and other community resources. Lee frequently serves as a referral agent, hooking up her older adult clients with skilled care providers and other needed services of the community. Additionally, Lee serves as a resource and educator for other professionals in the community who serve clients with arthritis.

Harriet Watkins, MS, COTA
Manager, Hebron House Senior
Center Plus Site, and Faculty
Member, COTA Program,
Catonsville Community College

Watkins has been influential within the Howard County Office on Aging's multiple community outreach programs. She developed and has managed for 10 years the daily operation of a social-model daytime program for community-based frail, older adults who need supportive services to remain in the community. Consultation has occurred throughout her involvement at this site and, in her other capacities, at the case, educational, and program and administration levels. In 1992, Watkins actively participated on the Professional Advisory Team during the development, planning, and implementation of the innovative program Operation Independence. This collaborative interdisciplinary effort was supported by the Maryland State Office and local Area Agency on Aging, the Maryland State Technical Assistance Program, Towson University and Catonsville Community College OT and occupational therapy assistant (OTA) programs, Volunteers for Medical Engineering local chapter, AOTA, Maryland Occupational Therapy Association, and others. The objectives of Operation Independence, which continue to be successfully met, include the following:

- Increasing the frequency of OT interventions for persons living in the community with difficulties in ADLs
- Educating potential consumers and caregivers
- Providing in-service training to professional staff working in community-based services.

That education focus directed attention toward heightening the awareness of the use of assistive technology and home modification as proven strategies for enabling older adults to maintain independence. The program has received national attention. It served as the basic foundation for Senior Tech in rural Maryland described below. It is currently being replicated at three sites in Georgia and California.

Pat Brokos, OTR
Maryland Easter Seal Society for Disabled Children and Adults

In 1993, Brokos directed the Senior Tech program, a collaborative agency effort that offered education and resource information on "low tech" devices to seniors and their caregivers so that seniors might stay in their homes safely and independently as long as possible. Included in their presentations at 15 local senior centers was an introduction to strategies about the use of assistive products to enable older adults to remain active in their communities. These same educational sessions were also informative for professionals and family caregivers. Hands-on opportunities to use over 60 products useful in daily routines, such as dressing, home management, grooming, eating, communication, health care, environmental control, and recreation, were made available to over 800 persons.

Jeannie Bires, OT
Housing Section, Philadelphia Corporation for Aging (PCA)

Using a combination of lottery, grants, and Medicaid funds, PCA (a nonprofit organization that serves as the city's agency on aging) operates three programs designed to assist older adults and others with disabilities in identifying and obtaining the home repairs, modifications, and functional architectural products that will enable them to stay safely and be functional in their own homes. PCA clients are initially seen by a social worker for a comprehensive needs assessment. Bires then visits the client's home to assess the client and his or her home, focusing on safety and accessibility. Depending on the funding available and the needs of the client, Bires may recommend a wide range of products, prac-

tices, and modifications. Bires meets with the Housing Section construction supervisor to review the current and future needs of the client. Bires and the supervisor also review the safety and structural condition of the client's home, repair needs, and costs. Bires identifies a major focus of her work as communicating effectively with housing department personnel. Her ability to adapt her language and explain client issues in simple terms of current and future needs is a major factor in her effectiveness. Bires, a strong proponent of occupational therapy practice in community-based, nonmedical settings states, "I could spend 10 hours with someone in acute care in the hospital, and it wouldn't be as valuable as the 1 hour I spend with them in their home."

Karen Barney, MS, OTR
Washington University

Barney is working with the local Geriatric Education Program on a multidisciplinary grant-funded project to prevent injuries among older adults in the St. Louis area. The project, entitled "Safe and Sound Through the Senior Years," provides for the following:

- Training of inner-city older adult volunteers to perform home safety assessments in their own homes and in the homes of others
- Training of professionals and para-professionals from surrounding rural areas in home safety
- Training of the trainer and trainer consultation.

In concert with this effort, the Geriatric Education Center sponsored a 2-day session on coalition building with a local disability center and the Division on Aging. Through that mechanism, the participating organizations established a violence prevention campaign that brings together resources and support from the aging and disability communities. In addition to developing strategies for violence prevention, the group works with persons who are older or disabled who become victims. As a spin-off of this effort, the consortium sponsored another initiative entitled "Door to Door," which educated hospital and nursing home staffs about safety and fall-prevention strategies for older adults.

Karen Seymour, COTA
Howard County Office on Aging

Seymour has assisted in the development of a new model social day program for adults over the age of 60. Called Senior Center Plus, the program is designed to provide a social alternative for those adults too frail for a regular senior center but as yet not needing the supervision of an adult day health center. OT is part of the unique focus of this program. Seniors who need assistance with two or more activities, such as meal preparation, medications, or getting in and out of wheelchairs, will participate in a personalized program of activities designed to promote wellness and delay institutionalization by focusing on maintaining function and health.

Seymour is collaborating with the program manager to develop activity schedules and formats for intake, evaluation, and documentation. She reports a challenging but exciting process of blending OT's functional focus with a schedule of traditional senior center activities.

Jean Kiernat, MS, OTR, FAOTA
Sun City Community Health Education and Resource Center

Last year alone, Kiernat and her staff at the center (a nonprofit community-based educational organization operated by Sun Health Corporation for the three Sun City, Arizona, communities) planned, coordinated, and provided health education and wellness programs to over 17,000 individuals. The program operates over 20 different support groups monthly and provides classes on topics ranging from cancer facts to memory enhancement strategies and Tai-Chi. They also sponsor and coordinate a large number of special events, such as "Convenience for the Inconvenienced" (a gizmo and gadget fair) and a "Fall Fair," where hundreds of visitors are assessed for gait, balance, medications, foot screenings, blood pressure, and a number of other factors that can contribute to increased fall risk in older adults. As a byproduct of their success, Del E. Webb, the national developer of Sun City, sees health promotion and wellness programs as an integral part of his retirement communities and will be using Kiernat and her staff to help plan the health education and wellness services for three new communities in California, Texas, and South Carolina. Kiernat, with coauthor Hasselkus, edited *Occupational Therapy and the Older Adult*. In their chapter, "Education for Empowerment," Hasselkus and Kiernat (1991) identify a number of factors to consider in the planning and delivery of education-oriented health promotion, wellness, and injury prevention programs:

- Teach what the group members say they want to learn.
- Plan to present information for no more than 30 minutes.
- Allow time for questions.
- Pay attention to the effect of the environment on your audience's ability to participate.
- Begin with an overview of your topic.
- Include opportunities that encourage participation.

- Use humor.
- Avoid jargon.
- Give handouts at the end of the presentation, not during.
- Summarize points at the end of your talk.
- Solicit feedback from the group at the end.

Shoshanna Shamberg, OTR
Abilities OT Services,
Baltimore, Maryland

Shamberg provides home assessments and accessibility consulting and training to individuals, organizations, and clients of organizations in the greater Baltimore–Washington, D.C., area. When providing individual client consultation, Shamberg works closely with architects and contractors in the selection of specific products to best meet her clients' needs. With sentiments similar to Bires, Shamberg identifies her ability to communicate effectively as a significant factor in her success. On a program level, after assisting a city housing department in surveying the abilities of its facilities to meet federal accessibility standards, Shamberg authored a training manual to be used for all Baltimore city housing department personnel. The manual not only reviewed disability awareness issues but highlighted products and practices that could make older adults and persons with disabilities more functional in their homes.

Mary Corcoran, PhD, OTR, and
Laura Gitlin, PhD
Faculty, Thomas Jefferson
University, Philadelphia,
Pennsylvania

Corcoran and Gitlin have taken steps to systematically evaluate the effectiveness of OT consultation in working with caregivers of persons with Alzheimer's disease. They are in the process of analyzing data gathered from a 3-year grant from the National Institute on Aging, during which Corcoran and Gitlin enrolled 200 caregivers of persons with Alzheimer's-type dementia. Of these caregivers, 100 were placed in a control group. The other 100 received five visits from an occupational therapist over a 2-month period. The occupational therapists were provided training in establishing partnerships with the caregivers, assisting the caregivers in looking at and analyzing problem-solving processes, and increasing the caregivers' use of environmental modifications in management of daily activities and behaviors. While the researchers believe that many OT practitioners do provide training and support for families of persons with dementia, it is often not provided over time in the home or in any systematized process that provides families with constructs for problem solving on their own. Corcoran and Gitlin perform outcome and cost-benefit analyses to increase potential for funding for this type of intervention.

Chris Cawley, OTR, and
Anne Morris, EdD, OTR

While employed by the Virginia Department of Health as consultants to Fairfax County Health Department, Cawley and Morris provided a wide range of both direct and consulting services to clients, caregivers, and staff of health and human service agencies in the Northern Virginia area. They provided training for home health aides, public health nurses, adult day care staff, senior center staff, and social services agencies staff on a number of topics related to the requirements and demands of those positions. Topics addressed included body mechanics, transfers, bathing processes, appropriate use of assistive products and resources to access technology, utilization of skilled care services, management of swallowing problems and feeding issues, home modification, products for daily living for those with arthritis, and products to minimize sensory losses (vision and hearing) in performance of daily activities.

Additionally, over the years, Cawley and Morris developed a wide range of educational programs targeted and designed to interest the older adult public in adopting successful aging strategies. They provided programs on home modification to meet special needs, memory enhancement, living with arthritis, fall prevention, wellness, bathroom safety, etc.

Cawley organized a hands-on demonstration center at a local retirement community. Over 400 older adults and their caregivers and professionals made appointments for a 2-hour, hands-on educational tour of an apartment that was filled with over 100 special products that had the potential to make daily living easier. The program provided older adults with the opportunity to recognize unique product design and to learn what assistive products are available, the factors to be considered in their selection, how and when to seek professional assistance in product selection, and where products may be purchased or ordered.

The knowledge and skills needed by an OT practitioner to function effectively in a consulting-oriented practice in the community are myriad. In addition to technical expertise and familiarity with the operations of community aging services, OT consultants in community settings must be expert communicators, analyzers, problem solvers, group facilitators, teachers, developers, etc. Even so, possessing these skills, attitudes, aptitudes, and knowledge does not ensure success in community settings.

Barriers to Community OT Practice

Certain stumbling blocks exist for occupational therapists looking for consultation or employment opportunities in the community. Some basic issues, if not understood and anticipated, may prevent success or create barriers. Each community is unique and may possess its own problems, but four issue areas are common:

1. Unexamined assumptions about the aging process among older people and their support systems
2. Differences between medical and social service models
3. Language
4. The solo nature of community-based practices that can isolate therapists to the degree that practice is unattractive.

UNEXAMINED ASSUMPTIONS ABOUT THE AGING PROCESS AMONG OLDER PEOPLE, FAMILIES, AND SOCIAL SERVICE PROVIDERS

In some ways, this is the most serious of barriers to OT practitioners who wish to serve older people in the community. OT practitioners work in a medical model where they are accustomed to viewing functional impairments caused by disease or chronic conditions that worsen with age.

For example, an OT evaluation of an older woman who no longer bathes independently might include an analysis of strength, range of motion, balance and mobility, vision deficits, and sensory and cognitive function (Levine & Brayley, 1991). OT intervention would be based on conclusions drawn in each of these areas and may include treatment, assistive devices, modification of the bathroom, and education of family members to provide verbal cueing. The result of the evaluation and intervention may be that the older woman resumes self-care in bathing with the supports described above. This positive result has flowed from the assumption that the problem in bathing had some physiological and environmental basis and could be addressed based on professional assessment and intervention.

But the outcome would have been different with another set of assumptions. It is not unusual for older adults and family members to think that decreased self-care capacity is a normal part of the aging process. The logic might seem clear to them: Many older people exhibit limited functioning; therefore, limitations in functioning are a normal consequence of aging. According to this pervasive and often unarticulated logic, older people, family members, and aging specialists unfamiliar with OT practice often do not address these areas with a physician (the gatekeeper in the medical model) and assume that these limitations are unavoidable. Energies and funds are then used to provide others to do "for" the older person, and self-care is assumed to be permanently limited.

As a result, the type of service that an OT practitioner is specifically trained to provide is never sought. For the woman who has stopped bathing herself independently, she and her family will assume that she is simply moving along the inevitable aging process and that someone else should or will do this function for her. Her spouse or daughter might now bathe her; her case manager might request public funds for an in-home aide several days a week, or the woman may simply stop bathing.

The seriousness of this barrier is the self-limitation it imposes on options for independent living. If one does not expect to be able to continue to care for oneself, then self-care options will not exist. Society's expectations regarding older people may also contribute to this unexamined assumption that loss of functioning should be accepted as a normal sign of aging, and rehabilitative efforts appropriate for younger people with disabilities are not applicable for older people with disabilities. With the older population, the emphasis on self-care and independence is often tempered with concern about risk and complicated by the presence of other multiple conditions, including dementia. With a well-intentioned desire to protect older people from a presumed future of functional decline, support services can sometimes be activated prematurely or too extensively because the expectation of self-care and independence is no longer seen as appropriate. These unexamined assumptions bear thinking about and offer a rich area for OT involvement.

For the OT practitioner wishing to expand practice into the community, these assumptions about the aging process can be addressed by enlightening older people, families, and the community service network about the methods for supporting self-care capacity. By developing partnerships with aging specialists in the community, OT practitioners enter the consumer network and the professional network for the benefit of the older population. Prevention programs, information about assistive technology and environmental modification, caregiver training, and many other areas are critical information to present to the community.

For example, the Howard County, Maryland, Area Agency on Aging developed an educational program called Operation Independence. The AAA developed a coalition with the American Occupational Therapy Association, occupational therapy departments in Maryland colleges, local volunteer occupational therapists, the Maryland Technology Assistance Program, and other state and local organizations. With a small amount of funding to purchase samples of low-technology assistive products, Operation Independence organizes ongoing presentations for seniors, caregivers, and professional agency staff. The presentations describe the work of occupational therapists, demonstrate common assistive devices, educate audiences on safety issues in the home environment and the value of modification, and direct individuals to where OT services can be obtained in the community.

DIFFERENCES BETWEEN HEALTH AND SOCIAL SERVICES MODELS

Methods of reimbursement create a fundamental difference between the health and social service models. In general, the health industry reimburses providers for medical services on a fee-for-service basis, with the physician acting as the gatekeeper. Services are provided for an individual patient during a specific period; in some settings, achievement of goals terminates the reimbursement and the service. The services provided to the patient are determined within the categories of reimbursable activities.

For instance, OT intervention in an acute care setting will be provided only in that setting and only for the duration of the hospital stay. The patient may be discharged to a home setting that the occupational therapist has never seen and which has environmental hazards unrecognized by the

family. Whether OT intervention is available to that older person in the community will depend on discharge policy, whether community-based OT services are available, whether the family voices concerns to the physician about the older person's functioning in the home setting, and whether the physician is knowledgeable about the full range of OT services.

In contrast, social service models, such as the public aging network of AAA, are funded to coordinate or directly provide a broad variety of nonmedical services to the older population in a geographic area. There may be a number of gatekeepers or no gatekeeper at all.

For instance, wellness and prevention are key areas for aging services. Although the level of funding may vary depending on the size of the service population and other factors, the funding in broad program areas is usually not specific to an individual client. An individual person may move among aging programs depending on need; funding is attached to the program function, not to the individual benefiting from that program. Fiscal restraints may result in a fee-for-service approach for selected services in the future, but the funding history of the network has moved it toward program development as opposed to the fee-for-service basis used in the health industry.

When community-based, long-term-care funds are tied to an individual, the physician may not play the same gatekeeper function as in the medical model. For example, many individual states have developed long-term care programs targeted to older adults who may be candidates for nursing home services. To prevent inappropriate or premature nursing home placement, assessments conducted by health and social service professionals in the community will determine the type of service most needed by the individual. Public funds for community-based services may then be authorized by a case manager for that individual. In these states, the funding will be specific to the individual. However, a medical diagnosis is usually not the determining factor for the publicly funded services. In many cases, the functioning level and the income status of the client will determine whether public funds will be used to maintain the person in the community.

In addition, the diverse funding streams in the community-based network result in fragmentation and great difficulty in determining exactly what a local community has to offer. For public programs, a complicated network of eligibility criteria exists because services are often provided by a variety of public agencies. It is not unusual for agencies to provide information and referral for the services specific to that agency, but not to the services of other agencies. Services for older people in the community come from a variety of sources, as described earlier in this chapter, and are spread across many sectors: public, private nonprofit, private for-profit, and voluntary. As a result, OT practitioners who wish to expand into community consultation must learn the network of services to fully understand how to work in the community.

While many organizations are attempting to maximize reimbursement through third-party sources, in the authors' informal survey, a number of therapists and COTAs reported that their funding comes from a blending of grant, city, county, state, and federal funding. Often funding must be renewed annually or biannually. While not as cost driven as acute care, many OT practitioners describe a focus on "count" that affects their decisions on whom to see and how to spend their

time. Therapists developing programs or seeking to expand programs often obtain assistance through grant funds. They find networking useful, with community-based nonprofit agencies long experienced in obtaining funding through a variety of funding mechanisms.

LANGUAGE BARRIER

All professions construct a specialized language that makes the exchange of information within that profession consistent and accurate. Professional dialogue or written material will also contain "shorthand" or acronyms that reduce frequently used phrases to abbreviations commonly understood by others in that profession.

The language of occupational therapy contains some words and acronyms used exclusively by OT practitioners and educators, such as the term *ATDs* for *assistive technology devices.* OT practitioners also use language common to health professionals that is not normally used by social service professionals, consumers, or family members, such as *COPD* for *chronic obstructive pulmonary disease,* in reference to the medical diagnosis that severely limits breathing abilities, which in turn limits energy and stamina for performing routine tasks. Finally, OT practitioners use words widely used by other health or social service professionals but with a meaning specific to occupational therapy. For instance, the word *deficit* will have a different meaning depending on whether it occurs in documentation produced by an OT practitioner or is written by an economist in an article on the U.S. balance of trade.

Now you can understand why something as invisible as language might present a barrier to forming partnerships outside a professional's usual sphere of activity. A skilled OT practitioner will automatically adjust language depending on whether the discussion is with hospital team members or with a patient reviewing assistive devices for the bathroom. However, professionals in all disciplines are often guilty of using specialized language across a variety of settings and not verifying if the meaning is understood by the audience. Lack of sensitivity to language differences could impede the expansion of OT services into nontraditional arenas. Not only could this lack of sensitivity be construed as professional arrogance, but also the potential partner may miss the value of OT services to the older client in the community.

Strategies for Reducing Language Barriers

The OT practitioner can reduce language barriers in many ways to be successful in consultation with community organizations. When consulting with other professionals outside the field, occupational therapists should keep a few points in mind:

1. Do not use specialized words or abbreviations and acronyms, unless you have verified that the words are familiar to the audience or you fully explain them at the time. Be prepared to use and describe full phrases with their explanations (for example, "activities of daily living for ADL") when they are first used and each time someone new joins the conversation. This technique educates your new partners and keeps each member of the coalition on equal footing. If your audience uses different words for the same concept, use those words, if appropriate.

2. Take time to learn the language of your partners, particularly if they work in a social service model and you come from a health model. Ask

questions when your potential partner uses unfamiliar words or acronyms, and identify an aging specialist in the community who can educate you on the structure and network in your community. For example, the staff of an area agency on aging may refer to the organization as a "triple A." Rather than think that these people work for the Automobile Association of America on the side, ask what the acronym "AAA" means. Instead of using professional terminology, describe OT services in familiar language, demonstrating your understanding of the kind of setting in which your potential partner relates to the client (not patient) in the community. Use descriptive examples that clearly explain to the audience how OT skills could benefit a functionally impaired client or a program that provides services to this population. The purpose is to be descriptive so your audience can understand the benefit of what an OT can offer individual clients or can contribute to the design of service.

ISOLATION

Many therapists who work with community-based social or human service organizations may be the only occupational therapy provider, rehab service personnel, or even health care practitioner within the organization or system. Congruent to Thomas Jefferson University's efforts to move students and practices into community-based settings, OT faculty at Thomas Jefferson are also dealing with the issues that face the often solo community-based practitioner. They identify the following problems as common to practitioners in community settings:

- Obtaining professional feedback and assistance in situational problem solving

- Dealing with supervisors who may have limited or no understanding of OT and how an OT practitioner works

- Pursuing continuing education opportunities in a system that does not recognize the need for continuing education

- Obtaining professional education that provides for the unique breadth and scope of skills an OT practitioner needs for practice in such a wide-open arena.

Kathy Swenson Miller, MS, OTR, OT Program, Thomas Jefferson University, is developing a model for supporting community-based OT practitioners who practice in diverse and solo settings. Basing the effort on a similar model developed for supporting fieldwork coordinators, Thomas Jefferson faculty are initiating a support group and network for providing peer and supervisory support, as well as investigating the potential for using the social work model of purchased supervision for occupational therapy.

Therapists working in community settings recognize the importance and benefits of forming peer relationships with therapists in like settings, often via telephone. AOTA offers extensive opportunities for networking through membership in the special-interest sections and through state and national conferences.

AOTA Documents Reflect Community Practice Issues

The recent AOTA membership update (AOTA, 1995b) identified primary practice sites. Growth was reflected in home health and private practice arenas reflecting increased application of the consultative approach to services delivery (AOTA,

1995b). Shifts were noted in primary work settings between 1990 and 1995. For OTRs, significant increases were noted in settings that typically use the medical model of services delivery. Included were home health, skilled nursing, intermediate care, and out-patient clinics.

For COTAs, increases were noted in skilled nursing, intermediate care, and home health. It is encouraging to see the data reflect that some practitioners report activity moving into nonmedical model service delivery approaches.

Documents adopted by the AOTA Representative Assembly define key concepts and offer further support to the focus assumed through consultative services provision to community programs. For example,

- The position paper "Occupational Therapy and Long-Term Services and Supports" (AOTA, 1996, pp. 167–170) emphasizes that occupational therapy practitioners are a major provider of services that enable persons of all ages and abilities to regain independence, assure autonomy, achieve their fullest potential, and attain optimal levels of wellness within their home and as fully integrated community contributors. Services may include assisting with basic routines of daily living; enabling the fullest level of function within the family, work, school, and leisure; as well as managing of chronic health concerns. The services may be delivered in institutions, an individual's home, or community-based agencies.

- Adoption of the document "Uniform Terminology, 3rd ed.: Application to Practice" (AOTA, 1996, pp. 287–294) emphasized the critical need to give consideration to context, that is, temporal and environmental aspects, as the linchpin to performance outcomes. Embedded in these performance contexts are features of performance in activities of daily living, work and productive activities, and leisure. The choice of specific intervention is a collaborative experience among the client or significant others and the OT practitioner, jointly identifying solutions to the performance area of client concern.

- Approval of the statement "Occupational Therapy Services for Persons With Alzheimer's Disease and Other Dementias" (AOTA, 1996, pp. 297–302) in 1994 clearly describes the role of occupational therapy across the continuum of services delivery aimed at managing irreversible dementias. Assessment in the early stages of cognitive decline directs attention toward routine daily tasks, such as driving, home management, and safety.

- Maintenance of the older person's ability to participate in functional activities is a core goal for community-based rehabilitation and long-term services delivery efforts (Nelson & Stucky, 1992; Oakley, 1994; Morris, Hunt, & Kolm, 1994; Epstein, 1991).

- The concept paper on service delivery (AOTA, 1996, pp. 363–368) recognizes that professional roles are expanding. Decisions about service delivery are grounded in thoughtful assessments of the "system, model, and context within which the client exists." The *client* is defined as the "person, group, program, or organization for whom the practitioner is providing services." It further defines *client-centered service delivery* as "an interactive approach to service that considers systems, models, and contexts in making decisions that focus on the client's needs and that engage the client as a participant." This approach to services

delivery clearly responds to dramatic societal change.

- In the position paper "Occupational Performance: Occupational Therapy's Definition of Function" (AOTA, 1996, pp. 154–158), a review of the historical roots of occupational therapy is provided. The commitment of the early founders of the profession to the importance of occupation and the preservation of function was clearly described. Although that commitment continues today, an even broader perspective has emerged that directs attention toward the dynamic interaction among the person, his or her occupation, and the environment.

- Occupational therapy practitioners use the term *occupational performance* to express function, emphasizing the interaction between the person and the environment wherein the activity occurs. It is commonly recognized that other disciplines are increasingly focusing on functional outcomes to indicate the efficacy of their interventions. The occupational therapy practitioner collaborates with the individual in an effort to facilitate enhanced occupational performance. Interventions direct attention toward role and occupation demands, personal skills, and environmental supports and barriers (AOTA, 1996, pp. 154–158).

- In the position paper "Broadening the Construct of Independence" (AOTA, 1996, pp. 165–166), independence is defined as "the ability to take responsibility for one's own role performance needs and desires." Personal autonomy is strongly valued and emphasized by practitioners, thereby encouraging self-determination, allowing the individual to decide what he or she wants and needs to do.

Summary

OT linkages already exist with the aging network. The OT practitioner interested in working in community settings should recognize that these community service providers share something with OT practitioners: They all have the goal of supporting the maximum independence of older people. Although there will always be a place for institutional medical facilities in the continuum of care for older adults, agencies such as AAAs, housing organizations, recreational facilities, senior apartments, churches, civic organizations, and others are dealing with increasing numbers of disabled older adults who wish to remain in the communities in which they have spent their lives or in which their adult children live. The target population that is served by the aging network in community-based, long-term care—the adult with physical or cognitive impairments whose capacity for self-care is changing—is the same population OT practitioners have been trained to assist. Moving from the medical treatment model to the community consultative model will amplify the impact of OT in promoting the health and wellness of older adults.

Case Studies

CASE STUDY 1

A local area agency on aging had referred a 66-year-old man, who has lived alone independently since having a CVA 14 years before, to the local health department, which sponsored a program that provided older adult residents with in-home assistance for bathing. The gentleman, when hearing that only female aides were available from the department to assist with bathing, declined health department assistance. The AAA and health department requested the OT practitioner assist the client in identifying the problem with bathing and make recommendations to the client for his follow-up.

The practitioner contacted the client, confirmed his interest in having a visit, clarified her objectives for her visit, and made arrangements for an appointment. During the visit, the two reviewed the client's functional history, surveyed the bathroom and the equipment, and observed the client's function. Together, the practitioner and client reviewed and discussed her observations, identified potential contributors to the gentleman's difficulty in bathing himself, and discussed options and pros and cons of different courses of action open to him. The practitioner reviewed resources. On the basis of the discussion, recommendations, and resources identified, the gentleman made an appointment with a physiatrist for an evaluation, obtained a referral for in-home OT and PT services from a local skilled care agency, and purchased a new transfer bench, a combination of activities that eventually enabled him to resume self-bathing.

CASE STUDY 2

The director of a local nonprofit in-home respite service contacted the OT practitioner to request OT consultation for the daughter of an 82-year-old woman with Alzheimer's disease. The respite service had been providing 8 hours per weekend of respite care but noted an increasing number of questions from the daughter regarding the management of the client's daily activities. The OT practitioner contacted the daughter, made an appointment, and reviewed the parameters and objectives of her visit. From the daughter, the practitioner obtained not only a history of the mother, but also an outline of the daughter's concerns, a review of the difficulties currently being experienced, and a snapshot of the daughter's situation regarding health, family resources, and plans for the future. The practitioner listened while the daughter described the procedures currently used to manage daily living activities. During the home visit, the practitioner surveyed the home and met the mother. The practitioner observed and assisted the daughter and client in performing a number of simple daily living activities. Afterwards, the daughter and practitioner reviewed ideas regarding services and modifications of procedures and the environment that could make performance of daily tasks simpler and safer for both mother and daughter. They reviewed the pros and cons of each strategy and discussed resources and methods of making each potential strategy happen. The daughter then selected four courses of action she wished to try to ease home access, transfers, bathing, and mealtime.

By the next month, the daughter had identified a resource for modifying the front door entry to ease access; had obtained nursing, PT, and OT services from a skilled care agency for training in transfers, skin care, and feeding techniques; had joined the local chapter of the Alzheimer's Association and a support group; and was using a senior day care center to provide herself with a much needed respite and her mother with additional stimulation.

Relationships of this type also allow the sharing of information about future functional limitations with family members. This sharing allows them to better monitor, plan for, and respond to their relatives' changing needs. The practitioner acts as a consultant to help caregivers explore different courses of action to promote the adoption of more successful aging-in-place strategies not only for the care receiver but for the caregivers themselves.

CASE STUDY 3

A public health nurse assigned to a local retirement community requested OT assistance in solving a problem for a resident of the community. A 72-year-old man with Parkinson's disease was having such difficulty rising from bed to go to the bathroom at night that he had begun sleeping in a living room chair. The nurse hypothesized that several other residents had taken similar courses of action. She wished to increase her knowledge of alternative strategies available to help residents deal with this problem.

The practitioner and nurse discussed the resident and the resident's functional and medical history. They reviewed the role the nurse plays in the community and the parameters and expectations associated with that role. They reviewed previous activities of the nurse and the resident in addressing the problem and the resident's response to suggested strategies. The practitioner described a number of factors that could be contributing to the client's difficulty and how those could be assessed during a home visit. The nurse requested the OT practitioner to accompany her on a home visit.

During the home visit, the practitioner guided the nurse through a look at different factors that could be contributing to the client's difficulty. By examining each factor together, they arrived at an agreement as to the primary factors contributing to the problem. The OT practitioner suggested several options for follow-up, including physical therapy (PT) and the use of assistive devices. Based on her knowledge of the couple, the nurse presented the recommendations to the couple. The practitioner provided the nurse information that the physician would want to consider when prescribing PT services, reviewed local resources for obtaining recommended PT services, and explained what to request to obtain the specific services needed. The OT practitioner also provided the nurse and the couple with a no-cost local source for trying out the recommended equipment in the company of the physical therapist, and later assisted the nurse in formulating a written request that resulted in use of excess funds for subsidy of the equipment purchase for the couple. As an outgrowth of the intervention, the nurse and the couple began discussing and solving other difficulties in performing daily activities, and the couple shared their "success" in remediating their problem with other residents in the building.

CASE STUDY 4

Practitioner A is employed by a state department of health to act as a consultant to a number of county organizations providing services to older adults in a metropolitan area. In addition to responding to calls, inquiries, and requests for assistance from service providers, she makes quarterly visits to a variety of center-based senior recreation and day health care programs to observe and meet with staff to discuss both participant and staff interests and needs. While visiting one of the adult day health care centers, the therapist noted a number of participants required 1:1 assistance when walking. Several participants were using assistive devices inappropriate for them, and one participant with osteoporosis was having increasing difficulty feeding herself. Meeting with the director and the center nurse, the therapist discussed her observations and explored their knowledge of the strategies at their disposal for improving the safety and function of the participants. The center staff was unaware that there were mechanisms for access to therapy evaluations and services for clients. The therapist provided the staff with information on services available from local therapy providers and reviewed the referral process and criteria for third-party payment. She guided the nurse through the process of communicating need for and objectives for therapy to the client's family, physician, and eventually the care provider. In addition to providing the nurse with experience she could draw on in the future, the therapist's visit established an ongoing relationship that ensured timely and appropriate access to skilled care services in the future. The therapist helped the nurses draw up a policy and procedure for referring participants to medical and rehabilitation service providers and explored strategies for maintaining staff awareness of such care services as a resource for participants. She assisted a committee of center directors in the process of assessing staff interests and needs regarding mobility, transfers, and mealtime management issues. She guided them through the process of arranging training on each topic. Sensitized to the limited level of familiarity with rehabilitation services possessed by many working in the social service system, the practitioner began routinely to disseminate information on rehabilitation services with each staff contact and incorporated similar information in later in-services to social service personnel.

CASE STUDY 5

The OT practitioner met with a group of 14 assistant directors of regional senior centers operated by a county recreation department. Having delivered a number of health promotion and injury prevention programs at their centers, she was familiar with the layouts and programs of the different centers. In her visits to the centers, she routinely discussed with the directors not only specific issues they were having with center participants but also the changing demographics of their neighborhoods and the increasing number of frail adults attending their activities. At the request of the centers' directors, she made a 2-hour presentation on sensory changes in older adults and products and practices available that could make task performance easier for older adults attending center activities.

The OT practitioner used props to allow the directors to experience how difficult it is to engage in tasks with sensory deficits. She then led the directors in a problem-solving exercise to explore their knowledge of alternative strategies for task performance. Together they reviewed products and simple seating, lighting, flooring, signage, acoustics, and other environmental changes that could make participation in center activities easier and more pleasant for persons with a wide range of abilities. The importance of integrating these changes into standard center operational procedures was discussed as a tool to diminish participant fear of being singled out for needing a "special" product or arrangement. The pivotal role senior center staff could play in assisting older adults in identifying the need for and obtaining special access to specialty services and products for easier daily living was discussed.

Copies of relevant articles on sensory changes and references were provided to the directors so they could obtain further professional information for consulting with OT, physical therapy, and specialists in the field of vision and hearing loss.

CASE STUDY 6

A 72-year-old woman with arthritis uses a scooter as her main method of mobilization. She has been living in the first floor of her two-story home for several years. She has recently applied for home repair services from the housing department. The client wishes to be able to either access her second-story full bath or have the half-bath on the first floor modified to incorporate a tub that she thinks she will be able to access independently. The department's architect requested OT consultation to help identify the functional abilities and priorities of the client that should be considered in project design and selection of products. The architect took this information into consideration when planning modification for the client.

CASE STUDY 7

A nurse working with the management of a local nonprofit, church-funded retirement community contacted an OT practitioner. The management was faced with an ever-increasing number of frail residents, many of whom had been living in the facility since it opened almost 20 years before. While the management believed it had done much to ensure residents' access to services through an active social service department and a busy health education and wellness program, it wanted to do something to encourage the use of assistive devices. It was the management's plan to develop a loan closet where residents could borrow devices, mainly commodes, walkers, or wheelchairs, as needed. On behalf of the management, the nurse was requesting OT assistance in identifying products to put in the loan closet.

The practitioner discussed with the nurse what outcomes she and the management would like to see from the operation of the closet. The practitioner also reviewed with the nurse other activities in place at the facility that could contribute to meeting the ostensible objective. The practitioner reviewed the pros and cons of operating a loan closet within a retirement community. After reviewing those, the practitioner briefly outlined a few other strategies that might be options for the facility to consider. The nurse believed the management had not considered other avenues to encouraging assistive device use. The practitioner offered to meet with the facility manager, social worker, and nurse to discuss their objectives and share with them an overview of other strategies they may wish to consider as alternatives or adjuncts to their plan.

During the meeting, the practitioner solicited input to clarify what the team saw as the problem; that is, that their residents "resisted" using assistive devices that could enhance function and safety. She then solicited their hypotheses as to why the residents resisted: Was it access, awareness, pride, fear, cost? She then reviewed the requirements and pros and cons of operating a loan closet. She briefly outlined a number of strategies that might be considered as alternatives to that and led the team through a rudimentary analysis of how each strategy might affect what they hypothesized were the reasons for the residents resisting the use of assistive devices. As the team discussed the issues, additional reasons for resistance were hypothesized, and additional strategies in response to those reasons were discussed.

As a result of using this problem-solving process, the team eventually elected to enact a number of strategies that ranged from a multi-agency, in-house educational campaign to broaden staff and resident awareness of and access to products to make daily living easier, to a change in policies regarding the use of facility vehicles for small group trips (like to a home center or to the low vision product information center).

Activities

1. Practitioner A was scheduled to visit three senior centers under a grant from a local area agency on aging. In her proposal to the agency, she had outlined objectives and formats for a coordinated series of programs focused on prevention of accidental injury and reduction of fall risk. Each program was to be no more than 1 hour long. Before developing her specific educational plan for each presentation, the therapist planned to call and speak to the center director. What questions should she ask the center director before formulating her plan for the series of presentations?

2. Contact your local agency on aging. Ask for materials outlining the scope of its services and programs. Present a brief summary of those services and programs to your colleagues. Identify two ways to integrate this information into materials available for use with your older adult clients.

3. Identify four sources of information on health promotion and wellness programming for older adults.

4. Identify three societal trends that will expand the opportunity and need for consultative occupational therapy services in the community.

5. Identify three models of consultation as outlined in Jaffe and Epstein.

6. Identify four barriers to occupational therapy consultation in the community.

7. Describe two differences between the medical and social services model of program delivery.

8. Identify two practitioners described in this chapter who are working in a situation that is similar to one where you work or would like to work. Contact them for more information.

Case Study Exercises

EXERCISE 1

The therapist received a call from the supervisor of a local respite service operated by a county health department. Title XX funds from the Department of Human Services now paid for 3 hours per week of respite services and 2 hours per week of assistance with morning care from a home health aide. This assistance enables a new client, a 70-year-old male with a history of alcoholism, diabetes, COPD, and CUA to attend a daily adult day health program.

The man lived with a 25-year-old tenant who provided some minor assistance in a.m. care in exchange for living space. The man's daughter lived across the street and functioned as the primary caregiver for her mother-in-law who had COPD and required assistance with many of her daily activities. She was physically unable to provide the personal assistance and supervision that her father needed to get ready to go out each morning. The father was on general relief without medical coverage and had just been assigned a social worker from the Department of Human Services.

The in-home respite coordinator identified problems with transfers as a primary concern of her companions. Twice, the father had refused to use his transfer bench to access the tub, citing falls at the rehab center during training in its use. The home health aide, employed by a second county agency, also cited concerns regarding transfers, reporting having to provide assistance in what she felt was an awkward and uncomfortable transfer for her and the client.

The adult day health center was considering discontinuing the client's attendance secondary to his chronic complaints about the activities, the food, the age of the other participants, and his desire to smoke. The client's social worker was concerned about the possible discharge from the day center. The daughter was willing to provide weekend help and evening assistance for her father, but would not be available all day long. She explained that when her father was at home during the day, he "calls for me twenty times a day. I go over in the morning to fix his breakfast, lunch, and supper. I also help him in and out of his chair, to and from the bathroom. But I can't do it all." The social worker was also concerned that the client had no physician or access to any medical care. He also had not yet obtained the orthosis, splint, and w/c recommended a year before by the outpatient therapists.

The client's tenant was willing to spend nights at home but was unavailable during the day. He was willing to stay as long as the situation did not deteriorate. The client disliked the day center and complained that previous therapy had no application to his current needs. Other comments included: "I can't get out of the couch; I'm sitting in a hole"; "People are always moving things, and I can't find anything"; "I can't do what I like"; and "The day care people are all old. They sit all day, but I can't!"

1. Identify five potential targets for your interventions.

2. Outline the consultation strategies and approaches you might use to work toward those targets.

EXERCISE 2

The therapist received a call from a local office of the public health department requesting assistance in formulating safe and appropriate bathing procedures and identifying the need for bathing-related equipment for a 91-year-old man. The nurse reported that the man had no specific medical diagnoses other than poor circulation. He was on no medications and had had no major changes in function over the past several years. The nurse's concern is that the man's current access for bathing requires him to step over the side of the tub, through a glass door enclosure, onto a shower bench with no back or side rails. The man requires no toileting assistance. However, in rising from sit to stand posture, he utilizes the towel bar to pull himself up.

His 89-year-old wife had been providing bathing and all other care. The wife herself lost vision in one eye a year ago. Glaucoma in the other eye severely limits her remaining vision. She feels that she can no longer physically provide the sponge bathing, which she has done for years. In addition to her husband's care, she cares for an adult son with mental retardation and a visual handicap. The son continues to spend his day at a local sheltered day program.

1. Identify factors to consider in analyzing the client's function, the environment, and recommended solutions to the concerns of the public health nurse.

2. Identify three other issues that have safety and functional implications for this family. Formulate strategies to explore those issues with the nurse.

References

Aging Design Research Program. (1993). *Design for aging: Occupational therapy and strategies for collaboration between architects and occupational therapists.* Washington, DC: Author.

American Occupational Therapy Association. (1996). *Reference manual of the official documents of the American Occupational Therapy Association, Inc.* Bethesda, MD: Author.

American Occupational Therapy Association. (1995a). *1995 Member Data Update.* Bethesda, MD: Author.

American Occupational Therapy Association. (1995b). Personal communication with Practice Department OT staff about phone inquiry notation (December 1995–April 1, 1996).

Bruhn, J. (1991). Occupational therapy in the 21st century: An outsider's view. *American Journal of Occupational Therapy, 45,* 775–780.

Compilation of the Older Americans Act of 1965 and the Native American Programs Act of 1974, As Amended Through December 31, 1992 (p. 1). (1993). Washington, DC: U.S. Government Printing Office.

Epstein, C. F. (1993). Long-term care. In H. L. Hopkins & H. D. Smith (Eds.), *Willard and Spackman's occupational therapy* (pp. 816–821). Philadelphia: J. B. Lippincott.

Epstein, C. F. (1991). Specialized restorative programs. In J. M. Kiernat (Ed.), *Occupational therapy and the older adult: A clinical manual* (pp. 285–300). Gaithersburg, MD: Aspen.

Gay, J. (1995). *Trainers manual: Small changes, big differences.* Iowa City, IA: Iowa Program for Assistive Technology.

Hasselkus, B., & Kiernat, J. (1991). Education for empowerment. In J. Kiernat (Ed.), *Occupational therapy and the older adult* (pp. 61–74). Gaithersburg, MD: Aspen.

Hettinger, J. (1995). New landscape, new models, new roles. *OT Week, 9*(42), 16–17.

Jaffe, E. (1992). Theories and principles of consultation. In E. Jaffe & C. Epstein (Eds.), *Occupational therapy consultation: Theory, principles and practice* (pp. 15–54). St. Louis, MO: Mosby-Year Book.

Joe, B. (1994). Operation independence, *OT Week.*

Kiernat, J. (Ed.) (1991). *Occupational therapy and the older adult.* Gaithersburg, MD: Aspen.

Leon, J., & Lair, T. (1990). *Functional status of the noninstitutionalized elderly: Estimates of ADL and IADL difficulties* (DHHS Publication No. [PHS] 90–3462). Rockville, MD: Public Health Service.

Levine, R. E., Corcoran, M. A., & Gitlin, L. N. (1993). Home care and private practice. In H. L. Hopkins & H. D. Smith (Eds.), *Willard and Spackman's occupational therapy* (pp. 370–371). Philadelphia: J. B. Lippincott.

Levine, R. E., & Brayley, C. R. (1991). Occupation as a therapeutic medium: A contextual approach to performance intervention. In D. Christiansen & C. Baum (Eds.), *Occupational therapy: Overcoming human performance deficits* (pp. 590–634). Thorofare, NJ: SLACK.

Morris, A. L., Hunt, G., & Kolm, D. (1994). *A part of daily life: Alzheimer's caregivers simplify activities and the home.* Bethesda, MD: American Occupational Therapy Association.

Morris, A. L., Connell, B. R., Sanford, J., & Kolm, D. (1996). *Changing needs, change homes: Adapting your home to fit you* [videotape]. Bethesda, MD: American Occupational Therapy Association.

Morris, A. L. (1995). *Listening to older adult learners: On the experience of using assistive technology in task performance and home modification.* Ann Arbor, MI: UMI Dissertation Services.

Nelson, D. L., & Stucky, C. (1992). The roles of occupational therapy in preventing further disability of elderly persons in long-term-care facilities. In J. Rothman & R. Levine (Eds.), *Prevention practice: Strategies for physical therapy and occupational therapy* (pp. 19–35). Philadelphia: W. B. Saunders.

Oakley, F. (1994). *The ABCs of Alzheimer's disease.* Bethesda, MD: American Occupational Therapy Association.

Price, G. D., & Fitz, P. (Eds.). (1990). *Cultural diversity and the allied health curriculum.* Hartford, CT: University of Connecticut, The Geriatric Education Center and Traveler's Center on Aging.

Rogers, J. C. (1990). Improving the ability to perform daily tasks. In B. Kemp, K. Brummel-Smith, & J. W. Ramsdell (Eds.), *Geriatric rehabilitation* (pp. 137–155). Boston: College Hill Press.

Stanton, S. (1995). Career enrichment strategies for a changing economic climate. *National, 12*(6), 6, 7, 20.

Swenson Miller, K. (1996). Personal communication.

U.S. Senate Special Committee on Aging, American Association of Retired Persons, Federal Council on the Aging, & U.S. Administration on Aging. (1991). *Aging America: Trends and projections* (DHHS Publication No. [FCoA] 91–28001). Washington, DC: Government Printing Office.

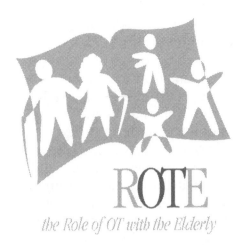

ROTE

the Role of OT with the Elderly

Adult Day Care

Kathleen H. Conyers, MEd,
OTR/L

Abstract

The ability to remain in one's own home and community, whether living alone or with family, is the desire of most elderly persons in this country. Despite numerous obstacles, most older persons prefer to "age in place," such as in their own homes or retirement communities, for as long as possible (Batchelder & Hilton, 1994; Macken, 1986). However, when disabling medical conditions, physical impairments, or psychosocial deficits hinder independent function in the home environment, elderly persons and their family members must look for assistance.

In years past, when problems arose concerning long-term care for the elderly, nursing home placement seemed to be the only choice, especially for working families. Fortunately, the provision of care for the elderly has been shifting from nursing homes, hospitals, and other medical facilities to the home and community setting. Maintaining the frail elderly in the community is a major goal of health care planners. Utilization of home health services by the elderly has grown tremendously over the past decade. However, growing restrictions on the duration of home health care and the relatively episodic or part-time nature of the service limit its ability to meet the older adult's long-term needs for socialization, health, personal care, and family respite (Osorio, 1991). Adult day care presents itself as a solution that allows the frail elderly individual and his or her family to maintain living at home while receiving those much needed health, medical, social, and rehabilitative services.

The field of adult day care is undergoing great growth, expansion, and change. Even

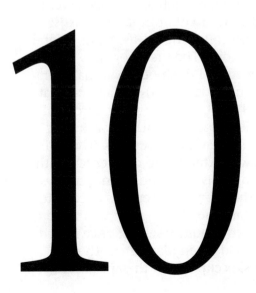

the name of this community-based program or service is undergoing change. Since its inception, these programs have been referred to as adult day health services, medical day care, senior day care, and adult day services, to name a few. Those in the field, however, prefer to use the terms adult day services or adult day programs because a wide range of services beyond day care are being provided at day centers (Cox & Reifler, 1994). It is also important to make clear the distinction between the provision of services to adults and day care services for children. The National Council on the Aging's (NCOA's) constituent unit, the National Institute on Adult Daycare (NIAD), supports this change in terminology. Therefore, for the purposes of this chapter, the terms *adult day services* or *adult day programs* are used. However, referenced sources will be quoted exactly as written.

The NIAD defines adult day care as a community-based group program designed to meet the needs of functionally impaired adults through an individual plan of care. It is a structured, comprehensive program that provides a variety of health, social, and related support services in a protective setting during any part of a day but less than 24 hours (NIAD, 1995). Adult day care is one of a number of rapidly growing long-term-care options that became available as health care expanded to encompass a variety of home- and community-based settings and services (Weissert, Elston, Bolda, Zelman, Mutran, & Mangum, 1990).

This chapter presents an overview of adult day services that are an integral part of the long-term-care delivery system serving the needs of the frail elderly. The historical and philosophical connections between adult day services and occupational therapy are explored and compared. A discussion and description of the classical models of care or types of day care settings are provided in an effort to classify the programs operating under the adult day services umbrella. A general description of adult day services, including staffing, program goals, services, funding sources, licensure, and certification are provided. Most important, a description of the variety of roles that occupational therapists and certified occupational therapy assistants can play in this setting are examined. Included are case studies, examples, and descriptions of the roles and functions of occupational therapy practitioners in these varied positions. Cultural, legal, and ethical concerns of occupational therapists will be reviewed regarding service delivery to this population. Implications for the future of occupational therapy and adult day services are explored as well.

Adult Day Care Development and Occupational Therapy: A Historical and Philosophical Connection

Adult day care began in psychiatric day hospitals, such as the Yale Psychiatric Clinic (1949), primarily to assist patients following release from mental institutions. The first programs were initiated by British occupational therapists in the late 1950s to help facilitate early hospital discharge for chronically ill elderly patients with a continuing need for restorative services. This concept was extended to day centers with an emphasis on stimulation, activity, and the supportive services needed to maintain the older person in a more social community setting once remediation had taken place. In both programs, occupational therapists comprised a major portion of the staff. Medical supervision, social work, nursing, and other rehabilitation specialists were available. However, occupational therapists and their early influence were a driving force in the development of this new type of day program (NIAD, 1995; Epstein, 1985b; Weiler & Rathbone-McCuan, 1978).

Americans became interested in establishing adult day care centers in the 1960s. At this time, further recognition was given to the growing needs of older persons through the Older Americans Act of 1965, Public Law 89–73. Subsequent legislation in the 1960s and early 1970s led to expanded health care services under amendments to the Social Security Act. These included Medicare (Title XVIII), Medicaid (Title XIX), and Social Service (Title XX) programs (Epstein, 1992). Recent statistics show that the number of adult day centers in the United States has grown from 15 in 1975 to 1,200 in 1985 (Von Behren, 1986) and from 2,100 in 1989 to 3,000 in 1994 (NIAD, 1994). Adult day centers are the fastest growing component of community-based long-term care. As the elderly population increases, adult day centers become a practical and appealing part of the solution to long-term-care needs (Partners in Caregiving, July 1995).

Most program participants in adult day care are older adults who need some assistance with their activities of daily living (bathing, dressing, eating, etc.) as a result of physical or emotional impairments. There are, however, an increasing number of young adults who find themselves in need of these services. Adult day care also provides support for the caregivers of these individuals in the form of respite from their daily responsibilities of care, emotional reassurance, educational training and assistance in obtaining additional services or supplies. NIAD estimates that the 3,000 or more adult day centers operating in the United States serve nearly 100,000 individuals and their caregivers (NIAD, 1995).

Philosophically, occupational therapy and adult day care both emphasize individual potential for growth and development, even in the face of disability, as well as a holistic integration of mental, physical, social, emotional, spiritual, and environmental aspects of well-being (Osorio, 1993; NCOA, 1984). A comparison of values underlying the practice of occupational therapy and the philosophy of adult day care shows striking parallels (Osorio, 1991). Yerxa (1983) described occupational therapy as concerned with the essential humanity of the individual and the quality of the individual's life despite his or her disability. Productivity, self-directedness, active participation, and faith in the patient's potential are all valued. An integrated view of the patient acknowledges the value of play and leisure and the importance of supporting the healthy aspects of the person so he or she can act on the environment rather than be determined by it. Adult day care is based on a philosophy that closely parallels the values underlying occupational therapy. As stated in NIAD's Standards for Adult Daycare (1984), adult day care

- Approaches each person as a unique individual with strengths and weaknesses, yet with a potential for growth and development

- Assumes a holistic approach to the individual, recognizing the interrelationship among the physical, social, emotional, and environmental aspects of well-being

- Promotes positive attitudes and a positive self-image, restoring, maintaining, and stimulating capacities for independence while providing supports for functional limitations (NIAD, 1984).

Types of Day Care Settings (Models of Care)

Von Behren (1988) states that, in early studies, attempts were made to classify adult day care centers into various models. These studies were static, often describing programs in early stages of development, and did not address the evolutionary growth of a new model. Usually the models were based on the primary service, target population, or services provided. Osorio (1991) states that these early efforts to develop a systematic method of classifying adult day care programs are understandable, given the wide variety of programs operating under the adult day care umbrella. She also states that although the issue of models of care is less visible now than a decade ago, some adult day care centers may continue to describe themselves or be perceived as based on a particular model. She describes the classical types of centers or models of care as follows:

I. Social Model:

    These centers provide supportive social and recreational services to a group of elders who have stable health conditions but who may be at risk due to social isolation, lack of family support, physical frailty or other similar characteristics. Services are primarily social and recreational, although screening or episodic health monitoring may be available. Prevention is a primary goal of social model programs.

II. Health Model or Medical Model:

    Serves participants with unstable health and specific functional impairments. Such centers generally offer on-site nursing care, one or more therapies on a consult or contract basis, medical social work, therapeutic recreation, and adapted social or recreational activities. Maintenance of function and, in some cases, restoration of function are the goals of these centers.

III. Restorative Model:

    These centers are more acute in orientation, serving those with rehabilitation potential who need shorter term nursing, occupational therapy, physical therapy or speech therapy. These restorative programs may be classified as day hospitals or day treatment centers and are usually located in hospitals, rehabilitation centers and skilled nursing facilities or as separate programs in medical model centers. Their goal is short-term treatment and timely discharge, frequently to a medical model center, where the participant can receive longer term maintenance and episodic restorative services (Osorio, 1991).

Osorio (1991) further suggests that it is probably more useful for occupational therapists (and other professionals) to conceptualize the universe of adult day care centers as a continuum from social to restorative. Although few centers correspond exactly to any detailed description of a particular model, all can be placed on a social-restorative continuum to facilitate appropriate referrals (Osorio, 1991).

In addition to the above mentioned "classical" models of care, centers providing a mix or combination of care have been established. For example, the health maintenance model incorporates both the social and medical models of adult day care. Whereas the social aspects of this program provide an environment that offers security, hot nutritious meals, socialization, meaningful activity, and respite for the caregivers, the medical aspects of this program focus on the provision of intense rehabilitation to meet the functional needs of the participants. The key in the health maintenance model is twofold: to maintain function and to rekindle interest in achieving new life goals (Howland & Gade-Schara, 1985).

These centers provide group involvement and promote wellness and independence, which in turn increases an individual's quality of life, contentment, mental functioning, and activity level (Neustadt, 1985).

The last decade has seen tremendous growth in the development of specialized or special-purpose centers, which are defined as those that serve a single type of clientele, such as the blind, mentally ill, or service veterans (Weissert et al., 1990). As well, specially designed programs for the elderly with Alzheimer's disease or dementia-related disorders have increased significantly as evidenced by the Dementia Care and Respite Services Program (DCRSP) —a $5.1 million initiative (1988–92) sponsored by the Robert Wood Johnson Foundation, with co-funding from the National Alzheimer's Association and the Federal Administration on Aging. Technical assistance and program direction were provided by the Bowman Gray School of Medicine of Wake Forest University. This demonstration project showed that nonprofit adult day centers could provide financially viable programs to people with dementia and their caregivers. This project resulted in establishing 18 centers in 13 different states specifically for people with dementia and their caregivers. As a result of the success of this project, Partners in Caregiving: The Dementia Services Program—a $2.5 million initiative (1992–96) sponsored by the Robert Wood Johnson Foundation—became the successor to the DCRSP in 1992. This replication project showed that the lessons learned from the DCRSP can be applied to a new group of sites quickly, economically, and with similar success. The Bowman Gray School of Medicine also provided technical assistance. As of July 1995, Partners in Caregiving: The Dementia Services Program, had established 50 centers in 31 states (Partners in Caregiving, 1995, July).

Special-purpose centers have also been established for individuals with acquired immunodeficiency syndrome (AIDS), multiple sclerosis, muscular dystrophy, and other special needs populations. Paulette Geller, chairperson of NIAD, speaking at a mini-conference of the 1995 White House Conference on Aging, stated:

> The spectrum of adult day services runs from care for children with chronic diseases, to young adults suffering from MS or MD, to people recovering from head trauma, to elders physically challenged by stroke, heart disease, lung disease, and dementia, such as Alzheimer's disease. Adult day centers have the opportunity to provide efficient care in a congregate setting which can respond to this broad spectrum of needs (Partners in Caregiving, Spring 1995a).

Description of Adult Day Services

PARTICIPANTS

Osorio (1991) states that adult day care clients are commonly called participants, a term that reflects the activity orientation and purposefulness characteristic of adult day care programs. Most adult day care participants have multiple chronic illnesses and specific functional impairment. Participants commonly come to adult day care on referral from an acute care hospital, a rehabilitation center, the family physician, or a community social services agency. Participants vary in their ability to safely spend periods of time alone, a measure of independence frequently involved in decisions about adult day care admissions, along with the level and type of day care provided (Osorio, 1991). Osorio presented the following participant descriptions in her chapter, "Adult Daycare Programs," in *Occupational Therapy and the Older Adult*:

> Mrs. J. is diabetic and has arthritis and congestive heart failure. She lives alone in a large senior housing development where she feels isolated and lonely. She comes to the daycare center twice a week for socialization and health monitoring. Staff help her access other services as needed. The center staff and participants are her extended family.

> Mr. L. lives with his widowed daughter. He has Parkinson's disease and depression and has had two heart attacks in the past 3 years. His unsteady gait and complex medication regime make it unsafe for him to be alone for more than an hour. He comes to daycare 5 days a week while his daughter works. A lifelong worrier, he not only needs the physical and health support but emotionally he feels safer with professional help readily available.

> Mrs. M. has late stage Alzheimer's and is aphasic, apraxic, and incontinent if not on a voiding schedule. She wanders and is disoriented to time, person and place. She requires constant supervision now, although when she enrolled in the center 5 years ago, she was independent in bathrooming, oriented to person and place, had only sporadic problems with word finding but became behaviorally disruptive over changes in her routine. She spends a full 10 hours at the center every week day. Her husband's goal is to minimize the length of time she spends in residential care. The staff supports his goal. Their daily plan of care has evolved over the years from one emphasizing maintenance of function and self-esteem to one that meets basic physiologic and safety needs. Mrs. M. is very comfortable in the daycare center, responding positively to the familiar staff and environment (Osorio, 1991).

These descriptions provide examples of the various levels of care and the range of needs of adult day service participants. They point out the importance of developing an individualized care plan to meet the unique needs of each participant and his or her caregiver. While much of this discussion has focused on the needs of the participant, the caregiver or family member's needs must also be addressed by adult day services staff. Padula (1992) explains that adult day care programs, concerned as they are with the whole person, are well aware of the influence that other persons in the participant's life may have on his or her well-being. Families and other caregivers are a mixed bag. Some have problems of their own. Some may be more caring or more skillful than others (Padula, 1992). Center staff members must maintain an awareness of family and caregiver needs.

Family members might include the spouse, children, siblings, grandchildren, or other extended family such as nieces or nephews. Rathbone-McCuan (1976) states that while the primary consumers of geriatric day care services are the elderly, another consumer group of almost equal importance is made up of the families that bear full or partial responsibility for their care. Recognition that the family is an important corollary consumer of geriatric day care services suggests that the family is a day care client and must be treated as such in program planning and service delivery. Family involvement with day care begins at the point at which the decision to seek care for the aging family member is made and continues until that service ends (Rathbone-McCuan, 1976). Adult day services may offer assistance to families in the form of family education programs, caregiver training programs, counseling sessions, and family support groups. Maintaining ongoing and open communication with the family is one of the keys to a successful experience for the participant.

SERVICES

Von Behren (1988) states that specific services provided in the adult day care setting can be divided into three categories:

1. Basic—meals, transportation, recreation, and personal care (dressing, grooming, toileting)
2. Professional—nursing services, social services, occupational therapy, and physical therapy
3. Medical—physical assessment and treatment, dentistry, podiatry, and psychiatry.

For adult day centers located in the United States, an overview of those providing specific services is as follows: 93% provide recreational therapy or activities, 92% meals, 90% social services, 81% transportation, 80% personal care (bathing, hair, and nail care), 77% nursing services, 60% rehabilitation therapy (speech, physical, and occupational), and 56% medical services (Adult Day Care Letter, 1989).

According to the National Institute on Adult Daycare, services provided by the adult day care center are designed to meet one or more of the following goals:

1. Promote the person's maximum level of independence.
2. Maintain the person's present level of functioning as long as possible, preventing or delaying further deterioration.
3. Restore and rehabilitate the person to the highest possible level of functioning.
4. Provide support, respite, and education for families and other caregivers.
5. Foster socialization and peer interaction (NIAD, 1984).

Services provided for an individual participant are based on a functional assessment and are developed through an interdisciplinary care planning process that may be well-defined and regulated in states where adult day centers are licensed or certified. Interdisciplinary functioning of staff is one of the key elements of a successful adult day care program, allowing for flexibility and collaboration in meeting participants' complex and interrelated needs (NIAD, 1990). Care plans are commonly problem oriented and cover in detail goals, activities, time frames, and responsible staff. The participant, caregiver, or both may be involved in developing the individual plan of care (Osorio, 1993).

Standards and Guidelines for Adult Daycare (NIAD, 1990) states that there are two key principles upon which all day care centers operate. The first is the interdisciplinary functioning of the staff. It is universally found in adult day care centers that programs are strengthened and services improved when participants' needs take precedence over rigid or artificial levels of responsibility. Because the program is client centered and the participants' needs are complex and interrelated, staff interactions and collaborations are required to respond to those needs.

The second common element in adult day care is the therapeutic milieu. The purpose of all activity in the center is to improve the participants' quality of life. Throughout the day, all actions and words center on participants' needs and the improvement of their well-being.

The setting of an adult day care program offers, first of all, a pleasant and enjoyable environment. There is music, conversation, activity, and much more. This setting by itself is actually therapeutic. It is within this environment that all of the various disciplines do their work, such as nursing, social work, therapies, and dietetics. The participants become part of a dynamic environment that adds a measure of satisfaction, involvement, and pleasant anticipation to their lives.

The unique blend of characteristics of the adult day care center as a mode of service delivery includes the following:

- A primary focus on the holistic needs of the participant
- An individualized plan of care for each participant
- Recognition of the significance of the family or caregiver
- Consideration of the sense of belonging that alleviates the isolation caused by the severe impairments experienced by the participants.

After a participant spends a few sessions in adult day care, comments from families often reflect the participant's change in attitude, new interest in life, and for the cognitively intact, renewed motivation to work toward his or her highest level of functioning. The therapeutic strength of adult day care is the blend of a structured health-oriented program with a relaxed environment (NIAD, 1990).

FUNDING SOURCES

In Von Behren's (1986) survey, 579 centers reported on their major sources of funding. Medicaid (48.6%) and participant fees (34%) were found to be the main funding sources in terms of total dollars. Sliding fee scales or other income-based fee structures are in place at many centers. In fact, 20% of adult day care centers report having no fee or asking for donations only (Von

Behren, 1986). Adult day care services are a reasonably priced long-term care service (Osorio, 1991).

NCOA published a summary report (NIAD, 1994/1995) with findings from a questionnaire with responses from 45 state adult day care associations regarding funding sources for adult day services in the United States. Those sources included the following:

- Medicaid (Title XIX) (through state health plans)
- Medicaid Home- and Community-Based Services (HCBS) waiver
- Title XX (social service block grant)
- Older Americans Act (Title III)
- Mental health
- M.R./D.D.
- Veterans' Affairs
- Other
- USDA Child and Adult Care Food Program (NIAD, 1994/1995).

At a White House Conference on Aging Mini-Conference held in Washington, D.C., on February 17, 1995, Pat Shull, Director of Adult Care of Chester County, West Chester, Pennsylvania, presented a provider's perspective on funding. She stated:

> The availability of Medicaid dollars for adult day programs varies with each state. Some provide sufficient reimbursement, others provide reimbursement that is far under the cost of adult day care, and others provide none at all.
> Funding through the Veterans Administration (VA) seems to vary almost as much as Medicaid funding. In the VA system, it seems to be almost specific to the particular facility that is administering funds. Medicare does not pay for adult day care services. If a person is discharged from the hospital and still has medical care needs, he or she has two options if Medicare is to pay. The person can either go to a

skilled nursing facility or be cared for in his or her home by visiting nurses or other professionals. Not only does Medicare not reimburse for adult day services, the regulations and the interpretations of those regulations make it nearly impossible for a person receiving in-home services under Medicare to attend adult day centers in most parts of the country.

In Shull's opinion, any plan regarding health care reform must include adult day services as a mandated service, not only in the text of custodial, long-term care but also in post-hospital care as well (Partners in Caregiving, 1995b). Her comments echo the concerns of providers in the field who believe that federal funding sources are currently inadequate. Providers want policy makers to consider preventive, community-based service options as cost-effective and efficient methods of service delivery when allocating health care funds.

LICENSURE AND CERTIFICATION

Weissert et al. (1990) in their study on adult day care found that requirements for licensure and certification regulate a substantial proportion of adult day care centers. State and local governments establish licensing standards expected of centers used by the public, and certification serves to align a center's operations with a funding agency's guidelines. State laws generally address standards for licensure, while state and federal grant regulations and statutes (such as the state or federal Medicaid program, the Older Americans Act, and the Social Services Block Grants) set certification standards (Weissert et al., 1990).

Licensure is a common requirement of funding and reimbursement sources, and it also provides a level of reassurance to participants, caregivers,

and other professionals that a center meets certain standards. State licensing standards address such issues as ratio of space to number served, accessibility, staffing, services provided, arrangements for meals and snacks, documentation and staff continuing education, and many other aspects of center operations.

Certification, however, is an established option for centers. It may be an independent process separate from licensing or an added credential for an already licensed center. Certification may qualify a center to receive reimbursement from a particular source (e.g., Medicaid) or serve a specific population (e.g., mentally retarded adults) (Osorio, 1991).

NIAD reports that, as of the winter of 1994–95, of the 45 states reporting from state adult day care associations, 21 states had licensure, 21 states had certification, 5 states had both licensure and certification, and 17 states had neither (NIAD, 1994/1995).

Although no national licensure or other method of establishing credentials is currently in place, NIAD publishes national standards that are available to centers that desire additional guidance in providing quality adult day care services (Osorio, 1991).

The Many and Varied Roles of Occupational Therapy in Adult Day Care

As stated earlier, the philosophy of occupational therapy is consistent with the total concept of care advocated in adult day services. The direct care services provided by an occupational therapy practitioner can help the day care participant to regain and retain meaningful life skills. The potential for continued involvement at home and in the community is enhanced by performing appropriate, purposeful activities. Family and other caregivers are also involved with occupational therapy personnel, thus ensuring the carryover of life tasks into the home environment (AOTA, 1986).

Occupational therapy roles can vary according to the emphasis of the day care center and may involve providing direct services, such as evaluation and treatment, or indirect services, such as consultation or education (Osorio, 1993). Occupational therapy practitioners working in adult day services can serve as direct care clinicians, activity program coordinators, case managers, consultants, administrators, educators, researchers, and board members.

DIRECT CARE CLINICIAN

As we examine each of these roles, we find that the most common role for the occupational therapist and the certified occupational therapy assistant is that of direct care clinician. These services are generally provided in a restorative or medical model center. Using the traditional occupational therapy model of service delivery, which includes screening, referral, assessment, treatment planning, reassessment, and discharge, is appropriate in adult day care (AOTA, 1986; Osorio, 1993).

As part of the adult day services multidisciplinary team, the occupational therapist, assisted by the certified occupational therapy assistant, performs a comprehensive assessment of the participant's cognitive, sensorimotor, and psychosocial skills, including the functional performance of self-care, work, and leisure roles. The assessment determines the need for therapy along with type, frequency, and duration of treatment. This initial assessment is the baseline by which the

participant's overall progress can be measured. It consists of standardized and nonstandardized measurements of cognitive, sensorimotor, and psychosocial skills in the functional performance domains of self-care, work, and leisure (AOTA, 1986).

This assessment should include (1) a home evaluation, (2) an assessment and modification of the day care center to maximize performance, and (3) an assessment of the participant's sense of mastery and control of the environment (Osorio, 1993). According to AOTA, following the initial assessment, recommendations for interventions, follow-up services, or further referral may be made (AOTA, 1986). The occupational therapist prepares a written report of the assessment results for the day care record and, when indicated, for the referring physician. Treatment planning and program implementation require that occupational therapy personnel use assessment findings and set long- and short-term goals in collaboration with the participant and his or her caregiver. These goals become a part of the multidisciplinary plan of care. The older adult's strengths, personality, and cultural background are considered in designing the appropriate program of therapeutic activities. In some cases, the occupational therapist may decide that direct treatment is not indicated. The therapist will then design a structured program for the center's staff to carry out to maintain the participant's present levels of function (AOTA, 1986).

NIAD's standards and guidelines for adult day care (NIAD, 1990) state the following:

> Depending on the occupational
> therapy assessment, interdiscipli-
> nary plan of care, and physician's
> orders, occupational therapy ser-
> vices that include but are not
> limited to the following shall

- Administer diagnostic and prognostic tests to determine integrity of upper extremities, ability to transfer, range of motion, balance, strength and coordination, endurance, activities of daily living and cognitive-perception functioning.

- Teach participants adaptive techniques to overcome barriers and impediments in activities of daily living.

- Teach and train other staff in the use of therapeutic, creative and self-care activities to improve or maintain the participant's capacity for self-care and independence and increase the range of motion, strength and coordination.

- Train the participant in the use of supportive and adaptive equipment and assistive devices.

- Evaluate home for environmental barriers and recommend changes needed for greater participant independence.

- Provide restorative therapy when indicated, establish a maintenance program when needed to prevent deterioration, and provide written and verbal instructions to center staff and the family/caregiver to assist the participant with implementation.

- Provide occupational therapy procedures that include these:

  — Training or retraining in activities of daily living (ADL)

  — Training in work simplification techniques

  — Exercises and graded activities to improve strength and range of motion

  — Sensory stimulation techniques to minimize sensory deficits

  — Coordination activities to promote increased manual dexterity

  — Evaluation and provision of needed slings or splints to increase or maintain functional use of upper extremities (NIAD, 1990).

While not totally inclusive, the above guidelines provide the basic range of restorative services provided by the direct care clinicians.

ACTIVITIES PROGRAM COORDINATOR

Occupational therapy practitioners may serve as activity program coordinators for adult day services. In contrast to the direct care occupational therapy program, which is time limited and problem specific, the activities program serves normal activity needs and is ongoing (AOTA, 1986). Activities programs as defined by Crepeau (1980) consist of planned events and tasks designed to provide incentive and opportunity to engage in continuing life experiences and, hence, satisfy interests and meet general activity needs. Activities programs contribute to the prevention of deterioration of mental, physical, and social abilities (Rogers, 1983).

In many instances, the success of the adult day services center itself is directly related to the success of its activities program. According to Rogers (1983), this program is designed to provide physical, intellectual, social, spiritual, and emotional challenges much the same as in everyday life. Participation is based on an assessment of interests and activity needs. As the activities coordinator, the occupational therapist, registered occupational therapist (OTR), or COTA assesses the interests of each participant to determine the activity needs and preferences. The interest survey may be conducted by observing, interviewing, or testing. Family members, friends, and staff may also be contacted for information. An activities plan is developed for each client. The plan identifies the client's interests, general activity needs, and stated goals and identifies the activities to be used to achieve these goals. Each participant's needs are reassessed regularly, and the activities plan is adjusted accordingly.

As the activities coordinator, the OTR or COTA collaborates with the participants to plan, execute, and evaluate a diversified program suited to identified needs and interests. Programs are planned to provide a balance of activities that the participants perceive as useful work and service as well as activities viewed as recreational, spiritual, and educational. Activities programs are varied so that individual as well as group activities are offered. This program is routinely evaluated by the OTR or COTA activities coordinator (Rogers, 1983).

In her article "Adult Day Care: A Model for Changing Times" (1985), Laurie Ellen Neustadt, COTA, describes the activities program at St. Mary's Day Health Center for older adults as central to the success of the Day Health Center program. She states that through an organized activities program, clients can develop their self-esteem and self-worth, establish support systems, engage in socialization, and become involved with purposeful activity. In adult day care activities, one must work with and meet the needs of an extremely varied population with problems ranging from multiple physical handicaps to acute psychological disorders. She explains that the COTA is trained to work with varying degrees of minimal to multiple handicaps and acute to chronic stages of disorder—both physical and psychological—and is competent in adapting activities for the problems encountered. The educational training program for COTAs—a strong focus on a variety of activities, the skills of needs

assessment, and activities adaptation—make the COTA a logical candidate for adult day care activity programmer (Neustadt, 1985).

Neustadt (1985) emphasizes the importance of an activity program designed by a COTA or an OTR being grounded and based on an occupational therapy frame of reference. She explains that the occupational behavior frame of reference is woven into the fiber of the activity program at St. Mary's. The activity program is comprehensive in that it addresses the physical, sensory integration, cognitive, psychological, and social performance components, as well as the occupational performance areas of self-care, work, homemaking, and play or leisure. She gives excellent examples of the activities used and the performance components they satisfy. She explains that the physical component is addressed in the daily group exercise program, the "Willing Walkers Club," and a daily informal exercise group. Clients presently receiving treatment from the registered occupational therapist do supportive exercises during this informal group with the COTA, using input from the OTR. Cards and table games, brain teasers, reminiscing groups, discussion groups, story reading, educational programs, and guest lecturers involve the cognitive component. Psychological and social components are touched upon in weekly membership group meetings. Specific issues that have come up with individuals or the groups are discussed. These components are also addressed in other group discussions, programs, and the daily interpersonal relationships that are an ongoing part of the center.

Neustadt further explains that center activities include the occupational performance areas of self-care, work, homemaking, and play or leisure. Most of the clients' self-care needs are addressed by the nursing and occupational therapy staff on an individual basis. Clients are involved in homemaking activities through cooking, sewing, and gardening groups. Clients also assist in home-making chores of the center such as watering plants, clearing the table, and helping with dishes. Clients have expressed a need to remain involved in work-oriented projects. Volunteer projects such as preparing mailings, sewing projects, and sorting stamps are brought in from community agencies like the American Red Cross and the Retired Senior Volunteer Program (Neustadt, 1985).

CASE MANAGER

An occupational therapist working as a case manager in adult day services is one of the newer roles. The definition of case management approved by the Case Management Society of America (CMSA) is that of a process directed at assessing needs, coordinating resources, and creating flexible, cost-effective options for catastrophically or chronically ill or injured individuals on a case-by-case basis to facilitate quality, individualized treatment goals (CMSA, 1995).

The role of case manager is to service clients by assessing, facilitating, planning, and advocating for health needs on an individual basis. The skills include, but are not limited to, positive relationship building, effective written or verbal communication, and the ability to effect change, perform critical analysis, plan, organize effectively, and promote autonomy. It is crucial to have knowledge of funding resources, services, and clinical standards and outcomes (CMSA, 1995).

In "The Occupational Therapist as a Case Manager," AOTA (1991) described minimum qualifications for occupational therapists and certified occupational therapy assistants. Occupational

therapists with 5 years of experience, of which 3 years are within a specific practice arena, are qualified to assume job positions as case managers. Advanced certified occupational therapy assistants with 5 years of experience, of which 3 years are within a specific practice arena, who have attained skills in management, communications, and systems, may assume a case management role with persons in a long-term care setting (AOTA, 1991). Occupational therapists interested in case management must also meet the criteria for eligibility to take the examination for certified case managers.

Snow states:

[O]ccupational therapists have a unique and exciting perspective to contribute to case management as a profession and as an activity. Therapists have the skills not only to see *what is*, but by virtue of their training, they can also envision *what might be*. Thus, therapists in the role of case manager can offer ideas and opportunities for changes that when enacted enhance the quality of life for their clients.... Our unique training and theory base make occupational therapists an excellent choice for the role of care coordinator, client advocate, resource allocator, and service evaluator (Snow, 1991).

As case manager in adult day services, the occupational therapist is the personal advocate for the participant. This is similar to primary nurse management of the hospitalized patient. The case manager performs an initial patient screen, leads the interdisciplinary team in preparing and regularly updating a comprehensive treatment plan, monitors intervention by other team members, and is the family or caregiver liaison. Case management means coordinating all information regarding medications, health, financial status, adequacy of home care, caregiver fatigue, ADL, and environment, and relaying that information to the appropriate staff person for intervention. Concerns regarding community resources are handled by the case manger in consultation with the social worker (Huff, 1988). Case management is clearly a profession that is having a profound effect on health care to older adults in this country. If they so choose, occupational therapists can be a major component in the case management profession (Snow, 1991).

CONSULTANT

For many years, occupational therapists have provided services to adult day centers as consultants. According to Epstein (1985b), the occupational therapy consultant can play an important role in the development and implementation of adult day care programs.

As a consultant, the occupational therapist does not provide direct treatment but uses occupational therapy expertise to help adult day care planners and staff (which may include occupational therapy personnel) mobilize internal and external resources needed to develop and effectively operate the program. This is achieved by communicating information, concepts, values, and skills from an occupational therapy perspective. Other key elements in consultation are an understanding of systems and of organizational theory and behavior, an ability to communicate and to listen effectively, and a capacity to diagnose a problem and offer appropriate strategies or recommend activities (Epstein, 1985a, 1985b).

According to Osorio (1991), consultant roles vary from traditional case consultation, a critical role in centers with no OT staff, to program consultation, where the occupational therapist is involved in defining programs, evaluating and resolving problems, and carrying out special projects. The occupational therapist may serve as consul-

tant to the board, director, or staff on a long-term or time-limited basis (Osorio, 1991).

Epstein (1992) maintains that adult day care programs are an important preventive strategy for maintaining frail elderly individuals in the community. Occupational therapy consultants can provide invaluable guidance and expertise to community groups establishing adult day care programs. They can facilitate the development of adult day care centers, help ensure their maintenance, and provide the case consultation necessary to develop individual plans of care for participants with special needs (Epstein, 1992).

Long-term care has extended its focus beyond institutional walls. Occupational therapy consultants must use their creative abilities in less traditional settings where older persons require health-related services. Adult day care programs, nutrition sites, senior centers, and congregate living sites are among those services to be considered. To improve the quality of life for this population, consultants must develop a diversified knowledge base, expanded resources, and broader systems skills. Today's aging population, with its multiple needs, will benefit from the expertise that such consultants can provide (Epstein, 1992).

As the number of adult day care programs continues to grow, so will the demand for occupational therapy services. Using a consultative model, particularly in social or health maintenance day settings, occupational therapists can make significant contributions in the delivery of day care services (Epstein, 1985b).

Epstein (1992) notes that this consultation occurred over a decade ago. The adult day care program is still housed in what was originally thought to be an interim "first" site. The program now runs 5 days a week, from 7:00 a.m. to 5:00 p.m. versus its original 3-day, 10:00 a.m. to 3:00 p.m. schedule. The clientele has expanded from 5 to 30 individuals. The program now arranges restorative services for its participants on an outpatient basis at the local hospital. Thus, it is now able to meet the needs of those participants who require a more medically oriented program while providing the necessary maintenance and social programs at the center. From the consultant's perspective, the program's growth and development have more than met initial expectations. From the community's perspective, the adult day care program is viewed as an important and necessary part of services provided for older persons in the county (Epstein, 1992).

ADMINISTRATOR

While few occupational therapists are currently serving as administrators of adult day programs, experienced occupational therapists with expertise in gerontology do possess the leadership and management skills to direct a program. Osorio (1985) explains that being the executive director of an adult day care center is similar to managing a large occupational therapy department or a private practice. Supervisory, planning, and documentation skills are essential. In other areas, the agency executive role is unique and can offer significant challenges to the experienced therapist seeking new opportunities in administration. Osorio summarizes the executive director's responsibilities, which include the following:

- Financial management
- Policy development and implementation
- Personnel functions, such as leadership and supervision of a multidisciplinary team

- Program planning and evaluation
- Maintenance of agency records, including documentation of services provided
- Compliance with licensing regulations, public relations, and marketing
- Preparation of operational reports
- Fund raising
- Long-range planning.

Other duties include student supervision, consultation to other agencies, and legislative advocacy.

According to Osorio (1985), the executive director is responsible for the total operation of the agency. A typical day may include the following:

- Conducting a team meeting
- Preparing a report for a funding source or a meeting with auditors
- Making face-to-face contact with current and prospective participants and families
- Negotiating a contract for meal service
- Responding to an unannounced visit by licensing staff
- Making personal contacts to recruit volunteers
- Raising funds for a needed piece of equipment.

Duties vary and require the development of new skills.

Osorio contends that the executive director's vision for the agency and relationship with the staff must be multidisciplinary. Although the director makes decisions based on the values in his or her profession of origin, the success of the agency depends on ability to hire, retrain, motivate, and supervise a multidisciplinary team capable of providing quality care. Territoriality has no place when one supervises professionals and students from other disciplines.

Osorio explains that contrary to the cardinal rule that each employee have only one supervisor, the executive director of a nonprofit agency is likely to have 20 or more. The board of directors sets policy for the agency, and the executive serves at the will of this board. In seeming contradiction, board members, who are volunteers, look to the executive director for guidance regarding the work that needs to be done to maintain the agency. The relationship between the board and the executive director can be described as one of dynamic tension, with each party challenging the other to uphold its responsibilities to the agency. Board members represent a broad cross section of the community served and offer each other and the executive continuous opportunities for learning. Education is a critical activity when attorneys and accountants are asked to make decisions about patient care issues, and human service professionals are involved in important financial decisions.

The successful executive director may spend as much time on activities away from the agency as on in-house responsibilities. He or she is responsible for marketing the services provided, maintaining productive relationships with other agencies, and participating in community-wide efforts to improve the health and social service delivery system. Just as the occupational therapist or executive director must think beyond occupational therapy within the agency, the executive director must think beyond the agency when serving on community committees, boards, and task forces (Osorio, 1985).

Osorio encourages occupational therapists to seek out adult day care centers as these centers offer a variety of opportunities to learn new skills and pose a challenge to therapists' existing administrative and personal skills

(Osorio, 1985). Given the philosophy of adult day care, occupational therapists with management skills are ideally suited for center administrator positions (Osorio, 1993).

EDUCATOR

Occupational Therapy Roles (AOTA, 1993) describes the major function of an educator as developing and providing educational offerings or OT training to consumer, peer, and community individuals or groups. The role of the OT educator is described as practitioners advancing along a continuum. The role ranges from providing informal education to individuals and small groups in the course of service provision to developing and providing comprehensive educational programs targeted to consumers and peers. At the entry level of the role, education typically occurs with peers and consumers within the individual's own service system (patient education department or school district in-service). At higher levels of expertise, provision of educational offerings may involve individuals or groups from multiple systems (e.g., provision of injury prevention programs to industry, caregiver education programs to community, and continuing education seminars).

Occupational Therapy Roles (AOTA, 1993) identifies the following key performance areas:

- Entry-level skills
- Intermediate skills
- High-proficiency skills
- Supervision.

Entry-Level Skills

The following skills are considered entry level:

- Implements strategies to assist the individual learner to identify his or her own learning needs

- Develops or collaborates with individual learner in establishing learning objectives
- Implements educational methods designed to support learner's objectives
- Responds to feedback about the teaching-learning process, and modifies his or her own educational strategies to support learning
- Supports the evaluation of educational effectiveness
- Monitors his or her own performance and identifies his or her own development needs.

The entry-level occupational therapist or working in adult day services would have the opportunity to educate participants, caregivers, and staff members on various topics, such as the role of occupational therapy, how to best assist a participant with specific ADL tasks, and teaching staff to follow a functional maintenance program designed by the occupational therapist.

Intermediate Skills

The following skills are considered intermediate:

- Selects or designs strategies to identify individual learner's needs
- Develops program plans and materials for formal program offerings (e.g., conferences, presentations, workshops, seminars)
- Uses a variety of teaching and learning methods appropriate to meet the learning objectives and learner's needs.

The occupational therapy practitioner as an educator with intermediate-level skills might present a workshop for adult day services staff, including experiential learning opportunities in which staff members simulate the impairments that their elderly participants must endure daily. The purpose of such a workshop would be to provide a setting for learners to develop a greater understanding of, appreciation for, and ability to relate empathetically to participants' needs.

High-Proficiency Skills

The following skills require high proficiency:

- Evaluates strategies to identify learning needs of individuals and groups
- Develops program plans and educational methods for extended or multiple program offerings
- Designs evaluation strategies to assess the impact of educational programs.

The occupational therapy practitioner serving as an educator with high-proficiency skills in the area of adult day services may find the need to present a seminar or series of seminars for local politicians on the efficacy and cost-containment value of adult day services as opposed to other long-term care options.

The qualifications to serve as an educator include the following:

- National Board for Certification in Occupational Therapy (NBCOT) certification as an OTR or COTA
- Progressive levels of expertise, which require combinations of self-study, continuing education, experience, and post-entry-level formal education
- Appropriate level of practice or service expertise as it relates to the provision of these educational services.

Supervision

Supervision depends on the nature of the project and the skills of the educator. COTAs at all levels usually will require OTR supervision for educational activities that occur related to occupational therapy consumers (AOTA, 1993).

In general terms, occupational therapists serve as educators by helping learners understand and value the promoting of health through activity (AOTA, 1986). Educator roles vary from fieldwork education supervisor to in-service, health, and community educator. Centers without occupational therapists would benefit from in-service education on topics such as environmental modification, adaptation of activities, and the impact of activity on health. Health education programs and support groups directed at participants and caregivers can stress various aspects of healthy behavior, coping, and caregiving skills. Community education activities involve developing public awareness of the potential needs of older adults and services available to them and their families (Osorio, 1991).

Occupational therapists use their expertise as educators through writing and producing books, pamphlets, audio cassettes, and videotapes to teach participants, caregivers, staff, and the community in general about issues pertaining to the needs of the frail elderly and how to address those needs. For example, Anne Morris and Gail Hunt have produced a 16-minute videotape and a 27-page companion booklet, *A Part of Daily Life: Alzheimer's Caregivers Simplify Activities and the Home* (Morris & Hunt, 1994). This educational resource provides instruction and demonstrates practical techniques that caregivers can use to manage family members with Alzheimer's disease in the home setting.

RESEARCHER

Occupational therapy practitioners working in adult day services are presented with unlimited opportunities to conduct research activities, especially in this era of health care reform where budget constraints and cost-cutting measures are widespread. In an article by Javernick (1993), Thibodaux states that with health care reform, occupational therapy practitioners are going to be called on to show outcomes for their services (Javernick, 1993). The only effective way to verify outcomes is through systematic scientific inquiry into the effects of occupational therapy intervention and clear dissemination of the results (Timmerman, Schmidt, & Heater, 1994). For research-oriented occupational therapy practitioners opportunities abound in day care centers in such areas as evaluating the effectiveness of center services and studying long-term outcomes of the rehabilitation, which frequently precedes adult day care referral (Osorio, 1993).

Occupational Therapy Roles (AOTA, 1993) describes the major function of a researcher as performance of scholarly work of the profession, including examining, developing, refining, and evaluating the profession's body of knowledge, theoretical base, and philosophical foundations.

The scope of the role of researcher ranges from the individual who critically examines and interprets empirical studies to the independent investigator. Key performance areas include the following:

- Entry-level skills
- Intermediate skills
- High-proficiency skills
- Qualifications.

Entry-Level Skills

The following are considered entry-level skills:

- Promotes and engages in research activities

- Reads, interprets, and applies scholarly information relative to occupational therapy
- Collects research data
- Assumes responsibility for the ethical concerns in research and complies with institutional bio-ethical committee protocols.

Intermediate Skills

The following are considered intermediate-level skills:

- Directs the completion of studies, including data analysis, interpretation, and dissemination of results
- Collaborates with others to facilitate studies of concern to the profession
- Monitors resources that facilitate research and scholarly activities.

High-Proficiency Skills

The following are high proficiency skills:

- Probes methods of science, theoretical information, or research designs to answer questions important to the profession
- Conceptualizes the body of knowledge in the profession to develop new theories, frames of reference, or models of practice
- Mentors novice researchers
- Participates at leadership level in professional volunteer organizations.

Qualifications

The following qualifications are required to be a researcher:

- NBCOT certification as an OTR or COTA
- A combination of self-study, continuing education, experience, and formal education for independent research or scholarly activities

- For COTAs, additional academic qualifications to be a principal investigator.

Supervision ranges from close to minimal, depending on the nature of the project and the skills of the researcher (AOTA, 1993).

Throughout the profession is genuine concern that research productivity has lagged behind that of other professions. Timmerman et al. (1994) state that a lack of occupational therapy research is a recognized and persistent problem that is often acknowledged throughout the literature but not addressed. Reasons for lack of research include the following:

- Occupational therapy clinicians, especially those entering professional practice with a bachelor's degree, appear not to believe that they possess the research expertise to design and implement studies (Taylor & Mitchell, 1990)
- Most therapists today believe that their workloads are too heavy to allow them to undertake research
- Most therapists have not been socialized into a profession that truly values research because few faculty members or clinical supervisors are engaged in research while they are serving as role models (Gillette & Mitcham, 1994).

Timmerman et al. strongly believe that action must be taken to involve clinicians in the effort to substantiate the efficacy of treatments through outcome studies. Timmerman et al. (1994) suggest that the following recommendations be implemented on a national level:

- Reward published research with continuing education units
- Institute low-cost seminars
- Increase American Occupational Therapy Foundation (AOTF) funds and accessibility

- Negotiate with employers for research support
- Incorporate research into all educational programs.

AOTF's Research Advisory Council is charged with overseeing the development of planning for the research needs of the profession. Gillette and Mitcham (1994), who are leaders at AOTF, report that they are in full agreement with recommendations made by Timmerman et al. and have even included additional strategies that are now under consideration by the AOTF's Research Advisory Council. In support of continued and increased occupational therapy research efforts, the long-range plan of the Research Advisory Council includes the following:

- Continue to foster the development of the profession's body of knowledge through direct and indirect support of research
- Support the recruitment, development, and retention of scholars for diverse roles in practice, education, and research
- Promote the dissemination, exchange, and use of knowledge derived through research
- Promote research competencies of practicing therapists
- Establish mechanisms that promote the valuing of research across the profession (AOTF, 1994).

With the support of the AOTF, the occupational therapy practitioner pursuing research in the adult day services setting can take advantage of all the educational, financial, and professional resources available. Important research projects in the area of adult day services can involve studies on program evaluation, quality assurance, and cost-effectiveness of the service.

BOARD MEMBER

Osorio (1991) states that every non-profit adult day care center has a board of directors that is legally responsible for the center. As a board member, an occupational therapist can play a role in setting policy and monitoring the business and programmatic aspects of the agency. Board members are volunteers, so it is ideal to combine this role with paid employment in other occupational therapy settings. For-profit and public centers usually have advisory boards, which have less legal authority but offer many of the same opportunities for involvement in program development and evaluation (Osorio, 1991).

REFERRAL SOURCE

Occupational therapists working with older adults in various settings can play a critical role in referring patients to adult day services. Although self-referral may occur with some frequency in the case of social model programs, it is more common for potential consumers to access adult day care on the recommendation of other care providers, such as physicians, therapists, social service agencies, health agencies, and hospitals. Family, friends, and word of mouth are common sources of referral, perhaps reflecting growing consumer awareness of the adult day care option and a high level of community satisfaction with the service. Occupational therapists and COTAs in a variety of settings should routinely screen their older adult patients for the appropriateness of adult day care referral (Osorio, 1991).

Cultural, Legal, and Ethical Considerations

CULTURAL CONSIDERATIONS

The OT practitioner working in adult day services must always consider the cultural background of the client in designing an appropriate program for direct care OT services. The elements of an individual's culture include morals, art, law, customs, speech patterns, interaction, economic and production patterns, goals, beliefs, and values (Krefting & Krefting, 1991). Occupational therapy assessment should begin with identifying the participant's valued goals and then proceed to determining the factors that interfere with the accomplishment of those goals. Whether functioning in direct care or as a consultant, case manager, activity program coordinator, administrator, researcher, educator, or board member, occupational therapists must be sensitive to the cultural background of the individual, group, or organization for which they are providing services.

According to Krefting and Krefting, the purpose of sensitizing therapists to cultural factors in human performance is to improve practice. The consequences of dismissing cultural factors in occupational therapy assessment and intervention are enormous, especially for the direct care clinician in adult day services. Without an understanding of cultural factors, establishing rapport will be difficult, thereby decreasing the patient's or client's (in this case, participant's) trust in the therapist. Poor rapport can develop into major communication problems, such as the two parties holding different treatment goals and priorities. Different goals and priorities can in turn result in a patient's or client's noncompliance and dissatisfaction with treatment. Moreover, by ignoring cultural factors, therapists can come to feel helpless or develop a dislike of an individual or a group. Family members may be affected by cultural problems and become antagonists rather than facilitators of treatment (Krefting & Krefting, 1991). Therefore, the following factors influenced by culture should be considered in the occupational therapy assessment:

- Use of time
- Balance of work and play
- Sense of personal space
- Values regarding finances
- Roles assumed in the family
- Knowledge of disability
- Sources of information
- Amount and level of assistance the client will accept from others
- Sense of control over events that happen to the client
- Typical or preferred coping strategies
- Style of expressing emotions (Krefting & Krefting, 1991).

What makes culture even more important is the increasing number and variety of cultural groups in North America. Changing immigration laws and refugee policies and increased mobility within regions of North America have created a situation in which a therapist may work with people from nearly every cultural group in the world. This growing cultural diversity shows no signs of slowing down, so cultural factors will undoubtedly continue to become more significant in occupational therapy practice (Krefting & Krefting, 1991).With adult day centers located in all parts of this country serving the needs of culturally diverse groups, sensitivity on the part of the OT practitioner, whether providing direct or indirect service, is required.

LEGAL AND ETHICAL CONSIDERATIONS

Occupational therapists and certified occupational therapy assistants must practice in accordance with state licensure laws, facility regulations, AOTA standards of practice (AOTA, 1983), and the Principles of Occupational Therapy Ethics (AOTA, 1984). Confidentiality should be maintained according to the AOTA Code of Ethics (AOTA, 1994b).

Conclusions

Adult day services are thriving and expanding to meet the needs of the rapidly increasing population of older adults and adults with special needs. Adult day service providers have found that their target population is currently older and more frail, has more impairments, has a greater incidence of Alzheimer's disease, and has more complex health care needs. Therefore, adult day services can be characterized as a growing, evolving program dedicated to meeting participants' needs. In many cases, the program is developed without external influence. The parameters, the services, the philosophy, and the participants all form an identifiable group. It is a program that provides a range of services in a structured, centralized setting designed to meet the restorative and maintenance needs of functionally impaired individuals and their families (NIAD, 1990).

When one considers adult day services, occupational therapy's historical and philosophical similarities, and the varied and challenging roles that occupational therapy practitioners can fulfill in adult day services, one would assume that significant numbers of occupational therapists and COTAs are practicing in this arena. Unfortunately, this is not the case. In 1976, Kiernat described adult day care as a "golden opportunity" for therapists. She wrote, "Day care is an exciting development for the profession of occupational therapy" (Kiernat, 1976). She expounded on all the opportunities that were available to therapists at that time to establish day care programs using various grants and other funding sources. "But where are the therapists?" she laments (Kiernat, 1976). In 1985, MacDonald, one of six committee members appointed to write a "roles and function" paper on the role of the occupational therapist in adult day care, stated that "committee members attempted to network with occupational therapists working in day care facilities, yet made surprisingly few contacts" (MacDonald, 1985). When these reports are combined with the data from AOTA's member data survey of 1990, not only are the numbers of occupational therapists and COTAs working in adult day service centers small, but also they are declining (see Table 10–1).

The reasons for the lack of OT practitioners in this setting are difficult to analyze. However, a combination of factors—such as the well-documented shortage of occupational therapists (Silvergleit, 1994), the lower percentage of OTRs specializing in geriatrics as opposed to other age groups (28.2% in geriatrics, 37.2% in adults, and 34.7% in pediatrics) (AOTA, 1990), and the limited resources of adult day centers to pay for OT services—may explain the low numbers. However, in spite of these facts and figures, with health care trends and funding moving toward community-based care, occupational therapists and COTAs working as clinicians, activities coordinators, consultants, case managers, administrators, and board members can still assume leadership positions in this ever-evolving practice arena.

Table 10–1. Occupational Therapy Practitioners Working in Adult Day Services*

	1973	1977	1982	1986	1990
OTRs	1.4	1.1	1.0	1.1	0.9
COTAs	1.2	2.4	2.0	4.3	1.7

*Numbers represent percentages.
Source: AOTA, 1990.

The field of adult day services is attempting to position itself as a major provider of long-term-care services along with nursing homes and home health care. The following categories, as published in *Respite Report: Special Issue* (Partners in Caregiving, Spring 1995c), constitute major areas of concern in the field with specific recommendations submitted to the 1995 White House Conference on Aging:

Financing/funding.

- Restructure the Medicaid program so that adult day services (both medical and social models) become a federally mandated benefit as opposed to coverage/ reimbursement at the discretion of each state.

- Restructure the Medicare program to include coverage/reimbursement for adult day services (both medical and social models).

- Mandate coverage/reimbursement for adult day services (both medical and social models) through the Department of Veteran's Affairs, as opposed to current contractual arrangements at the discretion of local VA medical centers.

Education/public awareness.

- Create an extensive educational campaign to inform consumers, service providers, and policy makers as to the existence of adult day services as a viable option to institutional care.

Tax credits and deductions.

- Expand current dependent care tax credits to include tax write-offs for the retired spouse using his or her own funds to purchase adult day services.

- Provide tax incentives to the private sector to encourage the creation of additional community-based adult day centers.

Private sector initiatives.

- Include adult day services as a vital component of all managed care and/or capitation models.

- Develop and mandate standardized adult day services benefits in long-term-care insurance products.

- Create consumer incentives to encourage the purchase of long-term-care insurance.

Research.

- Conduct research on the cost-effectiveness and long-term benefits/significance of adult day services, which would include the effect on hospital care and institutional care.

- Conduct research to quantify and qualify the belief that adult day services promote quality of life, which would include caregiver/ family and client/participant satisfaction.

Regulations.

- Adopt, as federal standards, the Standards and Guidelines for

Adult Day Care developed by the National Institute on Adult Day-care (Partners in Caregiving, 1995).

The preceding list of recommendations clearly identifies the goals and long-range plans of the adult day services movement in this country. Concerns regarding future funding sources represent the major areas of concern for this group.

The profession of occupational therapy, as well, shares these same concerns in this era of shrinking health care dollars. Mary Foto, President of the American Occupational Therapy Association, predicts that by the year 2000, 80% of reimbursement will be through some form of capitation or fixed rate. She states that change is the name of the game in health care. In the shift to managed care that is already under way, the profession confronts a number of critical issues regarding the allocation of educational and health care resources. She warns that unless occupational therapy practitioners commit themselves to improving their participation in the collection of outcome data, their understanding of reimbursement, and their personal involvement on behalf of the profession, other persons or entities will be making decisions for them (Joe, 1995).

Therefore, occupational therapists and COTAs need to support the adult day services movement and the profession of occupational therapy by taking on a proactive, leadership role. Actively supporting federal legislation that will cover and reimburse adult day services and occupational therapy services, especially those under managed care or capitation models, will ensure the growth and development of these vital community-based services for the elderly.

Yerxa (1995) states that today, the entire medical-industrial complex is searching for viable community-based alternatives to hospitalization and nursing home care. Adult day services and occupational therapy are both suited to fill this void and meet this need. Yerxa (1995) aptly explains that we are already developing and demonstrating new models of community-based practice that improve the health and life opportunities for persons with disabilities and keep persons out of institutions. These present and future needs require an army of occupational therapists steeped in the knowledge of whole people. The persons we serve are seen as open human systems, interacting with their environments, possessing strengths and capabilities to adapt to environmental challenges and attain health even in the presence of chronic conditions. Such knowledge, rather than being limited to the natural or physical sciences, is complex, sophisticated, interdisciplinary, and subtle. It requires a long period of professional education and an autonomous professional occupational therapist to apply it, individual by individual, in the real world of home and community.

Since the early 20th century, no other profession has focused on people's abilities to engage in their daily occupations with skill and satisfaction (Yerxa, 1995). According to history and philosophy, occupational therapy and adult day services are ideally suited to meet the complex needs of the growing frail elderly population utilizing a community-based model of service delivery.

Summary

Adult day services represent an idea whose time has come. This community-based group program, designed to meet the needs of the functionally impaired older adult, allows the participants to have the opportunity to remain living at home for as long as possible in a cost-effective manner. The adult day services movement is supported nationally by the National Council on Aging's constituent unit, the National Institute of Adult Daycare. The number of adult day care centers has risen from 15 in 1975 to 3,000 in 1994. As the elderly population has increased steadily and as health care delivery has shifted from institutions to the community, adult day services have become a practical and appealing part of the solution to long-term-care needs.

Occupational therapy and adult day services are closely related historically and philosophically. Adult day services have been classified into three basic models: social, medical, and restorative. However, it is more useful to conceptualize the world of adult day services into a continuum from social to restorative—stretching from limited direct services to intensive and extensive medical and therapeutic services. The development of health maintenance and special-purpose centers grew out of the desire to meet the combined needs of some frail elderly and the needs of special populations, such as those with Alzheimer's disease.

Most adult day services participants have multiple chronic illnesses and specific functional impairment. An individualized plan of care is established to meet the unique needs of each participant and his or her caregivers. It is very important that family member or caregiver needs be met by family education programs, caregiver training programs, counseling, and support groups. Services provided are divided into three categories: basic, professional, and medical. Interdisciplinary functioning of staff is one of the key elements of a successful adult day care program, allowing for flexibility and collaboration in meeting participants' complex and interrelated needs.

Adult day programs are funded mainly by Medicaid and participant fees. However, other federally mandated programs such as Title XX, the Older Americans Act (Title III), and others fund the centers. Some centers are licensed—a common requirement of funding and reimbursement sources. Certification is also an option. Certification may qualify a center to receive reimbursement from a particular source. Although no national licensure or other method of earning credentials is currently in place, NIAD publishes national standards for centers that desire additional guidance in providing quality care.

Occupational therapy practitioners working in adult day services assume a variety of roles. Those roles can vary according to the emphasis of the adult day services center and may involve the provision of direct services, such as evaluation and treatment, or indirect services, such as consultation or education. Occupational therapists and COTAs can serve as direct care clinicians, activity program coordinators, case managers, consultants, administrators, educators, researchers, and board members. They play the critical role of referral source—referring patients, clients, and residents to adult day centers.

A high-level of awareness pertaining to cultural issues must be maintained by occupational therapists and certified occupational therapy assistants serving adult day centers located in culturally diverse areas. Sensitivity on the part of the occupational therapy practitioner, whether providing direct or indirect service, is crucial. As well, occupational therapy professionals must always adhere to legal and ethical standards of practice. Respecting the rights of the elderly, treating them with respect and dignity, always enhances the practice of this profession, especially in adult day services.

Review Questions

1. Give a brief definition of adult day services.

2. Explain how adult day services may meet the needs of the frail elderly better than nursing home placement or home health services.

3. Describe the role of occupational therapy in the historical development of adult day services.

4. Note that the basic philosophy and values of occupational therapy and adult day services are similar in many ways. Identify and explain these similarities.

5. Name and describe the five types of adult day services settings (models of care).

6. Describe the importance of family members and caregivers in adult day service programs.

7. Identify and describe the three basic categories of services provided to adult day services participants.

8. Identify three funding sources for adult day services.

9. Discuss the difference between licensure and certification of adult day service centers.

10. Recall that occupational therapy practitioners working in adult day services can serve in a variety of roles. Name and describe four different occupational therapy roles.

11. Explain why it is important to consider cultural considerations when providing occupational therapy services in an adult day services setting.

12. In this era of decreasing health care dollars, funding, practitioners, and adult day services providers, identify approaches that each group can use to improve, increase, or enhance funding.

13. Pretend you are an occupational therapist who has been selected to serve as case manager to a group of participants at an adult day services center. Describe your role and functions in this setting.

14. Compare and contrast the role of the direct care OT practitioner providing services to participants in adult day centers to that of the consultant occupational therapist providing services to adult day centers.

15. Decide that you wish to take a more active role in advocating for increased funding for occupational therapy and adult day services. Plan and develop a strategy to promote your cause at the local, state, and federal levels.

Case Studies

CASE STUDY 1—E. R.

This case study describes the direct care clinician's focus with a day care participant (Damico, 1985).

E. R. is a 50-year-old man who had a cerebrovascular accident with resulting right hemiplegia and aphasia. On discharge from the hospital, his family closed his apartment and moved him to a more supervised environment. In this unfamiliar setting, he began to develop a pattern of isolation because of his communication deficits and lack of psychosocial skills. E. R. was admitted to the day care center. The occupational therapy plan over a course of years consisted of the following:

- Management of the right upper extremity, prevention of contracture. Modalities: Group exercise program, prescribed upper extremity activity program to be followed at the center, and development of a home program.
- Increasing psychosocial skills and independent living skills. Modalities: Participating in group lunch preparation sessions, homemaking training, and instruction in use of assistive devices.
- Establishing and increasing independence in apartment. Modalities: Home visits for safety equipment and environmental reorganization, laundry management, and shopping.

These goals could not have been accomplished in the relatively short period of time usually allotted in an acute rehabilitation setting or in a home care program (Damico, 1985).

CASE STUDY 2—ROLE OF THE CASE MANAGER

This case study describes how the occupational therapist in the role of a case manager interacts with a day care participant in a veterans' adult day health care center as described by Sherry Huff, OTR, RN, at the Portland Veterans Administration (VA) Medical Center in Portland, Oregon.

Mr. G, who is 95 years of age and a World War I veteran, is a widower with no children. His primary medical problem is severe congestive heart failure. He has decreased vision, is very hard of hearing, and has unstable ambulation and urinary incontinence. He is, however, fully alert and oriented. He has a brother who assists him managing his finances, but Mr. G writes his own checks.

After a long admission in the VA hospital for treatment of pneumonia and a urinary tract infection, Mr. G became so weak that it was necessary for him to relocate from his home of many years to foster care. He was referred by the hospital team to the newly opened adult day health center (ADHC) program for health monitoring, endurance building, and assistance in his transition and adjustment to his new home. The occupational therapist became his case manager.

From the outset, Mr. G complained of the care at his foster home, stating the food was not good as well as other complaints. The case manager listened to these problems, but consultation with the nurse practitioner assured the case manager that the patient was not losing weight or adding water weight in the form of pedal edema. Thus, combined with his grumbles at ADHC activities, the home problems were deemed to be minor and probably necessary in his readjustment to foster home living.

Incontinence, aggravated by the water pill Lasix, was another issue requiring the intervention of the case manager, with assistance and coordination of the team. Final resolution required experimentation with continence techniques and aides as well as phone conversations with the foster care provider concerning the recommended system.

The case manager also maintained communication with Mr. G's 88-year-old brother. The brother had no car and visited by bus on Sundays. He reported moderate satisfaction with the foster care, but he stated that he had nothing with which to compare it. Mr. G was asked about his care, but severe hearing loss made ongoing communication challenging and sometimes confusing, even with the use of amplification devices. Writing also proved to be laborious and frequently misunderstood. After approximately 2 months, it became apparent that Mr. G was not adjusting to his foster home and that indeed some of his complaints were valid. When asked, the brother and the transportation driver reported that at times Mr. G would be home alone. A visit by the case manager revealed that the home provided inappropriate stimulation and care for Mr. G and that the caregiver frequently left him alone. On the case manager's recommendation, the ADHC team agreed that Mr. G should move. The case manager then contacted the VA social worker in charge of foster home placement who arranged another home and also dealt with the defective home. The case manager then found a resource in a man with a pick-up truck who moves older people for a small fee. A case manager or occupational therapist visit to the new home confirmed the success of the move and provided an opportunity to demonstrate safe ambulation techniques and bathroom transfers, issue appropriate equipment, and recommend room rearrangement and lighting changes to optimize Mr. G's safe ambulation and optimum care. Mr. G is very happy in his new home.

CASE STUDY 3—ROLE OF THE CONSULTANT

The following case was excerpted from Epstein's article in the Gerontology Special Interest Section Newsletter (1985b) as well as highlighted in *Occupational Therapy Consultation: Theory, Principles, and Practice* (Epstein, 1992). This case study exemplifies the occupational therapist in a consultant role.

In a semirural part of New Jersey, a community organization committed to helping low-income elderly wanted to develop an adult day care program. Although the members of the organization understood the concept of adult day care and were sure of its validity for their population, they had no experience in delivering direct services. To develop the program and the appropriate health and social services, the board of directors decided to employ a health care consultant who was an occupational therapist. The consultant worked with the board of directors and the board's administrative assistant toward their goal of opening the center. The scope of the program was defined, and the necessary strategies for working with other community organizations were identified. Program guidelines, policies, and procedures were developed. Other important issues were funding and the search for space and staff (NCOA, 1984).

Initial consultation efforts focused on helping the board understand the variations possible in day care programming. The board had considered only the medical or restorative day care model prior to consultation and did not understand that social day care and social health maintenance day care were viable alternatives for their population (Padula, 1983).

The restorative model, while offering the most extensive rehabilitation services, is the most restrictive in terms of the amount of time a client is eligible to receive the service. It also requires broader compliance with a variety of health regulations which, in turn, severely limits the organization's options for space.

After much study and discussion, the model of choice was social-health maintenance. Here, the client would receive essential health monitoring services and would be able to participate for an unlimited amount of time. The choice of day care was a major decision, which then guided the planning for space, type of clientele, programming, and budgeting.

The consultant provided support and guidance as the group prepared to meet with potential community referral sources and the town planning board for permission to operate the day care center in a local church. The consultant also helped with the development of public relations materials and grant requests for funding. As planning progressed, the consultant devoted more time to designing a program plan and developing policies, procedures, budgets, and staff requirements.

The consultation culminated in the search for and hiring of a permanent director. The consultant's services were then gradually phased out, although the consultant remained available as needed.

The broad knowledge base and highly developed communication skills highlighted above are equally important when providing ongoing consultation to day care staff once a program is operational. Here the consultant's expertise helps the team identify and assess a client problem. A program plan is developed and carried out by the team. Through monitoring, the consultant periodically reassesses and modifies the plan.

References

Adult day care letter. (1989). Wall, NJ: Health Resources Publishing.

American Occupational Therapy Foundation. (1994a). Activities of the Research Advisory Council. *American Journal of Occupational Therapy, 44,* 659–661.

American Occupational Therapy Association. (1994b). Occupational therapy code of ethics. *American Journal of Occupational Therapy, 48*(11), 1037–1038.

American Occupational Therapy Association. (1993). *Occupational therapy roles.* Rockville, MD: Author.

American Occupational Therapy Association. (1991). *Statement: The occupational therapist as case manager.* Rockville, MD: Author.

American Occupational Therapy Association. (1990). *1990 member data survey.* Rockville, MD: Author.

American Occupational Therapy Association. (1986). Roles and functions of occupational therapy in adult day care. *American Journal of Occupational Therapy, 40*(12), 817–821.

American Occupational Therapy Association. (1984). Principles of occupational therapy ethics. *American Journal of Occupational Therapy, 38*(12), 799–802.

American Occupational Therapy Association. (1983). Standards of practice for occupational therapy. *American Journal of Occupational Therapy, 37*(12), 802–804.

Batchelder, J. M., & Hilton, C. L. (1994). Implications of the Americans with Disabilities Act of 1990 for elderly persons. *American Journal of Occupational Therapy, 48,* 73–80.

Case Management Society of America. (1995). *CMSA standards of practice.* Little Rock, AR: Author.

Cox, N. J., & Reifler, B. V. (1994). The future of adult day care in the nursing home. *Nursing Home Economics and Business Issues in Long Term Care, 1,* 7–11.

Crepeau, E. L. (1980). *Activities programming.* Durham, NH: New England Gerontology Center.

Damico, C. (1985). Adult day health care—A medical model. *Gerontology Special Interest Section Newsletter, 8,* 1–2.

Epstein, C. F. (1985a). Consultation: Communicating and facilitating. In J. Bair and M. Gray (Eds.), *The Occupational Therapy Manager* (pp. 299–221). Rockville, MD: AOTA.

Epstein, C. F. (1985b). The occupational therapy consultant in adult day care programs. *Gerontology Special Interest Section Newsletter, 8,* 3–4.

Epstein, C. F. (1992). Adult day care consultation in a rural community. In E. G. Jaffe & C. F. Epstein (Eds.), *Occupational therapy consultation: Theory, principles and practice* (pp. 419–430). St. Louis, MO: Mosby-Year Book.

Gillette, N. P., & Mitcham, M. D. (1994). Is it not always time for new research ideas? *American Journal of Occupational Therapy, 48,* 649–650.

Howland, S., & Gade-Schara, E., (1985). The Madison area adult day centers, inc.—A health maintenance model. *Gerontology Special Interest Section Newsletter, 8,* 1, 3.

Huff, S. (1988). The occupational therapist as case manager in an adult day health care setting. In E. Taira (Ed.), *Community programs for the health impaired elderly* (pp. 21–32). New York: The Haworth Press.

Javernick, J. A. (1993). Research 101. *OT Week, 7,* 16–17.

Joe, B. E. (1995). A president for our time. *OT Week, 9,* 16–17.

Kiernat, J. (1976). Geriatric day hospital: A golden opportunity for therapists. *American Journal of Occupational Therapy, 30,* 285–288.

Krefting, L. H., & Krefting, D. V. (1991). Cultural influences on performance. In M. Christensen and C. Baum (Eds.), *Occupational therapy: Overcoming human performance deficits* (pp. 102–122). Thorofare, NJ: SLACK.

MacDonald, K. C. (1985). Adult day care: Occupational therapy roles and function. *Gerontology Special Interest Section Newsletter, 8,* 2.

Macken, C. (1986). A profile of functionally impaired elderly persons living in the community. *Health Care Financing Review, 7,* 33–49.

Morris, A., & Hunt, G. (1994). *A part of daily life: Alzheimer's caregivers simplify activities and the home* [videotape]. Rockville, MD: American Occupational Therapy Association.

National Institute on Adult Daycare. (1984). *Standards for adult daycare.* Washington, DC: NCOA.

National Institute on Adult Daycare. (1990). *Standards and guidelines for adult day care.* Washington, DC: NCOA.

National Institute on Adult Daycare. (1994). *An adult day care chronology.* Washington, DC: NCOA.

National Institute on Adult Daycare. (1994/1995). *A summary report—Winter 1994/1995.* Washington, DC: NCOA.

National Institute on Adult Daycare. (1995). *Adult day care fact sheet.* Washington, DC: NCOA.

Neustadt, L. E. (1985). Adult day care: A model for changing times.

Physical and Occupational Therapy in Geriatrics, 4, 53–66.

Osorio, L. P. (1993). Adult day care. In H. L. Hopkins and H. D. Smith (Eds.), *Willard and Spackman's occupational therapy* (pp. 812–815). Philadelphia, PA: J. B. Lippincott.

Osorio, L. P. (1991). Adult daycare programs. In J. M. Kiernat (Ed.), *Occupational Therapy and the Older Adult* (pp. 241–258). Gaithersburg, MD: Aspen.

Osorio, L. P. (1985). Directing a day care center. *Gerontology Special Interest Section Newsletter, 8,* 5.

Padula, H. (1992). *Developing adult daycare—An approach to maintaining independence for impaired older persons.* Washington, DC: NCOA.

Padula, H. (1983). *Developing adult day care.* Washington, DC: NCOA.

Partners in Caregiving: The Dementia Services Program. (Spring 1995a). *Respite Report. Special Issue: White House Conference on Aging Mini-Conference, 7,* 3. Winston-Salem, NC: Author.

Partners in Caregiving: The Dementia Services Program. (Spring 1995b). Adult Day Services—Provider Perspectives. *Respite Report. Special Issue: White House Conference on Aging Mini-Conference, 7,* 4. Winston-Salem, NC: Author.

Partners in Caregiving: The Dementia Services Program. (Spring 1995c). *Respite Report. Special Issue: White House Conference on Aging Mini-Conference, 7,* 12. Winston-Salem, NC: Author.

Partners in Caregiving: The Dementia Services Program. (July 1995). *Life after diagnosis.* Winston-Salem, NC: Author.

Rathbone-McCuan, E. (1976). Geriatric day care: A family perspective. *The Gerontologist, 16,* 517–521.

Rogers, J. C. (1983). Roles and functions of occupational therapy in long-term care: Occupational therapy and activity programs. *American Journal of Occupational Therapy, 37*(12), 807–810.

Silvergleit, I. (1994). The high demand for OTRs and COTAs. *OT Week, 8,* 20–22.

Snow, T. L. (1991). Enriching lives by coordinating care. *OT Week, 5,* 10–11.

Taylor, E., & Mitchell, M. (1990). Research attitudes and activities of occupational therapy clinicians. *American Journal of Occupational Therapy, 44,* 350–355.

Timmerman, L., Schmidt, C., & Heater, S. L. (1994). Increasing occupational therapy research: Is it time to try something new? *American Journal of Occupational Therapy, 48,* 647–648.

Von Behren, R. (1988) *Adult daycare: A program of services for the functionally impaired.* Washington, DC: NCOA.

Von Behren, R. (1986). *Adult daycare in America: Summary of a national survey.* Washington, DC: NCOA.

Weiler, P. G., & Rathbone-McCuan, E. (1978). *Adult daycare: Community work with the elderly.* New York: Springer.

Weissert, W. G., Elston, J. M., Bolda, E. J., Zelman, W. N., Mutran, E., & Mangum, A. B. (1990). *Adult day care findings from a national survey.* Baltimore: Johns Hopkins University Press.

Yerxa, E. J. (1983). Audacious values: The energy source of occupational therapy practice. In G. Kielhofner (Ed.), *Health through occupation: Theory and practice in occupational therapy.* Philadelphia: F. A. Davis.

Yerxa, E. J. (1995). Nationally speaking—Who is the keeper of occupational therapy's practice and knowledge? *American Journal of Occupational Therapy, 49,* 295–299.

Related Readings and Resources

Melvin, J. A. (1993). *Working with the cognitively impaired: Adult-behavioral and environment considerations* [audio learning cassette]. Rockville, MD: American Occupational Therapy Association.

Oakley, F. (1993). *Understanding the ABCs of Alzheimer's disease.* Rockville, MD: American Occupational Therapy Association.

Module III

Lorraine Williams Pedretti, MS, OTR
Editor

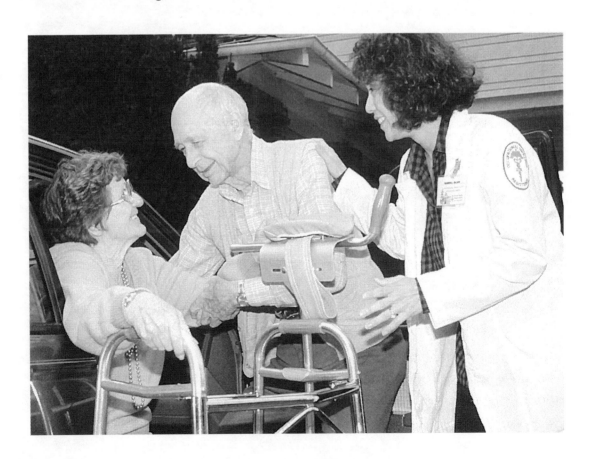

Author Biographies

Karen Allison, MOTR/L, of Austin, Texas, is a corporate clinical consultant for occupational therapy for Theracore Rehabilitation Services, based in Palm Harbor, Florida. She earned her bachelor's degree in psychology from Louisiana State University and her master's degree in occupational therapy from Texas Woman's University. As an occupational therapist for 13 years, Ms. Allison has served as an interdisciplinary manager for large groups of long-term-care facilities, been a guest lecturer at universities nationwide, and presented papers at conferences on management and geriatric rehabilitation.

Danielle N. Butin, MPH, OTR, is manager of health promotion and wellness at Oxford Health Plans, New York, and a clinical instructor in occupational therapy at Columbia University. She earned her bachelor's degree in occupational therapy from New York University and her master's degree in public health from Columbia University. Ms. Butin designs health promotion seminars and products as well as self-care models for disease management. She is also a consultant for research and training grants in geriatrics. She presented a workshop nationally on late-life depression, schizophrenia, and dementia, and she has published a number of articles in the *Journal of Occupational Therapy and Geriatrics.*

Amy Cook, MS, OTR, is coordinator of the Maturity Module for the Occupational Therapy Program at Dominican College in Orangeburg, New York, and also works as a geriatric practitioner in community health and long-term care. She received her bachelor's degree in elementary education from the State University of New York at Oneonta and her master's degree in occupational therapy from Columbia University. She is currently a doctoral student in health education at Columbia University's Teachers College. She is coauthor of an article on cancer and hand function and has conducted research on the prevention of falls among older adults.

Nikki D. Couloumbis, MS, OTR, received her master's degree in occupational therapy from Columbia University. At the time this chapter was written, she was a staff therapist at Pinecrest Rehabilitation Hospital in Delray Beach, Florida.

Diane Foti, MS, OTR, received her master's and bachelor's degrees in occupational therapy from San Jose State University. Her clinical practice has been in a variety of settings, with emphasis on the treatment of physical disabilities and gerontic occupational therapy. She is a part-time lecturer in the Department of Occupational Therapy at San Jose State University and a contributing author to *Occupational Therapy Practice Skills for Physical Dysfunction,* by Lorraine Pedretti.

Coralie H. (Corky) Glantz, OTR/L, FAOTA, is co-owner, with Nancy Richman, of Glantz/Richman Rehabilitation Associates, Ltd., in Riverwoods, Illinois, an agency providing nursing homes, retirement homes, and persons in home health and hospitals with occupational therapy, physical therapy, speech therapy, social services, and therapeutic recreation. Besides training and supervising staff members, she develops and teaches various workshops each year and gives presentations at professional conferences, organizational meetings, and universities nationally and internationally. Ms. Glantz has consulted in the development of innovative programming in geriatric service and has been extensively involved with staff training in long-term facilities. Active in AOTA and the Illinois Occupational Therapy Association, she also represents occupational therapy in non-occupational therapy organizations and advocates for the profession as well as the rights of the geriatric population.

Anne Birge James, MS, OTR/L, is an assistant professor in the College of Education, Nursing, and Health Professions at the University of Hartford in Connecticut. She received her master's degree in occupational therapy from Boston University and her bachelor's degree in occupational therapy from Western Michigan University. She has been a member of the clinical faculty in the School of Occupational and Physical Therapy at the University of Puget Sound in Tacoma, Washington, and in the School of Rehabilitation Medicine at the University of Washington in Seattle. She has worked in private practice and as a staff occupational therapist in various medical facilities. Ms. James has served as the supervisor of occupational therapy in the Burn Unit of Harborview Medical Center in Seattle, the assistant director of occupational therapy at Braintree Hospital in Massachusetts, and the unit supervisor of occupational therapy at Massachusetts General Hospital in Boston. She has presented lectures and workshops on therapeutic management and intervention outcomes for trauma disorders, fingertip amputations, rheumatoid arthritis, burn care, and hemiplegic shoulders and orthopedic shoulder injuries. She has also published several articles in the *American Journal of Occupational Therapy* and coauthored a chapter in *Orthopaedic Trauma Protocols,* edited by S. Hansen and M. Swiontkowski.

Barbara L. Kornblau, JD, OTR, DAAPM, CIRS, CCM, is a professor of occupational therapy at Nova Southeastern University, Ft. Lauderdale, Florida, and is an attorney at law. She earned her bachelor's degree in occupational therapy from the University of Wisconsin-Madison and her law degree from the University of Miami. Her experience also includes serving as a certified case manager, chairing AOTA's Work Programs Special Interest Section, holding membership in the National Association of Elder Law Attorneys, and being a lecturer and author on occupational therapy practice and the Americans with Disabilities Act.

Alison J. Laver, PhD, OT(C), DipCOT, SROT, is an assistant professor in the School of Rehabilitation Sciences, McMaster University, and associate researcher at St. Peter's Hospital, both in Hamilton, Ontario, Canada. She holds a diploma from the College of Occupational Therapists, Dorset House, Oxford, England, and earned her doctorate in psychology from the University of Surrey, Guildford, England. She has also worked in the United States and England as instructor, senior lecturer, and project supervisor, as well as occupational therapist. Currently she is a reviewer for the *Canadian Journal of Occupational Therapy* and is a mentor for AOTA's Partners for Professional Growth Program. In 1993, she was the winner in the education category of the Cosmopolitan Achievement Awards, which recognize outstanding women in Great Britain. Her areas of interest are assessment of occupational performance, especially self-care and productivity, assessment of neuropsychological functioning, and test design and psychometrics.

Linda L. Levy, MA, OTR/L, FAOTA, is an associate professor of occupational therapy at Temple University and a faculty associate of the Geriatric Education Center of Pennsylvania. She has a master's degree in social gerontology and health planning and a bachelor's degree in occupational therapy from the University of Pennsylvania. She has extensive clinical experience in psychiatric and geriatric issues, having directed occupational therapy programs at the Hospital of the University of Pennsylvania and the Philadelphia Psychiatric Center. She has published widely and presented numerous seminars on geriatric rehabilitation and the impact of dementia on individual behaviors, rehabilitation, and the family. Ms. Levy served as a health systems agency planner in mental health, developmental disabilities, and long-term-care services.

Ferol Menks Ludwig, PhD, OTR/L, FAOTA, GC, is a professor of occupational therapy at Nova Southeastern University, Ft. Lauderdale, Florida. She earned her bachelor's degree in occupational therapy and master of science degree in human development and family relations from Ohio State University. She earned her doctorate, as an occupational scientist, from the University of Southern California and is a certified gerontologist. Ms. Ludwig has served on occupational therapy faculties at the University of Florida, Texas Woman's University, and the University of Southern California. She has contributed to numerous publications and games regarding aging.

William M. Marcil, MS, OTR, FAOTA, president of Tidewater Occupational Therapy Associates, Inc., in Virginia Beach, Virginia, has been a practicing occupational therapist for 19 years, beginning as a COTA from Maria College in Albany, New York. He became involved in hospice work as an undergraduate student at the State University of New York at Buffalo. Mr. Marcil has continued to work with hospice care and, more recently, with HIV/AIDS, an area in which he is a recognized expert within the profession. He is the coauthor of three texts; has published in the *American Journal of Occupational Therapy, American Journal of Hospice Care, Advance for Occupational Therapists,* and *Home Healthcare Nurse;* and has contributed chapters to numerous professional texts. He has presented papers and workshops throughout the United States as well as in Guam, Australia, Canada, and New Zealand. He is currently pursuing his doctoral degree in leadership studies.

Pamela Maultsby, MS, OTR, is a therapist at St. Luke's Roosevelt Hospital and at a private practice in New York, New York.

Patricia A. Miller, MEd, OTR, FAOTA, is an assistant professor in clinical occupational therapy and public health and is the gerontology coordinator of the occupational therapy programs at Columbia University. She has published extensively in the areas of geriatric assessment and treatment of depression as well as interdisciplinary teamwork. Currently she is a consultant and lecturer at the Columbia University New York Geriatric Education Center. She received two grant awards from the Brookdale Institute on Aging and Adult Human Development for her work in gerontology curriculum development. Ms. Miller is a doctoral candidate in the Department of Higher Education at Columbia University.

Susan Pierce, OTR, CDRS, is president, driver rehabilitation specialist, and occupational therapy consultant for Adaptive Services, Inc., a company she founded in Orlando, Florida, in 1990. She received her bachelor's in occupational therapy from the University of Alabama in Birmingham. She has had over 17 years of experience in driver evaluation and education, including developing new driving programs in Georgia and Louisiana and working as a driver rehabilitation specialist at Humana Hospital-Lucerne Rehabilitation Center in Orlando. She has been active with the Association of Driver Educators for the Disabled, serving as secretary, association president, and chairperson of the Vocational Rehabilitation Committee, Certification Committee, and Test Development Committee.

Nancy Richman OTR/L, FAOTA, is co-owner, with Coralie H. Glantz, of Glantz/Richman Rehabilitation Associates, Ltd., in Riverwoods, Illinois, an agency providing nursing homes, retirement homes, and persons in home health and hospitals with occupational therapy, physical therapy, speech therapy, social services, and therapeutic recreation. Besides training and supervising staff members, she develops and teaches various workshops each year and gives presentations at professional conferences, organizational meetings, and universities nationally and internationally. Ms. Richman has consulted in the development of innovative programming in geriatric service and has been extensively involved with staff training in long-term facilities. Active in AOTA and the Illinois Occupational Therapy Association, she also represents occupational therapy in non-occupational therapy organizations and advocates for the profession as well as the rights of the geriatric population.

Kent Nelson Tigges, MS, OTR, FAOTA, FHIH, is professor emeritus of occupational therapy at the State University of New York at Buffalo and was formerly director of occupational therapy at Hospice Buffalo, Inc. He is credited with initiating, developing, and advocating the role of occupational therapy in hospice care. His most recent publications include *Oxford Textbook of Palliative Medicine*, published by Oxford University Press, as well as more than 40 articles in domestic and foreign journals and three textbooks. Mr. Tigges is a graduate of the University of Kansas and San Jose State University.

Learning Outline

Chapter 12
Evaluation and Interventions for the Performance Components . . .547

Chapter 13
Evaluation and Interventions for the Performance Areas

SECTION 1.

Evaluation and Interventions for the Performance Area of Self-Maintenance
Diane Foti, MS, OTR

Chapter 14
Palliative Medicine and Rehabilitation:
Assessment and Treatment in Hospice Care 743

Kent N. Tigges, MS, OTR, FAOTA, FHIH, and William M. Marcil, MS, OTR, FAOTA

Introduction to Module III

In Module III, assessment and evaluation, treatment planning, and treatment strategies are organized around the occupational performance model, and specific interventions for the performance components and performance areas are described. Several of the chapters include one or more case studies, which illustrate the application of the chapter content to occupational therapy intervention for the elderly.

Assessment and evaluation, treatment planning, and treatment approaches for older adults are presented in chapter 11. Assessment issues, the purposes and types of assessments, special considerations for assessment of older adults, and suitable assessment tools are described. Factors that are important for treatment planning and selecting appropriate treatment approaches are also discussed.

Chapter 12 reviews evaluation and interventions for the performance components. There is a comprehensive description of assessment and treatment methods for the sensorimotor component. Intervention for the cognitive/cognitive integrative component focuses primarily on dementia and is organized around cognitive disability theory and Allen's cognitive levels. An activity group model for caregivers and relatives with dementia, as one approach to occupational therapy intervention for persons with dementia, complements the theoretical data on cognitive disability. In presenting the psychological/psychosocial component, the author reviews the major psychiatric conditions seen in aging and then focuses on depression, the most common of these. Assessments for depression in the elderly and models for individual and group intervention are described.

The performance areas, self-maintenance, leisure, and work and productive activities, are covered in chapter 13. The chapter is divided into seven sections. Self-maintenance is treated in the first section. Assistive devices, mobility and transfers, and ambulation aids are just some of the topics covered. The causes and prevention of falls, falls assessment, and the important role that occupational therapy can play in this often neglected aspect of self-maintenance are discussed. The effects of age-related impairments on driving, driver assessment, assistance for older drivers, and the role of the occupational therapist as a driver rehabilitation specialist are some of the subjects included in section 3 on transportation for the elderly. Section 4 covers a seldom-discussed issue, sexual expression in later life. Real and imagined obstacles to sexual expression are explored and two models of treatment are described.

Transition to home after hospitalization or rehabilitation program, in section 5, gives a comprehensive picture of all the factors that require consideration for smooth transitions and continuity of care. Caregiver education, follow-up care, and environmental modification are some of the important issues.

Section 6 discusses evaluation and interventions for work and productive activities. Continuing to work, retirement, caregiving and care receiving, home management, and financial management by older adults are explored.

Interventions for leisure activities are reviewed in section 7. Leisure activity is an important aspect of adult life, and its continuity into late adulthood contributes to health and well-being. The role of occupational therapy in facilitating the development of leisure skills by the elderly in different treatment settings is described, including the special needs of persons with dementia.

Chapter 14, the final chapter of Module III, presents information about hospice and the role of occupational therapy in hospice care. The history of the hospice movement is traced. The tenets of hospice care and the role of occupational therapy in fulfilling these

tenets are presented. The authors describe the unique personal skills, attitudes, and approaches that are necessary when working with the terminally ill.

Module III underscores the fact that occupational therapy in gerontic practice encompasses almost all other specialty areas. The difference is that assessment, treatment approaches, and intervention strategies are adapted to meet the special needs of the elderly population.

It is apparent that there is a need for a greater number of assessment instruments that are designed and standardized for the elderly. Further development of teaching methods for persons experiencing the normal physical and mental changes of aging, based on current models of motor learning theory, is essential for more effective intervention. Learning how normal older adults adapt performance to accommodate declining sensorimotor, cognitive, and psychological functions is pertinent as a foundation for gerontic occupational therapy practice. Such measures can be important contributions of occupational therapy to the rehabilitation of the elderly.

As the number of older persons in the population increases, there will be an increasing need for occupational therapy practitioners specializing in gerontic practice. Adequate educational preparation and the development of better assessment instruments, teaching methods, and treatment approaches specialized for this population will be critical to practice excellence in the next 20 years.

Lorraine Williams Pedretti, MS, OTR

Competencies

OT Intervention for Older Adults

Lorraine Williams Pedretti, MS, OTR

Key: Competencies are italicized statements and performance objectives are numbered statements.

Chapter 11: The Occupational Therapy Intervention Process

Section 1: Occupational Therapy Assessment and Evaluation of Older Clients

Understand special needs and considerations of older adults in the occupational therapy assessment process.

1. Identify normal age-related changes in performance components' functions that can affect accurate assessment of older adults.

2. Identify cultural issues that can affect accurate assessment of older adults.

Identify the purposes of assessment, the suitable assessment tools, and their appropriate uses with the older adult population.

1. Identify and define six purposes of assessment.

2. Define six levels of function addressed by assessment data according to definitions of function developed by the National Center for Medical Rehabilitation Research.

3. Differentiate the top-down and bottom-up approaches to assessment and describe the advantages and disadvantages of each.

4. Identify resources for finding assessments for elderly clients.

5. Identify suitable assessment tools for assessing the performance areas and performance components in the older adult.

6. Identify which level(s) of function each assessment tool addresses.

Section 2: Treatment Planning and Treatment Approaches

Understand the treatment planning process and identify special considerations in treatment planning in gerontic practice.

1. Define treatment plan.

2. List the factors upon which a treatment plan is designed.

3. List some factors that especially affect treatment planning for the older adult.

4. Describe how the therapy setting and discharge destination affect the treatment plan.

5. Differentiate preventive, restorative, and compensatory approaches to treatment.

6. Describe how re-evaluation affects the treatment plan.

Chapter 12 : Evaluation and Interventions for the Performance Components

Understand the rationale for and develop effective occupational therapy programs for the performance components in gerontic OT practice.

Section 1: The Sensorimotor Component

1. Identify and describe methods of assessment and treatment for the sensorimotor component.

2. Describe how normal aging affects sensorimotor functioning.

3. Name two tests of manual dexterity that are suitable for the elderly.

4. Describe compensatory strategies for visual, tactile, hearing, and olfactory deficits.

Section 2: Cognitive Integration and Cognitive Components

1. Define cognition.

2. Define dementia.

3. List the cognitive impairments seen in dementia.

4. Name and define the three structural components of memory.

5. List three elements of long-term memory.

6. List and describe the cognitive and behavioral impairments that result from dementia.

7. Describe cognitive disability theory.

8. List and define the three dimensions of cognitions that are stages of a sensorimotor information-processing model described by Allen.

9. List and describe functional abilities at each of Allen's six levels of cognitive functioning.

10. Describe the kinds of activities that are suitable at each of the six cognitive levels.

11. Name assessment tools that are suitable for evaluating cognition.

12. Describe and discuss the activity group model for caregivers and relatives with dementia.

Section 4: Psychosocial and Psychological Components

1. List three major psychological dysfunctions found in the elderly.

2. Differentiate depression from dysthymia.

3. List at least four medical conditions that have been associated with depression.

4. List and define three clinical presentations of depression in the elderly.

5. Name and describe three personality disorders that may underlie depression in the elderly.

6. Describe appropriate approaches of health professionals to patients with each of these personality disorders.

7. List four assessment tools for measuring depression and describe each.

8. Describe the cognitive therapy approach to working with the depressed elderly.

Chapter 13: Evaluation and Interventions for the Performance Areas

Understand the rationale for and develop effective occupational therapy programs for the performance areas in gerontic OT practice.

Sections 1: Evaluation and Interventions for the Performance Area of Self-Maintenance

1. Define self-maintenance.

2. Describe normal and pathological factors that affect performance of self-maintenance tasks.

3. List and define the elements of the occupational therapy ADL evaluation.

4. Define continuum of care and discuss how continuity of treatment is affected by it.

5. Describe why the performance evaluation is critical to accurate treatment planning.

6. List six principles for the use of assistive devices in treatment.

7. List seven principles of energy conservation and work simplification.

8. Discuss the potential effects of poor posture on physiological function, safety, and performance.

9. Differentiate the roles of the physical therapist and the occupational therapist in mobility and transfer training.

10. Describe the principles for a safe sit-to-stand sequence and for stair climbing.

11. Discuss the role of the occupational therapist in nutrition of the elderly.

12. List the guidelines for a safe swallow.

13. Describe the environment that is conducive to independent eating.

14. Describe some treatment techniques that can be used to address problems in hygiene, toileting, bathing, and dressing.

15. Discuss the ways the occupational therapy practitioner can facilitate medication management.

Section 2: Prevention of Falls in the Elderly

1. List the causes of falls in the elderly.

2. Describe a three-level model for preventing falls.

3. Describe how occupational therapy can assess and treat problems related to falls.

Section 3: Transportation

1. Discuss the importance of driving for the elderly.

2. List the performance components used in driving.

3. Identify the sensory and perceptual functions on which most driving decisions are based.

4. Identify age-related impairments that can affect driving ability.

5. Describe the driving assessment and the role of the driver rehabilitation specialist in the assessment process.

6. List some methods to prevent accident and injury in the elderly.

7. Discuss how the driving environment can be adapted for the elderly.

8. List resources that provide assistance for older drivers.

9. Discuss the responsibility of the physician and other health professionals in protecting the public safety.

10. List the recommendations for facilitating the surrender of the driver's license.

11. Identify the resource for the occupational therapist who wants to become a driver rehabilitation specialist.

Section 4: Sexual Expression in Later Life

1. Justify why sexual expression is in the domain of occupational therapy.

2. Define sexuality.

3. Describe how satisfying sexual activity can contribute to a sense of independent function and personal well-being.

4. List the normal physical changes of aging that can affect sexual function.

5. Describe demographic factors that can affect sexual expression.

6. State the common stereotypes about the sexuality of the elderly.

7. List psychological conditions that affect sexual function.

8. List physical conditions and medications that can affect sexual function.

9. Describe two treatment approaches to dealing with sexual issues with the elderly.

Section 5: Transition to Home After Hospitalization or Rehabilitation Program

1. Define continuum of care.

2. Describe the CCRC model of continuum of care.

3. Define care management.

4. List the factors in the home situation that must be considered for effective discharge planning.

5. List the social dimensions that affect the patient's functioning on transition to home.

6. List the intrapersonal aspects, including cultural factors, of transition.

7. Describe the ethnographic perspective.

8. Describe the ethnographic interview process.

9. Describe the role of the occupational therapy practitioner in caregiver education.

10. Discuss why follow-up is important and how it can be carried out.

11. List community services and resources for the elderly.

12. Describe some common environmental modifications for ease, comfort, and safety.

13. List at least 10 principles for home safety, including safety in the kitchen, bathroom, and bedroom.

14. Discuss special safety issues for persons with dementia.

Section 6: Evaluation and Intervention for Work and Productive Activities

1. Describe the basic tenet of continuity theory.

2. Discuss how older adults interpret their own development.

3. Identify strategies that can keep older employees in the work force.

4. Identify the reasons that older workers may be unemployed.

5. Identify the role that occupational therapy can play to help maintain employment of older workers.

6. Discuss how the ADA gives the older disabled worker the backing needed to return to the workplace.

7. Describe the work visit and job analysis.

8. Discuss the psychosocial aspects of retirement.

9. Discuss the reasons that older persons retire.

10. Describe the impact of retirement on the marital relationship.

11. Identify work substitutes.

12. Describe the role of caregiver and identify who is typically found in this role.

13. Discuss how the burdens of caregiving can affect physical, social, and psychological functioning.

14. Describe the role of occupational therapy in relieving caregiver burden.

15. List assessment tools for evaluating home management and safety in the elderly.

16. Define conservatorship and guardianship.

17. Discuss some of the legal aspects of conservatorship and guardianship.

18. Define durable power of attorney.

19. Discuss ways that the elderly can be protected from theft and con games.

Section 7: Evaluation and Intervention for Leisure Activities

1. Define leisure.

2. Describe the role of recreation on adult life.

3. Define coordinated and complementary leisure and give some examples from your own life.

4. Discuss how the use of time changes with aging.

5. Discuss how assessment and programming for leisure activities can be combined with ADL skills and treatment that addresses physical dysfunction.

6. List some examples of leisure activities that can stimulate cognitive functions.

7. Describe how you would evaluate for leisure skills.

8. Describe the role of the occupational therapist in the development of activity programs in residential care facilities.

9. Identify the focus of leisure activity performance for patients with dementia.

10. Discuss how leisure activities can be adapted for patients with dementia.

Chapter 14: Palliative Medicine and Rehabilitation: Assessment and Treatment in Hospice Care

Understand the role of OT in the care of the terminally ill.

1. Define the concept of death.

2. Discuss three important issues on life and death.

3. Discuss the controversial aspects of voluntary euthanasia.

4. Trace the history of the hospice movement.

5. Compare and contrast traditional occupational therapy models in acute care and rehabilitation with occupational therapy in hospice care.

6. List five tenets of hospice care.

7. List two types of pain the occupational therapy practitioner is best suited to address.

8. Describe the essential attitudes and approaches necessary in treating the terminally ill.

9. Describe the components of the occupational therapy assessment in hospice.

10. List the goals of OT in hospice care.

11. Describe the role of OT in hospice treatment.

12. Describe communication with the professional team and the family in the hospice setting.

13. Describe the healthy professional relationship between the occupational therapy practitioner and the family in hospice care.

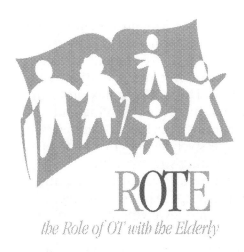

The Occupational Therapy Intervention Process

Section 1. Occupational Therapy Assessment and Evaluation of Older Clients

Alison J. Laver, PhD, OT(C), DipCOT, SROT

Abstract

Helping older clients with disabilities reach their potential calls for careful consideration of a variety of issues when selecting assessment methods and when assessing and evaluating older people. This unit examines those issues and reviews examples of promising assessments.

Introduction

The major tenet of geriatric occupational therapy is to help older clients with disabilities reach their highest attainable levels of skill and function (Katz, 1992). Occupational therapy practitioners have a primary concern with the maintenance and enhancement of an older person's quality of life, both during the normal process of the life span and following the onset of occupational dysfunction caused by trauma or disease. The purpose of occupational therapy evaluation and assessment for older clients is to gain a clear picture of the individual in order to develop effective treatment plans that will result in improved occupational function and enhanced quality of life. The role of evalua-

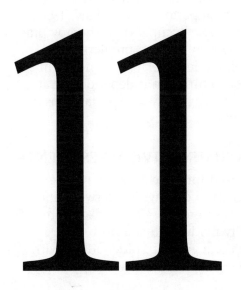

tion and assessment is of paramount importance to the occupational therapy intervention process for older adults, because it is used "to describe the client's problem, formulate a prognosis, and to evaluate the effects of occupational therapy intervention" (Law & Letts, 1989, p. 522).

This section is divided into three main parts. The first part provides an overview of issues that occupational therapy practitioners must consider when selecting assessment methods. The second part gives information related to special considerations that should be taken into account when assessing and evaluating older people. The third part will provide examples of assessments that can be used with older clients.

An Overview of Assessment Issues

Assessment can be viewed as a process involving the use of multiple methods of gathering and organizing information that is important to making specific clinical decisions (Haley, Coster, & Ludlow, 1991; Frey, 1988) and is "the planned collection, interpretation, and documentation of the functional status of an individual, related to the individual's capacity to perform valued or required self-care, work or leisure tasks" (Rogers & Holm, 1989, p. 6).

Before considering the specific requirements for the evaluation and assessment of older clients and reviewing potential assessment tools in this field, it is important to explore some general issues related to selecting occupational therapy assessments and applying them to the assessment of older clients.

PURPOSES OF ASSESSMENTS

When selecting an assessment for the evaluation of older clients, it is use-

ful to consider "the purpose for which assessment information is gathered and how it relates to function or performance of everyday activities, tasks, and roles. This is a complex problem because it involves observing and interpreting units of behaviour nested within progressively larger chunks of a person's ongoing stream of life activities" (Christiansen, 1993, p. 258). Identifying the purpose of an assessment is critical when reviewing its suitability for the older client. It is important to consider the intended purpose of an assessment during the critique and selection process because the content, methods, and utility of an assessment should be evaluated against its intended purpose. Assessments for older adults can be categorized into six main clinical purposes: predictive, discriminative, descriptive, evaluative, program evaluation and quality assurance, and reimbursement and policy issues (Haley et al., 1991).

PREDICTIVE ASSESSMENTS

Predictive assessments are used to classify older clients into predefined categories of interest. For example, predictive activities of daily living (ADL) assessments serve to predict an "event or functional status in another situation on the basis of the client's level of functional performance" (Law, 1993, p. 233). The occupational therapy practitioner may wish to predict future functional level related to the client's ability to function independently at home or eligibility for special housing or support services.

DISCRIMINATIVE ASSESSMENTS

Discriminative assessments are designed to distinguish between individuals or groups. Comparisons are usually made against a normative group or a group of older adults with similar diagnoses. Such comparisons may be made for diagnosis, placement, and determination of level of dysfunction, in relation to expectations of performance of healthy people of that age. The value of a discriminative assessment depends on the adequacy and generalizability of the normative sample or client population used to obtain reference data. Assessments that lack normative or comparative test data for older adult populations restrict the occupational therapy practitioner's ability to make accurate and valid comparative decisions on the basis of the assessment data.

DESCRIPTIVE ASSESSMENTS

Descriptive assessments provide information that describes the current functional status of the older client and focuses on the identification of the older person's functional abilities and limitations. For example, a descriptive ADL assessment is an evaluation of the client's function at one point in time and is often used to identify clients whose ADL performance is affected to a degree that merits intervention (Law, 1993). Functional status data from descriptive assessments are "important for clinical decision making, providing an information base for setting functionally oriented treatment goals, the identification of an appropriate treatment plan, and assisting individual decisions concerning admission and discharge" (Haley et al., 1991, pp. 694–695). One problem with many descriptive assessments relates to the level of descriptive data obtained. Many assessments simply address performance task domains (such as the ability to dress) by classifying the client in terms of the level of independence exhibited for each task. Descriptive functional assessments that are going to be used to provide a baseline for treatment planning must be sufficiently detailed and sensitive to determine the factors that are

limiting the client's performance of the task. For example, the descriptive assessment must help the therapist differentiate between the client who is dependent in dressing owing to a motor deficit and who has insufficient hand function to manipulate fastenings, versus the client who is impeded in dressing because of apraxia and who is unable to execute the appropriate motor plan.

EVALUATIVE ASSESSMENTS

Evaluative assessments are used to detect clinical change in the older person's occupational performance or performance component functioning over time. This type of assessment can be used to monitor the client's progress during rehabilitation and determine the effectiveness of a specific treatment intervention (Law, 1993). Evaluative assessments are used to examine changes in function on an individual basis and can be useful for single-case history and group research designs. Changes in the functional performance of older clients can be subtle and slow. When using an evaluative assessment with an older client it is important to consider the issue of sensitivity. Some assessments lack sensitivity because they do not have sufficient graduations to measure change, or because they do not include test items that are the focus of rehabilitation. When using an evaluative assessment it is also important to consider the test-retest reliability of the assessment.

PROGRAM EVALUATION OR QUALITY ASSURANCE ASSESSMENTS

Assessments used for program evaluation or quality-assurance purposes are becoming increasingly important because of changes in health care policy that emphasize the need for ongoing quality-assurance systems designed to review rehabilitation inputs, processes, and outcomes. Functional status has been identified as an important outcome measure for evaluating the merits of alternative treatment programs and service provision. Occupational therapy practitioners are being encouraged to evaluate the effectiveness of the interventions they provide and this type of assessment is going to become increasingly important in the field of geriatric occupational therapy. When using an assessment for purposes of quality assurance, the goals of the quality assurance or audit exercise must be carefully defined so that the outcome measures selected match the intended goals of the treatment provided.

REIMBURSEMENT AND POLICY ISSUE ASSESSMENTS

The quality of assessments used to address reimbursement and policy issues is of paramount importance to the occupational therapy profession because functional assessments are being used as outcome measures to address important questions related to service provision and outcome in geriatric rehabilitation. Policy-oriented disability studies require valid and reliable outcome measures to help establish appropriate eligibility criteria for social and insurance programs serving older adults with functional-performance deficits. If the profession wants occupational therapy services for older adults to be provided and paid for, it must clearly show the effectiveness of its intervention. The use of gross functional measures can indicate little change in a client's function following occupational therapy. More sensitive, targeted functional assessments are needed to identify small and subtle changes in performance. Research is

also required to explore the relationships between small gradations in functional change, quality of life, and monetary factors.

Of these six purposes, the most relevant to the occupational therapy practitioner carrying a caseload of older clients are the descriptive, discriminative, predictive, and evaluative assessments. These four types of assessment enable the occupational therapist to do the following:

1. Describe current functional status.
2. Differentiate between normal aging process and pathology.
3. Predict an individual's ability to function independently at home after discharge.
4. Evaluate changes in functional status over time.

No current assessment addresses all of these functions simultaneously and so occupational therapy practitioners must select a range of assessment methods to provide a comprehensive baseline of information from which to plan treatment. Information gathered from several assessment sources is evaluated and integrated into a single clinical image of the client's occupational performance status and environment through clinical reasoning processes.

DEFINING THE LEVELS OF FUNCTION ADDRESSED BY ASSESSMENT DATA

In addition to considering the purpose of the assessment selected for the evaluation of older clients, it is also important to clearly define the level of function that an assessment addresses. The most widely recognized and accepted system for defining function was developed by the World Health Organization (WHO) (World Health Organization, 1980) and is called the International Classification of Impairments, Disabilities, and Handicaps (ICIDH). This classification system has been described in previous sections of the ROTE (see chapter 4, sections I, II, and III). The WHO model has been widely implemented internationally; however, work has been undertaken in the United States to refine these definitions. The National Center for Medical Rehabilitation Research (NCMRR) drew on the expertise of an interdisciplinary group to review the WHO classifications and the Nagi (1991) model and to refine them specifically for professionals working in rehabilitation fields. The NCMRR (1992;

1993) has broadened the functional and dysfunctional hierarchy to include five levels. It differentiates pathophysiology, impairment, and functional limitation; retains disability; and re-conceptualizes handicap as a societal limitation (figure 11–1). The NCMRR model recognizes that the progression of dysfunction is not "always sequential or unidirectional" but should be viewed as a "complex feedback loop that integrates the whole person as an entity who must adjust to problems in many of these areas simultaneously" (1992, p. 31).

The NCMRR classification defines pathophysiology as the "interruption

Figure 11–1. The NCMRR Definitions of Function/Dysfunction

Hierarchy of Function/Dysfunction

Societal Limitation
Restriction, attributable to social policy or barriers (structural or attitudinal), which limits fulfillment of roles or denies access to services and opportunities that are associated with full participation in society

Disability
Inability or limitation in performing tasks, activities, and roles to levels expected within physical and social contexts

Functional Limitation
Restriction or lack of ability to perform an action in the manner or within a range consistent with the purpose of an organ or organ system

Impairment
Loss and/or abnormality of cognitive, emotional, or anatomical structure or function; including all losses or abnormalities, not just those attributable to the initial pathophysiology

Pathophysiology
Interruption of, or interference with, normal physiological and developmental processes or structures

of, or interference with, normal physiological and developmental processes or structures" (NCMRR, 1992, p. 32). The pathophysiological domain, therefore, focuses on "cellular, structural, or functional events subsequent to injury, disease, or genetic abnormality" (NCMRR, 1992, p. 32).

Impairment is defined at the level of organs and organ systems and is

> a loss or abnormality at the organ or organ system level of the body. Impairment may include cognitive, emotional, or physiological function, or anatomical structure, and includes all those losses or abnormalities, not just those attributable to the initial pathophysiology (NCMRR, 1992, p. 32).

Functional limitation considers the level of impact of dysfunction at the pathophysiology and impairment levels to the function of organs and organ systems. "Restriction or lack of ability to perform an action in the manner or within the range consistent with the purpose of an organ or organ system constitutes a functional limitation" (NCMRR, 1992, p. 33).

Disability is viewed at the individual level and is defined as "a limitation in performing tasks, activities, and roles to levels expected within physical and social contexts" (NCMRR, 1992, p. 33).

The highest level of dysfunction, societal limitation, is viewed at the level of society and is defined as "restrictions attributable to social policy or barriers (structural or attitudinal) which limit fulfillment of roles or deny access to services and opportunities associated with full participation in society" (NCMRR, 1992, p. 34).

The specification of these five major levels of function is an important advance within the field of rehabilitation because it assists clinicians and researchers in defining the domain of functional performance to be evalu-ated and clearly identifying which level or levels of function they are addressing in their assessment and intervention. These five levels of function will be referred to throughout this section, for example, in relation to the sample assessments. When using the NCMRR model from an occupational therapy viewpoint

1. Role disturbance and environmental barriers are viewed at the level of societal limitation.

2. Occupational performance domains (i.e., activities of daily living, work and productive activities, and play or leisure activities) are viewed at the level of disability.

3. Component task skills (e.g., reaching, grasping, sequencing) are viewed at the level of functional limitation.

4. Performance components (i.e., motor, neuromusculoskeletal, sensory, cognitive, and psychosocial) can be conceptualized at the level of impairment.

5. Specific deficits (e.g., visual object agnosia, memory loss, ideomotor apraxia) can be viewed at the level of pathophysiology.

The NCMRR hierarchy is particularly useful because it describes function in terms of interrelating levels. The focus of the occupational therapy practitioner's assessment can be targeted at any level and assessment data is then evaluated in a context of interrelationships among levels. However, despite its obvious uses the NCMRR model does not offer an adequate working model for clinical practice and research on its own, since it provides only broad descriptions of the levels of functional performance. A conceptual model of functional performance and performance dysfunction used as a basis of occupational therapy gerontic assessment also must encompass those per-

Figure 11–2. Conceptual Framework for Assessing Older Adults

	Disease Process				
Functional Performance Framework	**Patho-physiology**	**Impairment**	**Functional Limitation**	**Disability**	**Societal Limitation**
Life Span Framework	Age-related changes at cell and tissue level	Age-related changes to organ systems (e.g., visual acuity deficit)	Age-related changes in skill components (e.g., reduced speed and accuracy in reaching and grasping)	Age-related changes in performance of tasks and activities	Age-related changes in social roles (e.g., retirement, grandparent)
Contextual Framework				Physical environment and personal interaction that provides context in which tasks and activities are performed (e.g., supportive cues, lighting, and color contrasts of objects and background)	Physical and social environment in which roles are carried out
Assessment Domains	Specific deficits (e.g., apraxia, agnosia, spasticity)	Performance components: motor, sensory, cognitive, psychosocial, perceptual	Skill components of tasks (e.g., lift, reach, grasp, scan, name, sequence)	Performance of self-care activities, work, productive activities, play, leisure	Client's roles and physical and social environmental barriers to function

sonal factors (such as age, gender, and cultural, social, and educational backgrounds) that impact performance. Figure 11–2 shows the interrelating factors that must be encompassed in the occupational therapy practitioner's assessment of older clients.

A TOP-DOWN VERSUS A BOTTOM-UP APPROACH TO ASSESSMENT

There is debate about whether occupational therapists should conduct their assessment process using a "top-down" or a "bottom-up" approach. A "top-down assessment ... determines which particular tasks define each of the roles for that person, whether he or she can now do those tasks, and the probable reason for an inability to do so." A "bottom-up approach to assessment ... focuses on the deficits of components of function, such as strength, range of motion, balance, and so on, which are believed to be prerequisites to successful occupation performance" (Trombly, 1993, p. 253).

The bottom-up approach has been popular in the past and its advantage is that it provides the occupational therapist with important information about the underlying performance component functioning of the individual (i.e., information about the client's functioning at the impairment level). However, one of the problems with this approach is that the purpose of the assessment, and ensuing treatment plan, may not be obvious to the older person being assessed and may, therefore, lack meaning and relevance for the client.

> An example of the bottom-up approach is when the occupational therapist detects that a client who is referred to occupational therapy for remediation of occupational dysfunction (e.g., lack of independence in self-care) lacks sitting balance. Because sitting balance is considered to be an ability required to dress independently, the therapist may begin treatment by engaging the client in activities to improve balance. The occupational therapist may not make clear to the client the connection between the component deficit and occupational functioning. The outcome desired by the occupational therapist may or may not be congruent with important goals of the client or even with the client's

perceived reason for receiving occupational therapy services. Confusion and dissatisfaction may result (Trombly, 1993, p. 253).

In contrast, the top-down approach begins at the level of the person as a whole, not at the performance component level of organs and organ systems. The approach starts by investigating past and present role competency (societal limitation level) and by evaluating the client's current ability to perform meaningful tasks drawn from his or her previous daily activities (the disability level). When the client experiences a discrepancy between his or her previous role or task performance during the assessment process, then he or she can clearly see the need for treatment and will find meaning and relevancy in the resultant treatment plan. The top-down approach, thereby, helps to clarify the purpose of occupational therapy for the client. The approach also assists the therapist in forming accurate personal and clinical images of the client, critical for the identification of relevant and meaningful treatment goals.

Some recently developed occupational therapy assessments, such as the Structured Observational Test of Function (Laver & Powell, 1995), the Kitchen Task Assessment (Baum & Edwards, 1993), the Assessment of Motor and Process Skills (Fisher, 1992), and the Arnadottir Neurobehavioral Evaluation (Arnadottir, 1990), enable the occupational therapist to assess functioning at the disability level simultaneously to obtaining information about the client's functioning in at least one other level, often at the functional limitation level and even at the impairment and pathophysiology levels. These assessments will be described briefly in the discussion of assessment examples.

Special Considerations for Assessing Older Adults

Previous chapters outlined the changes that occupational therapy practitioners can anticipate as part of the healthy aging process. This knowledge is important, for it enables the practitioner to differentiate between pathology and normal aging processes and to understand how aging processes, especially those that occur to the sensory performance component area, can impact the administration of assessments to older clients and the quality and interpretation of the data obtained.

The performance of any client can be considered in the light of the variation in performance of representative normal subjects (Ellis and Young, 1988). One of the requirements of assessments for older adults is that they must take into account the life span developmental process and consider expected changes that arise in response to the aging process. Assessments used for the evaluation of older adults should be grounded in what is known about the order and timing of such changes in specific systems (e.g., visual, auditory, and motor systems) and in performance skills and occupational performance. The standard against which the older adult is assessed should be what is typically seen at that age, and the process through which the person accomplishes the assessment task must be evaluated against the process for that age. It is, therefore, important for occupational therapy practitioners to be familiar with current knowledge of primary (normal) aging to understand the variation in performance of older adults. It is important to review the representativeness and sample sizes of the normative data upon which assessments, developed for an older client population, are standardized.

Research and related literature on aging have tended to focus on describing changes in performance components (such as memory, vision, hearing, and motor function) rather than on the process of change in the performance of activities. There is a substantial body of literature that describes age-related changes occurring at the pathophysiology and impairment levels. Much of this literature comes from outside of the profession. However, some earlier occupational therapy articles provided descriptions of aspects of the normal aging process; for example, Hasselkus (1974) described "aging and the human nervous system," while Weg (1973) discussed the "changing physiology of aging." In the last decade research has become more applied and has explored the relationships between physiological, motor, sensory, cognitive, and perceptual changes associated with age and aspects of performance at the functional limitation and disability levels (e.g., Bernspang, Fugl-Meyer, & Viitanen, 1988; Poole, 1992).

In contrast to the wealth of literature concerning age-related changes at the pathophysiology and impairment levels, there is very little documentation of age-related change in occupational performance at the disability level. However, it is the latter that is of most interest to occupational therapists, who need to assess their clients' abilities to perform everyday activities. Of the few studies that have addressed the relationship between age and occupational performance, the majority have used batteries of experimental tasks as measurement tools. A few studies have attempted to use more ecologically valid test procedures. Dickerson and Fisher (1993) report that those "studies have demonstrated that when tested in familiar environments with ecologically valid tasks (i.e., naturalistic, familiar, meaningful tasks to a person) older adults perform as well as young adults" (p. 686). As a result of such findings, the use of traditional experimental psychometric assessments in clinical settings has been questioned. It appears that when the focus is on the performance of familiar, everyday tasks the detrimental effect of age is not always observed.

Dickerson and Fisher (1993) conducted a study to examine age difference in functional performance associated with normal aging. Their objective was "to compare the abilities of young adult and older adult women on meaningful and practiced daily living tasks on which they were expert, and on a less familiar, more contrived daily living activity that they had less opportunity to practice" (p. 686). Forty women were assessed performing familiar domestic (IADL) tasks, such as preparing food, and a less familiar task, wrapping up a package, on the Assessment of Motor and Process Skills (AMPS), (Fisher, 1992). Results indicated that older adult women had age-related motor and process deficits. The older women had lower performance on both the IADL and package tasks and did not benefit when the task was familiar and practiced. This finding suggests that even with ecologically valid and practiced tasks, age-related decline is still demonstrated. The implication of these results is that practitioners should not assume that persons can perform the tasks of daily living as efficiently or as competently as younger people just because tasks are done regularly. Occupational therapists are advised to observe the client performing familiar and practiced tasks, particularly ones in which safety may be an issue, in order to ensure safe independence (Dickerson & Fisher, 1993).

It is important to collect normative data on the performance of selected tasks in order to evaluate the extent to which performance will decrease as a result of increasing age. Performance is affected by how demanding the task is and by the individual's capacity, experience, and knowledge. Occupational therapists will need to take those factors into account when assessing and evaluating their elderly clients. An individual's capacity, defined in terms of the amount of information that the central nervous system can handle and process, is limited. For example, the auditory system can process only a certain amount of auditory stimulation at a time, and the brain has limits on how much sensory information, experienced through all the sensory systems (i.e., the visual, tactile, auditory, olfactory, gustatory, and proprioceptive systems), can be processed at any one point in time. All tasks place demands on the capacity of some or all of the sensory systems and on the brain's ability to process sensory stimulation.

If the demands of a task are within a person's capacity, then the level and quality of performance will be determined by the demands of the task. For example, a person may have the capacity to get dressed and to wash his or her own clothes, but he or she performs dressing with greater ease because it is a less demanding task. However, if the person reaches full capacity in a particular system, performance will be limited by that capacity regardless of the demand of a task. Thus, a person who develops motor and sensory deficits may be unable to perform either dressing or laundry. The difference in task demand is not the issue. Problems in task performance are related to the person's reduced capacity. For example, when a person practices a task over time the demands of that task are learned and the person becomes more efficient in the use of his or her capacities. Thus, a person who is familiar with a task should perform better than someone who is unfamiliar with the same task, even though their capacities might be the same. When a person performs a task he or she

1. Obtains factual information about the demands of the task

2. Develops ideas, insights, and beliefs related to the task

3. Develops strategies to perform the task more efficiently.

Occupational therapists need to be aware of how familiar or novel an assessment task is to the client. They also need to understand that capacity can alter in relation to both the normal aging process and pathology. Following reduction in capacity, occupational therapy practitioners can use practice and repetition to increase a client's skill and performance. When repeating an assessment procedure for evaluative purposes practitioners must be able to differentiate between changes that result because the assessment is now familiar and changes that have resulted in the actual capacity of the performance of the component or activity that they are assessing.

Experience, knowledge, and capacity are interrelated and are difficult to separate and assess in isolation. The relationship between experience, knowledge, capacity, and performance is also highly complex and subject to enormous individual variation. Although difficult to determine precisely, these factors must be considered when assessing and evaluating older clients. The demands of any task used in a performance-based assessment also require careful identification and should be considered when evaluating assessment data. In addition to demand, capacity, and experience issues, factors related to volition and societal expectations will have an impact.

The findings of Dickerson and Fisher (1993), described previously, challenge the view that many everyday tasks make relatively few demands. Performance on such tasks may or may not vary with age. The onset of any limitation depends on the nature of the task demands, on the individual's capacity, and on the rate at which capacities decline; i.e., the greater the capacity and the slower the rate of decline, the later performance will begin to decrease as a function of age (Welford, 1993).

It is thought that context may guide processing. For example, age-related memory differences are minimized if the demands of the task provide contextual support for retrieval. However, when contextual support is not available, and more self-initiated retrieval processes are demanded, then age-related differences are larger (Duchek & Balota, 1993). Practitioners, therefore, need to take the contextual environment in which assessments are administered into account when evaluating test data.

In order to be sensitive to pathology arising from neurological disorders, as opposed to decreased performance resulting from normal aging, practitioners are advised that any task selected as the foundation of a performance-based assessment should fall initially into the category of everyday low demand tasks. This level of assessment serves as a good starting point for an older client group. More complex, higher demand, familiar, and novel assessment tasks can then be introduced gradually if the client performs well on simple, everyday, low-demand tasks.

All these factors must be taken into account when the occupational therapy practitioner assesses and evaluates an older client. Some specific examples of how the aging process must be taken into account when assessing elderly people follow.

VISUAL ACUITY

Visual acuity has been shown to decrease with age because "the lens of the eye loses elasticity and cannot accommodate to enable the individual to see near objects. The lens also continues cellular growth throughout life, resulting in reduced transparency. Older adults require more illumination and have reduced dark adaptation, depth perception, color discrimination, and peripheral vision" (Poole, 1992, p. 59). This means that practitioners need to be aware of

1. The lighting in the test environment

2. The size of written instructions and test items

3. The color of both the test items

4. The background surface (Cooper, 1985; Cooper, Letts, & Rigby, 1993).

If demonstrated instructions are to be given, the positioning of the tester within the client's vision is also important.

Factors related to the visual system must be reviewed when practitioners select assessments. For example, the Rivermead Perceptual Assessment Battery (RPAB) (Whiting, Lincoln, Bhavnani, & Cockburn, 1985) is an occupational therapy assessment that has been standardized for adults and older adults. This assessment can be a useful test of perception; however, there is poor differentiation between the colors of some items on the color matching task. Color vision alters with aging owing to yellowing of the lens, which affects the perception of the blue-green end of the spectrum. The RPAB involves the differentiation of several pieces in blue and green shades. Clinical experience has shown that many older clients fail this subtest even though they can name and point to colors on command (Laver, 1990). Therefore, the RPAB color matching task has limitations for some elderly clients and the results from this subtest should be evaluated with caution.

Another example that illustrates the need to review the suitability of test materials for older clients is provided by critiquing the Middlesex Elderly Assessment of Mental State (MEAMS) (Golding, 1989). This assessment was developed as a screening test to identify gross impairment of cognitive skills. The MEAMS includes 12 subtests which assess orientation, comprehension, verbal language skills, short-term memory, arithmetic, visual perception, and motor perseveration. A useful screening test, it is quick and easy to administer and relatively well accepted by clients. Some subtests, such as name learning, are age appropriate. Photographs of older people are used for this test and the ability to remember names is a relevant skill. However, the line drawings used for the "remembering pictures" subtest are problematic, for they are very small and do not account for decreased visual acuity. Many clients have difficulty recognizing the objects from the line drawings and this problem can confound the evaluation of the item as a test of memory recall.

AUDITORY ACUITY

In addition to changes in the visual system, older adults also experience changes to the auditory system. Such changes can lead to decreased hearing acuity and reduced speech discrimination skills (Maguire, 1996). The practitioner needs to monitor the use of verbal instructions during assessment. Some clients may fail to perform assessments because of an inability to hear the instructions. As many older clients experience loss of both visual and auditory acuity, a combination of instruction formats is preferable. Some assessments do not permit the repetition of instructions or the use of additional verbal and visual cues; consequently, clients may not perform to the best of their ability because they do not comprehend the instructions.

TACTILE DISCRIMINATION AND MOTOR PERFORMANCE

Many assessments require the client to manipulate test items and to complete written and drawing tasks with pen and paper. Musculoskeletal system changes that occur with age include reduced flexibility and strength (Lewis, 1996). Both the sense of touch and the related sense of kinesthesia alter with aging (Maguire, 1996). This can be problematic when tests involving the manipulation of objects (including a pen and pencil) and the positioning of body parts are used to assess cognitive or perceptual functioning, as opposed to motor functioning, touch, or kinesthesia. For example, the Clifton Assessment Procedures for the Elderly (CAPE) is a useful assessment for older adults; however, the limiting aspect of the CAPE is the Psychomotor Maze subtest. Pattie (1988) acknowledged that "at a practical level some users have questioned the usefulness of the Gibson Spiral Maze" (p. 72), while Bender (1990a) refers to the maze as "the least successful element of the CAS [Cognitive Assessment Scale, a subtest of the CAPE]" and reports that "many clinicians manage without it" (p. 108). The maze is not drawn from the usual repertoire of activities carried out in everyday life by older people and lacks ecological validity. The score from the maze indicates level of impairment and does not identify causes for dysfunction. Fine motor performance and hand-eye coordination are complex skills based on the interaction of motor, sensory, cognitive, and perceptual functions. Performance on this test could be affected by a complex range of deficits including comprehension, apraxia, loss of visual acuity, and restricted range of movement. Therefore, practitioners need to observe the performance of the test informally to identify cues pertaining to performance component dysfunction. Further assessment is required to evaluate the specific type of neuropsychological dysfunction.

COGNITIVE FUNCTION AND SENSORY LOSS

Some research has explored the relationship between hearing and visual dysfunction and cognitive impairment. There is debate about whether older adults with sensory loss also experience cognitive deficits, or whether sensory loss impedes the assessment of cognitive function and results in reduced performance on tests related to poor sensory processing. Colsher & Wallace (1990) provided a brief literature review of this debate and have conducted research in this area. They found that "the relationship between performance measures of cognition and sensory function may be largely accounted for by age, educational attainment, and general physical and psychological health." Their results also indicated that "metamemory and metacognition may be more complexly related to sensory function. Possibly the relationship between the performance measures of cognition and sensory function is a more direct reflection of neurophysiological function (including sensory function) and the neurophysiological changes associated with illness and aging" (pp. 101–102). In the occupational therapist's evaluation of the client, the interpretation of assessment data is critically important. The practitioner must ensure that the client is assessed in the optimum test environment (e.g., good lighting, low background noise, no interruptions), that instructions are understood, and that test materials can be seen clearly.

CULTURAL ISSUES

Another very important factor that practitioners should consider when assessing an older client is the client's cultural background. Culturally diverse elders "are those older persons who belong to a group that has experienced discrimination and subordination within a dominant white society.... These older persons bear the burdens of aging and the historical effects of being a member of an ethnic minority group" (McCormack, Llorens, & Glogoski, 1991, p. 11). When assessing any older person it is important to establish a good rapport. This can be more challenging when dealing with language barriers and differences in accepted forms of nonverbal communication. When the practitioner and client cannot communicate directly, a bilingual interpreter, volunteer, or family member can be invited to participate as a translator during the assessment process. Family members can provide useful information but are not always the interpreter of choice "since they may be uncomfortable interpreting the intense personal feelings of elders or may distort what has been said due to their own interpretations" (McCormack et al., 1991, p. 21). Practitioners should try to use interpreters of the same sex as the client and be aware of generational differences. An older client who is an immigrant may have different beliefs and values than his or her children and grandchildren, who, as second- or third-generation offspring in the host culture, may have assimilated some of

its beliefs and values. "When children and grandchildren interpret, a lack of understanding of abstract concepts or in some cases a violation of cultural norms and role expectations can occur" (p. 21).

In addition to language barriers, the practitioner should be aware of other potential barriers that could impede the valid and reliable assessment of a culturally diverse client:

> These include a distrust of health care providers and health care systems, a strong sense that the health care system does not fit with cultural traditions, a lack of knowledge about or access to health care services ... a reliance upon family for care and support, and a possible lack of cross-cultural training and experiences with health care providers (McCormack et al., 1991, pp. 19–20).

When selecting appropriate assessments for culturally diverse elders, practitioners should take into account the client's health beliefs, values, roles, education, and experiences. The more complex the assessment activity, the greater the likelihood for cultural differences. The practitioner should be careful to select activities, tasks, test materials, and testing formats that will be relevant and meaningful for the client. Each assessment activity should be examined for relevance, meaning, and cultural bias. The majority of assessments described in this section have been developed for North American or British populations. When using any of these assessments, practitioners should be aware of the cultural biases of the tests. Clearly, second-language difficulties should be taken into account. Less obviously, "assessments will have subtle cultural weighting, and furthermore cannot be translated to suit the person being tested without compromising their validity" (Gravell, 1990, pp. 45–46).

A few test developers have considered cultural relevance. For example, Fisher, Liu, Velozo, and Pan (1992) have conducted research to explore the cross-cultural application of the Assessment of Motor and Process Skills (AMPS) scale. A translation of the AMPS was calibrated on a group of Taiwanese subjects and the authors concluded that the results "suggested that the AMPS could be applied to Taiwanese samples" (p. 876).

In another example, one of the criteria for the selection of the self-care tasks that form the basis of the Structured Observational Test of Function (SOTOF) (Laver & Powell, 1995) is stated, in the manual as being:

> To ensure ecological and face validity for a wide range of patients, the tasks selected are functional, purposeful, familiar and have relevance for both sexes and for people from different ethnic and social backgrounds; the tasks are also suitable for administration in the subject's own environmental context (Laver & Powell, 1995, p. 26).

The four tasks assessed using the SOTOF are feeding, drinking, washing, and dressing. Although the exact method of these tasks can vary from culture to culture they do have some universal applicability. For example, feeding oneself is both essential to life and a gratifying activity. Most cultures have some kind of food which is eaten from a bowl using a simple scooping implement such as a spoon. Eating from a bowl is the most common feeding activity through the life span. Drinking is a basic human activity essential for the maintenance of health. It is relevant throughout the life span. All cultures store liquid for drinking in some kind of vessel and decant into a smaller vessel for individual consumption.

Ultimately the validity of the assessment of a culturally diverse elder will depend on the skills of the practitioner. Occupational therapists should be sensitive to their client's culture, language, values, and beliefs. In addition, they should show "respect for the elder as an individual; and a recognition of the elder's cultural worth and uniqueness" (McCormack et al., 1991, p. 20).

Assessments developed for older populations should provide normative data so that results can be interpreted in the context of expected age-related changes. The ecological validity of assessments should be considered, particularly when assessing culturally diverse elders. As sensory changes occur with aging, they can impact the client's ability to perceive and understand instructions, and the practitioner should allow sufficient time and provide cues to facilitate the reception, processing, and response to test instructions. Furthermore, practitioners should consider the demand of the assessment tasks. Finally, assessment is needed across different stages of intervention and disease process to monitor progress or, in the case of degenerative disease, to monitor decline.

Examples of Assessment Tools Suitable for Older Clients

There are increasing numbers of assessments that are available to the occupational therapy practitioner for the assessment of older clients. As these tests are too numerous to review within the scope of this section, suggestions for resources that assist the identification of suitable assessments are presented. Examples of assessments that are relevant for occupational therapists to administer to elderly clients are then outlined briefly.

RESOURCES FOR IDENTIFYING ASSESSMENTS FOR ELDERLY CLIENTS

There are a number of useful texts and resources to which occupational therapy practitioners can refer when researching and selecting assessments to use with elderly clients. Texts that are specific to occupational therapy are Asher's (1989) *An Annotated Index of Occupational Therapy Evaluation Tools,* which lists and critiques a number of tests, some of which are appropriate for older adults. Another useful text is Lewis's (1989) *Elder Care in Occupational Therapy,* which contains a comprehensive section (pp. 255–280) that provides references and brief descriptions for a wide range of specific assessment tools.

Interprofessional gerontology texts can also provide useful information for occupational therapists, for example, Israel, Kozarevic, & Sartorius (1984) have assembled the *Source Book of Geriatric Assessment,* a two-volume compilation of references and descriptions for more than 120 assessment instruments for older people. Wattis and Hindmarch's (1988) *Psychological Assessment of the Elderly* provides a general introduction to assessment with some specific information about a variety of tests that have been used in the field of gerontology over the last 20 years. Tests described in depth include the Clifton Assessment Procedures for the Elderly (CAPE) (Pattie & Gilleard, 1979) and the Comprehensive Assessment and Referral Evaluation (CARE) interview schedule (Gurland et al., 1977).

Another useful text is *Assessment of the Elderly* (Beech & Harding, 1990). It has some general chapters on different areas of assessment (such as memory, communication, mobility, and mental health) and a section of test reviews that provide detailed test critiques for 16 different assessments, including CAPE; Mini Mental State Examination (Folstein, Folstein, & McHugh, 1975); Kendrick Cognitive Scales for the Elderly (Kendrick, 1972); the Rivermead Behavioural Memory Test (Wilson, Cockburn, & Baddeley, 1991); and the Rivermead Perceptual Assessment Battery (RPAB) (Whiting et al., 1985).

SPECIFIC EXAMPLES OF ASSESSMENTS FOR ELDERLY CLIENTS

No one test provides information at all five levels of function or dysfunction (societal limitation, disability, functional limitation, impairment, and pathophysiology). The occupational therapist needs to select a range of assessment methods in order to obtain a full picture of the client's function and dysfunction. Some assessments provide data at one level of function, many offer data across two levels of function, and a few assess across several levels. The following text describes a top-down approach to assessment, beginning with tests that focus the assessment of function at the societal limitation level.

Societal Limitation Level

At this level the practitioner is interested in factors that restrict the client's functioning in the social and physical environment and that impact the ability to maintain roles. Required are assessments of barriers to functioning (both structural and attitudinal) that limit fulfillment of roles or restrict access to services and opportunities associated with full participation in society. The practitioner can begin by exploring the client's previous and current roles through the use of assessments such as The Role Checklist

(Oakley, Kielhofner, Barris, & Reichler, 1986) and the Role Adaptation, Bereavement Inventory (Larson, 1992). Since many older adults experience significant role changes with the onset of retirement, it is important to assess previous, current, and anticipated future roles.

The Role Checklist (Oakley et al., 1986) is a written assessment that helps practitioners to obtain valid and reliable information about their clients' roles. "The instrument provides data on individual perception of participation in roles throughout the life span and on the degree to which each role is valued" (Oakley et al., 1986, p. 158). The Checklist covers four different role dimensions:

1. Perceived incumbency, which relates to the person's belief that he or she occupies a role

2. Occupational role career, which documents the progression of roles throughout the life span

3. Role balance

4. Role value, which assesses the degree of value that the client attaches to each role and which incorporates the issue of volition.

The Role Checklist is appropriate for use with older clients who have physical or psychosocial dysfunction.

The Role Adaptation Bereavement Inventory (RABI) (Larson, 1992) was developed for use with clients who are grieving the death of a spouse or primary life partner and who are having difficulty adapting to new roles and lifestyles as a result of atypical grief reactions or depression. The RABI is used to identify how well a client functions in role performance and in which areas he or she has assets or deficits related to the grieving process. The Inventory is an occupational therapy observational assessment in which 50

behavioral items are scored on a five-point scale. Research has been conducted to examine aspects of reliability (Larson, 1992).

The Life Experiences Checklist (LEC) (Ager, 1990) is another tool that provides useful information at the societal limitation level. The LEC can be used to assess the "range and extent of life experiences enjoyed by an individual and, where appropriate, comparing it with that afforded the general population" (Ager, 1990, p. 5). The measure was developed for a range of client groups, including older adults, and can be used for "quality assurance, programme planning, individual therapy and staff training" (p. 5). Normative data is available for urban, suburban, and rural populations. The LEC is administered using a self-rated survey or an interview format and can be completed by the client or by an informant who knows the client well. The measure comprises a series of statement items grouped into five assessment domains: home, leisure, relationships, freedom, and opportunities.

At the societal limitation level the practitioner will also need to assess the client's physical environment, particularly in relation to safety issues. Three useful assessments in this area include:

1. The Functional Assessment and Safety Tool (FAST) (Darzins et al., 1994)

2. The Safety Assessment of Function and the Environment for Rehabilitation (SAFER) tool (Oliver, Blathwayt, Brackley, & Tamaki, 1993; Letts & Marshall, 1995)

3. The Home Occupation-Environment Assessment (HOEA) (Baum, Edwards, Bradford, & Lane, 1995).

All three assessments provide information related to function at both a societal limitation and a disability level.

The FAST was developed to assist practitioners in discharge planning by "providing a comprehensive assessment that addresses both clients' function and the support systems in their living environment" (Darzins et al., 1994, p. 1). The client, key informants, and the occupational therapist can all provide input into the data collection process. A key informant is defined as "any person who is prominently involved in the day to day care of the client" (p. 1). Client and key informant data are obtained through interview. The practitioner records information from direct observations of the client's functioning and the client's environment. The FAST covers the following broad assessment domains, each of which is further subdivided into specific assessment tasks: clothing, hygiene, nutrition, mobility, safety, residence, and supports.

The SAFER tool can be used to evaluate an older person's ability to manage functional activities safely within the home. It enables occupational therapy practitioners to "identify risk factors before an accident occurs, make recommendations to improve safety, and improve overall quality of life and perhaps reduce the risk of injury, hospitalization, chronic disability, and death" (Letts & Marshall, 1995). The SAFER tool comprises 97 items that review both personal and environmental safety factors. Items are grouped into the following assessment domains: living situation, mobility, kitchen, fire hazards, eating, household, dressing, grooming, bathroom, medication, communication, wandering, memory aids, and general. The tool was developed by a group of therapists working for the Community Occupational Therapists and Associates (COTA) in Toronto, Canada. This assessment package comprises item guidelines, recommendations, and record forms.

The item guidelines outline a series of questions for each item. These questions are not given to the client verbatim but provide cues to the practitioner to identify problem areas. For example, under the domain of "living situation," the seventh item is labeled "Environment cluttered." In the guidelines for this item, the practitioner is asked to assess the following:

- Are items placed in such a manner that they may inhibit safe mobility throughout the home, e.g., plants, newspapers, furniture narrowing a walkway?
- Are there any pets in the home that the client finds are underfoot?
- Does the placement of food/water dishes for pets interfere with a clear walkway?

The SAFER tool offers recommendations to practitioners who identify problems in any of the safety items. For example, recommendations for the Environment cluttered item include: "Remove unnecessary clutter; remove objects no longer in use; ensure clear walkways; remove unsteady furniture; eliminate piles of paper (fire hazard)." On the record form items are checked on a three-point categorical scale: addressed, not applicable, and problem. Studies have been conducted to examine the internal consistency and aspects of the validity of the tool (Letts & Marshall, 1995), and research is being undertaken to examine inter-rater and test-retest reliability.

The Home Occupation-Environment Assessment (HOEA) (Baum et al., 1995) has been developed for use with clients with dementia. The assessment covers several domains, including living situation, social supports, nature of social activities, use of equipment, general condition of the home, potentially hazardous situations, support of mobility, kitchen safety and functionality, bedroom functionality, bathroom safety and functionality, living area functionality, behaviors, performance, other observations, and action needed. Each domain is further divided into individual items, for example, the "support of mobility" domain comprises the following items: rooms accommodate equipment; furniture arrangement allows unobstructed moves; access to out of doors; can transfer to car; can access public transportation; and can get up and down from chair, bed, toilet. The record form provides space to indicate whether the item was assessed (yes or no) and the majority of items are rated on a three-point scale (no problem or requires monitor or requires attention).

Caregiver support is often critical to maintaining an older client in the community. A caregiver's ill health and experience of burden can, therefore, become a barrier to a client's function at the societal limitation level. Occupational therapy practitioners can involve the caregiver in assessment on two levels. First, a caregiver can provide information about the client's functioning in the home environment. This reported information might relate to performance of activities (disability level), performance of skills (functional limitation level), and performance component functioning (impairment level). Second, a caregiver can serve as the focus of an assessment to identify the caregiver's level of burden in order to highlight families at risk and to prioritize families for respite care (to identify barriers to the client's function at a societal limitation level). Several assessments use caregiver reports to obtain information about a client, for example, the Memory and Behavior Problem Checklist (Zarit, Reever, & Bach-Peterson, 1980) and the Functional Behavior Profile (Baum, Edwards, &

Morrow-Howell, 1993). There are a few measures of caregiver burden, including the Zarit Burden Interview (Zarit et al., 1980) and the Supports section of the FAST (Darzins et al., 1994). Two of these assessments are described in more detail to illustrate the type of information that they offer to the practitioner.

The Memory and Behavior Problem Checklist (MBPC) and the Zarit Burden Interview provide methods for reporting the caregiver's observation of the client's current functioning and behavior, and the perceived burden experienced by the caregiver in managing the person with impairment. The MBPC "was developed to report problems identified by the carer in managing the person with impairment. The instrument has two sections, one documenting the presence of the behavior and the second, documenting the carer's tolerance for the behavior, if it is observed" (Baum, 1993, p. 32). The Burden Interview provides a picture of the caregiver's perceptions of both emotion-focused and demand-focused stress. "The instrument is scored on a 5-point scale according to how the caregiver feels about the item presented. The score 0 indicates no feeling; 1. they feel a little; 2. they feel moderately; 3. feel quite a bit; 4. feel extremely" (Baum, 1993 p. 35). While these measures were initially developed as research tools for use with subjects with dementia, they have also been used successfully to assess older clients with stroke. Research is in progress to standardize the two measures for stroke populations in the United States (Personal communication, Dr. Carolyn Baum, Director for the Program in Occupational Therapy, Washington University School of Medicine, St. Louis, April 21, 1995) and the two have been used as outcome measures in Canada (Laver, 1995). The measures can be administered as a survey or in an interview format and take no longer than 20 minutes to administer.

Disability Level

At the disability level the practitioner is concerned with assessing the client's limitation in performing tasks, activities, and roles to levels expected for someone of the same age; sex; and educational, cultural, and socioeconomic status. This assessment is conducted within the context of the client's physical and social environment. At this level the practitioner examines the activities and tasks associated with the client's roles. Assessment domains can include ADL, work and productive activities, and leisure activities. ADL assessment should cover grooming; oral hygiene; bathing or showering; toilet hygiene; personal device care; dressing; feeding; medication routine; health maintenance; socialization; functional communication; functional mobility; community mobility, including driving and the use of public transport; emergency response; and sexual expression. Assessment of work and productive activities can include assessment of home management, including clothing care, cleaning, meal preparation, shopping, money management, household maintenance, and safety procedures; care of others, such as a spouse who has a disability or grandchildren; educational activities, such as new learning opportunities; and vocational activities, including paid employment, volunteer work, and retirement planning. Assessment of leisure involves the exploration of leisure interests, skills, and opportunities, as well as the evaluation of the performance of specific leisure tasks.

Many ADL and IADL assessments developed for adult populations have also been used with older adults. For example, the Functional Independence Measure (FIM) (Center for Functional Assessment Research, 1993), which

"measures traditional ADL associated with basic skills such as dressing, bathing, toileting, and mobility... is an 18-item instrument that uses a seven-point scale graded from 1 (dependent) to 7 (independent). It includes 13 motor items and 5 cognitive social items" (Ottenbacher et al., 1994, pp. 1297, 1299).

Some ADL and IADL assessments have been developed specifically for an older client group. For example, Oakley and colleagues have developed a Daily Activities Questionnaire (Oakley et al., 1992), which is a functional assessment for people with Alzheimer's disease. The work of Lawton and Brody (1969) has provided a foundation for several other assessments of older adults' IADL performance, such as Tappen's (1994) Refined ADL Assessment Scale (RADL) for clients with Alzheimer's and related conditions; the Assessment of Living Skills and Resources (ALSAR) (Williams et al., 1991); and the Older Americans Resources and Services (OARS) (Pfeiffer, 1975).

Other examples of assessments that focus evaluation at the disability level include the Activity Card Sort (Baum & Edwards, 1995); the Canadian Occupational Performance Measure (COPM) (Law et al., 1994); the Interest Check List (Matsatsuyu, 1969); the Structured Observational Test of Function (Laver & Powell, 1995); the Kitchen Task Assessment (Baum & Edwards, 1993); the Assessment of Motor and Process Skills (Fisher, 1992); and the Arnadottir OT-ADL Neurobehavioral Evaluation (Arnadottir, 1990). Some of these assessments are described briefly below.

The Activity Card Sort (Baum & Edwards, 1995) involves photographs of 75 activities: 20 ADL and IADL activities, 44 leisure activities, and 11 social activities. The client or caregiver views the photographs and sorts them into four categories:

1. Have never participated in the activity

2. Participate in the activity now

3. Participate in activity less than before

4. Have given up activity (Baum, 1993).

The client is given the opportunity to discuss the activities in each photograph. The test originally was developed for clients with Alzheimer's disease. It has now been adapted for clients with stroke. The stroke version comprises a checklist that describes 78 activities, which are grouped into three domains:

1. Home management

2. Leisure activities

3. Social activities.

The assessment is conducted during the acute phase, when activities are rated on a two-point scale: "done prior to illness" or "not done," and as a follow-up, when activities are rated on a three-point scale: "gave up due to illness," "beginning to do again," and "do now."

The Canadian Occupational Performance Measure (COPM) (Law et al., 1994) is an individualized measure of a client's self-perception in occupational performance and covers the constructs of self-care, productivity, and leisure. The area of self-care includes personal care, functional mobility, and community management. The area of productivity includes paid or unpaid work, household management, and school or play. Leisure includes quiet recreation, active recreation, and socialization. Function is rated in terms of importance, performance, and satisfaction on three 10-point scales. The test has several advantages: it has acceptable levels of test-retest reliability; it encompasses the broad domain of occupational performance by covering all three areas of self-care, productivity,

and leisure; it incorporates the roles and role expectations of the client; it considers the importance of performance areas to the client; it considers the client's satisfaction with present performance; it focuses on the client's own environment, thereby ensuring the relevance of the problems to the client; and it allows for input from members of the client's social environment if the client is unable to answer on his or her own behalf. Studies have been undertaken to examine the psychometric properties of the COPM and it has been shown to be a reliable and sensitive measure (Law et al., 1994).

The Structured Observational Test of Function (SOTOF) (Laver & Powell, 1995) provides assessment of the impact of neurological deficits on older adults' ability to engage in daily tasks. The SOTOF offers a structured way to administer an assessment of activities of daily living to assess underlying neuropsychological deficit in addition to the client's level of independence in self-care. The SOTOF involves observation of performance of four personal activities of daily living (feeding, drinking, washing, and dressing) and asking clients questions about what they are doing and perceiving. The clinician indicates on a score sheet whether the client is able to perform the task independently; which skills (e.g., reaching, sequencing) are intact; which problems are evident (e.g., perceptual, motor); and what the underlying dysfunction (e.g., ideomotor apraxia, agnosia) might be. Studies have been undertaken to evaluate the psychometric properties and clinical utility of SOTOF (Laver & Powell, 1995; Laver 1994a; Laver 1994b). Results indicate the SOTOF is a valid, reliable, and clinically useful tool that provides information regarding the relationship between an individual's neurological deficits and ADL performance.

The SOTOF identifies information related to several different levels of functioning: the disability level, through the identification of the client's residual occupational performance in the domain of ADL (by examining ability to perform simple ADL tasks such as feeding and dressing); the functional limitation level, through the breakdown of the client's residual and deficit skills and abilities within ADL performance (e.g., reaching, scanning, grasping, and sequencing); the impairment level, by identifying which performance components (perceptual, cognitive, motor, and sensory) have been affected; and the pathophysiology level, through the postulation of specific neuropsychological deficits (e.g., apraxia, agnosia, aphasia) that are impacting self-care function.

The Arnadottir OT-ADL Neurobehavioral Evaluation (A-ONE) (Arnadottir, 1990) is a comprehensive test that addresses four levels of function (disability to pathophysiology) and has good ecological validity. The A-ONE is "a clinical test intended for the evaluation of patients who have neurobehavioral dysfunctions of cortical origin.... The test format involves the primary ADL with items that address neurobehavioral deficits. The evaluation yields objective scores regarding functional independence and neurobehavior" (p. 217). As a test based on personal ADL tasks, the A-ONE can be used relatively early in the intervention of clients with neurological deficits impacting function. The test involves the completion of full-body washing and dressing and requires the patient to move to a sink for washing, so stamina and some degree of mobility are required. The test was developed for both adults and older adults.

The Kitchen Task Assessment (KTA) (Baum & Edwards, 1993) was developed specifically for an older adult population. It addresses three levels of function (disability, functional limitation, and impairment). At the level of impairment the KTA focuses on cognitive function; at the disability level it addresses the IADL task of preparing cooked pudding. Other tasks, such as preparing soup, are being added to the test. The KTA initially was developed for clients with dementia to determine the level of help needed to perform a task; and "the results allow the clinician to help caregivers understand the level of support the impaired person needs to perform daily living tasks" (p. 431). Research is in progress to standardize the assessment for stroke populations.

Functional Limitation Level

At the functional limitation level the practitioner assesses the client's ability to perform skill components of tasks, for example, scans, reaches, coordinates, lifts, grips, sequences, and manipulates. Occupational therapists are well trained in activity analysis and are able to analyze the components of a task and assess the client's ability to perform each component. This is particularly useful when no standardized assessment is available for a task important to a client, for example, an unusual leisure activity. Several of the assessments described previously provide information about the subcomponent skill performance of tasks. For example, the AMPS provides a structured way to assess observable motor and process skills associated with a range of IADL tasks and the KTA assesses the component skills of a meal preparation task. Both the SOTOF and the A-ONE were developed using activity analysis to provide a structured method for assessing the component skills of self-care tasks.

IMPAIRMENT LEVEL

At the impairment level the practitioner assesses performance component functioning, including the sensorimotor, cognitive, and psychosocial components. The assessment of sensorimotor function covers the testing of sensory, perceptual, neuromusculoskeletal, and motor function. Cognitive assessment includes the testing of areas such as level of arousal, orientation, initiation, memory, and sequencing. When assessing psychosocial skills the practitioner should consider psychological functioning (including values, interests, and self-concept). Assessment should identify those losses or abnormalities attributable to the normal aging process in addition to the impairment that has arisen as a consequence of trauma or disease.

Function at the impairment level can be assessed in older adults using a wide variety of assessment methods, many of which have been developed by psychologists or physicians. Examples are the Clifton Assessment Procedures for the Elderly (CAPE) (Pattie & Gilleard, 1979); the Cognitive Competency Test (Wang & Ennis, 1986); The Middlesex Elderly Assessment of Mental State (MEAMS) (Golding, 1989); and the Kendrick Cognitive Tests for the Elderly (Kendrick, 1972). The following tests have been developed by a research team that included occupational therapists: the Rivermead Perceptual Assessment Battery (RPAB) (Whiting et al., 1985); the Ontario Society of Occupational Therapists (OSOT) Perceptual Evaluation (Boys, Fisher, Holzberg, & Reid, 1988); the Chessington Occupational Therapy Neurological Assessment Battery (COTNAB) (Tyerman, Tyerman, Howard, & Hadfield, 1986); and the Cambridge Assessment Battery (Fraser & Turton, 1986). In addition, three of the assessments

that were described above as related to assessment at the disability level also provide information at the impairment level. They are the Structured Observational Test of Function (SOTOF) (Laver & Powell, 1995); the Kitchen Task Assessment (KTA) (Baum & Edwards, 1993); and the Arnadottir OT-ADL Neurobehavioral Evaluation (A-ONE) (Arnadottir, 1990). The SOTOF and the A-ONE provide assessment of cognitive, perceptual, sensory, and motor function; the KTA provides assessment of cognitive function.

The KTA, SOTOF, CAPE, MEAMS, and Kendrick were developed specifically for an older adult population. However, despite the increasing recognition of the effect of age on neuropsychological function and the high incidence of neuropsychological deficit in the older population, none of the other assessments was developed specifically for an older adult population. Studies have been conducted to standardize the RPAB and the COTNAB for older populations (Lincoln & Clarke, 1987; Laver & Huchison, 1993). There continues to be a need for assessments that are developed specifically for an older population and that take normal aging processes into account. Reviews of many of these assessments are available (e.g., Pattie, 1988; Crammond, Clark, & Smith, 1989; Arnadottir, 1990; Bender, 1990a and 1990b; Laver, 1990; Grieve, 1993). Several of these tests are discussed below to provide examples of this type of assessment.

The Cognitive Competency Test (Wang & Ennis, 1986) is an observational test comprising "a variety of items simulating skills required in daily life functioning [and assesses] very basic cognitive functions which are considered fundamental to the maintenance of safe and independent living" (p. 131). The test contains eight subtests to assess the domains of personal information; card arrangement, which involves sequences of everyday activities such as making a phone call, laundry, and meal preparation; picture interpretation, in which the client describes what is currently happening in a picture and draws conclusions about preceding or subsequent events; memory; practical reasoning skills; management of finances; verbal reasoning and judgment; and rote learning and spatial orientation.

RPAB (Whiting et al., 1985) was designed to assess deficits in visual perception following stroke or head injury. Normative data enable the occupational therapist to evaluate whether a person has greater difficulty with visual perceptual tasks than might have been expected prior to brain damage. The aspects of visual perception addressed by the battery can be summarized under eight headings:

1. Form constancy
2. Color constancy
3. Sequencing
4. Object completion
5. Figure ground discrimination
6. Body image
7. Inattention
8. Spatial awareness.

The test is composed of 16 short subtests. Fifteen of them are timed activities administered at a table on a layout guide. They include activities such as picture cards, block designs, jigsaws, and drawing.

CAPE is designed to evaluate cognitive and behavioral functioning. It consists of two parts: the Cognitive Assessment Scale (CAS) and the Behavioural Rating Scale (BRS). These two scales can be used separately or together. The CAS comprises three sections:

1. An information and orientation subtest, which includes an interview covering 12 questions pertaining to orientation of time, place, and person and 3 questions on current information

2. A mental ability test involving counting, reading, writing, and reciting the alphabet

3. A psychomotor task requiring the completion of the "Gibson Spiral Maze" to assess fine motor performance and hand-eye coordination.

The Behavioural Rating Scale is administered as a survey to the client's primary caregiver (such as a nurse or relative). Questions on this scale relate to four main areas: physical disability, apathy, communication difficulties, and social disturbance. Reviews of the research potential and clinical utility of CAPE have been undertaken by Bender (1990a) and Pattie (1988).

The Kendrick Cognitive Test for the Elderly assesses the cognitive abilities considered to be most sensitive to age changes (Bender, 1990b). It involves the evaluation of immediate recall of briefly presented data and the speed of processing and storing information. The test has two parts: the Kendrick Object Learning Test (KOLT) and the Kendrick Digit Copying Test (KDCT). The KOLT involves the presentation of four picture cards depicting common objects. Clients are given a limited time to recall the pictures seen. The KDCT assesses the client's speed at copying 100 random numbers.

Pathophysiology Level

Finally, at the pathophysiology level the practitioner is interested in the interruption of normal physiological and developmental processes or structures. Assessment at this level focuses, therefore, on cellular, structural, or functional events subsequent to injury or disease or related to expected aging processes. This level is not the prime focus of occupational therapy assessment, and information about functioning at this level is often provided by other professionals, such as doctors. However, some occupational therapy assessments do provide the practitioner with information at this level. For example, the Arnadottir OT-ADL Neurobehavioral Evaluation (A-ONE) (Arnadottir, 1990) can be used to postulate both the specific deficit (such as apraxias, spatial-relations impairment, and body scheme disorders) and the location of the cortical dysfunctions.

Summary

The primary purpose of occupational therapy evaluation and assessment for older clients is to get a clear and comprehensive picture of the individual and develop treatment plans that will result in improved occupational function and quality of life.

Occupational therapy assessments are used for

1. Predicting a client's future functional level

2. Comparing clients' function to that of normative groups

3. Describing the current functional status of clients

4. Evaluating clinical change in occupational performance or performance component functioning

5. Evaluating the occupational therapy program and quality assurance systems

6. Providing valid and reliable outcome measures to help establish appropriate eligibility criteria for social and insurance programs.

The levels of function addressed by assessment data are defined by the International Classification of Impairments, Disabilities, and Handicaps (ICIDH) developed by the World Health Organization. The National Center for Medical Rehabilitation Research refined the original classification for professionals working in rehabilitation fields, broadening the functional and dysfunctional hierarchy to include five levels: social limitation, disability, functional limitation, impairment, and pathophysiology. These five major levels of function assist clinicians and researchers to identify the functional performance to be evaluated and the level or levels of function they are addressing in their assessment and intervention.

When assessing older adults, there are several special considerations that the clinician must take into account. They include effects of the normal aging process and their impact on occupational performance, as well as pathology that limits occupational performance. Cultural issues must also be considered.

There are many assessment tools suitable for older clients. Useful texts that identify assessments for elderly clients are available. This section concludes with summaries of specific assessments that address the five levels of function and dysfunction.

Review Questions

1. How is a predictive assessment different from a descriptive assessment?

2. What is the purpose of evaluative assessments?

3. Differentiate between functional limitation and disability. Give an example of each.

4. What is the advantage of the "top-down" approach to assessment?

5. List some considerations for assessing older adults.

6. What are the disadvantages of using a family member to interpret?

7. If you are evaluating a client at the societal limitation level and wish to assess data on occupational roles and their value throughout the life span, which assessment tool would you select?

8. At the societal limitation level, which assessment tools could you use to evaluate the physical environment and safety issues?

9. Which assessments can be used to evaluate caregiver support and caregiver burden?

10. What types of assessments are used to address the disability level? Give at least three specific examples.

11. If you wished to assess the impact of neurological deficits in an older adult's ability to engage in daily tasks, which test would you use?

References

Ager, A. (1990). Life experiences checklist. Windsor, UK: NFER-NELSON.

Arnadottir, G. (1990). *The brain and behavior: Assessing cortical dysfunction through activities of daily living.* St. Louis: C. V. Mosby.

Asher, I. E. (1989). *An annotated index of occupational therapy evaluation tools.* Rockville: The American Occupational Therapy Association.

Baum, C. M. (1993). The effect of occupation on behaviors of persons with senile dementia of the Alzheimer's type and their carers. Unpublished doctoral thesis, Washington University, St. Louis.

Baum, C., & Edwards, D. (1995). *The Activity Card Sort.* St. Louis: Occupational Therapy Program, Washington University.

Baum, C. M., & Edwards, D. F. (1993). Cognitive performance in senile dementia of the Alzheimer's type: The Kitchen Task Assessment. *American Journal of Occupational Therapy, 47,* 431–436.

Baum, C., Edwards, D., Bradford, T., & Lane, R. (1995). *Home Occupation-Environment Assessment (HOEA).* St. Louis: Occupational Therapy Program, Washington University.

Baum, C. M., Edwards, D. F., & Morrow-Howell, N. (1993). Identification and measurement of productive behaviors in senile dementia of the Alzheimer's type. *Gerontologist, 33,* 403–408.

Beech, J. R., & Harding, L. (Eds.). (1990). *Assessment of the elderly.* Windsor: NFER-NELSON.

Bender, M. P. (1990a). Test review—Clifton Assessment Procedures for the Elderly. In J. R. Beech & L. Harding (Eds.), *Assessment of the elderly.* (pp. 107–109). Windsor: NFER-NELSON.

Bender, M. P. (1990b). Test review—Kendrick cognitive tests for the elderly. In J. R. Beech & L. Harding (Eds.), *Assessment of the elderly.* (pp. 117–119). Windsor: NFER-NELSON.

Bernspang, B., Fugl-Meyer, A. R., & Viitanen, M. (1988). Perceptual function in the elderly and after stroke. *Scandinavian Journal of Caring Science, 2,* 75–79.

Boys, M., Fisher, P., Holzberg, C., & Reid, D. W. (1988). The OSOT Perceptual Evaluation: A research perspective. *American Journal of Occupational Therapy, 42,* 92–98.

Center for Functional Assessment Research. (1993). *Guide for uniform data set for medical rehabilitation (Adult FIM)* (Version 4.0). Buffalo: Center for Functional Assessment Research and Uniform Data System for Medical Rehabilitation.

Christiansen, C. (1993). Continuing challenges of functional assessment in rehabilitation: Recommended changes. *American Journal of Occupational Therapy, 47,* 258–259.

Colsher, P. L., & Wallace, R. B. (1990). Are hearing and visual dysfunction associated with cognitive impairment? A population-based approach. *Journal of Applied Gerontology, 9,* 91–105.

Cooper, B. A. (1985). A model for implementing color contrast in the environment of the elderly. *American Journal of Occupational Therapy, 39,* 253–258.

Cooper, B. A., Letts, L., & Rigby, P. (1993). Exploring the use of color cueing on an assistive device in the home: Six case studies. *Physical and Occupational Therapy in Geriatrics, 11,* 47–59.

Crammond, H. J., Clark, M. S., & Smith, D. S. (1989). The effect of using the dominant or non-dominant hand on performance of the Rivermead Perceptual Assessment Battery. *Clinical Rehabilitation, 3,* 215–221.

Darzins, P., Edwards, M., Lowe, S., McEvoy, E., Rudman, D., Taipale, K., & Vertesi, A. (1994). *Functional assessment and safety tool user's manual.* Hamilton: McMaster University/Hamilton Civic Hospitals.

Dickerson, A. E., & Fisher, A. G. (1993). Age differences in functional performance. *American Journal of Occupational Therapy, 47,* 686–692.

Duchek, J. M., & Balota, D. A. (1993). The impact of normal aging on memory functioning. In J. Morley (Ed.), *Cowdry's geriatrics.* New York: Manning.

Ellis, A. W., & Young, A. W. (1988). *Human Cognitive Neuropsychology.* London: Lawrence Erlbaum Associates.

Fisher, A. G. (1992). Assessment of motor and process skills. Unpublished test manual. Colorado State University, Fort Collins, CO.

Fisher, A. G., Liu, Y., Velozo, C. A., & Pan, A. W. (1992). Cross-cultural assessment of process skills. *American Journal of Occupational Therapy, 46,* 876–885.

Folstein, M. F., Folstein, S. C., & McHugh, P. (1975). Mini-Mental state: A practical method for grading the cognitive state of patients for the clinician. *Journal of Psychiatric Research, 12,* 189–198.

Fraser, C. M., & Turton, A. (1986, August). The development of the Cambridge Apraxia Battery. *Occupational Therapy, 248–252.*

Frey, W. D. (1988). Functional outcome: Assessment and evaluation. In J. A. DeLisa (Ed.), *Rehabilitation medicine: Principles and practice* (pp. 158–172). London: J. B. Lippincott.

Golding, E. (1989). *The Middlesex Elderly Assessment of Mental State.* Suffolk: Thames Valley Test.

Gravell, R. (1990). The assessment of communication. In J. R. Beech & L. Harding (Eds.), *Assessment of the elderly* (pp. 41–52). Windsor: NFER-NELSON.

Grieve, J. (1993). *Neuropsychology for occupational therapists—Assessment of perception and cognition.* London: Blackwell Scientific Publications.

Gurland, B. J., Kuriansky, J. B., Sharpe, L., Simon, R., Stiller, P., & Birkett, P. (1977). Comprehensive Assessment and Referral Evaluation (CARE)—Rationale, development and reliability. *International Journal of Aging and Human Development, 8,* 9–42.

Haley, S. M., Coster, W. J., & Ludlow, L. H. (1991). Pediatric functional outcome measures. *Physical Medicine and Rehabilitation Clinics of North America, 2,* 689–723.

Hasselkus, B. R. (1974). Aging and the human nervous system. *American Journal of Occupational Therapy, 28,* 16–21.

Israel, L., Kozarevic, D., & Sartorius, N. (1984). *Source book of geriatric assessment* (2 volumes). Basel: Karger/World Health Organization.

Katz, N. (1992). *Cognitive rehabilitation: Models for intervention in occupational therapy.* London: Andover Medical Publishers.

Kendrick, D. (1972). *Kendrick cognitive tests for the elderly.* Windsor: NFER-NELSON.

Larson, K. O. (1992). Initial study for internal reliability of the "Role Adaptation Bereavement Inventory." Unpublished master's thesis, New York University. Provided by author.

Laver, A. J. (1990). Test review—Rivermead Perceptual Assessment Battery. In J. R. Beech & L. Harding

(Eds.), *Testing people* (pp. 134–138). Windsor: NFER-NELSON.

Laver, A. J. (1994a). The development of the Structured Observational Test of Function (SOTOF). Unpublished doctoral thesis, University of Surrey, Guildford, U.K.

Laver, A. J. (1994b). The Structured Observational Test of Function (SOTOF). AOTA *Gerontology Special Interest Section Newsletter, 17 (1),* 1–3.

Laver, A. J. (1995). The evaluation of a short-term conductive education programme for a sample of twelve adults with a primary diagnosis of stroke. Unpublished manuscript. McMaster University, School of Occupational Therapy and Physiotherapy, Hamilton, Ontario.

Laver, A. J., & Huchison, S. (1993). *The performance and experience of normal elderly people on the Chessington Occupational Therapy Neurological Assessment Battery (COTNAB)—65+ Standards.* Nottingham: Nottingham Rehab.

Laver, A. J., & Powell, G. E. (1995). *The Structured Observational Test of Function (SOTOF): Test manual.* Windsor: NFER-NELSON.

Law, M. (1993). Evaluating activities of daily living: Directions for the future. *American Journal of Occupational Therapy, 47,* 233–237.

Law, M., Baptiste, S., Carswell, A., McColl, M. A., Polatajko, H., & Pollock, N. (1994). *Canadian Occupational Performance Measure* (2nd ed.). Toronto: CAOT Publications ACE.

Law, M., & Letts, L. (1989). A critical review of scales of activities of daily living. *American Journal of Occupational Therapy, 43,* 522–528.

Lawton, M. P., & Brody, E. M. (1969). Assessment of older people: Self-maintaining and instrumental activities of daily living. *Gerontologist, 9,* 179–186.

Letts, L., & Marshall, L. (1995). Evaluating the validity and consistency of the SAFER tool. *Physical and Occupational Therapy in Geriatrics, 13(4),* 49–66.

Lewis, C. B. (1996). Musculoskeletal changes with age: Clinical implications. In C. B. Lewis (Ed.), *Aging: The health care challenge* (3rd ed.). Philadelphia: F. A. Davis.

Lewis, S. C. (1989). *Elder care in occupational therapy.* Thorofare, NJ: SLACK.

Lincoln, N., & Clarke, D. (1987). The performance of normal elderly people on the Rivermead Perceptual Assessment Battery (RPAB). *British Journal of Occupational Therapy, 50,* 156–157.

Maguire, G. H. (1996). The changing realm of the senses. In C. B. Lewis (Ed.), *Aging: The health care challenge* (3rd ed.) Philadelphia: F. A. Davis.

Matsatsuyu, J. S. (1969). The interest check list. *American Journal of Occupational Therapy, 23,* 323–327.

McCormack, G. L., Llorens, L. A., & Glogoski, C. (1991). Culturally diverse elders. In J. M. Kiernat (Ed.), *Occupational therapy and the older adult* (pp. 11–42). Gaithersburg, MD: Aspen Publishers.

Nagi, S. Z. (1991). Disability concepts revisited: Implications for prevention. In A. M. Pope & A. R. Tarlov (Eds.), *Disability in America* (pp. 309–327). Washington, DC: National Academy Press.

National Center For Medical Rehabilitation Research (NCMRR). (1992). *Report and plan for medical rehabilitation research to Congress.* National Center for Medical Rehabilitation Research, Bethesda: National Institute for Child Health and Human Development, National Institutes of Health.

National Center For Medical Rehabilitation Research (NCMRR). (1993). *Research plan for the National Center for Medical Rehabilitation Research.* (NIH Publication no. 93–3509.) Bethesda: U.S. Department of Health and Human Services, National Institutes of Health.

Oakley, F., Kielhofner, G., Barris, R., & Reichler, R. K. (1986). The Role Checklist: Development and empirical assessment of reliability. *Occupational Therapy Journal of Research, 6,* 157–170.

Oakley, F., Sunderland, T., Hill, J. L., Phillips, S. L., Makahon, R., & Ebner, J. D. (1992). The Daily Activities Questionnaire: A functional assessment for people with Alzheimer's Disease. *Physical & Occupational Therapy in Geriatrics, 10,* 67–81.

Oliver, R., Blathwayt, J., Brackley, C., & Tamaki, T. (1993). Development of the Safety Assessment of Function and the Environment (SAFER) tool. *Canadian Journal of Occupational Therapy, 60,* 78–82.

Ottenbacher, K. J., Mann, W. C., Granger, C. V., Tomita, M., Hurren, D., & Charvat, B. (1994). Inter-rater agreement and stability of functional assessment in the community-based elderly. *Arch. Phys. Med. Rehabil., 75,* 1297–1301.

Pattie, A. (1988). Measuring levels of disability—The Clifton Assessment Procedures for the Elderly. In J. P. Wattis & I. Hindmarch (Eds.), *Psychological assessment of the elderly* (pp. 61–75). London: Churchill Livingstone.

Pattie, A., & Gilleard, C. (1979). *Clifton assessment procedures for the elderly.* London: Hodder & Stoughton.

Pfeiffer, M. (1975). *Multidimensional functional assessment: The OARS methodology.* Durham, NC: Duke University Center for the Study of Aging and Human Development.

Poole, J. L. (1992). Age-related changes in sensory system dynamics related to balance. *Physical and Occupational Therapy in Geriatrics, 10,* 55–66.

Rogers, J. C., & Holm, M. B. (1989). The therapist's thinking behind functional assessment. In C. B. Royeen (Ed.), *AOTA Self Study Series—Assessing Function* (lesson 1). Rockville: The American Occupational Therapy Association.

Tappen, R. M. (1994, June). Development of the Refined ADL Assessment Scale for patients with Alzheimer's and related disorders. *Journal of Gerontological Nursing,* 36–42.

Trombly, C. (1993). Anticipating the future: Assessment of occupational function. *American Journal of Occupational Therapy, 47,* 253–257.

Tyerman, R., Tyerman, A., Howard, P., & Hadfield, C. (1986). *The Chessington O.T. Neurological Assessment Battery Introductory Manual.* Nottingham: Nottingham Rehab.

Wang, P. I., & Ennis, K. E. (1986). Competency assessment in clinical populations: An introduction to the Cognitive Competency Test. In B. Uzzell & E. Gross (Eds.), *Clinical neuropsychology of intervention* (pp. 113–133). Boston: Martinus Nijhoff Publishing.

Wattis, J. P., & Hindmarch, I. (1988). *Psychological assessment of the elderly.* London: Churchill Livingstone.

Weg, R. B. (1973). The changing physiology of aging. *American Journal of Occupational Therapy, 27,* 213–217.

Welford, A. T. (1993). The gerontological balance sheet. In J. Cerella, J. Rybash, W. Hoyer, & M. L. Commons (Eds.), *Adult information processing: Limits on loss* (pp. 3–10). London: Academic Press.

Whiting, S., Lincoln, N., Bhavnani, G., & Cockburn, J. (1985). *RPAB— Rivermead Perceptual Assessment Battery—Manual*. Windsor: NFER-NELSON.

Williams, J. H., Drinka, T. J. K., Greenberg, J. R., Farrell-Holtan, J., Euhardy, R., & Schram, M. (1991). Development and testing of the Assessment of Living Skills and Resources (ALSAR) in elderly community-dwelling veterans. *Gerontologist, 31,* 84–91.

Wilson, B., Cockburn, J., & Baddeley, A. (1991). *The Rivermead Behavioural Memory Test*. Suffolk: Thames Valley Test.

World Health Organization. (1980). *International classification of impairments, disabilities, and handicaps*. Geneva: World Health Organization.

Zarit, S. H., Reever, K. E., & Bach-Peterson, J. (1980). Relatives of the impaired elderly, correlates of feeling of burden. *Gerontologist, 20,* 649–655.

Section 2. Treatment Planning and Treatment Approaches

Karen Allison, MOTR/L

Abstract

All treatment begins with a plan and is based on several factors. This unit examines various approaches to planning and the factors that go into a successful treatment plan.

Treatment Planning

A treatment plan is a statement of the proposed therapeutic program. It is based on:

1. An analysis of data gathered in the evaluation
2. The identified performance deficits
3. The treatment context
4. The circumstances of the individual patient.

The treatment plan includes the long- and short-term objectives, treatment methods, and intended progression of treatment. Ongoing reevaluation, intrinsic to the treatment process, is used to modify the treatment plan in accordance with the patient's progress toward stated goals and objectives. After evaluation and data analysis, the therapist engages in a problem-solving process to develop a treatment plan suited for the individual patient (Hopkins, 1993; Pedretti, 1996; Trombly, 1989).

Building the treatment plan, then, is a vital first step in providing occupational therapy services. Regardless of the diagnosis, every patient needs the benefit of an organized plan, formulated with successful outcomes in mind. Only a registered occupational therapist (OTR) can write an occupational therapy plan of care. However, diverse factors and people must be considered when formulating the treatment plan. People who might contribute to development of the plan are the patient, the patient's family, other health care professionals, and the patient care coordinator. Factors internal and external to the rehabilitation process also require consideration. Internal factors include information in the medical history and about the patient's condition, such as diagnosis, date of onset, prior existing conditions, and results of the therapist's initial evaluation. External factors include the setting for therapy, payer source, discharge placement, and designated caregiver (figure 11–3).

DIAGNOSIS

The therapist usually learns the diagnosis before seeing the patient. The diagnosis gives clues about the possible rehabilitation process. For example, what might a therapist assume from the diagnosis of uncomplicated total hip replacement? Left hemisphere cerebral vascular accident (CVA)? Chronic obstructive pulmonary disease (COPD)?

Although not exclusive to geriatrics, it is much more common with the elderly that a patient entering rehabilitation presents with multiple diagnoses. An elderly patient who has had a recent CVA, for example, may also have a history of hearing loss, arthritis with multiple joint replacement, and congestive heart failure (CHF). The medical and rehabilitation diagnoses are therefore frequently different. The physician treats a primary diagnosis such as a CVA, and the therapist treats the secondary hemiparesis, while addressing ADL in the context of the multiple complicating conditions.

Figure 11–3. Factors Internal and External to the Rehabilitation Process

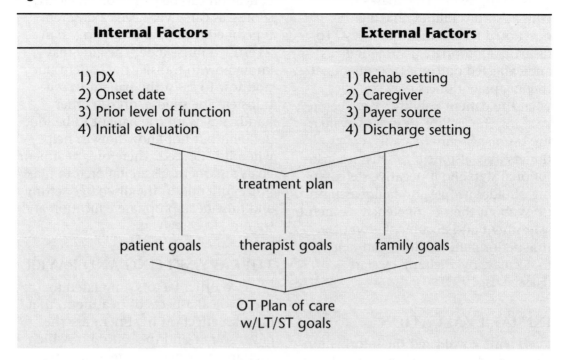

Internal Factors	External Factors
1) DX	1) Rehab setting
2) Onset date	2) Caregiver
3) Prior level of function	3) Payer source
4) Initial evaluation	4) Discharge setting

treatment plan

patient goals   therapist goals   family goals

OT Plan of care
w/LT/ST goals

When treating the elderly, a pitfall is to regard age as a diagnosis or complication of a diagnosis. Having lived a long time, in itself, does not mean that a person necessarily has decreased motivation or potential for rehabilitation. Such an assumption should be avoided and basing a denial of treatment on age is inappropriate.

DATE OF ONSET

The elderly patient may be seen for therapy immediately after the onset of an acute condition, or therapy may be ordered to deal with the long-term-effects of an insidious disease process. The latter is especially true for the custodial patient of a long-term-care residence. Such patients are frequently seen for therapy after a documented change of function while in the nursing home. Residential facilities must ensure that each resident's ADL abilities do not diminish unless the clinical condition causes an unavoidable decline. It is the occupational therapy practitioner's responsibility to understand how a change of condition, even for a quality-of-life patient, demands therapy. If there is acute onset of a clinical condition, therapy may be ordered routinely by the doctor. If a functional decline occurs the therapist may need to request the order, with the date of onset being the day the decline was noted and documented in the medical record.

PRIOR LEVEL OF FUNCTION

For the patient with an acute onset condition who is living at home, premorbid function is usually the standard level on which treatment goals are based and which therapy works to regain. However, for a nursing home resident, prior level of function is often unclear. Nursing home residents sometimes experience a condition known as "learned helplessness," a dependency caused by the staff's underestimation of competence and social stereotyping that results in overhelping

(Hasselkus, 1993). This masks the patient's true abilities, making the functional level difficult to assess. To develop appropriate treatment goals and expected outcomes, occupational therapy practitioners may consider what the patient's abilities were before entering the facility, as well as evaluating his or her current status. Practitioners may also help to sensitize institutional staff about negative stereotyping of older people and faulty assumptions about their competencies. Careful assessment and documentation of true performance abilities can help to decrease overhelping by staff (Hasselkus, 1993).

INITIAL EVALUATION

Having considered the information about the diagnosis and associated medical conditions, date of onset, and prior level of function, the practitioner proceeds with a comprehensive initial evaluation. This is the occupational therapist's record of the baseline of function from which to plan treatment outcomes. The results of treatment are influenced by the patient's medical progress and by the external factors.

WHERE TO AND WITH WHOM

Determining where the geriatric patient will go when rehabilitation is completed is very important for the therapist. Whether the patient will return home where there are stairs, throw rugs, and a cat, or will live in a residential facility where safety is paramount but independence is not encouraged, will affect the treatment plan. Each setting has specific needs that should be addressed by occupational therapy. Likewise, whether the patient needs continued assistance with ADL when discharged and who will provide that assistance must be identified so that appropriate caregiver

education can be planned. An elderly spouse as caregiver needs a different type of education and training than a certified nurse aide. The aide may know how to transfer the patient but not how to assist the patient in self-transfer. The spouse, on the other hand, may want the patient to be independent but not know how to help when it is needed. Therefore, treatment goals and methods are tailored to maximize function in the discharge setting and provide appropriate education and training to caregivers.

THERAPY SETTING AND PAYER

Two other factors, unrelated to the medical aspects of treatment, that have an effect on treatment are the payer source and the setting in which therapy takes place. A treatment plan formulated to be carried out in a spacious gym with modern rehabilitation equipment will be different from one carried out in a patient's small apartment. Goals for functional outcomes may be the same, but the way in which goals are reached is different. For example, an exercise program using bar weights, appropriate positioning, and postural support, carried out under the watchful eye of the therapist can take place in a clinic gym. At home, the patient may be given resistive elastic bands, use food cans as weights, and be supervised by the caregiver, who is following written instructions for a home exercise program.

With the rapid spread of managed care, the length of time a therapist has to carry out a plan of care is usually quite short. As plans are compressed to meet time constraints, every treatment in the rehabilitation process must be goal directed. The treatment plan itself should be objective and outcome driven. A realistic rehabilitation potential should be determined and shared with the appropriate people. Rehabilitation potential is very important because it determines whether the patient receives therapy. If a physician does not believe the patient will benefit from occupational therapy, he or she will not write an order for it. If the case manager does not understand what occupational therapy does, treatments will not be approved. If the nurse believes that the patient is too old for help, therapy screening will not be requested. Communication with other health professionals and patient care coordinators concerning the patient's ability to benefit from occupational therapy is imperative.

While the potential for benefiting from rehabilitation may be immediately apparent in some cases, the issue is very complex in the care of the elderly. It is necessary to understand that the rehabilitation potential of a patient is directly reflected in the long- and short-term goals set for the patient. Goals should reflect a patient's rehabilitation potential within the scope of his or her capabilities and environment, and have meaning to the patient and family as well. Rehabilitation potential is always good if the goals are within the scope of the patient's functional capacities, regardless of how narrow that scope is. Case study 1 illustrates this point.

Treatment

As with other patient populations, treatment for the elderly may be preventive, restorative, or compensatory. A brief look at each treatment approach illustrates its possibilities and appropriateness for occupational therapy intervention.

PREVENTION AND RESTORATION

A practitioner's primary role in a preventive approach is the prevention of deterioration beyond that expected in the normal aging process. To achieve that, aging must be regarded as a normal part of the developmental process with its own demands and needs, just as in the earlier stages of life. Ideally, primary prevention is practiced before the onset of disease or injury. Smoking cessation, exercise, and staying within normal weight parameters are examples of primary prevention. The use of joint protection principles to prevent the deformities of rheumatoid arthritis is another example.

A secondary preventive approach is used in occupational therapy to plateau decline or prevent further injury after the onset of injury or disease. Frequently, prevention is discussed during the education process of therapy. Case study 2 illustrates the secondary prevention process.

COMPENSATION

When function will not be restored, compensatory activities and methods should be taught. Unfortunately, compensatory learning comes more easily to the young. For the older person with a lifetime of well-established habits, learning methods of compensation and accepting helpful assistive devices is often met with resistance, frustration, and disgust. The premorbid condition, motivation for self-reliance, degree of dysfunction, and realistic attainable goals all contribute to the success of a compensatory treatment program.

Assistive devices may be indicated for some activities. The rule for the use of such equipment is that the device should allow the patient to do a desired activity that cannot be performed without the device. For example, spending treatment time teaching an elderly man, who has lost the use of one upper extremity, to use a button hook may be a priority to the practitioner. However, if the patient and his wife are perfectly happy with her buttoning his shirt and he expresses no interest in the button hook, it is best put away. Allowing the man's wife to help with the task may appear counterproductive to the goal of functional independence. But it is the patient's treatment plan, not the practitioner's, and neither the button hook nor independence for buttoning the shirt is important to him. Independence is highly valued in American culture but it should not be pursued on that basis or because the occupational therapy practitioner values it. Independence must be important to the patient and within the scope of his or her capacities (Foti, Pedretti, & Lillie, 1996).

Discharge Planning

Occupational therapy is begun with the end in mind. Discharge planning begins on day one of treatment. A baseline is established with the initial evaluation and the practitioner reevaluates regularly, noting progress weekly or more often if needed. The treatment plan is modified on the basis of the ongoing reevaluation. Measurable goals in the plan of care expedite the reevaluation and discharge process. Once discharged, the custodial patient may benefit from restorative nursing with the occupational therapy practitioner checking periodically to see that function is maintained. For the patient who is returning to a private residence, a home program may be appropriate along with patient and caregiver education and follow-up as needed.

Accurate and thorough documentation is an important part of occupational therapy for the elderly. No case is closed until the evaluation, plan of care, charge sheet, progress notes, and discharge summary are completed and filed in the permanent medical record.

Summary

Providing occupational therapy services for the elderly consists of three main phases:

1. Identifying appropriate patients
2. Planning treatment and rendering treatment as necessary
3. Documenting accurately.

Designing an occupational therapy treatment plan is a vital first step in providing treatment. The plan is based on internal and external factors and contains goals that are realistic for the patient's capacities, treatment context, discharge setting, and caregiver needs. The diagnosis, associated complications and other medical conditions, date of onset, and prior level of function are factors that must be considered in writing a plan of care. Rehabilitation potential is always good if goals are achievable within the patient's capacity.

Treatment of older persons may be preventive, restorative, or compensatory, depending on the diagnoses and expected outcomes. A combination of approaches is used in many cases.

Consideration of discharge setting and planning for discharge begins on the first day of treatment. There is ongoing reevaluation of the treatment plan, and the patient's progress is recorded regularly. Measurable goals in the care plan expedite the reevaluation and discharge process. Accurate documentation of the evaluation, treatment plan, charge sheet, progress notes, and discharge summary in the permanent medical record is critical to comprehensive occupational therapy services.

Activity

1. Write a plan of care for a 64-year-old male patient. Be creative. From your clinical knowledge, select the following:
   - Diagnosis
   - Date of onset
   - Prior level of function
   - Results of the initial evaluation. Use an abbreviated report for this exercise, including four functional areas related to the diagnosis.
   - Therapy setting and discharge setting
   - Four goals. Indicate whether each goal was contributed mainly by the patient, family, or occupational therapist.

Review Questions

1. Who are the people and what are the factors that must be considered in treatment plan development?
2. What can be a pitfall when treating the elderly?
3. How do complications and preexisting conditions affect the treatment plan and rehabilitation program?
4. When is a custodial client in a long-term care residence likely to be referred for occupational therapy?
5. For a custodial patient seen for occupational therapy secondary to functional decline, what is the date of onset?
6. How is the prior level of function determined for a patient who is living at home?
7. What is the problem that may mask a patient's true functional abilities in nursing homes?
8. What may the practitioner use to estimate potential for regaining function in nursing-home patients?
9. Why is knowing the discharge setting and designated caregiver important in treatment planning?
10. Why are the payer source and treatment setting important factors in treatment planning?
11. How would an occupational therapy treatment program differ for a geriatric patient seen through a home health agency and the same patient seen at a rehabilitation clinic?

Case Studies

CASE STUDY 1

This case illustrates the importance of setting realistic goals for reimbursement purposes, and the value of occupational therapy at all levels of care.

The physical therapist is seeing a patient for wound care. At the rehabilitation team meeting the PT asks for an OT referral for positioning to relieve the pressure area. The occupational therapy evaluation shows a 94-year-old male resident of a nursing home who is bed-bound secondary to a massive CVA six years ago, with late-stage dementia. The patient is incontinent and syringe fed. If the occupational therapy goals are ADL independence with minimum assistance of one and independent bed mobility, then the potential for achieving rehabilitation goals is poor. If, however, the plan of care states goals for education of caregivers in appropriate bed positioning and provision of positioning devices as needed, and emphasizes decreasing the risk of skin breakdown for safety from infection, then rehabilitation potential is good. The goals of the latter treatment plan are within this patient's capabilities and the environmental context. That is, his skin and underlying tissue will remain intact if relief from pressure is provided and this can be accomplished in his environment, the bed. The practitioner is, of course, making assumptions that freedom from pain and infection is meaningful to the patient. Also, the practitioner makes a professional determination that the patient's functional capabilities are very limited and that he would benefit most from a quality of life approach: educating caregivers in performing vital tasks to give comfort such as bed positioning that he can no longer perform independently.

CASE STUDY 2

This case illustrates how the secondary preventive approach is used in occupational therapy to prevent further decline.

An occupational therapist receives an order to restore mobility to the right upper extremity of a 64-year-old female outpatient. The patient fell one week prior to the order, requiring open reduction at the wrist. Before the accident she was an active, independent retiree. She is a widow who lives alone and is now very concerned about the possibility of future falls. Her conversation is dominated by references to fear of becoming dependent on others. She is especially fearful because she is right-hand dominant and her fingers are stiff and sore. The primary goal is to restore the use of the injured extremity, the undertaking of which is normally an immensely rewarding task for the patient and the therapist. With appropriate therapeutic intervention, restoration of function is an expected outcome for this patient. However, along with treatment to restore joint mobility and muscle function, the plan should specify education to reduce the chance of future falls outside the home and a home survey to identify fall risks in the home. Thus, restoration of function and prevention of further falls are addressed in the treatment program.

References

Foti, D., Pedretti, L. W., & Lillie, S. (1996). Activities of daily living. In L. W. Pedretti (Ed.), *Occupational therapy: Practice skills for physical dysfunction* (4th ed., pp. 463–506). St. Louis: Mosby-Yearbook.

Hasselkus, B. R. (1993). Functional disability in older adults. In H. L. Hopkins & H. D. Smith (Eds.), *Willard and Spackman's occupational therapy* (8th ed., pp. 742–752). Philadelphia: J. B. Lippincott.

Hopkins, H. L. (1993). Tools of practice: Sec. 4. Problem solving. In H. L. Hopkins & H. D. Smith (Eds.), *Willard and Spackman's occupational therapy* (8th ed., pp. 292–294). Philadelphia: J. B. Lippincott.

Pedretti, L. W. (1996). Treatment planning. In L.W. Pedretti (Ed.), *Occupational therapy: Practice skills for physical dysfunction* (4th ed., pp. 43–54). St. Louis: Mosby-Yearbook.

Trombly, C. A. (1989). Treatment planning process. In C.A. Trombly (Ed.), *Occupational therapy for physical dysfunction* (3rd ed., pp. 3–12). Baltimore: Williams and Wilkins.

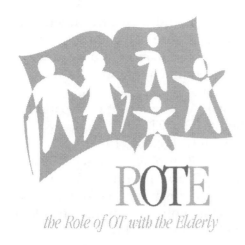

ROTE

the Role of OT with the Elderly

Evaluation and Interventions for the Performance Components

Section 1. The Sensorimotor Component

Anne Birge James, MS, OTR/L

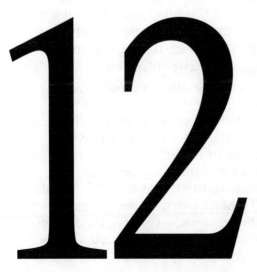

Abstract

Older adults have had a lifetime to develop adaptations to functional limitations resulting from sensorimotor deficits. Therefore, the most successful approach to treatment is to focus on assessment of performance components within a functional context. Top-down evaluations using a task-oriented approach will facilitate remediation and the transference of components to occupational tasks.

Assessment and Treatment of Sensorimotor Components Within a Functional Context

Assessment and treatment of sensorimotor deficits within the practice of occupational therapy must be aimed at those performance component deficits that cause a limitation in occupational performance. While the skilled clinician can base some accurate predictions about occupational performance on an assessment of performance components, the variability in use of adaptations and coping strategies by individuals makes it impossible to get a reliable assessment of occupational performance without addressing it specifically (Trombly, 1993). The geriatric population, in particular, seems to demonstrate significant heterogeneity in its behavior for both performance components and performance areas (Bonder & Goodman, 1995; Levy, 1993). It is, therefore, necessary to use a top-down approach to assessment, beginning first by exploring the client's roles (Trombly, 1995c).

The tasks that make up an individual's life roles will vary greatly from person to person. Identification of important tasks should be a collaborative effort between the occupational therapist and client, but ultimately the roles and tasks must be defined by the client (Clark, 1993; Trombly, 1995c). For clients with cognitive dysfunction, family members and significant others can assist the therapist with this step in the evaluation process. Once tasks are identified, careful observation of the client performing these selected activities will help the occupational therapist focus the assessment of performance components on those deficit component skills that most probably caused the observed functional limitations. This will maximize the efficiency of the evaluation, so that treatment can be initiated promptly. Additionally, Medicare requires that therapists measure and report functional outcomes, so that documentation of treatment aimed at remediation of performance components must specifically link gains made in those skills to the functional task(s) it has enhanced. The top-down approach will facilitate that process.

Historically, many occupational therapists have used a bottom-up approach to evaluation, initiating the process with an assessment of performance components. In a bottom-up approach it is more difficult to structure the evaluation because assessments may be selected on the basis of pathology, rather than the individual's needs and skills. Beginning with a performance component assessment may also make it difficult for clients to understand the relationship between

isolated skills and their own functional potential. The use of a client-centered approach to evaluation and treatment has received much attention in recent occupational therapy literature (Canadian Association of Occupational Therapists [CAOT], 1991; Nelson & Payton, 1991; Pollock, 1993; Townsend, Brintnell, & Staisey, 1990; Trombly, 1995b). This approach suggests that occupational performance is an individual phenomenon, dependent on the individual's culture, environment, and valued roles (CAOT, 1991; Trombly 1993), thereby requiring a top-down assessment approach. Additionally, recent literature suggests that motivation is an important element for participation, learning, and recovery (Arnadottir, 1990; Craik, 1991; Montgomery, 1991; Shumway-Cook & Woollacott, 1995). To treat sensorimotor dysfunction without establishing its relevance to an individual's performance priorities may result in poor follow-through and unreached functional potential. Use of a client-centered approach will help the therapist and client collaborate to establish treatment priorities, enhancing potential for desired outcomes. Educating the client regarding the relationship between the sensorimotor skills being addressed in treatment and the established functional goals is particularly critical. If this relationship is not apparent to the client, it may negatively impact motivation; follow-through; and, ultimately, outcomes.

Recent studies in motor learning also support the use of assessment and treatment of sensorimotor skills within the context of functional activities because of the importance of contextual cues and the task-specificity of motor control (Gordon, 1987; Horak, 1991; Mathiowetz & Bass Haugen, 1995a; Shumway-Cook & Woollacott, 1995). Use of a task-oriented approach is particularly appropriate in the accurate evaluation and treatment of the elderly for at least three reasons. First, the elderly seem to utilize a wider variety of contextual cues during motor tasks compared with younger adults who seem to attend to information from fewer afferent sources to guide performance (Bennett & Castiello, 1994; Proteau, Charest, & Chaput, 1994). Contextual cues are often minimized for performance component testing to help improve test validity. It is important to remember that the validity of an instrument is relative *only* to the construct(s) the test purports to measure; therefore, the relationship to function is not typically a part of validity testing for tools designed to measure only at the performance component level.

Second, another advantage to using a task-oriented approach with the elderly is the relatively low complexity of most performance component assessments compared with the task requirements of daily living skills. Degradation of motor performance in response to increased complexity of the task occurs earlier in the elderly population (Cerella, Poon, & Williams, 1980; Shumway-Cook & Woollacott, 1995). Therefore, performance on a sensorimotor assessment may accurately indicate the skill is intact, yet the skill may degrade when used in the context of a complex functional task. For example, testing a client in a clinical setting free of distraction reveals that she has intact stereognosis. The task demands, however, of maintaining standing balance at the grocery store while trying to distinguish coins from keys in the bottom of a pocket book with a line of customers waiting may overwhelm the capacity of her sensorimotor system, making it difficult or impossible for her to access her "intact" stereognosis within the context of a task.

Third, performance components other than sensory or motor skills may

have a significant impact on the functional performance of tasks thought to be primarily sensorimotor in nature (Shumway-Cook & Woollacott, 1995). For example, a person may demonstrate intact balance reactions but does not participate in community activities because of a fear of falling.

While the top-down approach begins with a focus on functional skills, the assessment and treatment of isolated performance components is a crucial part of the process. Enhancement of component skills may play a key role in maximizing the functional outcome, since capability in performance areas is dependent on more basic abilities (Christiansen, 1991; Fleishman, 1972; Trombly, 1995c). Treatment aimed at performance component deficits may, in some cases, be the most effective approach if remediation will enhance functional outcomes across several performance areas. Treatment at the task level relies primarily on compensatory strategies that tend to be more task specific, requiring customized adaptations for each task.

It is crucial that one take into account the effect of specific pathologies and their precautions and contraindications on the safety, reliability, and validity of any assessment prior to using it. Similarly, treatment techniques are often developed to meet the needs of a specific client population. The appropriateness of an assessment tool or treatment technique for specific diagnostic categories is beyond the scope of this text.

Assessment of Sensorimotor Skills

If therapists are to best determine the sensorimotor areas that require further testing, the assessment of performance areas should be structured to give the therapist a broad view of the client's underlying performance component skills. This can be done through careful selection of performance-based assessment of work, self-care, and leisure. There are some assessment tools aimed at identifying subtask deficits within the context of functional tasks, which help the examiner determine potential limitations in sensorimotor skills. They include the Assessment of Motor and Processing Skills (AMPS) (Fisher, 1992); the A-One Evaluation (Arnadottir, 1990); and the TEMPA (Desrosiers, Hébert, Dutil, & Bravo, 1993; Desrosiers, Hébert, Dutil, Bravo, & Mercier, 1994). As the framework for a task-oriented approach continues to develop within the practice of occupational therapy, it is anticipated that more of these types of assessment tools will be developed.

Once the occupational therapist has established those performance components that require further assessment, the most appropriate test instruments and procedures must be selected, taking into account the client's expected roles; functional capacity; anticipated performance context (including both the human and non-human environment); and the extent of occupational therapy services it is anticipated that the client will receive. There are many assessment tools commonly used by occupational therapists for the evaluation of sensorimotor skills in the adult population. Any of these tools may be appropriate for use with the older adult, though some special considerations with this population warrant discussion.

There is ample literature suggesting a decline in the performance of motor skills with age (Bennett & Castiello, 1994; Desrosiers, Hébert, Bravo, & Dutil, 1995; Williams, 1990). Most of these studies examined reaction time or some other speeded measure as the dependent variable, though the tasks typically included some degree of precision, such as a target. The data were

collected primarily from "healthy older adult" sample populations. While the criteria used to determine "healthy" varied, all subjects were reportedly independent in activities of daily living. Researchers disagree about the cause for this apparent slowing of response or performance in the elderly. Many researchers suggest that the demands of the task exceed the information-processing capacity of the aging central nervous system and the older adult's performance is driven by this slower system (Birren, Woods, & Williams, 1980; Botwinick, 1984; Williams, 1990). An alternative theory has suggested that component skills deteriorate with age and any one of several compromised systems may impact reaction times (e.g., poor vision may require an individual to slow performance in order to reach a target) (Botwinick, 1984). Williams (1990) reported that deterioration in performance was greater with age when tasks involved a significant accuracy component compared with tasks in which precision was not a major component. This may be because older adults seem to be more cautious, favoring accuracy at the expense of speed (Botwinick, 1984). Regardless of the cause of the decline in motor skill, care should be taken when interpreting the results of timed tests, particularly those with a significant accuracy component, when the subject is compared with normative data. Many of the coordination and hand function tests used in occupational therapy fall into that category.

When using tests that have normative data, one must investigate the sample used to establish norms in order to determine whether a comparison of an individual with those norms would reveal useful and relevant information. While it is always prudent to use caution when comparing clients with normative data, the variability in the elderly population may limit the usefulness of that data when evaluating older adults. Careful use of normative data in the assessment of the elderly is crucial to ensure that accurate interpretation of test results leads to sound clinical judgments. Some normed tests, particularly those designed to test manual dexterity, were developed for specific populations and normative data cannot be generalized to an elderly population. For example, norms for the Purdue Pegboard data come from a sampling of applicants and workers in various manual-labor jobs. While the test may be a useful tool for assessing change in an older person over time, comparing the performance of an elderly client with the published norms would not provide the occupational therapist with valid assessment data. Many normed tests of sensorimotor function have grouped the sample population into specific age ranges and have published norms for older adults. Often, however, the oldest age group represents a broader range than the other groups (e.g., norms may be determined for each decade of age up to 59 years and the last category of normative data is for ages 60 and up). Studies of eye-hand coordination suggest that performance continues to decline in each decade (i.e., one would expect performance of someone in the 80s to be slower than that of someone in the 60s) (Welford, 1982; Williams, 1990). Because these larger groupings represent greater age ranges, the variability will be higher in these groups as compared with the sample populations used for the younger age groups. Whenever possible, it is desirable to identify the age range and distribution of the subjects in the sample population before making judgments based on comparison of the client's performance to the norm. It is also important to investigate other characteristics of the sample population because of the general variability in performance

among the elderly, even those in a relatively narrow age range. Samples for normative data can come from a variety of sources and it may not be possible to generalize to other segments of the population. For example, normative data from a group of individuals living in a retirement community that provides daily meals for residents may be quite different from data collected from individuals of a comparable age living independently in their own homes.

Normative data do not exist for many occupational therapy assessments (e.g., cutaneous sensory tests and manual muscle tests). Lack of normative data may be due to one or more reasons:

1. Many assessments use ordinal scales limiting the use of descriptive statistics.

2. Wide variability in the healthy population would make comparison with the norms of little clinical use even if they did exist (e.g., passive range of motion measurements).

3. Establishment of normative data requires testing large samples of the population and the data may not exist.

Many criterion-based tests have a ceiling that is considered "normal" (e.g., 100% accuracy for identification of pain sensibility), so sampling a large normal population to examine a range of normal behaviors would not provide clinically useful information. Many criterion-based measurements of sensorimotor function can be useful in the assessment of the older adult if the measurements are carefully chosen and the criteria critically analyzed for appropriateness to the individual client. The criteria are commonly established on young or middle-aged adults and may not be a valid standard for the elderly. Passive range of motion measurements provide a good example. Most texts consider normal shoulder flexion and abduction passive range of motion to be 0–180 degrees (Norkin & White, 1995; Trombly, 1995c). Bassey, Ebrahim, Dallosso, and Morgan (1989) evaluated shoulder passive range of motion in the elderly. Four hundred and seventy-nine subjects were 65 to 74 years of age and 474 subjects were 75 years of age and over. Mean shoulder abduction ranges were analyzed separately for men and women in the two age groups and ranged from 112 to 128 degrees. All means were well below the typically cited "normal" range for shoulder abduction.

Older adults with recent and regular participation in physical activities seem to perform better than their more sedentary peers on motor skills tests, suggesting that regular practice of sensorimotor skills helps to minimize the age-related deterioration of these skills (Lord & Castell, 1994; Salthouse, 1985; Tse & Bailey, 1992). It is therefore important to consider the client's history and life experience when making clinical decisions regarding motor skills. The potential error that seems most likely to occur when a client's sensorimotor history is not explored is that of underestimating that client's treatment needs. For example, an assessment of a 76-year-old man 12 weeks after suffering a Colles fracture revealed that grip and pinch strength and performance on the Jebsen-Taylor Hand Function Test were within normal limits for the client's sex and age. His history, however, included taking daily walks, sailing his 30-foot sailboat twice a week in the summer, and routinely completing small woodworking projects. Identifying such strength and dexterity performance components as "intact" may lead the therapist to discontinue treatment, when in fact the client is quite "impaired" by his own standards and may achieve more optimal functional outcomes if treatment

were continued and if strength and dexterity were specifically addressed.

The following is a summary of tools for sensorimotor assessment of older adults. The specific testing procedures are beyond the scope of this text and may be found in the references. Special considerations for their use with the older adult are included.

SENSORY TESTING

Tactile Sensory Processing and Sensory Awareness

There are many assessments designed to examine an individual's ability to interpret light touch, pressure, temperature, pain, and vibration through skin receptors and the ability to differentiate these sensory stimuli. The purpose of sensory testing is typically either to identify the presence of sensory deficits that may contribute to impaired manipulatory function or to determine the status of protective sensation. Sensory testing is time consuming and the vast array of assessments make it necessary to select a few tests that will yield the most useful data, given the goal of testing and the client's functional deficits. In the case of certain pathologies (e.g., peripheral nerve injuries) more extensive testing may be indicated.

Tactile sensory tests involve the successive applications of a stimulus to determine the presence, absence, or impairment of a specific sensory function, including light touch, pressure, pain, temperature, and vibratory sensibilities. Discriminatory tests include static two-point discrimination, moving two-point discrimination, and sharp or dull discrimination. Most lack a standardized testing protocol, though various procedures have been described in the literature (Bentzel, 1995a; Callahan, 1990b; Pedretti, 1996b; Tan,

1992). For touch awareness (light touch), pain, and temperature sensibility, it is generally expected that subjects with normal sensation will identify 100% of the stimuli; however, normative data are not available. A few tests of tactile sensation have undergone reliability studies and have established norms. Normal values were established for moving and stationary two-point discrimination in 467 subjects, aged 4 to 92 years (Louis et al., 1984). Linear regression analysis of their data showed a significant increase in both moving and stationary two-point discrimination scores for older adults. Most normal thresholds, however, are not given for varied age groups (Bentzel, 1995a; Callahan, 1990b). The Semmes-Weinstein monofilaments to test touch and pressure sensibility have been shown to have a consistently repeatable application force (Fess, 1990) and good inter-rater reliability (Bowen, Griener, & Jones, 1990). Normal thresholds of sensation were established on 24 "young adults" (Weinstein, 1993) and then reestablished on a group of 70 adults (Bowen et al., 1990). Their results confirmed the original normal thresholds; however, no ages were reported for the subjects in their sample population.

While the Semmes-Weinstein monofilament test is probably the most reliable and sensitive measure of sensibility available, the normal threshold criteria should be used cautiously with older adults. It is also more expensive to purchase than most other instruments and is time consuming to administer. The "mini-kit," which is less expensive, may be useful in determining the presence or absence of protective sensation, which has important treatment implications for teaching the client protective strategies to prevent injuring the limb.

Stereognosis

Testing the ability to interpret tactile sensation may provide information regarding the relationship between an individual's tactile sensation and functional limitations. The test for stereognosis requires the client to manipulate small objects, so motor function must be relatively intact (Bentzel, 1995a). Pedretti, Zoltan, and Wheatley (1996) described standardized objects and procedures for this test. Bentzel (1995a) indicated that familiar objects should be used but did not specify which ones. Objects with varying sizes and shapes can be selected to reflect a range of discriminatory abilities. For example, a test including a paper clip and safety pin of approximately the same size or two different coins requires finer discriminatory abilities than a selection that includes only dissimilar objects.

Pain Response

There is clinical evidence to suggest that responses to pain may change with aging, resulting in increased pain tolerance in the older population (Botwinick, 1984). Visual analog scales and behavioral assessments are often used to assess pain (Engel, 1993). Pain is a subjective experience; therefore, use of such assessment tools is not likely to be influenced by the age of the client. Caution may be indicated, however, if one is measuring pain as an indicator of soft tissue pathology in an older adult whose pain threshold may be higher. For example, in a client with carpometacarpal (CMC) osteoarthritis of the thumb, pain may be one criterion used to identify those activities that put undue stress on the joint and, therefore, should be altered. If an individual's pain threshold seems high, activity analysis that examines the direction and extent of forces acting on the CMC joint may provide a safer and more appropriate measure for guiding the modification of activities of daily living.

Vestibular Function

Vestibular function plays a key role in maintaining balance and may warrant focused assessment in older adults, since falls represent a significant health risk. Balance, however, is a more complex phenomenon than simply a response to vestibular input. Visual and proprioceptive input provide the central nervous system with critical information for maintaining balance. Functional balance assessments may identify balance deficits; however, they do not identify the specific performance components that contribute to the problem. Adults with vestibular deficits can often compensate well by using other sensory input for balance and often have no apparent functional deficit (Shumway-Cook & Woollacott, 1995). Determining the type of afferent information an individual relies on for balance may help the occupational therapist plan treatment by targeting the impaired system, if remediation is thought feasible, or teaching compensatory strategies individually designed to rely on intact afferent systems. The Clinical Test for Sensory Interaction in Balance (CTSIB) is an assessment tool designed to identify the sensory strategies used in balance (Horak, 1987; Shumway-Cook & Horak, 1986). This test examines standing balance under six different sensory conditions that either eliminate or distort visual input or somatosensory input from the surface (floor). It can help the examiner establish the presence of a vestibular loss pattern. As with any balance testing, this test is likely to destabilize the client and extreme care should be taken to ensure the safety of the client. The client should wear a gait belt and be guarded closely. Since fear of falling can have a negative impact on performance, it is critical that the purpose and procedures of the test be explained to the client, particularly those procedures intended to ensure safety.

Visual Perception

Careful assessment of visual perceptual function of the older adult is important for several reasons. Studies have shown a decrease in visual perception with age, including a decrease in contrast sensitivity (Owsley, Sekuler, & Siemsen, 1983), visual acuity (Fozard, 1990), light sensitivity (Fozard, 1990), depth perception, and the speed of visual information processing (Fozard, 1990; Williams, 1990). Additionally, 7.8% of the population over 65 years of age experience visual loss due to age-related diseases (Nelson, 1987). Visual perception plays a key role in sensorimotor function, including hand-eye coordination (Williams, 1990) and balance (Shumway-Cook & Woollacott, 1995). Lastly, the selection of an effective treatment approach designed to enhance visual input or provide compensatory strategies is dependent on accurate information regarding the client's visual perceptual status.

Warren (1994) has described the limitations of the traditional approach to the evaluation of visual perception, which is divided into independent assessments of the optic system, typically done by physicians and optometrists, and the perceptual process, traditionally evaluated by psychologists and occupational therapists. Perceptual function, however, is dependent on the optic system and Warren (1993a; 1994) proposes a hierarchical model for evaluation and treatment. She has outlined a comprehensive and systematic approach to evaluation of visual perceptual function in adults that is appropriate for the elderly (Warren, 1993a, 1993b, 1994, 1996). Special considerations for the assessment of clients with neurological dysfunction are discussed, making it particularly applicable to adults who have had a cerebrovascular accident.

Auditory, Olfactory, and Gustatory Sensation

Occupational therapists frequently include assessment of visual perception in the initial evaluation of clients because of the obvious effect of vision on occupational performance. Other special senses, such as hearing, olfaction, and gustation are often absent from the typical occupational therapy evaluation. In the elderly population, these special senses merit focused assessment. Limitations in these areas may have a significant impact on safety and daily living skills. The decline of these sensory functions may be gradual, going unnoticed by the individual.

Many studies have reported that hearing declines throughout adulthood (Fozard, 1990). Perception of the higher frequencies declines more quickly than the speech frequencies through age 60. After age 60, however, hearing loss of the speech frequencies accelerates (Fozard, 1990). Typically, the therapist will suspect a hearing loss during the evaluation of performance areas. Follow-up should begin with a review of the client's history to determine the presence of documented pathology. For clients with suspected hearing loss who have not been evaluated recently, the occupational therapist has an obligation to refer the client to the appropriate professional for evaluation (American Occupational Therapy Association, 1992).

A reduction in hearing threshhold is not the only significant age-related change that impacts the comprehension of speech. Gordon-Salant (1987) studied the comprehension of words with varied background noise. She found that there was not a uniform age effect for comprehension of words presented in a quiet environment; however, in the presence of background noise, there was a significant decline in comprehension with increasing age. Additionally, Fozard (1990) reported that older adults rely more heavily on contextual cues for speech comprehension when compared with younger adults. When comprehension of various types of speech was analyzed, interrupted and speeded speech showed the largest decline with age (Fozard, 1990). While the occupational threrapist may not be involved in the direct assessment of hearing, accommodating for typical age-related changes can enhance the assessment of older adults. Evaluations should occur in an environment with minimal background noise. The therapist should avoid interruptions when speaking and keep the rate of speech slow. Use of contextual cues when presenting evaluation materials and giving directions may enhance the patient's performance. Keeping communications focused on the task at hand is important for maintaining contextual cues. Therapists often, for example, break up the "formality" of an evaluation session by gathering information about the individual (interests, family, etc.) throughout the session. This informal "chatting" provides the therapist with useful information and helps facilitate rapport. For the older adult, however, such "chatting" may actually reduce comprehension and degrade performance. It may be best to gather information about interests or family at a separate time when, again, contextual cues can be enhanced (e.g., discussing family and friends while looking at photographs or cards).

The sense of smell is important for pleasure and serves as a warning device. A decline in smell functioning with age has been well established in the literature (Nordin, Monsch, & Murphy, 1995). When a loss occurs slowly over time, as is seen with aging adults, the individual does not typically perceive declining function. Doty, Shaman, and Dann (1984) developed the Smell Identification Test and gathered normative data on a large sample. Scores were reported by decade from the second through the tenth decades. The test has 40 scents in "scratch and sniff" booklets and is available from Sensonics, Inc. (P.O. Box 112, Haddon Heights, NJ 08035). Smaller versions of the test are also available and may be more appropriate for screening olfaction in an occupational therapy assessment.

Gustatory sensation (taste) tends to decrease with age. After about age 50, the ability to discriminate taste sensation declines. By age 80, there is considerable difficulty distinguishing between the four basic tastes: sweet, sour, salty, and bitter (Levy, 1988; Lewis, 1979; Pedretti, 1996b). The taste receptors for sweet and salt flavors at the front of the tongue seem to atrophy first and there may be an increased sensitivity to bitterness. This can have an impact on nutrition of the elderly who may complain that food is tasteless, or tastes sour or bitter (Levy, 1988; Lewis, 1979). Smoking can also contribute to a decrease in taste sensation (Levy, 1988; Pedretti, 1996b). There is a strong relationship between taste and smell. Much taste sensation depends on the possession of an intact sense of smell. A decline in olfactory functioning can contribute to a decrease in taste sensitivity and, consequently, the enjoyment of food (Levy, 1988).

Compensation for diminished sense of taste through the use of heated foods and pungent herbs and spices can enhance the pleasure of eating. Food should also be prepared to be attractive (Levy, 1988). Taste is not only essential to the enjoyment of food but it stimulates salivation and swallowing. Therefore, the occupational therapist is concerned with taste sensitivity as part of an oral-motor evaluation and for planning feeding training programs (Pedretti, 1996b).

Pedretti (1996b) described a test for taste sensation based on the work of Silverman and Elfant (1979). The test involves application of the four basic tastes to the appropriate areas of the tongue. The standard given for normal adults is the ability to identify all of the tastes accurately. Standards for older adults are not described.

TESTS OF MOTOR FUNCTION

Neuromusculoskeletal Functions

Range of motion (ROM) should be evaluated initially through a gross functional assessment by asking the client to demonstrate movements of the limbs in all planes. A comparison of this active ROM with the demands of the individual's activities of daily living is vital. If movement is adequate *for this individual's functional needs* no further assessment is indicated and ROM can be recorded as within functional limits (WFL). If discrepancies exist between the individual's ROM needs and the abilities demonstrated during gross functional assessment, goniometric measurements of both passive and active ROM should be completed. Procedural information is available from many sources, including Pedretti, 1996a; Norkin & White, 1995; and Trombly, 1995a. Average ranges for each joint are cited in the texts and are not broken into age groups. Caution should be used when comparing the older adult with these average ranges, because information is not included regarding the establishment of the published comparisons. Norkin &

White (1995) discussed the impact of age on ROM and cited several studies; however, the studies focused on isolated joints or motions and did not report typical ranges for all joints.

A manual muscle test (MMT) may be used to identify strength deficits and is typically indicated in the elderly only when a suspected imbalance in muscle strength is thought to interfere with function. The MMT allows treatment aimed at increasing strength to be appropriately focused. It is a criterion-referenced test, with normal strength defined thus: "The part moves through full range of motion against maximum resistance and gravity. Normal differs for each muscle group and in persons of different ages, sex, and occupation" (Trombly, 1995a, p. 109). The difficulties inherent in defining "normal" for an individual limits the reliability of this test with the elderly unless the pathology causes a muscle imbalance. In such cases, a comparison can be made between impaired muscles and analogous intact muscles.

Grip and pinch strength can be tested using dynamometers and pinch meters. Norms are available for age groups of five years, beginning at age 20, the oldest age group representing the population 75 and over (Mathiowetz, Kashman, et al., 1985).

Motor Dexterity

There are many tests of manual dexterity described in the occupational therapy literature (e.g., Mathiowetz & Bass Haugen, 1995a; Smith, 1993). The purpose of the test must first be examined, because many, designed to predict work potential for industrial jobs, would have limited applicability to the older adult. Many of the prevocational tests take a substantial amount of time to administer and are likely to include a significant endurance component. Two tests, however, seem particularly suited for evaluating manual dexterity in the elderly. The Box and Block Test requires the client to transfer 1-inch blocks from one side of a divided box to the other and norms were initially established on 628 normal subjects aged 20 to 75+ (Mathiowetz, Volland, Kashman, & Weber, 1985). Following a brief practice session, the client is timed for 1 minute with each hand, so the test duration is fairly brief. Desrosiers, Bravo, Hébert, Dutil, and Mercier (1994) completed reliability, validity, and norms studies of the Box and Block Test with an elderly population. Their norms include 5-year age groupings up to age 84, providing more detailed norms for the elderly population than the data presented by Mathiowetz, Volland, et al. (1985). The scores for men and women in the study by Desrosiers et al. (1994), however, were combined, as the examiners found no gender differences. Therefore, data from this study cannot be compared with Mathiowetz, Volland, et al. (1985), who reported different norms for men and women. The Nine Hole Peg Test (Mathiowetz, Weber, Kashman, & Volland, 1985) is another test of manual dexterity that can be administered quickly and is normed on adults aged 20 to 75+. It is inexpensive to construct and compact, making it easy to use in treatment settings where the therapist must carry tools to the client (e.g., for bedside treatment or consulting). The Nine Hole Peg Test requires a finer pinch and greater accuracy component compared with the Box and Block Test.

Treatment of Sensorimotor Skills

Occupational therapy, ultimately, must provide clients with the strategies necessary to function independently whenever possible. It is possible to focus treatment on narrowly defined performance components (e.g., strength or range of motion). There is, however, much evidence to suggest that in order to enable individuals with motor impairment to regain function, treatment must occur within the context of the functional task (Carr & Shepherd, 1987b; Horak, 1991; Mathiowetz & Bass Haugen, 1994; Mathiowetz & Bass Haugen, 1995b; Sabari, 1991; Shumway-Cook & Woollacott, 1995). Carr and Shepherd (1987a; 1987b) recommend practicing "missing components" of a task, that is, a small component of the task or an impairment in a performance component, only when the client is unable to complete the task. Treatment at the performance component level is always practiced within the context of a task as soon as possible, preferably within the same treatment session.

Motivation and client participation seem to be enhanced when the client is involved in a task carefully designed to remediate a specific impairment, as compared with a rote exercise program targeting the same performance component deficit (Lang, Nelson, & Bush, 1992). Participation in activities may be more motivating than rote exercise for some elderly individuals. Zimmerer-Branum and Nelson (1995) presented two programs to increase or maintain active shoulder flexion to elderly nursing home residents. One was rote exercise, the other a targeted ball-throwing task. When given a choice between the task and rote exercise, a significantly higher number selected the task. Motivation is a critical element for the success of a therapeutic intervention. Maximizing the use of tasks that are meaningful to the client is an important step in establishing a therapeutic relationship with the client and creating an environment that facilitates participation (CAOT, 1991). While many people appear to find participation in

activities motivating, one cannot rely on group data to make treatment decisions for an individual client. The individual must always be involved in the process of defining roles and tasks with personal meaning. In the United States, for example, rote exercise for strengthening is an activity of daily living for many people, particularly for problems of strength and endurance. Many clients may believe this to be an effective strategy and enjoy the challenge of "beating" yesterday's number of repetitions, even when their history did not include a rote exercise routine. In this case, however, the challenge to the occupational therapy practitioner will be to help the client transfer gains made doing rote exercise into performance areas.

Some impairments may be difficult to remediate within the context of a task because either it is difficult to structure a task in a way that eliminates undesirable compensatory strategies or the person is simply unable to perform the task given the impairments. Under these circumstances, it is crucial that the client understand how treatment of the performance components will make it possible to participate in those tasks identified as most meaningful. At the first possible opportunity, the occupational therapy practitioner must structure activities that require the gains made in performance components to be used in a functional context. The practitioner must analyze the task within the performance context. The environment can then be altered as needed to enhance performance. As performance component skills improve, the occupational therapy practitioner must facilitate the practice of tasks in a more natural context to make the skill accessible to the client in daily life. For example a client with a right hemiparesis would like to don his winter coat while standing so that he can participate in weekly Bingo games without having to ask for assistance with the coat. He lacks adequate grip strength in the right hand to initiate donning the left sleeve. He practices the dressing task in standing, with assistance from the therapist to initiate the left sleeve, and begins putty exercises for strengthening grip in the right hand. As soon as the client has adequate grip to lift a button-down shirt while standing, the therapist has the client begin practicing upper body dressing with a light-weight shirt while standing. Strengthening exercises continue while practice of the task is graded to increase the weight of the garment as grip strength improves. This strategy facilitates motor learning by having the client practice progressively stronger muscle contractions within the context of the task and provides a therapy program that includes a clear connection for the client between the strengthening exercises and the functional goal.

Careful integration of treatment aimed at performance components with intervention at the task level also makes it easier for the occupational therapy practitioner to link all treatment to functional outcomes, facilitating the reevaluation process and meeting documentation requirements.

TREATMENT OF SENSORY DEFICITS

Some sensory deficits are not amenable to remediation because of the underlying pathology or because the treatment aimed at remediation falls outside the scope of occupational therapy practice (e.g., a hearing aid prescription). The use of compensatory techniques focuses treatment at the performance areas and is covered in chapter 13; however, some of the compensatory strategies for sensory deficits have been included here, as they often enable performance across several tasks.

Treatment of Tactile Sensory Awareness Deficits

Sensory reeducation is a treatment approach that teaches clients with sensory impairment to reinterpret altered sensory perception. These techniques have been used for clients with peripheral and central nervous system deficits (Bentzel, 1995b; Dellon, 1988). The effectiveness of these techniques seems to be best documented in studies of clients who sustained a peripheral nerve injury (Bentzel, 1995b; Callahan, 1990a). No studies were found that looked at the impact of age on the effectiveness of sensory reeducation for peripheral nerve injury and this diagnostic group does not compose a significant portion of the occupational therapy practitioner's caseload in geriatric practice. Results of studies that explored the effectiveness of sensory reeducation for clients who have sustained a cerebral vascular accident (CVA) are mixed (Bentzel, 1995b), and further study is needed before the efficacy of this treatment can be established. One important consideration in using this technique is that it requires intense concentration and active participation in order to be successful (Bentzel, 1995b; Callahan, 1990a; Dellon, 1988). Clients who have even mild cognitive impairment or who lack the initiative to be active participants and follow through with independent programs between therapy sessions are not appropriate candidates for sensory reeducation. This may limit its applicability to some geriatric populations.

Compensatory strategies must be used when sensation is severely impaired or absent in order to avoid injury to the insensate areas. Intact senses may be used for compensation, for example, using vision to monitor the insensate part in relation to sharp or hot objects, or using a body part with intact sensation to test water temperature. This approach depends on adequate cognitive function for learning new skills and generalizing them quickly into functional activities. This may be difficult for clients with cognitive deficits and for tasks that are strongly habituated. Another strategy is to protect the insensate part when it may be at risk. Like the use of alternative sensory input, these strategies require the client to initiate the compensation, such as putting on protective gloves when near hot objects or always wearing shoes when walking. Changing the environment to reduce potential dangers requires little active participation from the client once hazards are identified and eliminated. Turning down the temperature of the hot water heater and wrapping exposed hot water pipes with insulation are examples.

Vestibular Retraining

Clients with vestibular dysfunction can undergo a training program that seems to be effective in reducing the symptoms of vertigo and disequilibrium (Cohen, 1994; Herdman, 1994). Individuals often compensate well for declining vestibular function by relying on visual and somatosensory input. Many elderly individuals, however, experience multisensory deficits, which makes it impossible to compensate with alternative systems because all systems for postural control are impaired (Herdman, 1994; Shumway-Cook & Woollacott, 1995). For example, a client with recent macular degeneration was beginning to experience increasing falls with episodes of vertigo. While macular degeneration

did not cause vestibular dysfunction, in this case the vestibular dysfunction was probably present prior to the visual loss and presented no functional problem as long as the client could rely on visual input. Given the diagnosis, restoring vision was not feasible, but treatment aimed at enhancing vestibular function reduced vertigo, disequilibrium, and the risk of falls for this client.

Visual Perceptual Retraining

Decreased pupil size, loss of transparency, and increased thickness of the lens occur with aging, allowing less light in to the retina (Fozard, 1990; Levy, 1993). Older adults need twice the illumination of younger persons (Levy, 1993) and may benefit from environmental adaptations to enhance contrast, simplify the visual field (e.g., minimize clutter and use solid rather than patterned objects), and improve lighting. When lighting is increased, care should be taken to minimize glare by using halogen or fluorescent lighting (Warren, 1994). Such strategies may be important for the older adult even when the referring diagnosis does not suggest a new visual impairment. Often a new illness or injury will require an individual to rely more heavily on visual input. For example, a client who recently developed lower extremity weakness resulting in limited mobility skills may have reduced capacity to recover from small challenges to balance. The client may need more visual input from the environment in order to avoid obstacles and prevent falls. Often individuals are unaware of the simple and inexpensive environmental adaptations that can facilitate functioning in the visually impaired. These adaptations to enhance visual input may deserve attention in treatment whether or not the diagnosis that prompted referral resulted in a change in the person's visual status.

Occupational therapy practitioners often focus treatment of visual perceptual dysfunction at the performance component level, using a variety of activities to develop skills in visual scanning, figure-ground perception, right-left discrimination, and topographical orientation (Quintana, 1995). Few studies have been done to support the efficacy of this treatment for the improvement of functional performance (Quintana, 1995). Ross (1992) examined the impact of computer-based treatment to enhance visual scanning skills on a functional visual scanning task (locating items on a grocery shelf). She found that while scanning skills improved on the computer task, there was no generalization of these skills to a different visual scanning task.

Compensatory strategies for visual perceptual deficits may be a more effective treatment approach. A systematic approach to visual scanning, for example, can be applied to several activities of daily living and practice should occur within the context of each of the relevant tasks. Warren (1993a; 1993b; 1994; 1996) described treatment strategies that are consistent with the hierarchical assessment model she has proposed. This systematic approach helps the therapist structure treatment that is focused initially on basic skills with a progressive increase in the complexity of skill acquisition.

Compensatory Strategies for Hearing Deficits

Remediation of hearing deficits lies outside the scope of occupational therapy practice; however, compensatory strategies may be essential for successful treatment because practitioners rely heavily on verbal communication within the treatment setting. Slowing the rate of speech and minimizing interruptions can facilitate comprehension (Fozard, 1990). Depending on the severity of the deficit, reducing the ambient noise level or limiting treatment to rooms with better acoustic qualities may be adequate to overcome the hearing deficit. If the environment is not adaptable (e.g., when working on community skills) or hearing loss is severe, the client with adequate visual function can rely on written language. Reading comprehension skills should always be assessed first, since they may vary significantly from auditory comprehension skills and are more sensitive to educational background. Demonstration may be most effective for communication of motor tasks, whereas more complex content, for instance, the identification of client roles, may be best assessed with written language. Written communication is significantly slower than verbal communication and preplanning may facilitate treatment, such as giving the client a written outline of the next session's treatment plan before he or she comes to the clinic. An overview of the purpose of the session and the activities to be used will frame the context, making it easier to interpret gestural and other contextual cues. This strategy may also be useful for clients who rely primarily on verbal communication, but the severity of the hearing loss necessitates frequent repetition, and comprehension is often limited or difficult to determine.

Hearing is used for more than communication, for auditory cues, such as doorbells, timers, alarm clocks, fire alarms, or the noise of a dropped item, provide important information for daily living. Other activities, such as watching television or listening to radio, have an inherent auditory component. Amplification or adaptive devices are available for many household items with auditory signals. Clients who enjoy the companionship of a dog can get a service animal trained to meet the needs of hearing-impaired individuals. These animals are professionally trained and information is available through The Delta Society, P.O. Box 1080, Renton, WA 98057.

Compensatory Strategies for Olfactory Deficits

Individuals with reduced sensibility to smell must be made aware of the deficit so that they can rely on other methods to identify invisible hazards, such as gas leaks and hidden burning material. Functioning smoke detectors should be standard in any home, but client education will help assure that the individual trusts the smoke detector alarm rather than "following his nose." Careful use of timers can reduce the risk of kitchen fires resulting from burning food. Dating food items and relying on visual inspection can be used to evaluate food spoilage. While these strategies would be useful for any person with olfactory loss, they are particularly pertinent for the elderly population because of the prevalence of reduced smell sensitivity. Nordin, Monsch, & Murphy (1995) studied 80 normal elderly subjects and reported that 48.8% had hyposmia and 6.2% had anosmia. Of the 39 subjects with hyposmia, 33 reported they had normal smell sensitivity, suggesting they were unaware of their deficit.

ORTHOTICS

Orthotics can be used to support a painful joint, position to prevent deformity, position to enhance function, correct deformities, and to restore function (Hunter, Schneider, Mackin, & Callahan, 1990; Linden & Trombly, 1995; Schultz-Johnson, 1992).

Extensive resources exist on design and fabrication (Fess & Philips, 1987; Linden & Trombly, 1995; Lowe, 1995; Malick, 1985; Tenney & Lisak, 1986), but they do not specifically address the needs of the geriatric population. Age-related changes in the skin, such as thinning of the epidermis, collagen changes, and decreased vascularity make the skin more prone to breakdown from pressure, shear, or friction forces (Matteson, 1988). These forces may occur with splint usage. Protection of the skin under a newly made splint may be enhanced by reducing initial wearing times, increasing the number of daily skin inspections, and increasing wearing schedules more slowly.

Managing the use of orthotics in institutional settings can be a frustrating experience for the occupational therapy practitioner, since orthotics are frequently lost or damaged. Riveting straps to splints can help keep all the parts together. Collaboration with the client (when able), nursing staff, laundry department, and dietary services can help reduce loss and facilitate the return of lost items.

STRENGTHENING PROGRAMS

Muscle strength is one sensorimotor performance component that may be difficult to treat effectively within the context of a task, for two reasons. First, the muscle must be stressed to facilitate the recruitment of more motor units (Zemke, 1995) and adjusting the parameters used to increase strength may be difficult to do without significantly altering the task. Second, when the focus of treatment is on task completion, the individual logically uses "whatever works" to get the job done, making it difficult to eliminate or minimize the use of compensatory strategies without making the task seem unnatural or contrived.

Several parameters can be adjusted to increase muscle strength, including the amount of resistance, duration of a contraction, type of contraction, velocity of contraction, and frequency of exercise (Zemke, 1995). Comparing the individual's pattern of muscle weakness with performance area deficits is crucial in the development of an optimal strengthening program for the individual client, that is, one that will have a positive impact not only on strength but also on function.

There is evidence that the muscles of older adults respond to strengthening programs (Grimby, 1990; Lord & Castell, 1994). The increase in muscle strength with training seems to be primarily the result of neural factors, for example, motor unit activation patterns as opposed to muscle hypertrophy (Grimby, 1990). This means that exercises to increase strength should be specific to the type of strength gain desired (Grimby, 1990). For instance, if a client cannot take items from and return items to a shelf at shoulder height because of weakness in the shoulder flexors, concentric strengthening exercises will enhance the reaching-up function, but eccentric strengthening exercises will also be needed to facilitate retrieving items from the shelf. The length-tension relationship should also be assessed relative to the task deficit so that strengthening exercises can focus on strengthening the muscle in the ranges in which it will be used.

Care should be taken to assess the cause of weakness, since generalized muscle weakness with evidence of reduced cardiovascular function suggests that weakness is due to lack of cardiovascular nutrients. In these cases treatment should be focused on aerobic activity (Lewis & Bottomley, 1990), discussed in the section that follows.

ENDURANCE TRAINING

Limitations in endurance may interfere significantly with an individual's ability to participate in all of the tasks that define his or her roles. A newly acquired physical disability typically has an impact on endurance, even in the absence of cardiopulmonary pathology. A limitation in strength or sensation, change in muscle tone, decrease in range of motion, or a visuospatial impairment typically requires the client to expend more energy for the completion of self-care tasks than was required prior to the disability. Older adults often lead a more sedentary life style than they did in their younger years, which causes a resultant decline in cardiovascular fitness (Lewis & Bottomley, 1990). As a result, they may have few reserves for the extra demands of a newly acquired disability.

When endurance limits ability to participate fully in tasks that the person finds meaningful, treatment should begin with a graded program to increase endurance by progressively increasing the number and duration of activities completed in each day. Once this goal has been reached, an endurance program to enhance general conditioning is indicated to raise the endurance threshold above that which is needed to complete daily tasks. This will allow the individual to complete the daily routine without feeling exhausted at the end of the day. It will also provide some reserves so that if the person becomes ill, deconditioning effects will not impact daily functioning (Dean, 1994).

There are a variety of traditional and adapted aerobic exercise programs that may be used effectively with the elderly (Herring, 1991). Individual or group programs can be used to suit the needs of the client. The addition of a new activity or resumption of a long-lost task that requires the cardiopulmonary output needed to increase endurance can also be used, such as badminton, T'ai Chi, or washing and waxing the car. Adaptations to activities can often be made to enable participation by individuals with disabilities, taking care to preserve the cardiovascular demands of the task so that endurance is increased.

COORDINATION TRAINING

The literature suggests that while there may be temporal changes in coordination skills of older adults, the patterning of reach and prehension typically remain unchanged (Bennett & Castiello, 1994; Shiffman, 1992). Treatment aimed at specific deficits in prehension patterns or isolated coordination skills, such as in-hand manipulation of objects, may respond to focused, repetitive treatment of the missing components. Transfer of skills gained into functional tasks, however, should not be expected to occur spontaneously and must be carefully crafted into the treatment program.

USE OF SENSORY INPUT TO REMEDIATE MOTOR SKILLS

Traditional treatment approaches for the remediation of motor control were based largely on the work of Rood, Bobath (Neurodevelopmental Treatment), Brunnstrom, and Kabat & Voss (Proprioceptive Neuromuscular Facilitation). The theories and techniques vary among the approaches; however, all use specific sensory inputs to facilitate motor skills. These techniques have been used for many years in the remediation of motor deficits following cerebrovascular accident and so are commonly used with the elderly population. A lack of efficacy studies

linking the use of these approaches in the treatment of neurologically impaired adults to functional outcomes, and recent research in the movement sciences are calling these theories and treatment techniques into question. Many clinicians can demonstrate the improvement of their clients' performance through the use of these techniques within the clinical setting. The difficulty has been to get clients to carry over improvements in performance immediately following treatment to daily living skills. Retaining and being able to generalize a motor skill are dependent on learning the skill, effecting a relatively permanent change of behavior (Schmidt, 1988). Performance is, of course, a prerequisite to learning. If a client is unable to perform a skill, it cannot be carried over into activities of daily living. The use of traditional treatment techniques can be useful by providing clients with an opportunity to practice and develop the ability to perform movements. The learning must take place within the context of tasks and treatment must move into the performance areas.

USE OF FEEDBACK IN THE REMEDIATION OF MOTOR SKILLS

The remediation of motor skill deficits within the context of a task may be facilitated by the application of some principles of motor learning. Feedback, or knowledge of results, is important in acquiring a skill. Occupational therapy practitioners commonly give their clients feedback in all aspects of treatment. The literature supports the theory that frequent feedback facilitates performance; however, studies suggest that intermittent feedback results in better retention of the skill over time (Jarus, 1995; Schmidt, 1991; Shumway-Cook & Woollacott, 1995). It is suggested that this occurs because individuals learn to rely on extrinsic feedback from the therapist when it is available. When extrinsic feedback is intermittent or summarized, individuals must learn to rely on intrinsic feedback, facilitating retention of the skill. Much of the motor-learning research has been done on young adults; however, Jarus (1995) looked at the effect of varied feedback schedules on performance and learning in young adults (aged 20 to 30 years) and older adults (aged 50 to 70 years). Reduced frequency of feedback improved retention for both groups, with no difference between the groups.

Summary

Evaluation and treatment of the older adult can present a challenging puzzle to the occupational therapy practitioner. The older adult has the time and experience to develop an array of adaptations over the course of a lifetime, making it difficult to link sensorimotor impairments to their resulting functional limitations. Treatment aimed at the performance component level is often easier to plan and carry out. Progress within the component may even be measurable. The challenge to the occupational therapy practitioner, however, is to link the performance components to performance areas, so that gains made in performance components are quickly transferred to occupational tasks.

Review Questions

1. State two reasons why the "top-down" approach to assessment is recommended.

2. List two assessment tools that identify subtask deficits within the context of functional tasks.

3. What are two of the factors that might contribute to the decline in speed of performance of motor-skills with age?

4. What is the primary goal for testing tactile sensory functions?

5. What kinds of objects are most desirable as test items when testing stereognosis?

6. Which systems provide information that is critical to vestibular functions?

7. Name an assessment that is designed to identify the sensory strategies used in balance.

8. List five visual functions that tend to decrease with normal aging.

9. How did Warren propose that the evaluation of visual perception be tested?

10. How is the sense of smell important to occupational performance?

11. Do older adults have the same ranges of motion in all joints as those published on charts of average ROM?

12. Name two tests that are suited for evaluating manual dexterity in the elderly.

13. When is it desirable to practice a small component of a task rather than the entire task?

14. If treatment is done at the performance component level, what should the practitioner do to ensure better motor learning?

15. List three compensatory strategies that can be used to avoid injury of insensate parts.

16. Describe environmental adaptations that can be used to enhance visual contrast and accommodate the need for increased illumination with age.

17. What are some strategies that can be used to compensate for olfactory deficits?

18. Why are orthotics more likely to cause skin breakdown and maceration in the elderly?

19. Why is it difficult to treat muscle weakness in the context of task performance?

20. How should muscle strengthening programs be designed?

21. How can an endurance training program be progressed for the older adult?

References

American Occupational Therapy Association. (1992). Standards of practice for occupational therapy. *American Journal of Occupational Therapy, 46,* 1082–1085.

Arnadottir, G. (1990). *The brain and behavior: Assessing cortical dysfunction through activities of daily living.* St. Louis: C. V. Mosby.

Bassey, E. J., Ebrahim, S. B. J., Dallosso, H. M., & Morgan, K. (1989). Normal values for range of shoulder abduction in men and women aged over 65 years. *Annals of Human Biology, 16,* 249–257.

Bennett, K. M. B., & Castiello, U. (1994). Reach to grasp: Changes with age. *Journal of Gerontology: Psychological Sciences, 49,* P1–P7.

Bentzel, K. (1995a). Evaluation of sensation. In C. A. Trombly (Ed.), *Occupational therapy for physical dysfunction* (4th ed., pp. 187–199). Baltimore: Williams & Wilkins.

Bentzel, K. (1995b). Remediating sensory impairment. In C. A. Trombly (Ed.), *Occupational therapy for physical dysfunction* (4th ed., pp. 423–431). Baltimore: Williams & Wilkins.

Birren, J. E., Woods, A. M., & Williams, M. V. (1980). Behavioral slowing with age: Causes, organization, and consequences. In L. W. Poon (Ed.), *Aging in the 1980s: Psychological issues* (pp. 293–308). Washington, DC: American Psychological Association.

Bonder, B. R., & Goodman, G. (1995). Preventing occupational dysfunction secondary to aging. In C. A. Trombly (Ed.), *Occupational therapy for physical dysfunction* (4th ed., pp. 391–404). Baltimore: Williams & Wilkins.

Botwinick, J. (1984). *Aging and behavior* (3rd ed.). New York: Springer Publishing.

Bowen, V. L., Griener, J. S., & Jones, S. V. (1990). Threshold of sensation: Inter-rater reliability and establishment of normal using the Semmes-Weinstein monofilament. *Journal of Hand Therapy, 3,* 36–37.

Callahan, M. D. (1990a). Methods of compensation and reeducation for sensory dysfunction. In J. M. Hunter, L. H. Schneider, E. J. Mackin, & A. D. Callahan (Eds.), *Rehabilitation of the hand: Surgery and Therapy* (3rd ed., pp. 611–621). St. Louis: C. V. Mosby.

Callahan, M. D. (1990b). Sensibility testing: Clinical methods. In J. M. Hunter, L. H. Schneider, E. J. Mackin, & A. D. Callahan (Eds.), *Rehabilitation of the hand: Surgery and therapy* (3rd ed., pp. 594–610). St. Louis: C. V. Mosby.

Canadian Association of Occupational Therapists. (1991). *Guidelines for the client-centered practice of occupational therapy.* Toronto: CAOT Publications ACE.

Carr, J. H., & Shepherd, R. B. (1987a). A motor learning model for rehabilitation. In J. H. Carr & R. B. Shepherd (Eds.), *Movement science: Foundations for physical therapy practice* (pp. 31–91). Rockville, MD: Aspen.

Carr, J. H., & Shepherd, R. B. (1987b). *A motor relearning programme for stroke* (2nd ed.). Rockville, MD: Aspen Publishers.

Cerella, J., Poon, L. W., & Williams, D. M. (1980). Age and the complexity hypothesis. In L. W. Poon (Ed.), *Aging in the 1980s: Psychological issues* (pp. 332–342). Washington, DC: American Psychological Association.

Christiansen, C. (1991). Occupational therapy: Intervention for life performance. In C. Christiansen & C. Baum (Eds.), *Occupational therapy:*

Overcoming human performance deficits (pp. 3–43). Thorofare, NJ: Slack.

Clark, F. (1993). Occupation imbedded in a real life: Interweaving occupational science and occupational therapy. *American Journal of Occupational Therapy, 47,* 1067–1078.

Cohen, H. (1994). Vestibular rehabilitation improves daily life function. *American Journal of Occupational Therapy, 48,* 919–925.

Craik, R. L. (1991). Recovery processes: Maximizing function. In Foundation for physical therapy, contemporary management of motor problems: *Proceedings of the II step conference* (pp. 165–173). Alexandria, VA: Foundation for Physical Therapy.

Dean, E. (1994). Cardiac development. In B. R. Bonder & M. B. Wagner, *Functional performance in older adults* (pp. 62–92). Philadelphia: F. A. Davis.

Dellon, A. (1988). *Evaluation of sensibility and reeducation of sensation in the hand.* Baltimore: Lucas.

Desrosiers, J., Bravo, G., Hébert, R., Dutil, E., & Mercier, L. (1994). Validation of the Box and Block Test as a measure of dexterity of elderly people: Reliability, validity, and norms studies. *Archives of Physical Medicine and Rehabilitation, 75,* 751–755.

Desrosiers, J., Hébert, R., Bravo, G., & Dutil, E. (1995). Upper–extremity motor co-ordination of healthy elderly people. *Age and Aging, 24,* 108–112.

Desrosiers, J., Hébert, R., Dutil, E., & Bravo, G. (1993). Development and reliability of an upper extremity function test for the elderly: The TEMPA. *Canadian Journal of Occupational Therapy, 60,* 9–16.

Desrosiers, J., Hébert, R., Dutil, E., Bravo, G., Mercier, L. (1994). Validity of the TEMPA: A measurement instrument for upper extremity performance. *Occupational Therapy Journal of Research, 14,* 267–281.

Doty, R. L., Shaman, P., & Dann, M. (1984). Development of the University of Pennsylvania Smell Identification Test: A standardized microencapsulated test of olfactory function. *Physiology and Behavior, 32,* 489–502.

Engel, J. M. (1993). Pain management. In L. Hopkins & H. D. Smith (Eds.), *Willard and Spackman's occupational therapy* (8th ed., pp. 596–604). Philadelphia: J. B. Lippincott.

Fess, E. (1990). Assessment of the upper extremity: Instrumentation criteria. *Occupational Therapy Practice, 1,* 1–11.

Fess. E. W., & Philips, C. A. (1987). *Hand splinting: Principles and methods* (2nd ed.). St. Louis: C. V. Mosby.

Fisher, A. G. (1992). *Assessment of motor and processing skills.* Fort Collins, CO: Three Star Press.

Fleishman, E. (1972). On the relation between abilities, learning, and human performance. *American Psychologist, 27,* 1017–1032.

Fozard, J. L. (1990). Vision and hearing in aging. In J. E. Birren & K. W. Shaie (Eds.), *Handbook of the psychology of aging* (3rd ed., pp. 150–170). San Diego: Academic Press.

Gordon, J. (1987). Assumptions underlying physical therapy intervention: Theoretical and historical perspectives. In J. H. Carr & R. B. Shepherd (Eds.), *Movement science: Foundations for physical therapy practice* (pp. 1–30). Rockville, MD: Aspen.

Gordon-Salant, S. (1987). Age-related differences in speech recognition performance as a function of test format and paradigm. *Ear and Hearing, 8,* 277–282.

Grimby, G. (1990). Muscle changes and trainability in the elderly. *Topics in Geriatric Rehabilitation, 5,* 54–62.

Herdman, S. J. (1994). *Vestibular rehabilitation.* Philadelphia: F. A. Davis.

Herring, C. L. (1991). Maintaining fitness in later life. In J. M. Kiernat, *Occupational therapy and the older adult* (pp. 43–60). Gaithersburg, MD: Aspen.

Horak, F. (1987). Clinical measurement of postural control in adults. *Physical Therapy, 67,* 1881–1885.

Horak, F. (1991). Assumptions underlying motor control for neurologic rehabilitation. In *Foundation for physical therapy, contemporary management of motor problems: Proceedings of the II step conference* (pp. 11–27). Alexandria, VA: Foundation for Physical Therapy.

Hunter, J. M., Schneider, L. H., Mackin, E. J., & Callahan, A. D. (Eds.). (1990). *Rehabilitation of the hand: Surgery and therapy* (3rd ed.). St. Louis: C. V. Mosby.

Jarus, T. (1995). Is more always better? Optimal amounts of feedback in learning to calibrate sensory awareness. *Occupational Therapy Journal of Research, 15,* 181–197.

Lang, E. M., Nelson, D. L., & Bush, M. A. (1992). Comparison of performance in materials-based occupation, imagery-based occupation, and rote exercise in nursing home residents. *American Journal of Occupational Therapy, 46,* 607–611.

Levy, L. L. (1988). Sensory change and compensation. In L. J. Davis & M. Kirkland. *The role of occupational therapy with the elderly* (pp. 49–67).

Rockville, MD: American Occupational Therapy Association.

Levy, L. L. (1993). Knowledge bases of occupational therapy: Late adulthood. In H. L. Hopkins & H. D. Smith (Eds.), *Willard and Spackman's occupational therapy* (8th ed., pp. 130–137). Philadelphia: J. B. Lippincott.

Lewis, C., & Bottomley, J. (1990). Musculoskeletal changes with age: Clinical implications. In C. Lewis (Ed.), *Aging: Health care's challenge* (2nd ed. pp. 135–160). Philadelphia: F. A. Davis.

Lewis, S. C. (1979). *The mature years: A geriatric occupational therapy text.* Thorofare, NJ: Slack.

Linden, C. A., & Trombly, C. A. (1995). Orthoses: Kinds and purposes. In C. A. Trombly (Ed.), *Occupational therapy for physical dysfunction* (4th ed., pp. 551–581). Baltimore: Williams & Wilkins.

Lord, A. R., & Castell, S. (1994). Physical activity program for older persons: Effect on balance, strength, neuromuscular control, and reaction time. *Archives of Physical Medicine and Rehabilitation, 75,* 648–652,

Louis, D. S., Greene, T. L., Jacobson, K. E., Rasmussen, C., Kolowich, P., & Goldstein, S. A. (1984). Evaluation of normal values for stationary and moving two-point discrimination in the hand. *Journal of Hand Surgery, 9A,* 552–555.

Lowe, C. T. (1995). Construction of hand splints. In C. A. Trombly (Ed.), *Occupational therapy for physical dysfunction* (4th ed., pp. 583–597). Baltimore: Williams & Wilkins.

Malick, M. H. (1985). *Manual on static hand splinting: New materials and techniques* (5th ed.). Pittsburgh: Harmarville Rehabilitation Centers.

Mathiowetz, V., & Bass Haugen, J. (1994). Motor behavior research: Implications for therapeutic approaches to central nervous system dysfunction. *American Journal of Occupational Therapy, 48,* 733–745.

Mathiowetz, V., & Bass Haugen, J. (1995a). Evaluation of Motor Behavior. In C. A. Trombly (Ed.), *Occupational therapy for physical dysfunction* (4th ed., pp. 157–185). Baltimore: Williams & Wilkins.

Mathiowetz, V., & Bass Haugen, J. (1995b). Remediating of Motor Behavior: Contemporary task oriented approach. In C. A. Trombly (Ed.), *Occupational therapy for physical dysfunction* (4th ed., pp. 510–527). Baltimore: Williams & Wilkins.

Mathiowetz, V., Kashman, N., Volland, G., Weber, K., Dowe, M., & Rogers, S. (1985). Grip and pinch strength: Normative data for adults. *Archives of Physical Medicine and Rehabilitation, 66,* 69–74.

Mathiowetz, V., Volland, G., Kashman, N., & Weber, K. (1985). Adult norms for the Box and Block Test of manual dexterity. *American Journal of Occupational Therapy, 39,* 386–391.

Mathiowetz, V., Weber, K., Kashman, N., & Volland, G. (1985). Adult norms for the Nine Hole Peg Test of finger dexterity. *Occupational Therapy Journal of Research, 5,* 24–38.

Matteson, M. A. (1988). Age-related changes in the integument. In M. A. Matteson & E. S. McConnell (Eds.), *Gerontological nursing: Concepts and practice* (pp. 153–169). Philadelphia: W. B. Saunders.

Montgomery, P. C. (1991). Perceptual issues in motor control. In Foundation for physical therapy, contemporary management of motor problems: *Proceedings of the II step conference* (pp. 175–184). Alexandria, VA: Foundation for Physical Therapy.

Nelson, C. E., & Payton, O. D. (1991). A system for involving patients in program planning. *American Journal of Occupational Therapy, 45,* 753–755.

Nelson, K. A. (1987). Visual impairment among elderly Americans: Statistics in transition. *Journal of Visual Impairment and Blindness, Statistical Brief #35,* 331–333.

Nordin, S., Monsch, A. U., & Murphy, C. (1995). Unawareness of smell loss in normal aging and Alzheimer's disease: Discrepancy between self-reported and diagnosed smell sensitivity. *Journal of Gerontology: Psychological Science, 50B,* p187–p192.

Norkin, C. C., & White, D. J. (1995). *Measurement of joint motion: A guide to goniometry.* Philadelphia: F. A. Davis.

Owsley, C., Sekuler, R., & Siemsen, D. (1983). Contrast sensitivity throughout adulthood. *Vision Research, 23,* 689–699.

Pedretti, L. W. (1996a). Evaluation of joint range of motion. In L. W. Pedretti (Ed.), *Occupational therapy: Practice skills for physical dysfunction* (4th ed., pp. 79–107). St. Louis: Mosby-Year Book.

Pedretti, L. W. (1996b). Evaluation of sensation and treatment of sensory dysfunction. In L. W. Pedretti (Ed.), *Occupational therapy: Practice skills for physical dysfunction* (4th ed., pp. 213–230). St. Louis: Mosby-Year Book.

Pedretti, L. W., Zoltan, B., & Wheatley, C. J. (1996). Evaluation and treatment of perceptual and motor deficits. In L. W. Pedretti (Ed.), *Occupational therapy: Practice skills* for *physical dysfunction* (4th ed., pp. 231–239). St. Louis: Mosby-Year Book.

Pollock, N. (1993). Client-centered assessment. *American Journal of Occupational Therapy, 47,* 298–301.

Proteau, L., Charest, I., & Chaput, S. (1994). Differential roles with aging of visual and proprioceptive afferent information for fine motor control. *Journal of Gerontology: Psychological Sciences, 49,* P100–P107.

Quintana, L. A. (1995). Remediating perceptual impairments. In C. A. Trombly (Ed.), *Occupational therapy for physical dysfunction* (4th ed., pp. 529–537). Baltimore: Williams & Wilkins.

Ross, F. L. (1992). The use of computers in occupational therapy for visual scanning training. *American Journal of Occupational Therapy, 46,* 314–322.

Sabari, J. S. (1991). Motor learning concepts applied to activity-based intervention with adults with hemiplegia. *American Journal of Occupational Therapy, 45,* 523–530.

Salthouse, T. A. (1985). Speed of behavior and its implications for cognition. In J. E. Birren & K. W. Schaie, *Handbook of the psychology of aging* (2nd ed., pp. 400–426). New York: Van Nostrand Reinhold.

Schmidt, R. A. (1988). *Motor control and learning: A behavioral emphasis.* Champagne, IL: Human Kinetics Publishers.

Schmidt, R. A. (1991). Motor learning principles for physical therapy. In Foundation for Physical Therapy, Contemporary management of motor problems: *Proceedings of the II step conference* (pp. 49–63). Alexandria, VA: Foundation for Physical Therapy.

Schultz-Johnson, K. (1992). Splinting: A problem-solving approach. In

B. G. Stanley & S. M. Tribuzi (Eds.), *Concepts in hand rehabilitation* (pp. 239–271). Philadelphia: F. A. Davis.

Shiffman, L. M. (1992). Effects of aging on adult hand function. *American Journal of Occupational Therapy, 46,* 785–792.

Shumway-Cook, A., & Horak, F. (1986). Assessing the influence of sensory interaction on balance. *Physical Therapy, 66,* 1548–1550.

Shumway-Cook, A., & Woollacott, M. H. (1995). *Motor control: Theory and practical applications.* Baltimore: Williams & Wilkins.

Silverman, E. H., & Elfant., I. L. (1979). Dysphagia: An evaluation and treatment program for the adult, *American Journal of Occupational Therapy, 33,* 6, 382–392.

Smith, H. D. (1993). Assessment and evaluation: An overview. In H. L. Hopkins & H. D. Smith (Eds.), *Willard and Spackman's occupational therapy* (8th ed., pp. 169–191). Philadelphia: J. B. Lippincott.

Tan, A. M. (1992). Sensibility testing. In B. G. Stanley & S. M. Tribuzi (Eds.), *Concepts in hand rehabilitation* (pp. 92–112). Philadelphia: F. A. Davis.

Tenney, C. G., & Lisak, J. M. (1986). *Atlas of hand splinting.* Boston: Little, Brown.

Townsend, E., Brintnell, S., & Staisey, N. (1990). Developing guidelines for client-centered occupational therapy practice. *Canadian Journal of Occupational Therapy, 57,* 69–76.

Trombly, C. (1993). Anticipating the future: Assessment of occupational function. *American Journal of Occupational Therapy, 47,* 253–257.

Trombly, C. A. (1995a). Evaluation of biomechanical and physiological aspects of motor performance. In C. A. Trombly (Ed.), *Occupational* therapy for physical dysfunction (4th ed., pp. 73–156). Baltimore: Williams & Wilkins.

Trombly, C. A. (1995b). Planning, guiding, and documenting therapy. In C. A. Trombly (Ed.), Occupational therapy for physical dysfunction (4th ed., pp. 29–40). Baltimore: Williams & Wilkins.

Trombly, C. A. (1995c). Theoretical foundations for practice. In C. A. Trombly (Ed.), Occupational therapy for physical dysfunction (4th ed., pp. 15–27). Baltimore: Williams & Wilkins.

Tse, S. K., & Bailey, D. M. (1992). T'ai Chi and postural control in the well elderly. American Journal of Occupational Therapy, 46, 295–300.

Warren, M. (1993a). A hierarchical model for evaluation and treatment of visual perceptual dysfunction in adult acquired brain injury, part 1. American Journal of Occupational Therapy, 47, 42–54.

Warren, M. (1993b). A hierarchical model for evaluation and treatment of visual perceptual dysfunction in adult acquired brain injury, part 2. American Journal of Occupational Therapy, 47, 54–66.

Warren, M. (1994). Visuospatial skills: Assessment and intervention strategies. In C. B. Royeen (Ed.), American Occupational Therapy Association Self-Study Series: Cognitive Rehabilitation (Lesson 7) (pp. 1–76). Bethesda, MD: American Occupational Therapy Association.

Warren, M. (1996). Evaluation and treatment of visual deficits. In L. W. Pedretti (Ed.), Occupational therapy: Practice skills for physical dysfunction (4th ed., pp. 193–212). St. Louis: Mosby-Year Book.

Weinstein, S. (1993). Fifty years of somatosensory testing: From the Semmes-Weinstein Monofilaments to the Weinstein Enhanced Sensory Test. Journal of Hand Therapy, 6, 11–22.

Welford, A. T. (1982). Motor skills and aging. In J. A. Mortimer & P. J. Pirozzolo (Eds.), The aging motor system (pp. 152–187). New York: Praeger.

Williams, H. G. (1990). Aging and eye-hand coordination. In C. Bard, M. Fleury, & L. Hay (Eds.), Development of eye-hand coordination across the life span (pp. 327–357). Columbia, SC: University of South Carolina Press.

Zemke, R. (1995). Remediating biomechanical and physiological impairment of motor performance. In C. A. Trombly (Ed.), Occupational therapy for physical dysfunction (4th ed., pp. 405–422). Baltimore: Williams & Wilkins.

Zimmerer-Branum, S., & Nelson, D. L. (1995). Choice between occupational forms by elderly nursing home residents. American Journal of Occupational Therapy, 49, 397–402.

Section 2. Cognitive Integration and Cognitive Components

Linda L. Levy, MA, OTR/L, FAOTA

Abstract

Cognitive disability theory is used by occupational therapists to help cognitively impaired older adults to reach their highest level of function, to participate in many activities, and to compensate for limitations.

Introduction

Cognition is a basic, universal human trait that underlies nearly all aspects of individual performance. The abilities to interact; communicate; and maintain independence, autonomy, and quality of life all depend upon higher-order cortical functions. When cognitive function is impaired, all aspects of daily living are affected.

Occupational therapy has developed theoretical foundations for intervention with cognitively impaired populations. These theoretical approaches integrate our most current understandings of cognition with occupational therapy's basic tenets and principles (Katz, 1992). This section provides an overview of the most established cognitive theoretical approach in occupational therapy, Allen's cognitive disability theory (1985). Allen's theory is particularly useful for gerontic practitioners because it has been adopted by Medicare to guide documentation of the functional consequences of cognitive impairment (Allen, Foto, Moon-Sperling, & Wilson, 1989; Health Care Financing Administration [HCFA], 1989). The cognitive disability approach is conceptualized to address the functional consequences of neurologically based cognitive impairments experienced by individuals from any variety of neurocognitive and neurodegenerative disorders, such as stroke, brain injury, Pick's disease, Parkinson's disease, Jakob-Creutzfeldt disease, multiple sclerosis, dementias, or major depression. This discussion, however, emphasizes the application of this approach to the cognitive limitations presented by dementia, the single most common and well-defined cause of cognitive impairment in the aged (National Center for Health Statistics [NCHS], 1993; U.S. Senate, 1991).

Dementia is an acquired organic syndrome in which there is progressive deterioration in global cognitive function of such severity that it interferes with the individual's occupational and social performance (American Psychiatric Association [APA], 1994). It is all too common in the aging population. Survey data report an overall prevalence of 5 to 10% among persons aged 65 and older (Jorm, 1990). The prevalence roughly doubles with every five years of age, reaching a level of at least 16% in persons aged 80 and over (Breteler, Claus, Van Duijn, Launer, & Hofman, 1992), and there is evidence that it can reach 47% among those 85 and older (Evans, Funkenstein, Albert, Scherr, & Cook, 1989). Dementia is also the most common diagnosis in nursing homes, affecting 50% to 65% of all residents (NCHS, 1993; U.S. Senate, 1991). The most common cause of dementia is Alzheimer's disease, accounting for 60% or more of dementing illness. There are two other types of dementing illnesses: multi-infarct dementia, now called "vascular dementia" in DSM-IV, and mixed (Alzheimer's and multi-infarct/"vascular"). The course of dementia, while inexorably deteriorating, is unpredictable, lasting an average of 10 years. Treatment possibilities are still limited and care for the basic illness is unknown.

Clinical Characteristics of Dementia

Dementia is characterized by an irreversible and progressive decline in all cognitive and functional abilities. Clinical characteristics of dementia are common to all types. In general, they can be collapsed into three categories: cognitive impairment, functional impairment, and behavioral impairment.

COGNITIVE IMPAIRMENT

The most common cognitive impairment seen in dementia is progressively worsening memory impairment, but over time all cognitive subcomponents are affected. Memory is a complex function. It builds upon attention (information needs to be attended to before it can be remembered). When memory is impaired, as in dementia, it compromises all higher-order cognitive functions (i.e., learning, reasoning, planning, problem solving, judgment, abstraction, and social awareness).

Memory can be described from a number of perspectives. From a processing perspective (Best, 1989), memory is conceptualized in terms of three information-processing stages: the ability to attend and take in new information through the senses (encoding), retain it for variable periods of time (storage), and then to access it when it is needed (retrieval). In dementia, we know that even from the earliest stages individuals experience difficulty in all three information-processing stages. Significant impairment is demonstrated early on in learning (encoding), retaining (storing), and retrieving information, especially with regard to new information that must be remembered for more than a very brief period of time (Duchek, Cheney, Ferraro, & Storandt, 1991; Welsh, Butters, Hughes, Mohs, & Heyman, 1991).

Memory can also be described in terms of its structural components. The most frequently cited model (Atkinson & Shiffrin, 1968) proposes that memory is made up of three basic structures: sensory memory, short-term memory, and long-term memory. Sensory memory retains raw uninterpreted sensory information for up to 3 seconds. Short-term memory retains knowledge currently in use for up to 30 seconds. It is limited to 7 (plus or minus 2) chunks of information (Miller, 1956) and is closely related to attentional capacity (Nissen, 1986). In dementia, deficits are clear in both short-term memory and attentional capacity (Botwinick, Storandt, & Berg, 1986; Storandt, Botwinick, Danzinger, Berg & Hughes, 1984). Long-term memory is vast and complex. It retains information permanently, has an unlimited capacity, and requires further elaboration.

Tulving (1972; 1983) proposed a framework to help define the nature of long-term memory. He conceptualized long-term memory as either episodic or semantic and later added a third form that he termed procedural (Squire, 1989; Tulving, 1985). Episodic memory involves the ability to recall information and personally experienced events to a specific time and place. Semantic memory is more conceptual and involves general knowledge about the meanings of words, numbers, symbols, and their interrelationships irrespective of time. Procedural memory involves recall of the necessary skills or procedures to perform an activity. It relies upon retained connections between stimuli and action responses. Hence, both episodic and semantic memory involve remembering what, whereas procedural memory involves remembering how. Research demonstrates that even in the earliest stages of dementia, both episodic and semantic memory are severely affected (Nebes, 1989). Procedural memory does not appear to be as affected by the disease. Just as the most basic sensory and motor abilities are spared by the disease process, it appears that remembering how to perform familiar motor behavior is likewise spared, at least until the later stages of the disease. (Dick, 1992; Dick, Kean, & Sands, 1988; Dick, Shankle, et al., 1996; Eslinger & Damasio, 1986; Knopman & Nissen, 1987; LaBarge, Smith, Dick, & Storandt, 1992; Levy, 1986a, 1989, 1992). Procedural memory was recognized much earlier in the occupational therapy literature (Allen, 1982, 1985; Levy, 1974). It remains an important source of cognitive capacity that is capitalized upon in rehabilitation for elderly clients with cognitive limitations.

Although progressively worsening memory deficits are the hallmark cognitive impairments of dementia, higher-order cognitive functions, such as reasoning, problem solving, judgment, and abstraction have already been significantly affected. Other cognitive components are also affected. Early in the course of the disease, individuals can experience aphasia, anomia, and language difficulties (Faber-Langendoen et al., 1988). This appears to be associated with a more rapid course of deterioration (Yasavage, Brooks, Taylor, & Tinkleberg, 1993). Word-finding and word-fluency difficulties are especially common and are considered to be largely secondary to memory deficits. And yet, auditory comprehension appears to be retained at least until late stages of the disease. Agnosia presents as difficulties in the individual's ability to recognize objects or people (Mendez, Mendez, Martin, Smyth, & Whitehouse, 1990; Yasavage et al.,

1993). It is particularly difficult for caregivers to cope with.

Apraxia is well documented in the advanced stages of the disease (Edwards, Deuel, & Baum, 1991; Geschwind & Damasio, 1985; Yasavage et al., 1993), and there is evidence that it can be present in earlier stages (Foster, Chase, Patronas, Gillespie, & Fedio, 1986). Other visuospatial difficulties are common; for example, one of the most frequent first-reported manifestations of the disease is becoming lost in a familiar neighborhood. And although visuospatial difficulties are most often considered to be secondary to memory impairment, lesions in the visual association cortex have also been reported (Hof, Bouras, Constantinidis, & Morrison, 1990). Such lesions produce impairments in figure ground discrimination, visual recognition, and spatial localization (Mendez et al., 1990). By the end stage of the disease, all cognitive components (i.e., judgment, reasoning, planning, problem solving, learning, memory, visuomotor organization, praxis, perception, orientation, and attention) are profoundly impaired. It should also be noted that at this stage of the disease, motor control has been significantly affected, resulting in incontinence, ataxia, altered proprioception, gait changes, myoclonus, and Parkinsonism (Bucher & Larson, 1987; Visser, 1983).

FUNCTIONAL IMPAIRMENT

A key component in the diagnosis of dementia is impairment in functional performance. For diagnostic and statistical purposes, functional impairment is defined in terms of the ability to perform basic activities of daily living (ADLs) and instrumental activities of daily living (IADLs). ADLs consist of seven personal care activities: dressing, bathing, toileting, grooming, eating, transfers, and ambulating. IADLs consist of six home management activities: preparing meals, shopping for personal items, managing finances, using the telephone, doing heavy housework, and doing light housework. In dementia, the most common first manifestation of the disease is difficulty in performing IADLs, which progresses over time to the inability to manage any ADL functions (Levy, 1986b; Reisberg, Ferris, & Franssen, 1985). Decline in functional abilities is one of the most difficult aspects of dementia for both patients (Cottrell & Schultz, 1993) and their caregivers (Green, Mohs, Schmeidler, Aryan, & Davis, 1993).

Although there is an implicit relationship between functional capacity and the extent of cognitive impairment (Allen, 1985; Bassett & Folstein, 1991; Josephsson, Backman, Borell, Brenspang, Nygard, & Ronnberg, 1993; Zanetti, Bianchetti, Frisoni, Rozzini, & Trabucchi, 1993), the precise nature of the relationship has yet to be determined. To date, attention and memory deficits have been implicated in predicting functional decline (Vitaliano, Breen, Albert, Russo, & Prinz, 1984; Vitaliano, Russo, Breen, Vitiello, & Prinz, 1986). Allen's work (1985) has made important contributions in conceptualizing some of the essential information-processing components underlying IADL–ADL functional performance. The cognitive disability approach differs from that employed by other disciplines in its focus on the degree to which particular deficits in information-processing capabilities compromise performance of functional activities (Burns, Mortimer, & Merchek, 1994), rather than the more limited focus on the ability versus the inability to perform specific IADL–ADL tasks. Clearly, functional impairment is an area in which occupational therapy offers considerable assistance.

BEHAVIORAL IMPAIRMENT

Unlike cognitive and functional impairments, there is considerable variability in the extent to which individuals experience behavioral problems. In general, behavioral problems occur in response to cognitive impairments, especially the steadily worsening memory impairments. Individuals with progressive memory loss will become increasingly disoriented. They will first forget what time it is, then where they are and where they have placed their belongings. As the disease worsens, they will even forget their own names, which leads to increasing agitation and confusion. Not knowing what time it is (or even the right decade) or where they are, they tend to wander (it appears in search of familiar cues) and often get lost. Because they cannot remember where they have put their belongings, they may accuse caregivers of stealing and paranoid features may emerge. Significant relationships between the presence and severity of behavioral problems and the severity of the disease have been demonstrated (Rovner, Kafonek, Filipp, Lucas, & Folstein, 1986; Swearer, Drachman, O'Donnell, & Mitchell, 1988).

Agitation is the most frequently documented behavioral problem experienced in persons with dementia, and it usually presents in the middle to late stages of the disease (Cohen-Mansfield, Marx, & Rosenthal, 1990). Agitated behaviors are categorized as verbally "non-aggressive" (complaining or whining, negativism, constant requests for attention); verbally aggressive (cursing, temper tantrums, screaming); physically "non-aggressive" (general restlessness, wandering, repetitious mannerism); or physically aggressive (hitting, pushing, scratching, kicking). "Non-aggressive" agitated behaviors are the more frequent responses to the dementing disease (Cohen-Mansfield et al., 1990; Deutch & Rovner, 1991). When it occurs, physical aggression is more frequent in institutions than in home care settings (Rovner et al., 1986). It is important to recognize that falls, associated with substantial morbidity and mortality, are common in agitated elderly individuals (Cohen-Mansfield et al., 1990).

Increasingly, it is becoming recognized that agitated behaviors emanate from a variety of causes and have diverse meanings. They are considered to reflect ineffective attempts to communicate feelings of pain, discomfort, fear, boredom, distress, loneliness, or other basic needs that need to be disentangled by responsive caregivers. They are often triggered or exacerbated by environmental stimuli, most typically, sensory overload. Sensory overload is related to the frequency, intensity, and quantity of unpredictable stimuli and can cause markedly increased agitation and "catastrophic reactions" (the overreactions or excessive upsets precipitated by situations that overwhelm the limited thinking capacity of the brain). Moreover, activities such as bathing and changing clothes are commonly cited by caregivers as circumstances that trigger agitation (Mace & Rabins, 1991). In all cases, agitated behaviors are most effectively addressed in light of their underlying causes or meanings (Burgener, Jirovec, Murrell, & Barton, 1992; Cohen-Mansfield & Billig, 1986; Cohen-Mansfield, Werner, Marx, & Lipson, 1993; Feil, 1992, 1993). It should also be noted that there is evidence that agitated behaviors in both home and institutional settings decrease when therapeutic activity programs are available (Baum, Edwards, & Morrow-Howell, 1993; Rabinovich & Cohen-Mansfield, 1992; Rovner, 1994; Rovner & Katz, 1992).

Behavioral symptoms can also involve mood disturbances, including depression (both major depression and other less severe depressive states); affective lability; manic or hypomanic states; and what are broadly described as personality changes. (It is ironic that although personality changes are among the most common behavioral symptoms reported in patients with dementia, they have been the least intensively investigated.) In the early to mild stages of the disease, the most frequently reported behavioral symptoms are minor depression and personality changes (Rubin & Kinscherf, 1989). The prevalence of major depression in dementia is reported to be between 10% and 30% (Burns, 1991; Teri & Wagner, 1992), although there are also studies that suggest prevalence rates as high as 40% (Lazarus, Newton, Cohler, Lesser, & Schweon, 1987) and 86% (Merriam, Aronson, Gaston, Wey, & Katz, 1988). The evidence is clear that depression should be treated (Teri & Wagner, 1992). Cognitively impaired depressed patients respond to antidepressant therapy as well as those without cognitive impairment. However, they require a longer and more aggressive course of treatment (Reifler, Larson, & Teri, 1986; Reynolds et al., 1987). Note also that relationships have been demonstrated to exist between activity involvement and lowered incidence of depression (Rabinovich & Cohen-Mansfield, 1992; Teri & Logsdon, 1991).

Behavioral symptoms may also include overtly psychotic phenomena, such as delusions and hallucinations, although they are rarely seen until the late stages of the disease (Rubin & Kinscherf, 1989). When experienced by patients, psychotic symptoms appear to be more important determinants of behavioral problems than severity of cognitive impairment (Rovner et al., 1986). This finding suggests that psychiatric interventions aimed at ameliorating psychotic symptoms should be carefully considered to reduce behavioral problems and to improve function for those patients with hallucinations and delusions.

Caregivers consistently identify the behavioral disturbances of dementia as the most significant sources of caregiver stress, exceeding the level of cognitive impairment (Swearer et al., 1988; Teri, Borson, Kiyak, & Yamagishi, 1989; Zarit, Reever, & Bachman-Peterson, 1980). Clearly, the need for around-the-clock supervision necessary because of patients' wandering or impaired judgment can exhaust even the most stable and caring of caregivers. And ultimately, long-term stress places caregivers at high risk for clinical depression (Teri & Wagner, 1992). There is evidence that it depresses immune system functioning and the caregiver's overall physical health as well (Kiecolt-Glaser et al., 1987). Rehabilitation and care for the individual with cognitive impairment requires active participation of the caregiver. For that reason, preservation of the overall health of the caregiver, with particular attention to the treatment or prevention of depression, is essential.

It is not the cognitive, functional, or behavioral problems associated with dementia per se that cause caregivers to become severely stressed, depressed, or physically ill, but rather the caregivers's inability to cope with them. (Chiu & Smith, 1990; Kemp, 1988; Zarit et al., 1980). Recent studies indicate that family members who cope better with the problems associated with dementia have higher levels of self-efficacy, the belief that one is capable of addressing a problematic behavior because one has the requisite skills, knowledge, and physical capacity (Cummings, 1987; Gallagher, Lovett, & Zeiss, 1987; Teri & Logsdon, 1991). Hence, there is a need for strategies to help caregivers develop a sense of self-efficacy to cope with the cognitive, functional, and behavioral

problems they encounter. This too is a primary objective of the cognitive disability approach to intervention.

Factors Specific to Rehabilitation for Dementia

A number of factors are specific to rehabilitation for dementia. As of now, there is no medical treatment for dementia. However, there is compelling evidence that, although the biological aspects of the disease are not currently treatable, some of the cognitive, functional, and behavioral problems are amenable to intervention (Kamholz & Gottlieb, 1992; Kahn, 1975; Kemp, 1988; Larson, Reifler, Featherstone, & English, 1984; Levy, 1986a; Teri, Rabins, et al., 1992). It is not reasonable to assume that intervention will restore cognitive functioning or reverse organic brain damage (Gottlieb, 1990; Levy, 1986a).

The major tenet of gerontological rehabilitation, to help the disabled elder to reach his or her highest attainable level of function, is no less applicable to the care of persons with dementia (Chiu & Smith, 1990; Gottlieb, 1990; Reifler & Teri, 1986). In 1987, this position was codified in the Omnibus Budget Reconciliation Act (OBRA) (P.L. 100–203, 1987), federal legislation that mandated a comprehensive rehabilitative and restorative philosophy for all in geriatric health care. The overall goals of intervention are to maintain or restore functional capacity, to promote participation in activities that maximize physical and mental health, and to ease the burdens of caregiving activities (Rovner, 1994). Historically (prior to 1987), patients with dementia have not been viewed as viable rehabilitation candidates.

From the earliest stage of the disease process, elders with dementia suffer such severe cognitive and functional impairments that they are only minimally able to participate in the formulation and implementation of the rehabilitation plan. As a result, an adaptive approach (Mosey, 1994) to rehabilitation must be employed (Levy, 1989; 1992). An adaptive approach places emphasis on changing the task, level of cuing, or aspects of the environment to compensate for the effects of cognitive deficits on areas of occupational performance, when no change in impairment can be expected. It requires active participation of the caregiver to implement recommended intervention strategies (Chiu & Smith, 1990; Levy, 1986b, 1989, 1992). In this role, the caregiver needs guidance, support, and assistance from knowledgeable and supportive health professionals (Edwards & Baum, 1990; Zarit, Orr, & Zarit, 1985).

Dementias are dynamic diseases. They produce progressive declines in function, and different functional issues arise in different stages of the disease. Caregivers must be educated about the trajectory of disability imposed by the disease in order to maximize the capabilities that remain, to recognize and address potentially remediable "excess disabilities" that may emerge, and to prepare themselves for the changes to come (Baum, 1991; Chiu & Smith, 1990; Edwards & Baum, 1990; Gottlieb, 1990; Levy, 1986b, 1989).

Dementia not only affects the older adult; it also significantly affects the family or caregivers who deal with frustration, grief, anger, exhaustion, and psychological burnout while they care for the patient over a long period (Mace & Rabins, 1991). Rehabilitative goals have a dual focus: to maximize the affected individual's level of functioning and quality of life and to maximize the quality of life of the family or caregivers (Mace & Rabins, 1991; Pearlin, Mullar, Semple, & Skaff, 1990; Zarit, Orr, & Zarit, 1985).

The concept of rehabilitation of patients with cognitive impairments is relatively new, and the few strategies that have been reported have yet to be evaluated systematically (Chiu & Smith, 1990; Rentz, 1991). Allen was the first to propose a comprehensive rehabilitation theory to address the functional problems experienced by elders with dementia (in Levy, 1986b), and her approach has already made benchmark contributions to this rapidly developing area of rehabilitation (Allen et al., 1989; Burns et al., 1994; Chiu & Smith, 1990; HCFA, 1989; Kemp, 1988; Levy, 1986b, 1989; Rentz, 1991). Her approach provides practitioners with a conceptual framework that

- Identifies the causes of the functional impairments of dementia.

- Provides guidelines for assessing the specific nature of the cognitive, functional, and behavioral difficulties experienced by the individual.

- Describes viable intervention strategies to assist individuals and their families or caregivers in coping with the wide range of physical, psychological, and social problems that occur as the disease progresses.

- Provides guidance on how best to enable the individual to live as normal a life as possible despite the disability that exists throughout the course of the disease.

- Proposes a comprehensive and humanistic approach to care.

The following is an overview of the cognitive disability approach to rehabilitation of the cognitive, functional, and behavioral impairments experienced by the elder with dementia. For a more comprehensive discussion the reader is referred to Allen (1985); Allen, Earheart, and Blue (1992); and Allen and Robertson (1993); and Levy (1986a, 1989, 1992).

Cognitive Disability Theory

Neuropsychologists approach the problem of cognitive impairment in dementing diseases by analyzing the difficulties in terms of specific cognitive components (perception, attention, memory, orientation, praxis) that deviate from test norms. And although relationships between impairments and functional performance have been reported (Backman, Josephsson, Herlitz, Stigsdotter, & Vitanan, 1991; Camp & McKitrick, 1992; Josephsson et al., 1993; Vitaliano et al., 1984; Vitaliano et al., 1986; Zanetti et al., 1993), findings have not led to useful intervention strategies. In contrast, the cognitive disability approach considers cognition from a global or multi-component perspective that is specifically addressed to the functional and behavioral consequences of cognitive impairment. It provides an information-processing model of the etiology of the functional impairment that identifies different information-processing patterns revealed by different patterns of functional performance. Critical cognitive components such as memory and attention are woven into the model; however, they are more broadly conceptualized as components of information-processing patterns that vary throughout a hierarchy of functional levels.

The primary intent of cognitive disability theory is to identify information-processing capacities that determine whether an individual can perform a functional activity safely and successfully, and the specific nature of the cognitive impairments that need to be compensated for in the event of cognitive limitations. To that end, Allen (1985, 1987, 1992) proposed a hierarchy of six cognitive levels that describe the dimensions of information processed in pursuing normal life activities, as well as qualitative differences in functional capacities and limitations. Given the focus on functional activity, the six levels are considered to represent information processing that is regulated by sensorimotor associations in the brain (Allen et al., 1992; Miller, 1981). Allen views three dimensions of cognition as stages of a sensorimotor information-processing model that are considered at each of the six hierarchical cognitive levels.

STAGE 1: ATTENTION TO SENSORY CUES

All information processing begins with the ability to attend to sensory input from the environment. Allen orders sensory cues that capture and sustain attention from internal cues (subliminal and proprioceptive); to external concrete cues (tactile, visual, and verbal); to complex abstract cues (related visual cues, verbal hypotheticals, symbols or ideas). At lower cognitive levels, attention is limited to internal cues, such as musculoskeletal and proprioceptive sensations. At more advanced cognitive levels, individuals can respond to progressively wider ranges of cues, including tactile, visual, auditory, and eventually complex symbolic cues from the environment. In order to maximize functional capacities, therapists must adapt activities both to capitalize on the cues that the individual is able to attend to and to limit exposure to activities that require attention to cues that are beyond the individual's range of comprehension.

STAGE 2: SENSORIMOTOR ASSOCIATIONS

Sensorimotor associations are the interpretive processes that follow from attention to sensory cues and reflect the capacity to translate cues into functional performance. They can also be conceptualized as the goals implicit in initiating an action response. Levy (1974) and Allen (1982) were the first to recognize that the implicit goal of the individual performing an action may not be consistent with the explicit goals in performing an action. Individuals pursue activities with varying goals in mind, ranging, for example, from the simple pleasure of moving, to an interest in the effects of actions, to an investment in producing a high-quality end product. The problem to be recognized is that at lower cognitive levels, an individual may be able to comprehend only the motions involved in a desired activity, such as the familiar sensory sensations elicited by the motion of pushing a vacuum back and forth, and would not be able to comprehend the more conventional goal—or the result—that would be expected from an individual with higher cognitive capacities, namely, a clean rug. Consequently, at lower cognitive levels, unintentional results become commonplace. It is important to recognize that the inability to comply with the traditional goals and expectations of an activity reflects a specific cognitive impairment. Caregivers can compensate for this impairment by adjusting conventional norms and expectations for activity performance.

STAGE 3: MOTOR ACTIONS

Actions are elicited by attention to sensory cues (input); guided by sensorimotor associations (throughput); and can be observed in activity performance (output). They are the final stage of Allen's information-processing model. There are two types: spontaneous (self-initiated from memory stores) and imitated (cued through visual and motor channels by demonstration from another person). At lower cognitive levels, individuals are able to initiate and imitate only motor actions that are near reflexive or already very familiar behavioral actions. (Note: neuropsychologists would describe this as the capacity to initiate and imitate procedural memory responses.) At more advanced cognitive levels, self-initiated motor actions extend beyond the well-rehearsed and familiar, to planned actions that reflect attention to visual and ultimately abstract cues. Here, individuals use conceptual information, including episodic and semantic memory, to produce solutions to everyday problems and are able to participate freely in a broad range of activities.

Consistent with all occupational therapy approaches, the cognitive disability model relies on activity analysis as a primary means of intervention. Cognitive disability theory provides a means for analyzing the relative difficulty of any desired activity in terms of requisite information-processing demands. From this analysis, environmental factors can be identified that facilitate or constrain the production of each cognitive dimension. Rehabilitation strategies are derived from conceptualizing how the environmental elements associated with each cognitive dimension might best be adapted or modified within the structure of a desired activity to capitalize on remaining cognitive capacities and to compensate for cognitive limitations. The intent is to place desired activities within an individual's range of comprehension and control. Specifically, therapists modify the structure of a desired activity to capitalize on, and to compensate for the following:

1. The *sensory cues* that the individual is able to attend to while performing an activity at any given cognitive level

2. The quality of *sensorimotor association* that the individual is able to conceptualize, or the *goal* that the

individual is able to act on at any given level

3. The degree of assistance required to enable the individual to complete a desired *motor action* at any given level, whether the desired motor action can be productively self-initiated or must be imitated from the therapist to elicit a productive motor response.

Cognitive Levels in Rehabilitation

In order to conceptualize rehabilitative intervention, the therapist must identify first the individual's cognitive capacities and limitations and must identify second the environmental factors that can be modified to enable successful participation in desired activities. Regardless of the level of cognitive function, cognitive processes are maximized and behavioral responses become more effectively organized when environmental stimuli are presented to the impaired individual in a manner that matches his or her level of cognitive functioning (Levy, 1986a). The discussion that follows provides a brief overview of the three information-processing dimensions as they are revealed at each level and the environmental factors associated with each dimension. Guidelines for conceptualizing environmental modification strategies that capitalize on cognitive capacities and compensate for limitations, at each of the cognitive levels, are presented (Levy, 1989, 1992). In addition, Medicare assistance codes for each level (Allen et al., 1989; HCFA, 1989) are identified. These codes provide therapists with the means to document levels of cognitive assistance required to maximize functional performance capabilities throughout the debilitating course of the disease.

COGNITIVE LEVEL 6: PLANNED ACTIONS (MEDICARE ASSISTANCE CODE: INDEPENDENT)

Attention is captured by abstract and symbolic cues. The *goal* is to use abstract reasoning to plan action sequences and to anticipate errors. *Motor actions* are those that have been planned in advance. Individuals can use complex information to carry out activities with accuracy and safety. Problems are anticipated, errors are avoided, and consequences of actions are considered. Theoretically, this level represents the absence of cognitive disability. Interventions to compensate for cognitive limitations are not required. This is the only level where planning, problem solving, and learning do not depend on overt visuomotor activity, external cues, or both.

COGNITIVE LEVEL 5: EXPLORATORY ACTIONS (MEDICARE ASSISTANCE CODE: STAND-BY/SUPERVISION COGNITIVE ASSISTANCE)

At this level, *attention* is captured and sustained by external cues, specifically the interesting properties of concrete objects. The *goal* of action is to explore the effects of self-initiated motor actions on physical objects and to investigate those effects through the use of planning and overt trial-and-error problem solving. (Covert problem solving requires symbolic memory. It is absent.) *Motor actions* are exploratory, to produce interesting effects on material objects, and extend through visual memory to the ability to follow through on a concrete four- or five-step process. The individual is able to learn through concrete, visible, and meaningful stimuli.

Many activities can be accomplished successfully at this level, because in concrete activities (those involving familiar four- to five-step motor actions with visibly perceivable results), individuals function relatively independently. However, the cognitive limitations experienced by individuals at this level become apparent when they attempt activities that require attention to abstract and symbolic cues (such as those that involve verbal and written instructions, diagrams, or drawings). Activities requiring attention to such cues will accentuate the disability and should be avoided.

Caregivers find that individuals can complete grooming, dressing, and eating activities without assistance. Household tasks are carried out relatively independently, although the individual may require assistance in the abstract reasoning required to establish safety procedures and to anticipate hazardous situations. Difficulties are observed with memory (semantic and episodic), judgment, reasoning, and planning ahead, as well as with the performance of complex daily activities, such as reading, writing, job peformance, managing finances, shopping, and driving.

This level parallels stage 4 (the "late confusional"-predementia stage) of the Global Deterioration Scale for the assessment of primary degenerative dementia (Reisberg, Ferris, Leon, & Cook, 1982), one of the most frequently used medical scales for staging the progression of the disease. Although there are significant differences in the rate of progression through the various stages of the disease, duration in this stage has been estimated to be 2 years.

COGNITIVE LEVEL 4: GOAL-DIRECTED ACTIVITY (MEDICARE ASSISTANCE CODE: MINIMUM COGNITIVE ASSISTANCE)

Attention at this level is directed to visible as well as tactile cues, and it is sustained throughout familiar short-term activities to their completion. The *goal* in performing a motor action is to perceive a concrete cause-and-effect relationship between a visible cue and a desired outcome. Problem-solving abilities are absent. *Motor actions* are limited to the ability to follow a two- to three-step, highly familiar motor process that leads to the accomplishment of visible predictable goals. Individuals can learn two- to three-step procedures that have visible and predictable results.

Activities that can be accomplished successfully at this level are (1) those that are adapted to capitalize on the capacity to use two- to three-step familiar motor actions that have predictable visible results and (2) activities that compensate for the individual's inability to comprehend unpredictable results or notice mistakes when they occur. Individuals use what they see in the environment for cues as to what to do. Decisions are made on the basis of limited, visual information. Assistance is required with abstract components of concrete tasks such as procuring and setting up supplies and scheduling activities. At this level, individuals should be provided with opportunities to engage in simple, relatively error-proof, concrete activities that support desired social roles. This goal is best accomplished by incorporating into the individual's daily routine yard work, household chores (e.g., laundry, simple meal preparation, shopping for a few familiar purchases), familiar sports and dance activities, simple board games and puzzles, letter writing or typing, and walks to familiar destinations.

Despite significant cognitive impairment, the individual appears to be less confused at this level than at the succeeding level because activities are pursued with specific outcomes in mind. Therapists and caregivers should encourage individuals to engage in comprehensible concrete activities that will protect personal dignity and enable social role retention. However, they should not expect the individual to notice mistakes or solve problems when they occur, to retain directions out of context, to plan beyond the immediate situation, to generalize learning to new situations, or to anticipate safety hazards.

Memory (semantic and episodic) is significantly impaired at this level. Instructions cannot be remembered, and patients are disoriented to time and sometimes to place. Clocks with the date, day, and year may assist orientation. Calendars, notes, labels, or pictures may serve as reminders of daily activities and locations of objects. Memories of long-distant past events are retained longer than more recent memories, which adds to the individual's confusion and lack of understanding about current situations. Environmental consistency is particularly important. Predictable routines allow individuals to perceive a greater sense of control.

Ensuring safety is an important concern at this level. Many accidents can be avoided by preventive measures. The home environment should be carefully scrutinized for potential safety hazards. Particular attention should be paid to clutter, loose rugs, lighting, door locks, electrical appliances, hot water pipes, cigarettes, matches, firearms, power tools, knives, detergents, polishes, chemicals, medications, and the tub and shower. Should the individual wander and become lost, caregivers should consider purchasing an identification bracelet and should ensure that identifying photographs are available.

It is important to be especially sensitive to the fear and frustation that accompany the confusion. At this stage of the disease, individuals are beginning to recognize that their environments are less manageable and understandable, because of their significant memory impairments. Depression and anxiety are frequent and reasonable reactions. Individuals should be guided to unvarying surroundings or involved in success-oriented (manual) activities when they become agitated.

Caregivers find that individuals can complete familiar grooming activities, although they frequently neglect areas that are not completely visible. For example, the back of the body may remain unwashed, shampoo may not be rinsed from the back of the head, and the individual may neglect to shave under the chin unless redirected. Dressing can be accomplished relatively independently, especially with task set-up. The individual can eat independently but may require assistance to season foods, share a limited quantity of food, open unfamiliar containers, or avoid burns. Again, individuals should be protected from invisible hazards from sources such as heat, chemicals, and electricity. Twenty-four-hour supervision is recommended to ensure safety.

This level parallels stage 5 (the "early dementia" stage) of the Global Deterioration Scale (Reisberg et al., 1982). There are significant differences in the rate of progression through the various stages of the disease, although the duration of this stage has been estimated at approximately 18 months.

COGNITIVE LEVEL 3: MANUAL ACTIONS (MEDICARE ASSISTANCE CODE: MODERATE COGNITIVE ASSISTANCE)

At this cognitive level, *attention* is directed to tactile cues that can be acted on and to familiar objects that can be manipulated. The *goal* in performing a motor action is limited to tactile exploration of the kinds of effects one's actions have on the environment. Actions are typically repeated to verify that similar results occur. *Motor actions* are limited to the ability to follow a one-step, highly familiar, action-oriented direction that has been demonstrated for the individual to follow. It is unrealistic to expect the individual to learn new behavior.

Level-three functional activities are caregiver intensive. Activities that can be successfully accomplished are those that are adapted to capitalize on the individual's capacity to be cued to imitate one-step, familiar, repetitive actions that provide predictable tactile effects and that compensate for the inability to follow multi-step directions or to initiate actions required to achieve a goal (conceptualize a predictable result). The individual should be provided with opportunities to participate in adapted activities that reinforce the relationship between one's actions and predictable tactile effects on the environment. Some possibilities include sports activities (such as swimming, biking, and playing catch); household maintenance activities (such as washing the car, mowing lawns, cultivating gardens, hand-washing laundry); kitchen activities (such as washing and drying the dishes, peeling and chopping vegetables, and cleaning counter tops); and IADLs demonstrated one step at a time. As in the previous level, functional performance can be maximized by teaching the caregivers how to present activities to the individual in a manner that will best promote productive motor actions. To that end, caregivers must initiate, sustain, and guide the individual through the steps of a functional activity.

Spontaneous motor actions include such unproductive behaviors as click-

ing dials on and off, using keys indiscriminately in locks, and pouring soup in the coffee maker. The individual will be drawn to anything that can be touched and manipulated. Hence, potentially dangerous appliances like toasters, blenders, and coffee makers should be hidden from view; if possible, stove knobs should be removed, or push buttons on the stove covered, and lawn and garden tools and chemicals should be hidden. It is no less critical at this level for the caregiver to provide the individual with opportunities for more productive "face-saving" and acceptable uses of familiar tactile movement patterns to enable a sense of competence, dignity, and role investment within his or her social environment. To reiterate, however, the goal of an activity is not related to a specific outcome or end product but rather to the relationship between actions and their predictable effects. Consequently therapists and caregivers need to appreciate the need for the individual to do the same thing over and over again, even though by traditional standards this behavior might appear to be apraxic or perseverative. Opportunities to engage in activities that appear to have no specific outcome, such as vacuuming the same spot over and over again and polishing the same spot on the car door, should be encouraged. Such activities are comprehensible to the individual and should also be deemed acceptable.

It is important to keep the environment as routine and predictable as possible, because at this cognitive level, it is no longer possible to separate out unnecessary stimuli. The plethora of impinging stimulation can easily overwhelm someone who is already struggling to make sense out of an incomprehensible world. Decreasing unnecessary sources of stimulation can help him or her cope more effectively. Since individuals at this level can respond to the environment in terms of procedural memories only, adjusting to novelty is difficult. Changes in the environment must be accompanied by reassurance and increased emotional support. Relocation is particularly detrimental and is likely to result in precipitous decline in function.

Caregivers find that individuals are able to brush teeth, wash hands and face, and use familiar table utensils independently, although they need to be reminded to perform these activities. In the absence of a concomitant physical disability, they are also able to manage dressing. However, if the caregiver does not present clothing and hand items to the individual one at a time, errors are frequent. For example, underwear may be placed over trousers, clothes may be donned inside out or backwards, and nightclothes may be selected for daytime wear. Most self-maintenance activities must be broken down into one-step motor actions, and supplies for activities such as brushing teeth, shaving, bathing, and washing hair should be presented one at a time. Twenty-four-hour supervision is necessary to ensure safety.

This level parallels stage 6 (the "middle dementia" stage) of the Global Deterioration Scale (Reisberg et al., 1982). The duration of this stage is estimated to be 2 1/2 years.

COGNITIVE LEVEL 2: POSTURAL ACTIONS (MEDICARE ASSISTANCE CODE: MAXIMUM COGNITIVE ASSISTANCE)

At this level, *attention* has shifted from external to internal cues. It is now limited to internal proprioceptive cues from muscles and joints that are elicited by one's own highly familiar body movements. The *goal* in performing a motor action is to repeat the one-step motor action component of the

activity for the pleasure of its effect on the body alone (i.e., on one's sense of position and balance, or on sensory input to muscles and joints). *Motor actions* are limited to the ability to imitate, albeit inexactly, a one-step direction only if it involves the use of a highly familiar, near-reflexive, gross motor pattern. The individual is severely apraxic, agnosic, and no longer attends to objects (other than perhaps eating utensils) in the task environment.

Activities that can be successfully accomplished at this level are those that are adapted to capitalize on the capacity to imitate one-step familiar, repetitive, gross motor actions, and that compensate for the inability to comprehend a purpose beyond the sensation of movement. Therapists and caregivers will find that providing opportunities to imitate simple movement, calisthenics, and modified sports activities are most often useful, but one-step activities (such as folding laundry, chopping vegetables, and polishing furniture) can be imitated if these activities were nearly habitual prior to the onset of the disability. Similarly, most IADLs can be accomplished if the individual is provided with a model to follow. For instance, to enable the individual to wash his or her arms, the caregiver should take a washcloth and demonstrate washing his or her own arms (the washcloth can be dry). Spontaneous behaviors are largely unproductive or bizarre (e.g., sitting backward on the toilet and "driving" it like a car—flushing to shift gears, constantly disrobing and redressing, reapplying the same lipstick over and over again). It appears as though individuals are searching for opportunities to apply very familiar, gross motor patterns (i.e., procedural memories) to the environment regardless of the context. Hence it is critical that therapists and caregivers provide individuals with opportunities to imitate actions that are appropriate to the environmental context to encourage functional performance and to enable the retention of dignity and role investment within the task environment.

It is important to remember that dementing diseases affect the cognitive structures most directly, yet leave the emotions largely intact. Caregivers should not expect individuals to participate in complex conversations, but should not exclude them from family communications either, for they will understand the emotional overtones. Simple sentences should be used when addressing them, as well as simple questions, one at a time, repeated, as necessary. One needs to try to communicate with the individual on an emotional level and to be especially sensitive to the emotional tones that words and actions are communicating. When verbal abilities deteriorate further, persons at this cognitive level often substitute familiar and somewhat related words for those names they can no longer remember, whether of objects or of people. For instance, they may substitute the word "mom" for the name of a close female friend, daughter, or sister. Later, when they are no longer able to respond with words, nonverbal communication and gestures such as familiar body movements become the essential modes of communication. Building trust and emotional connection is far more important than communicating to "make sense."

Therapists and caregivers find that with demonstration, individuals at this level may cooperate by moving body parts to assist in activities such as grooming, dressing, and eating but that maximal assistance and direct supervision are still essential. Requests related to actions (for example, raise your arm, sit, stand) may be followed, but may also require repetition and demonstration of the movement. Awareness is largely limited to movement within the environment and to items that directly contact the individual's body (e.g., washcloths, clothing, hand lotion). With supervision, but otherwise unassisted, individuals may be able to eat foods that can be eaten with fingers, and this should be encouraged. They may also be able to use spoons and non-slip scoop-edged plates or bowls, although other utensils are used incorrectly. It is helpful to serve all food in bowls at this level, because they are easier to manage with one–step motor actions. It is also important to recognize that individuals are not able to determine what is edible and what is not. Hence, anything that could be mistaken for food, such as decorative artificial fruit and poisonous house plants, should be removed.

Aimless pacing is common, but the individual will walk in directions guided by companions. However, the environment should be structured to provide a safe space for wandering, with two- to three-step push-button or combination locks on the doors and an unobstructed walkway within the living environment. To prevent voiding in unacceptable locations (or to manage incontinence), individuals should be escorted to the bathroom every two hours while they are awake, and wastebaskets or any other receptacles that could be mistaken for a toilet should be removed. Individuals at this level are easily confused when objects are hidden by doors, drawers, or closets. Whenever possible it is helpful to leave bathroom and bedroom doors open and to place frequently used objects or treasured possessions on furniture surfaces or hangers where they can be seen easily. Twenty-four-hour supervision is required.

This level parallels stage 6 (the "middle dementia" stage) of the Global Deterioration Scale (Reisberg et al., 1982). Depending upon factors such as health status and age at the onset of the disease, the duration of this stage can extend to 6 years.

COGNITIVE LEVEL 1: AUTOMATIC ACTIONS (MEDICARE ASSISTANCE CODE: TOTAL COGNITIVE ASSISTANCE)

At the first cognitive level, *attention* is limited to subliminal internal cues, such as hunger, taste, and smell. Individuals, while conscious, appear to stare and are largely unresponsive to external stimuli. There is no *goal*, or reason, for performing motor actions; hence, few motor actions are being performed. *Motor actions* are limited to the potential to follow near-reflexive one-word directives, such as "sip" or "turn." With little (if any) purpose and few (if any) motor actions available, the individual has few cognitive capabilities to capitalize on. It is unrealistic to attempt to modify activities, although the environment can be modified to elicit orienting responses.

Therapists and caregivers find that an orienting response can be elicited by familiar gustatory and olfactory stimuli, such as favorite foods and spices, fragrant plants, hand lotion, or aftershave, and gentle touch, massage, or a family pet. They also find that the individual either actively resists or is at best uncooperative in efforts to provide required maximal assistance in grooming, bathing, and feeding. The individual may need to be fed or allowed to eat with the fingers. Walking and transfers from bed to wheelchair may be achieved with physical guidance. Assisted ambulation and, later, regular turning and passive, active, and assistive range of motion are necessary in order to forestall the secondary complications of the disease, such as bed sores, contractures, osteoporosis, and infection.

This level parallels stage 7 (the "late dementia" stage) of the Global Deterioration Scale (Reisberg et al., 1982). Although it marks the terminal phase of the disease, medical comorbidities and secondary complications of dementia (i.e., aspiration, pneumonia, malnutrition, trauma, or infection) frequently cause death prior to this stage.

In summary, rehabilitation for the cognitively impaired elder requires familiarity with the information-processing dimensions identified in Allen's cognitive disability model. The environmental elements associated with these information-processing dimensions are identified for each of the cognitive levels, including

1. The cues that should be provided by the therapist or caregiver

2. What is interpreted on the basis of those cues

3. The type and complexity of assistance and directions to be given to elicit productive motor actions.

To maximize functional performance throughout the deteriorating course of the disease, therapists provide caregivers with guidance on how to capitalize on the cognitive capabilities of the individual and compensate for specific cognitive limitations by modifying both the demands and the structure of desired life activities.

Evaluation and Assessment

Therapists use a variety of methods to assess cognitive functional capacities and limitations, defined in this model in terms of the three dimensions of cognition (attention to sensory cues, goal-directed behavior, and self-initiated actions) processed in the course of pursuing functional activities. (Note: traditional neuropsychological or mental status instruments fail to elicit cognitive functions such as attention, procedural learning, or imitation, and are therefore limited in providing information useful for assessing rehabilitation potential as revealed by this model.)

The most frequently used assessment method is informal, and involves guided observation of the individual engaged in any desired motor task, using the concepts and profiles described above to determine level of cognitive function. More comprehensive profiles of the quality of functional activities associated with each cognitive level are also available (Allen, 1985; Allen et al., 1992; Levy, 1992).

Formal assessments include the Allen Cognitive Level Test (ACL) (Allen, 1985), which is a standardized leather-lacing task used as a screening tool. Scoring is based on the complexity of the lacing stitch that the elder is able to imitate, and a numerical score is assigned that represents the elder's cognitive level. An "enlarged" ACL (Allen et al., 1992; Kehrberg, 1993) compensates for the visual and fine motor demands of this task. Heying (1985) demonstrated a significant correlation between the ACL score of patients with dementia and caregiver's ratings of ADL performance.

Perhaps the most useful tool to assess levels of cognitive capacities and limitations in the elderly is the Routine Task Inventory (RTI) (Allen, 1985; Allen et al., 1992). The RTI was designed as a practical observational measure of performance within Allen's framework for describing cognitive disabilities and serves to identify qualitative differences in functional performance. It also provides a comprehensive listing of behaviors indicative of function and dysfunction to be observed in the performance of physical and instrumental daily living tasks that are specific to each of the cognitive levels. This assessment methodology has been developed further in the Cognitive Performance Test (CPT), an instrument for assessing cognitive functional capacities and limitations in patients with dementia (Allen et al., 1992; Burns et al., 1994). The CPT is made up of six tasks: dressing, shopping, making toast, using the phone, washing, and traveling. Consistent with Allen's theoretical approach, the deficits observed in the CPT predict functional capabilities on a wide variety of daily life activities. The CPT holds enormous promise for future research in this area of rehabilitation. It provides a single standardized instrument to assess functional impairment across the deteriorating course of the disease and may thereby address a well-recognized need within the health care system. It provides a means to educate caregivers about the effects of the disease on functional abilities of older adults and appropriate intervention strategies. It may provide a means to evaluate the effects of intervention on functional status, institutional placement, or disease progression.

Summary

Cognitive disability theory presents an adaptive approach (Mosey, 1994) to rehabilitation that helps the cognitively impaired older adult reach his or her highest attainable level of function and maintain active participation in as many preferred activities as possible, given the significant deficits that exist. Using principles derived from Allen's model, therapists knowledgeably modify the multi-dimensional information-processing demands of functional activities to enable the older adult with cognitive impairments to still meet activity demands.

Occupational therapy has an essential role in the treatment of the ever-increasing numbers of older people experiencing the functional consequences of cognitive impairments presented by diseases such as dementia. By modifying activities appropriately, they help to optimize these individuals' remaining capacities and to compensate for their limitations. They can help cognitively disabled individuals to retain a sense of competence, comprehension, and control throughout the deteriorating course of their disease.

Review Questions

1. List the three categories of clinical characteristics of dementia.
2. What is the most common cognitive impairment seen in dementia?
3. Why is memory so critical to other cognitive functions?
4. Name and define the three information-processing stages of memory.
5. Name three forms of long-term memory and define each.
6. Besides memory impairment, what are some of the other cognitive components affected by dementia?
7. What is the focus of the cognitive disability approach to treatment of cognitive deficits?
8. What is the most frequently documented behavioral problem experienced by persons with dementia? How might it be manifested?
9. List other behavioral symptoms that might be seen in dementia.
10. How do cognitively impaired depressed patients respond to antidepressant therapy?
11. What is the most significant source of caregiver stress?
12. Which strategies are most effective in helping caregivers to cope?
13. The treatment approach recommended for persons with dementia is the adaptive approach. Summarize the principles of this approach.
14. How are activities analyzed in cognitive disability theory?
15. What is the goal of the cognitive disability approach?
16. How is that goal accomplished?
17. Which cognitive level theoretically represents the absence of cognitive disability?
18. At which cognitive level is the individual able to learn through concrete, visible, and meaningful stimuli?
19. At which cognitive level can activities that use two- or three-step familiar motor actions with predictable visible results be accomplished successfully?
20. Your patient is at cognitive level 3. Describe the characteristics of appropriate activities and give some examples.
21. At which cognitive level would you use activities with one-step motor actions with highly familiar, near reflexive gross motor patterns that can be imitated?
22. How is an individual's cognitive level determined?

References

Allen, C. K. (1982). Independence through activity: The practice of occupational therapy. *American Journal of Occupational Therapy, 36,* 731–739.

Allen, C. K. (1985). *Occupational therapy for psychiatric diseases: Measurement and management of cognitive disabilities.* Boston: Little, Brown.

Allen, C. K. (1987). Activity: Occupational therapy's treatment method. *American Journal of Occupational Therapy, 41,* 563–575.

Allen, C. K. (1992). Cognitive disabilities. In N. Katz (Ed.), *Cognitive rehabilitation: Models for intervention in occupational therapy* (pp. 1–21). Boston: Andover Medical Publishers.

Allen, C. K., Earheart, C. A., & Blue, T. (1992). *Occupational therapy treatment goals for the physically and cognitively disabled.* Rockville, MD: American Occupational Therapy Association.

Allen, C. K, Foto, M., Moon-Sperling, T., & Wilson, D. (1989). A medical review approach to Medicare outpatient documentation. *American Journal of Occupational Therapy, 43,* 793–800.

Allen, C. K., & Robertson, S. (1993). *Study guide for occupational therapy treatment goals for the physically and cognitively disabled.* Rockville, MD: American Occupational Therapy Association.

American Psychiatric Association (APA). (1994). *Diagnostic and statistical manual of mental disorders* (4th ed.) (DSM-IV). Washington, DC: American Psychiatric Association.

Atkinson, R. C., & Shiffrin, R. M. (1968). Human memory: A proposed system and its control processes. In K. Spence & J. Spence (Eds.), *The psychology of learning and motivation* (Vol. 2, o.p.). New York: Academic Press.

Backman, L., Josephsson, S., Herlitz, A., Stigsdotter, A., & Vitanan, M. (1991). The generalizability of training gains in dementia: Effects of imagery-based mnemonic on face-name retention duration. *Psychology and Aging, 6,* 489–492.

Bassett, S. S., & Folstein, M. F. (1991). Cognitive impairment and functional disability in the absence of psychiatric diagnosis. *Psychological Medicine, 21,* 77–84.

Baum, C. M. (1991). Addressing the needs of the cognitively impaired elderly from a family policy perspective. *American Journal of Occupational Therapy, 45,* 594–606.

Baum, C., Edwards, D., & Morrow-Howell, N. (1993). Identification and measurement of productive behaviors in senile dementia of the Alzheimer's type. *Gerontologist, 33,* 403–408.

Best, J. B. (1989). *Cognitive Psychology.* St. Paul: West Publishing.

Botwinick, J., Storandt, M., & Berg, L. (1986). A longitudinal, behavioral study of senile dementia of the Alzheimer's type. *Archives of Neurology, 43,* 1124–1127.

Breteler, M. M. B., Claus, J. J., Van Duijn, C. M., Launer, L. J., & Hofman, A. (1992). Epidemiology of Alzheimer's disease. *Epidemiology Review, 14,* 59–82.

Bucher, D. M., & Larson, E. B. (1987). Falls and fractures in patients with Alzheimer's type dementia. *Journal of the American Medical Association, 257,* 1492–1495.

Burgener, S., Jirovec, M., Murrell, L., & Barton, D. (1992). Caregiver and environmental variables related to difficult behaviors in institutionalized, demented elderly persons. *Journal of Gerontology, 47,* 242–249.

Burns, A. (1991). Affective symptoms in Alzheimer's disease. *International Journal of Geriatric Psychiatry, 6,* 371–376.

Burns, T., Mortimer, J., Merchek, P. (1994). Cognitive performance test: A new approach to functional assessment in Alzheimer's disease. *Journal of Geriatric Psychiatry and Neurology, 7,* 46–54.

Camp, C., & McKitrick, L. (1992). Memory interventions in Alzheimer's-type dementia populations: Methodological and theoretical issues. In R. West & J. Sinnot (Eds.), *Everyday memory and aging: Current research and methodology* (pp. 155–172). New York: Springer.

Chiu, H. C., & Smith, B. A. (1990). Rehabilitation of persons with dementia. In B. Kemp, K. Brummel-Smith, & J. Ramsdell (Eds.), *Geriatric Rehabilitation* (pp. 389–405). Boston: Little, Brown.

Cohen-Mansfield, J., & Billig, N. (1986). Agitated behaviors in the elderly I: A conceptual review. *Journal of the American Geriatrics Society, 34*(10), 711–721.

Cohen-Mansfield, J., Marx, M. S., & Rosenthal, A. S. (1990). Dementia and agitation in nursing home residents: How are they related? *Psychology and Aging, 5,* 3–8.

Cohen-Mansfield, J., Werner, P., Marx, M. S., & Lipson, S. (1993). Assessment and management of behavior problems in the nursing home setting. In L. A. Rubenstein & D. Wieland (Eds.), *Improving care in the nursing home: Comprehensive reviews of clinical research* (275–313). Newbury Park: Sage Publications.

Cottrell, V., & Schultz, R. (1993). The perspective of the patient with Alzheimer's disease: A neglected dimension of dementia research. *Gerontologist, 33,* 205–211.

Cummings, J. L. (1987). Neuropsychiatric aspects of multi-infarct dementia and dementia of the Alzheimer type. *Archives of Neurology, 44,* 389–394.

Deutch, L. H., & Rovner, B. W. (1991). Agitation and other noncognitive abnormalities in Alzheimer's disease. *Psychiatric Clinics of North America, 14,* 341–351.

Dick, M. (1992). Motor and procedural memory in Alzheimer's disease. In L. Backman (Ed.), *Memory functioning in dementia* (pp. 135–150). Amsterdam: North Holland.

Dick, M., Kean, M., & Sands, D. (1988). The preselection effect on recall facilitation of motor movement in Alzheimer-type dementia. *Journal of Gerontology, 43,* 127–135.

Dick, M., Shankle, R., Bet, R., Dick-Muehlke, C., Cotman, C., & Kean, M. (1996). Acquisition and long-term retention of a gross motor skill in Alzheimer's disease patients under constant and varied practice conditions. *Journal of Gerontology, 51B,* 103–111.

Duchek, J. M., Cheney, M., Ferraro, F. R., & Storandt, M. (1991). Paired associate learning in senile dementia of the Alzheimer type. *Archives of Neurology, 48,* 1038–1040.

Edwards, D., & Baum, C. (1990). Caregiver burden across stages of dementia. *Occupational Therapy Practice, 2,* 17–31.

Edwards, D. F., Deuel, R. K., & Baum, C. M. (1991). Constructional apraxia in senile dementia: Contributions to functional loss. *Physical and Occupational Therapy in Geriatrics, 9,* 53–59.

Eslinger, P. J., & Damasio, A. R. (1986). Preserved motor learning in Alzheimer's disease: Implications for anatomy and behavior. *Journal of Neuroscience, 6,* 3006–3009.

Evans, D. A., Funkenstein, H. H., Albert, M. S., Scherr, P. A., & Cook, N. R. (1989). Prevalence of Alzheimer's disease in a community population of older persons. *Journal of the American Medical Association, 262,* 2551–2556.

Faber-Langendoen, K., Morris, J. C., Knesevich, J. W., LaBarge, E., Miller, J. P., & Berg, L. (1988). Aphasia in senile dementia of the Alzheimer type. *Annals of Neurology, 23,* 465–370.

Feil, N. (1992). Validation therapy. *Somatics, Autumn-Winter,* 44–51.

Feil, N. (1993). *The validation breakthrough.* Baltimore: Health Professions Press.

Foster, N. L., Chase, T., Patronas, N., Gillespie, M., & Fedio, P. (1986). Cerebral mapping of apraxia in Alzheimer's disease by positron emission tomography. *Annals of Neurology, 19,* 139–143.

Gallagher, D., Lovett, S., & Zeiss, A. (1987). *Interventions with caregivers of frail elderly persons.* Palo Alto, CA: Caregiver Research Program.

Geschwind, N., & Damasio, A. (1985). Apraxia. In J. Frederik (Ed.), *Handbook of Clinical Neurology (Vol. 45,* pp. 423–341). New York: Wiley.

Gottlieb, G. (1990). Rehabilitation and dementia of the Alzheimer's type. In S. Brody & L. G. Paulson (Eds.), *Aging and rehabilitation 2: The state of the practice* (pp. 255–271). New York: Springer.

Green, C. R., Mohs, R. C., Schmeidler, J., Aryan, M., & Davis, K. L. (1993). Functional decline in Alzheimer's disease: A longitudinal study. *Journal American Geriatric Society, 41,* 654–661.

Health Care Financing Administration (HCFA). (1989). Outpatient occupational therapy Medicare part B guidelines (DHHS Transmittal No. 55). In *Health insurance manual* (pp. 5-71–5-83). Baltimore: Author.

Heying, L. M. (1985). Research with subjects having senile dementia. In C. K. Allen (Ed.), *Occupational therapy for psychiatric diseases: Measurement and management of cognitive disabilities* (pp. 339–365). Boston: Little, Brown.

Hof, P. R., Bouras, C., Constantinidis, J., & Morrison, J. H. (1990). Selective disconnection of specific visual association pathways in cases of Alzheimer's disease presenting with Balint's syndrome. *Journal of Neuropathology and Experimental Neurology, 49,* 168–184.

Jorm, A. F. (1990). *The epidemiology of Alzheimer's disease and related disorders.* London, UK: Chapman & Hall, 1990.

Kahn, R. (1975). The mental health system and the future aged. *Gerontologist, 15* (1, Pt. 2), 24–31.

Kamholz, B., & Gottlieb, G. (1992). The nature and efficacy of interventions for depression and dementia. In B. S. Fogel, A. Furino, & G. Gottlieb (Eds.), *Access and financing of neuropsychiatric care for the elderly American* (pp. 39–67). Washington, DC: American Psychiatric Association Press.

Katz, N. (1992). *Cognitive rehabilitation: Models for intervention in occupational therapy.* Boston: Andover Medical Publishers.

Kehrberg, K. (1993). The larger Allen Cognitive Level Test. Test kit and instructions. Colchester, CT: S & S.

Kemp, B. (1988). Eight methods family members can use to manage behavioral problems in dementia. *Topics in Geriatric Rehabilitation, 4,* 50–59.

Kiecolt-Glaser, J., Glaser, R., Shuttleworth, E., Dyer, C., Ogrocki, P., & Speicher, C. (1987). Chronic stress and immunity in family caregivers of Alzheimer's disease victims. *Psychosomatic Medicine, 49,* 523–535.

Knopman, D. S., & Nissen, M. J. (1987). Implicit learning in patients with probable Alzheimer's disease. *Neurology, 37,* 784–788.

LaBarge, E., Smith, D. S., Dick, L., & Storandt, M. (1992). Agraphia in dementia of the Alzheimer type. *Archives of Neurology, 49,* 1151–1156.

Larson, E. B., Reifler, B. V., Featherstone, H. J., & English, D. J. (1984). Dementia in elderly outpatients: A prospective study. *Annals of Internal Medicine, 100,* 417–423.

Lazarus, L. W., Newton, N., Cohler, B., Lesser, J., & Schweon, C. (1987). Frequency and presentation of depressive symptoms in patients with primary degenerative dementia. *American Journal of Psychiatry, 144,* 41–45.

Levy, L. L. (1974). Movement therapy for psychiatric patients. *American Journal of Occupational Therapy, 28*(6), 354–357.

Levy, L. L. (1986a). Cognitive treatment. In L. J. Davis & M. Kirkland (Eds.), *Role of occupational therapy with the elderly* (pp. 289–324). Rockville, MD: American Occupational Therapy Association.

Levy, L. L. (1986b). A practical guide to the care of the Alzheimer's disease victim. *Topics in Geriatric Rehabilitation, 1,* 16–26.

Levy, L. L. (1989). Activity adaptation in rehabilitation of the physically and cognitively disabled aged. *Topics in Geriatric Rehabilitation, 4*(4), 53–66.

Levy, L. L. (1992). The use of the cognitive disability frame of reference in rehabilitation of cognitively disabled older adults. In N. Katz (Ed.),

Cognitive rehabilitation: Models for intervention in occupational therapy (pp. 22–50). Boston: Andover Medical Publishers.

Mace, N. L., & Rabins, P. V. (1991). *The thirty-six hour day: A family guide to care for persons with Alzheimer's disease, related dementing illnesses, and memory loss in later life* (rev. ed.). Baltimore: Johns Hopkins University Press.

Mendez, M. F., Mendez, M. A., Martin, R., Smyth, K. A., & Whitehouse, P. J. (1990). Complex visual disturbances in Alzheimer's disease. *Neurology, 40,* 439–443.

Merriam, A. E., Aronson, M. K., Gaston, P., Wey, S., & Katz, I. (1988). The psychiatric symptoms of Alzheimer's disease. *Journal of the American Geriatrics Society, 36,* 7–12.

Miller, G. A. (1956). The magical number seven, plus or minus two: Some limits on our capacity for processing information. *Psychological Review, 63,* 81–97.

Miller, R. (1981). *Meaning and purpose in the intact brain: A philosophical, psychological, and biological account of conscious processes.* New York: Clarendon Press.

Mosey, A. (1994). Working taxonomies. In C. B. Royeen (Ed.), *AOTA self-study series: Cognitive rehabilitation* (pp. 23–35). Rockville, MD: American Occupational Therapy Association.

National Center for Health Statistics (NCHS). (1993). *Chartbook on Health Data on Older Americans: United States 1992* (DHHS Publication No. [PHS] 93–1413). Washington, DC: U.S. Government Printing Office.

Nebes, R. D. (1989). Semantic memory in Alzheimer's disease. *Psychological Bulletin, 106,* 377–394.

Nissen, M. J. (1986). Neuropsychology of attention and memory. *Journal of Head Trauma Rehabilitation, 1,* 13–21.

Pearlin, L. I., Mullar, J., Semple, S., & Skaff, M. (1990). Caregiving and the stress process: An overview of concepts and their measures. *The Gerontologist, 30,* 583–594.

P.L. 100–203. (1987). *Omnibus Budget Reconciliation Act, Subtitle C, Nursing Home Reform.* Washington, DC: U.S. Government Printing Office.

Rabinovich, B., & Cohen-Mansfield, J. (1992). The impact of participation in structured recreational activities on the agitated behavior of nursing home residents: An observational study. *Activities, Adaptation, and Aging, 16,* 89–98.

Reifler, B. V., Larson, E., & Teri, L. (1986). Dementia of the Alzheimer's type and depression. Journal of the *American Geriatric Society, 34,* 855–859.

Reifler, B. V., & Teri, L. (1986). Rehabilitation and Alzheimer's disease. In S. J. Brody & G. E. Ruff (Eds.), *Aging and rehabilitation: Advances in the state of the art* (pp. 241–254). New York: Springer.

Reisberg, B., Ferris, S. H., & Franssen, E. (1985). An ordinal functional assessment tool for Alzheimer's-type dementia. *Hospital and Community Psychiatry, 36,* 593–595.

Reisberg, B., Ferris, S. H., Leon, M. J., & Cook, T. (1982). The global deterioration scale for the assessment of primary degenerative dementia. *American Journal of Psychiatry, 139,* 1136–1139.

Rentz, D. (1991). The assessment of rehabilitation potential: Cognitive factors. In R. Hartke (Ed.), *Psychological aspects of geriatric rehabilitation* (pp. 97–112). Gaithersburg, MD: Aspen.

Reynolds, C. F., Perel, J. M., Kupfer, D. J., Zimmer, B., Stack, J. A., & Hoch, C. H. (1987). Open trial response to anti-depressant treatment in elderly patients with mixed depression and cognitive impairment. *Psychiatry Research, 21,* 111–122.

Rovner, B. W. (1994). What is therapeutic about special care units? The role of psychosocial rehabilitation. *Alzheimer's disease and associated disorders, 8,*(1), 355–359.

Rovner, B. W., Kafonek, S., Filipp, L., Lucas, M. J., & Folstein, M. F. (1986). Prevalence of mental illness in a community nursing home. *American Journal of Psychiatry, 143,* 1446–1449.

Rovner, B. W., & Katz, I. R. (1992). Psychiatric disorders in the nursing home: A selective view of studies related to clinical care. *International Journal of Geriatric Psychiatry, 7,* 75–82.

Rubin, E. H., & Kinscherf, D. A. (1989). Psychopathology of very mild dementia of the Alzheimer's type. *American Journal of Psychiatry, 146,* 1017–1021.

Squire, L. R. (1987). *Memory and brain.* New York: Oxford University Press.

Storandt, M., Botwinick, J., Danziger, W. L., Berg, L., & Hughes, C. P. (1984). Psychometric differentiation of mild senile dementia of the Alzheimer type. *Archives of Neurology, 41,* 497–499.

Swearer, J. M., Drachman, D. A., O'Donnell, B. F., & Mitchell, A. L. (1988). Troublesome and disruptive behaviors in dementia: Relationships to diagnosis and disease severity. *Journal of the American Geriatrics Society, 34,* 784–790.

Teri, L., Borson, S., Kiyak, A., & Yamagishi, M. (1989). Behavioral disturbance, congitive dysfunction, and functional skill: Prevalence and relationship in

Alzheimer's disease. *Journal of the American Geriatrics Society, 37,* 109–116.

Teri, L., & Logsdon, R. (1991). Identifying pleasant activities for Alzheimer's disease patients: The pleasant events schedule-AD. *The Gerontologist, 31,* 124–131.

Teri, L., Rabins, P., Whitehouse, P., Berg, L., Reisber, B., Sunderland, T., Eichelman, B., & Creighton, P. (1992). Management of behavior disturbance in Alzheimer's Disease: Current knowledge and future directions. *Alzheimer's Disease and Related Disorders, 6,* 77–88.

Teri, L., & Wagner, A. (1992). Alzheimer's disease and depression. *Journal of Consulting Clinical Psychology, 60,* 379–391.

Tulving, E. (1972). Episodic and semantic memory. In E. Tulving & W. Donaldson (Eds.), *Organization of memory* (o.p.). New York: Academic Press.

Tulving, E. (1983). *Elements of episodic memory.* New York: Oxford University Press.

Tulving, E. (1985). How many memory systems are there? *American Psychologist, 40,* 385–398.

U.S. Senate, Special Committee on Aging (1991). *Aging America, trends and projections, 1991 edition* (DHHS Publication No. 91–28001). Washington, DC: U.S. Government Printing Office.

Visser, H. (1983). Gait and balance in senile dementia of Alzheimer's type. *Age and Aging, 12,* 269–299.

Vitaliano, P. P., Breen, A. R., Albert, M. S., Russo, J., & Prinz, P. N. (1984). Memory, attention, and functional status in community residing Alzheimer type dementia patients and optimally healthy individuals. *Journal of Gerontology, 39,* 58–64.

Vitaliano, P. P., Russo, J., Breen, A. R., Vitiello, M. V., & Prinz, P. N. (1986). Functional decline in the early stages of Alzheimer's disease. *Journal of Psychology and Aging, 1,* 41–46.

Welsh, K., Butters, N., Hughes, J., Mohs, R., & Heyman, A. (1991). Detection of abnormal memory decline in mild cases of Alzheimer's disease using CERAD neuropsychological measures. *Archives of Neurology, 48,* 278–281.

Yasavage, J. A, Brooks, J. O., Taylor, L., & Tinkleberg, J. (1993). Development of aphasia, apraxia, and agnosia and decline in Alzheimer's disease. *American Journal of Psychiatry, 150,* 742–747.

Zanetti, O., Bianchetti, A., Frisoni, G., Rozzini, R., & Trabucchi, M. (1993). Determinants of disability in Alzheimer's disease. *International Journal of Geriatric Psychiatry, 8,* 581–586.

Zarit, S., Orr, N., & Zarit, J. (1985). *The hidden victims of Alzheimer's disease: Families under stress.* New York: University Press.

Zarit, S., Reever, K., & Bachman-Peterson, S. (1980). The burden interview. *Gerontologist, 20,* 649–656.

Section 3:
COPE (Caregiver Options for Practical Experiences): An Activity Group for Caregivers with Relatives with Dementia

Danielle N. Butin, MPH, OTR
Patricia A. Miller, MEd, OTR, FAOTA
Pamela Maultsby, MS, OTR
Nadine Winter, MS, OTR

The authors gratefully acknowledge Colleen Heany and the Westchester Chapter of the New York State Alzheimer's Association.

Abstract

As the elderly population increases, there will be more people in need of services for dementia and related conditions, and studies suggest that most of these people will be living at home. A pilot program from the New York Department of Health made use of four theoretical models to guide therapists' interventions and enable caregivers to facilitate their family member's participation in meaningful activities.

Introduction

Alzheimer's disease (Senile Dementia, Alzheimer's Type [SDAT]), the most common form of dementia, currently affects over 2.6 million people in the United States and is expected to rise to 4 million by the year 2000 (Berila, 1994). Dementia is the fifth leading cause of total disability in the United States and the fourth leading cause of death. It is an organic brain syndrome that results in a progressive failure of the person in all activities of daily living, global failure of cognitive function, and a disruption in the personality structure. Specifically, Alzheimer's disease is a dementing disorder of unknown etiology; it includes a gradual decline in mental status and language skills, and changes in mood and often personality (Buckwalter, Abraham, & Neuendorfer, 1988). Many studies document that between one-half and two-thirds of all patients with dementia live at home (Bergmann, Foster, & Justice, 1978), with their families providing more than 80% of the long-term care and support (Pepper Commission, 1990).

Although caregivers are equipped with varying skills in caring for loved ones with dementia, the progressive aspect of this disease creates changing needs for both. Accordingly, caregivers often seek ways in which to improve upon their management and coping skills in order to enhance the lives of their loved one residing at home (Hasselkus, 1988). Family caregivers with older, impaired relatives frequently request help from health professionals in order to manage their emotional and financial burdens, manage conflicts, and to solve problems arising from acute and ongoing concerns (Gessert, 1987).

The function and coping strategies of caregivers and their relatives with Alzheimer's and related dementias improved after they took part in a pilot demonstration program that combined a participative model of problem solving (Miller, 1993) with renewed involvement in activities. Caregiver Options for Practical Experiences (COPE) explored and attempted to meet the functional and psychosocial needs of both caregivers and care recipients. Six caregivers and their relatives with dementia met weekly for 10 weeks for an activity group conducted in two parts. The first component was for caregivers alone and consisted of a participative model of problem solving designed to enhance coping strategies and empower participants in managing their relative's daily care. The second activity-based group involved both caregivers and care recipients and was specifically tailored to the needs of each pair in order to improve communication and reestablish involvement in daily activities. After the 10-week period, activity levels of both caregivers and care recipients increased, and caregivers reported a decrease in disruptive behaviors in their relatives.

Theoretical Foundation

Four theoretical models guided the therapists' interventions with this population: a competence-environmental press model, a group dynamics model, an activities health model, and a cognitive-behavioral psychotherapeutic model. In the competence-environmental press model (Ansello, King, & Taler, 1986), both the human and physical environment has a profound effect in either enhancing or limiting the independent behavior of the individual with dementia (Barris, Kielhofner, Levine, & Neville, 1985). A hands-on approach that involves the collaboration of the occupational therapist and families in modifying the environment to increase the competence of their relatives with dementia is congruent with the knowledge and skills of occupational therapists. This approach enhances problem solving, which better enables the caregiver to address future difficulties, thereby increasing a sense of efficacy and mastery (Bandura, 1977).

Corcoran and Gitlin (1992) evaluated intervention strategies designed for home-based treatment and the extent to which these strategies were accepted

and carried out by caregivers over five intervention visits. According to Corcoran and Gitlin (1992), providing problem-solving opportunities to the caregiver enabled the caregiver to modify the care recipient's behavior by manipulating and grading tasks or sociocultural components of the environment. They concluded, with the therapist and independently, that a majority of the subjects did develop effective solutions to improve the quality of life of both caregiver and care recipient. The competence-environmental press model fosters within the family a consistent positive cycle and enhances interactions.

This demonstration project was carried out in a group format. Therefore, Yalom's (1985) theoretical model served to guide treatment because it elaborates on the various group factors that help to facilitate therapeutic change. The eleven curative factors are interdependent and may represent different components of the change process. Certainly, the universality of concerns, opportunities for interpersonal learning, and the instillation of hope are positive aspects of group work with this population (Yalom, 1995).

Activities health, the third model utilized, is manifested in the ability of the individual to participate in socioculturally delineated and directed activities with satisfaction. An activity that has no meaning to the individual also lacks therapeutic value. Activities not only define human existence but are also the means and ends for the development or restoration of function (Cynkin & Robinson, 1990). According to Baum (1991),

> We as occupational therapists have a body of knowledge to bring to this problem. We cannot only help caregivers acquire the skills for their role in care giving, but also help caregivers balance their activi-

ties to maintain a more healthful role for themselves.

The literature emphasized the importance of continued participation in activities in the face of disabilities associated with Alzheimer's disease, despite compromised participation (Gordon, Gaitz, & Scott, 1976).

The fourth model utilized was the cognitive-behavioral model developed by Aaron Beck (Beck, 1967). This theory is based on the premise that an individual's behavior and affect are governed by the manner in which experiences are cognitively structured. Beck proposed that negative emotions generally result from distorted perceptions about the self, the future, and the individual's experience. Once individuals discover connections among their beliefs, affective state, and behavior, they are more likely to change maladaptive behavior in order to cope with routines of daily living more effectively. The aim of therapy was to enable caregivers of individuals with Alzheimer's disease to facilitate their family member's participation in meaningful activities. By learning to structure tasks in a way that draws upon remaining competencies, the person's cognition is changed to focus on abilities, purposeful use of time, and a sense of belonging. The opportunity to reinforce positive behavior, to decrease resistive behavior, and enhance communication skills promote positive experiences (Florsheim, 1991), thereby altering negative cognitions.

Subjects

The subjects were 12 individuals representing 6 families, each consisting of a caregiver and care recipient. The sample selected were Caucasian and all participants were from a middle- to upper-class community. The caregivers were four male spouses, one female spouse, and one daughter. Ages of care-givers ranged from 52 to 83 with a mean age of 67.7. Ages of care recipients were 54 to 81 with a mean of 70. Caregivers and their relatives with dementia were recruited from the Alzheimer's Association. Families were interviewed by the association social worker to determine whether they met the specific entry criteria for the group.

The criteria for participation in COPE required that the person with dementia be able to do the following:

1. Follow one- or two-step directions

2. Concentrate on a simple task for ten minutes

3. Display a tolerance for spending time with others

4. Not exhibit overtly psychotic symptoms.

These skills generally represent individuals in the moderate to severe stages of the disease process (Reisberg, 1986). The care recipient needed to have a caregiver who was interested in learning ways to manage daily routines more easily and to structure the day more pleasurably through the use of activities.

Method

The method was designed to learn more about the characteristics of this population by observing and listening to the expressed needs of the caregiver and the individual with dementia (care recipient) while providing occupational therapy. A grant, written by these authors, from the New York State Department of Health, funded the Westchester Chapter of the New York Alzheimer's Association for the implementation of this study.

Prior to the initiation of the group, caregivers were asked to complete an Activities Health Assessment (Cynkin & Robinson, 1990) and Interest Check

List (Matsutsuyu, 1969) for themselves and their care recipients. This provided group leaders with information about past activity interests and current activity patterns, and identified potential areas for therapeutic activity selection.

Each family was also asked to complete the COPE Assessment Form in order for the group leaders to identify primary areas of concern and to determine content areas to address in Group 1 (the caregiver meetings). All pre-group assessments were repeated at the end of the group to ascertain changes.

Format of Groups and Objectives

The group, held in a church rectory in Westchester, New York, met once a week in the late afternoon for 10 weeks. The two hour-long sessions consisted of two groups: Group 1 for discussion with the caregivers only and Group 2 for activity involvement with the care recipients and caregivers together.

The caregivers met with two occupational therapists, a rehabilitation counselor, and a social worker. The social worker was the liaison person to the group from the Alzheimer's Association. The purposes of Group 1 (the caregiver meeting) were as follows:

1. To address problems concerning safety and daily living skills

2. To offer suggestions on ways to enhance communication between the caregiver and the care recipient

3. To discuss stress reduction and time management techniques

4. To learn cognitive methods to restructure automatic thoughts that had a negative impact upon behavior and affect

5. To select individually tailored activities to pursue in Group 2 and at home for future weeks

6. To discuss community resources and any remaining issues from the previous week.

In order to facilitate a problem-solving model, each caregiver discussion group began with the following questions, "What worked for you last week, what didn't, and why?" and, "What could be done differently this week?" This process served to empower caregivers as partners in the problem-solving process. Unlike traditional Alzheimer support groups, COPE had as a primary objective to produce better carryover at home of activities that would produce more positive behavioral changes for both the caregiver and care recipient.

While the caregivers were participating in Group 1 for 45 minutes in one room, their relatives with dementia were in an adjoining room engaged in gentle exercises, balloon volleyball, and informal discussion. One occupational therapist trained two volunteers from the Alzheimer's Association to conduct this group.

The purposes of Group 2 (the caregiver and care recipient activity group) were the following:

1. To provide individualized activities to be engaged in by the caregiver and the family member

2. To role-model constructive interactions for the caregivers to apply with their care recipients

3. To practice individually selected activities for transfer to the home environment

4. To assist caregivers in practicing ways to change negative thoughts and behaviors to more positive ones to reduce disturbing behaviors and to increase the activity level of their relatives.

All activities, supervised by the occupational therapists and rehabilitation counselor, were simple, repetitive in nature, and had a predictable outcome.

Many activities resulted in a finished product, a tangible reward for completing the activity. Activities were designed to enable the leader to grade the instructions and the task for individuals functioning at different levels. The activities implemented were identified by the caregivers in the COPE Assessment Form or were adaptations of previously enjoyed activities discussed in the caregiver discussion group. The therapists analyzed the value component inherent in activities previously enjoyed by the care recipients in order to select and match a related valued activity with current functional ability. For example, one care recipient had enjoyed working as a teacher for many years. Having been generative with children made the activity of creating Halloween bags for homeless children a gratifying, valued experience for her. Teaching caregivers how to identify realistic, purposeful activities and to simplify them were major objectives of the learning process. Each family was provided a choice between two different activities to engage in weekly. The stations for the activities were in different parts of the house and each station had a leader to supervise the activity. One or two couples were assigned to each station according to their choice.

Results

According to the Activities Schedule and the Post-Group Interviews, five out of six care recipients' activity levels increased as a result of caregiver restructuring of the environment, grading activities, adapting verbal and gestural behaviors, and greater acceptance of the care recipient's condition. It was noted by some of the caregivers that when their relative's activity level improved, the emotional outlook of both improved. This was especially evident in Group 2, where the leaders observed their improved affect while engaged in an activity together. This is consistent with the work of Fidler and Fidler (1978), who stated that through achievement and feedback people acquire self-esteem, confidence, and merit.

Discussion

According to Doble (1991), the aim of therapy is to enable the caregiver to facilitate a family member's participation in meaningful activities. COPE assisted the caregivers by heightening their awareness of the care recipients' remaining strengths. Importantly, since dementia compromises the capacity to maintain participation in activities (Doble, 1991; Gordon et al., 1976; Levy, 1989), the group leaders designed and adapted individually tailored activities to increase the care recipient's activity level. Caregivers were able to carry over a number of these activities at home.

The positive finding that care recipients developed fewer disturbing behaviors is attributed to their caregivers' willingness to learn and apply recommendations. Gender may also have had an impact on the caregiver's coping ability, expectations, and sense of burden. This was evident when female caregivers said that they were not troubled by their husbands' behavior (e.g., losing objects, not helping with the housework), while the male caregivers stated that they were having a difficult time handling similar behaviors in their wives. One of the female caregivers explained the difference by stating that while the women had always managed the household, the men are experiencing a change in roles. The authors recognized that gender can cause dissonance with activity patterns when they are not consistent with lifelong values and roles. Role identity differences that affect caregivers' willingness and comfort in assuming responsibility for tasks that are unfamiliar to them should not be taken for granted but should be made explicit in the group. For example, the men tended to utilize a task-oriented method for caregiving. This approach can be facilitated and reinforced by teaching specific adapted strategies to different components of caregiving. Alternately, the women tended to use a parental approach, integrating new activities into their repertoire of existing tasks. While the nurturing aspects of this style can be beneficial, women might find themselves more quickly overextended and overwhelmed than men. Therefore, teaching recognition of boundaries and setting appropriate limits can be extremely helpful in promoting a daily routine, including respite time for the caregiver (Corcoran, 1992).

Occupational therapists treat caregivers and their relatives with dementia by teaching about the illness and instructing in "hands on" interventions, such as practicing activities of everyday living skills, modeling appropriate interactions to improve communication, and enabling caregivers and care recipients to work and play together. Caregivers and care recipients had an opportunity to learn by doing, which is consistent with the theoretical foundation of occupational therapy.

Summary

This pilot project for caregivers and their relatives with dementia was a nontraditional, community occupational therapy intervention, from the New York State Department of Health, made possible by a small grant to the Alzheimer's Association. As the elderly population increases there will be more people in need of services for dementia and related conditions. The researchers hope that this project will heighten awareness of the need for services for both caregivers and their relatives with dementia. Providing caregivers with options for practical experiences (COPE) may respond to a gap identified by these leaders and voiced by this population. Occupational therapists are in a unique position to empower caregivers to improve the quality of life for their family members.

Case Studies

CASE STUDY 1

The care recipient was a woman, 76 years old and diagnosed with Parkinson's disease with dementia. The caregiver, her husband, was 77 years of age.

Reasons for Referral

Although the caregiver did not specify one specific reason for attending the COPE group, he did list numerous difficulties he was experiencing in caring for his wife. He had responsibility for most of her activities of daily living and found it quite frustrating.

Moreover, he identified numerous concerns with his wife's behavior on the COPE Assessment Form:

1. Restlessness
2. Suspiciousness
3. Anxiety in the absence of the caregiver.

The caregiver also expressed concern with the symptoms that his wife had been exhibiting: poor appetite, sleeplessness, irritability, and diminished energy. In addition to the description of the care recipient's possible depression, the caregiver appeared depressed. Therefore, it appeared that both the caregiver and care recipient required further evaluation and intervention for depression.

Participation and Progress in the Group

Both the caregiver and the care recipient steadily attended and participated in the group. From the beginning, the caregiver appeared defeated and made many self-derogatory comments. He repeatedly said that he was the one to blame for their lack of involvement in activity, because he found himself short-tempered and impatient. He recognized the effect of his behavior on his wife, but found it difficult to change his behavior despite his desire to make a change. Importantly, the caregiver displayed excellent self-observation skills and insight into his feelings and behavior with his wife. He was encouraged by group leaders to "see" the positive aspects of his wife's performance in activities, as opposed to seeing only her liabilities. He required ongoing encouragement to do this in order to experience some of the benefits of activity participation. He also learned the importance of encouraging only those activities that his wife could clearly perform and of helping her with those she could not do safely. Altering expectations had been difficult for both of them. Although they experienced success with a number of activities (sports, cooking), they were both perfectionists. Therefore, the potential for enjoying the process appeared to lose out to the need for a perfect outcome. They had both acknowledged this and found it difficult to change. One explanation is certainly the impact of a depression on functional performance and activity interests. Both the caregiver and the care recipient accepted the recommendation of the occupational therapist to seek psychiatric interventions for depression. When treated, both found renewed energy and interest in changing the self-defeating inactivity cycle. Despite feeling depressed, both had a sense of humor that was worth noting. When stressed, they were able to respond to humor, serving as a source of strength. The caregiver had improved his ability to collaborate with his wife in an effort to engage in activities jointly. His ability to encourage her had improved and he was able to solve problems arising from the difficult aspects of a task so that he could help her appropriately when an activity was genuinely too difficult. He needed to see this as an area of improvement in order to interrupt the cycle of negative perceptions and subsequent inactivity.

Recommendations to the Caregiver for Aftercare

1. Continue to follow up with psychiatric interventions to ameliorate depressive symptoms.
2. Remember to look for positive aspects of the care recipient's performance and encourage her to engage only in tasks that are safe and appropriate for her functional level.
3. Try to engage in one activity per day together, to break the inactivity cycle.
4. Use a lot of positive reinforcement.
5. Activities: physical sports—beanbag toss, exercise tape, horseshoes, Velcro darts; baking or cooking—ready-made pie crusts and cookie dough, salads, stirring; simple, repetitive crafts—go to craft store for simple ideas.

When the COPE questionnaire was administered to the caregiver at the end of the group, he stated that the COPE group had increased his understanding of his wife's dementia, increased his tolerance, and helped him realize that he was "not alone." However, he admitted to still becoming frustrated and overreacting to behavior exhibited by his wife. He hoped this would change when his depression cleared and his abilities to use recommended strategies would improve.

CASE STUDY 2

The care recipient was a woman diagnosed with senile dementia of the Alzheimer's Type. She had been a school teacher for 40 years and had a master's degree in education. The caregiver was her husband. The ages of this couple were not disclosed.

Reasons for Referral

The caregiver stated that his main reason for attending the COPE group was to try to gain an "understanding" of his wife's illness and behaviors resulting from it. The caregiver reported the following concerns with his wife's behavior on the COPE Assessment Form:

1. Restlessness
2. Anxiety in the absence of the caregiver
3. Hiding or misplacing things
4. Suspiciousness
5. Not recognizing familiar people
6. Inability to concentrate on a task or activity
7. Reliving situations from the past
8. Unable to stay alone
9. Unable to follow simple written or verbal directions.

He commented that his wife needed help with dressing because she did not recognize her own clothes and took them off frequently. The caregiver was not only concerned about her behavior when she was left alone but also noted concerns of burden for himself. He noted feeling stressed and burdened by having to take care of his wife all the time, that this constant supervision did not allow him much privacy or time for himself. Relationships with other family members and friends were being compromised by the decreased amount of time available to spend with them. Despite his frustration, the caregiver did not indicate that he was feeling depressed.

Participation and Progress in the Group

Both the caregiver and care recipient consistently and actively participated in all aspects of the group program. During the caregiver group, the caregiver was initially quite verbal about his frustrations and did not believe that activities appropriate to his wife's functional level could be developed. The husband required encouragement from group leaders to "give it a chance" and was reassured throughout the group session that, if activities were presented at the right level, both he and his wife could experience success. The care recipient was very social during the group and was easy to engage in activities. She clearly enjoyed being with her husband and therefore was receptive to most activity suggestions he offered. The caregiver succeeded at simplifying tasks and learned how to identify and share the appropriate components of an activity with his wife. He also mastered the process of helping her to perform most of an activity, which he facilitated by setting up the task and completing it with finishing touches. By the end of the group, the caregiver was extremely supportive of the care recipient and was motivated to find activities that were mutually enjoyable. His optimism, willingness to try new things, and renewed interest in activities were wonderful strengths that he brought to the group and to his wife.

Recommendations to the Caregiver for Aftercare

1. Remember to set up simple 1–2 step activities and intervene only when the care recipient has difficulties. Provide her with repetitive, guided directions for each step and then let her try the task.

2. Remain involved in theatrical pursuits such as videos of shows and audio tapes of show tunes. Review local papers and *The New York Times* for announcements and consider subscribing to a local theater newsletter that covers all fine arts announcements.

3. Continue to engage in craft projects to be made for others (such as candy bags for children, wrapping paper, dough ornaments or magnets). Go to a craft store and ask for simple craft ideas. Remember, keep things simple!

4. Do simple, repetitive cooking tasks together. Some successful and enjoyable tasks might be making a pie with ready-made crusts and canned filling, making cookies from ready-made cookie dough (roll out and cut out shapes), stirring, and making salads.

5. Continue to exercise daily together, using the exercise tape and video made during the COPE group.

6. Dancing! Continue to dance together to your favorite music.

7. Find a day care center for your wife to go to in Florida while residing there for the winter.

In the post-group assessment, the caregiver reported that he enjoyed the COPE group and felt it taught him how to persevere with daily activities and helped him improve his patience. He particularly found the identification and modification of activities to be interesting and planned on using some of the suggestions. He stated that the COPE group helped him to "cope with the disease and realize that he was not alone in the world." He, like others, felt that the group should have been longer in length.

At the end of the 10-week program, leaders presented written recommendations and goals to each caregiver, individualized to meet each caregiver and care recipient's specific needs. The recommendations were written in layman's terms and in a nonthreatening manner. Caregivers gave feedback, presenting areas of agreement and disagreement. Practicality of goals was reviewed. Here are some of the recommendations of the group:

1. Post daily schedule on refrigerator.
2. Find a local group of children to make crafts for: candy bags, cookies, sachets, wrapping paper.
3. Walk on a daily basis.
4. Exercise together.
5. Include care recipients in daily outings to grocery store, running errands, etc.
6. Acknowledge verbal expression barriers; reinterpret and clarify, use gestures and touch, and respond to latent meaning of what is being communicated.
7. Help care recipients with hygiene by setting out exactly what is needed for showering, dental care, and so on, and keep extraneous items out of sight.
8. Continue to follow up with psychiatric interventions to ameliorate depressive symptoms.
9. Engage in one activity per day together to break the inactivity cycle.

Because the caregivers expressed such sadness about ending the group, a reunion session for the caregivers and the leaders only was planned to take place one month later.

Reunion Session

The reunion session, comprising only the caregivers and leaders of the group, revealed examples of problems that had changed since the Alzheimer's COPE group began. One caregiver had expressed frustration during the group sessions prior to the reunion that his wife's incontinence problem had been increasing to the point where he no longer wanted to leave the home with her. He stated that her anxiety and fear increased during outings and that he often needed to take her to the bathroom. At the reunion, he stated that he had tried all of the recommendations presented by the leaders and that they worked. One recommendation was to ask another woman to help his wife while she was in the bathroom. Another suggestion was to ask another woman to stand by the bathroom door to tell others entering the bathroom that a man was inside assisting his ill wife. The caregiver stated that he now felt more confident going places with his wife.

During the reunion, three caregivers stated that their spouses continually misplaced or lost things. One male caregiver in particular stated that he was having a difficult time handling this behavior because prior to her getting Alzheimer's disease his wife had been very neat and a fine housekeeper. Two female caregivers replied that they were not troubled by similar behavior in their husbands. One stated, and the two caregivers agreed, that a reason for the differences in outlook was that they had always cleaned up and put things away for their husbands and that now they were just doing more of it. Therefore, the differences between male and female caregiver reactions could be explained, in part, by societal role differences.

Three male caregivers during the original COPE sessions had expressed similarities in feeling public embarrassment when having to fill in for their spouse's word-finding difficulties and make excuses for their social behavior. During the reunion session, they all commented that they had become better able to cope with this problem and felt more comfortable in social situations. One reason the caregivers gave for their enhanced ability to cope was the networking achieved through the Alzheimer's COPE group, as many caregivers had exchanged numbers and spoke on the phone.

During the reunion, two male caregivers stated that they continued to have a problem telling their adult children that their mother's condition was progressing and that they sometimes had difficulty coping. They stated that discussing ways to tell their children and being able to express their concerns during the group made it somewhat easier to talk to their children honestly. A female caregiver expressed no difficulty in letting her children know everything, but found their support to be overprotective.

Increased activity between caregiver and care recipient and identification of care recipient strengths were also discussed. The caregivers stated that the COPE group introduced activities that they had never thought of and that performing activities within the group sessions acted as a catalyst in initiating their own ideas for activities at home. A caregiver, who was a daughter, commented that she was finally able to identify her mother's strengths by watching her participate in simple and repetitive activities during the sessions. She also commented that engaging in activities enabled her mother to maintain a sense of dignity.

During the reunion, three caregivers stated that the recommendations of the leaders for a psychiatric referral had helped them realize that they, too, had been affected by the difficulty of caring for someone with dementia. Before the Alzheimer's COPE group, one caregiver mentioned that he used to attach a stigma to individuals who were being treated for depression, but that now he had become more understanding. Through therapy, one of the caregivers was working on coming to terms with the reality of preparing for institutionalization for his wife, which was an immobilizing concept before receiving psychiatric help.

Another caregiver stated that before the Alzheimer's COPE group, she was in denial about her mother having Alzheimer's disease. She added that the Alzheimer's COPE group had increased her awareness and acceptance of the illness and helped her find ways to manage more easily.

References

Ansello, E., King, N. R., & Taler, G. (1986). The environmental press model: A theoretical framework for intervention in elder abuse. In K. Pillemar & R. S. Wolf (Eds.), *Elder abuse: Conflict in the family* (pp. 314–329). Dover, MA: Auburn House.

Bandura, A. (1977). Self-efficacy: Toward a unifying theory of behavioral change. *Psychological Review, 84*, 191–215.

Barris, R., Kielhofner, G. C. Levine, R. E., & Neville, A. (1985). In G. Kielhofner (Ed.), *A model of human occupation: Theory and application* (pp. 42–62). Baltimore, MD: Williams & Wilkins.

Baum, C. M. (1991). Addressing the needs of the cognitively impaired elderly from a family policy perspective. *American Journal of Occupational Therapy, 45*(7), 594–606.

Beck, A. T. (1967). *Depression—Clinical, experimental and theoretical aspects.* New York: Harper & Row Publisher.

Bergmann, K., Foster, E., & Justice, A. (1978). Management of the demented elderly patient in the community. *British Journal of Psychiatry, 132*, 441–449.

Berila, R. A. (1994). Dementia. In B. R. Bonder & M. B. Wagner (Eds.), *Functional performance in older adults* (pp. 240–255). Philadelphia: F. A. Davis.

Buckwalter, K. C., Abraham, I. L., & Neuendorfer, M. M. (1988). Alzheimer's disease: Involving nursing in the development and implementation of health care for patients and families. *Nursing Clinics of North America, 23*(1), 1–9.

Corcoran, M. A., & Gitlin, L. N. (1992). Dementia management: An occupational therapy home based inter-vention for caregivers. *American Journal of Occupational Therapy, 44*(9), 4801–4808.

Corcoran, M. A. (1992). Gender differences in dementia management plans of spousal caregivers: Implications for occupational therapy. *American Journal of Occupational Therapy, 46*(11), 1006–1012.

Cynkin, S. A., & Robinson, A. M. (1990). *Occupational therapy and activities health: Toward health through activities.* Boston: Little, Brown.

Doble, S. E. (1991). A home-based model of rehabilitation for individuals with SDAT and their caregivers. *Topics in Geriatric Rehabilitation, 7*(2), 33–44.

Fidler, G., & Fidler, J. (1978). Doing and becoming: purposeful action and self-actualization. *American Journal of Occupational Therapy, 32*, 305–310.

Florsheim, G. (1991). An expansion of the a-b-c approach to cognitive/behavioral therapy. *Clinical Gerontologist, 10*(4), 65–69.

Gessert, V. G. (1987). Living room: A support group for families with aging relatives. *Gerontology Special Interest Section Newsletter, 10*(4), 1–3.

Gordon, C., Gaitz, C. M., & Scott, J. (1976). Leisure and lives. In R. H. Binstock & E. Shanas (Eds.), *Handbook of aging and the social sciences.* New York: Van Nostrand Reinhold.

Hasselkus, B. R. (1988). Meaning in family caregiving: Perspectives on caregiver/professional relationships. *Gerontologist, 28*, 686–690.

Levy, L. L. (1989). Activity adaptation in rehabilitation of the physically and cognitively disabled aged. *Topics in Geriatric Rehabilitation, 4*(4), 53–56.

Matsutsuyu, J. (1969). The interest checklist. *American Journal of Occupational Therapy, 23,* 323.

Miller, P. A. (1993). Problem solving in long-term care: A systematic approach to promoting adaptive behavior. In J. Toner, L. Tepper, & B. Greenfield (Eds.), *Long-term care—Management, scope and practical issues* (pp. 107–122). Philadelphia: Charles Press.

Pepper Commission (U.S. Bipartisan Commission on Comprehensive Health Care). (1990). *A call for action* (pp. 101–114). Washington, DC: U.S. Government Printing Office.

Reisberg, B. (1986). Dementia: A systematic approach to identifying reversible causes. *Geriatrics, 41*(4), 30–46.

Yalom., I. D. (1985). *The theory and practice of group psychotherapy.* New York: Basic Books.

Yalom, I. D. (1995). *The theory and practice of group psychotherapy.* New York: Basic Books.

Section 4. Psychosocial and Psychological Components

Danielle N. Butin, MPH, OTR

Abstract

As the number of elderly individuals in the United States increases, a concurrent increase is expected in the prevalence of late-life psychiatric disorders. Occupational therapists have long played an important role in the field of psychiatry and their involvement in geriatric mental health treatment settings will continue to expand. This section introduces some of the psychiatric illnesses that affect older adults, with a special focus on the assessment and treatment of depression.

Major Psychiatric Conditions

DEPRESSION

Depression can be an extremely debilitating condition because of its dramatic impact on both functional and social activities. The Epidemiological Catchment Area Program (ECA), a well-known community-based study sponsored by the National Institute of Mental Health (NIMH), found that approximately 27% of all people over 60 years of age reported depressive symptoms (ranging from dysphoria to major depression) (Small, 1991). However, most older adults with a depressive disorder do not seek treatment (National Institute of Mental Health [NIMH], 1993), despite the fact that 80% of all people with a clinical depression can be treated successfully with medication and therapy (NIMH, 1995). This phenomenon in older adults might be attributed to the stigma associated with mental illness and the tendency of many older adults to be stoic and minimize emotional pain. This denial may, in part, contribute to the high rate of suicide in the elderly in the United States (Blazer, Bachar, & Hughes, 1987). There are numerous causes of depression in the elderly, including genetic predisposition; poor self-esteem leading to increased vulnerability; chronic illness; changed life patterns; or a combination of genetic, psychological, and environmental factors (NIMH, 1993).

ANXIETY

Pure anxiety disorders are seen less frequently in older adults, compared with a younger adult population. However, in an elderly population, anxiety seen with medical or psychiatric conditions can contribute significantly to a person's diminished ability to function. (Smith, Sherrill, & Colenda, 1995). A challenge for health professionals may be the identification of anxiety disorders in older adults based on patterns of service utilization. For example, one study (Katerndahl & Realini, 1995) found that older adults who frequent the emergency room regularly may have an underlying anxiety disorder. Unfortunately, most of these individuals do not seek out psychiatric care. Katerndahl & Realini (1995) found that 35% of people with panic disorders sought care in their family physician's office, followed by visits to the emergency room. People with anxiety disorders need access to psychiatric care in order to secure the best treatment and resources possible. Relaxation training and nonpharmacological agents have provided success with the adult population (Smith et al., 1995) and may have continued utility with an older adult population. One self-help book yielding excellent results for older adults with anxiety disorders is Hope and Help for your Nerves (Weekes, 1990). It provides a straightforward and informative approach, and most older adults can read and benefit from this resource with minimal effort.

SCHIZOPHRENIA

Older adults with schizophrenia continue to experience psychotic and nonpsychotic symptoms. In a study that assessed age-related differences between people who were older and younger with schizophrenia (Davidson et al., 1995), the positive symptoms (e.g., delusions, hallucinations) were moderately less severe for older patients, but the negative symptoms (e.g., apathy, poor ADL skills) and cognitive impairments were more severe than those of younger patients. This creates an interesting framework for treatment in occupational therapy with this population.

CRITERIA FOR DEPRESSION AND DYSTHYMIA

Many older adults with major depression or dysthymia are not properly identified or treated, because the DSM-IV criteria may not be sensitive enough to recognize depression in the elderly (Hendrie & Crossett, 1990).

While a number of symptoms in depression and dysthymia may be similar, the latter involves longer term symptoms that are generally not as disabling as those observed in major depression. However, people with dysthymia can also experience a superimposed major depression (NIMH, 1993). The specific characteristics and differences of these disorders can be seen in figure 12–1. Five basic symptoms of depression are often missed, because they are misinterpreted as signs of physical illness. These symptoms

include appetite loss, insomnia or hypersomnia, psychomotor agitation or retardation, and fatigue or complaints of loss of energy. If patients are not asked about other target symptoms of depression the disease is often unrecognized. These symptoms include irritability, sad mood, loss of interest in favorite activities, anhedonia (inability to experience pleasure), preoccupation with guilt, feelings of worthlessness, inability to concentrate or make decisions, and recurring thoughts of suicide and death (Coleman, 1995). These symptoms are also seen in dysphoria, described as a state of unpleasant mood. Here, the pervasive symptoms include somatic complaints, feelings of failure, loneliness, nighttime wakefulness with brooding thoughts and worrying. Excessive worrying is one of the strongest indicators for dysphoria (Gurland & Toner, 1983). Although not classified as a separate condition in DSM-IV (American Psychiatric Association, 1994), dysphoria is commonly treated in the elderly and many geriatric psychiatrists find this condition worth treating with medication or therapy.

COMORBIDITY OF DEPRESSION AND PHYSICAL ILLNESS

Some medical conditions, for example, coronary artery disease, neurological disorders, metabolic disorders, and cancer have been associated with depression (Sunderland, Lawlor, Molchan, & Martinez, 1988). Depression can be seen as the primary presenting symptom in some conditions (for example, hypothyroidism), and depression has been observed in up to 50% of people after a cerebral vascular accident (CVA) (Popkin & MacKenzie, 1980; Robinson, Starr, Kubos, & Price, 1983). Approximately one-third of medically ill adults have been found to have depressive symptoms and up to one-quarter of those assessed met the criteria for a major depression

Figure 12–1. DSM–IV Criteria

Major Depressive Illness		Dysthymic Disorder	
Symptoms*	Period of Time	Symptoms*	Period of Time
Depressed mood, sad, blue, down in the dumps	Every day for 2 weeks	Depressed mood for most of the day, for more days than not, as indicated by subjective report or objective observations	Depressed mood occurs during most of the day for more days than not for at least 2 years.

Major Depressive Illness (continued)

OR

Loss of interest or pleasure in all or almost all things the person usually does

AND

4 of the following:

- Poor appetite or increased appetite (weight loss or gain of at least 5% body weight in a month)
- Sleeping difficulty (too much or too little)
- Loss of energy, fatigue, tiredness
- Poor concentration, difficulty making decisions nearly every day
- Feelings of worthlessness or excessive or inappropriate guilt (which may be delusional) nearly every day
- Restlessness (mental or physical) or clearcut slowing down physically
- Recurrent thoughts of death, recurrent suicidal ideation without a specific plan, or a suicide attempt or specific plan

Dysthymic Disorder (continued)

AND

2 (or more) of the following present while depressed:

- Poor appetite or overeating
- Sleeping difficulty—too much or too little
- Loss of energy, fatigue, tiredness
- Poor concentration, difficulty making decisions
- Low self-esteem
- Feelings of hopelessness

Period of Time (Dysthymic): Any symptom-free intervals last no longer than 2 months.

Initial 2-year period must be free of major depressive episodes.

*Symptoms cannot meet criteria for a mixed episode. These symptoms must cause clinically significant distress or impairment in social, occupational, or other important areas of functioning. The symptoms cannot be due to direct physiological effects of a substance (e.g., drug of abuse, medication) or a general medical condition (e.g., hypothyroidism). The symptoms will not be better accounted for by bereavement (i.e., after the loss of a loved one). The symptoms persist for longer than 2 months or are characterized by marked functional impairment, morbid preoccupation with worthlessness, suicidal ideation, psychotic symptoms, or psychomotor retardation.

*Cannot be diagnosed if a person has had a manic or hypomanic episode. Symptoms cannot be due to direct physiological effects of a substance (e.g., drug of abuse, medication) or a general medical condition (e.g., hypothyroidism).

Differences in diagnosis are made by examining factors of onset, duration, persistence, and severity.

Source: Adapted from American Psychiatric Association, DSM–IV, 1994.

(Clark, Cavanaugh, & Gibbons, 1983; Nielsen & Williams, 1980).

Case study 1 illustrates the clinical challenge of comorbidity. The symptoms of depression in an individual who is medically ill must be separated and recognized, and then the challenge of making a functional diagnosis must be faced.

It is the clinician's responsibility to understand and recognize these complex presentations of depression and to become comfortable with making appropriate referrals when indicated. Mr. L's physician and home health care team missed his symptoms of depression. Unfortunately, such symptoms are commonly overlooked by health care practitioners. The occupational therapist's potential contribution to the treatment team is unique because occupational therapy can assess and recognize the impact of mood on function. By increasing the ability to recognize this syndrome, occupational therapists can have a dramatic impact on quality of life.

Clinical Presentations of Depression in the Elderly

The functional presentation of depressive disorders (major depression, dysthymia, dysphoria) can vary considerably.

SOMATIZATION

First, many older adults somaticize, possibly because physical pain may be more tolerable and socially acceptable than psychic pain or mental illness. Among others, the somatic symptoms may include diminished energy, sleep problems, and constipation (Gurland & Toner, 1983). Ultimately, depressed feelings can lead to physiological changes and can suppress one's immune system.

DEPRESSIVE PSEUDODEMENTIA

Depressive pseudodementia is a syndrome that resembles dementia but is actually secondary to depression. Here, the individual appears confused and, unfortunately, can be mistakenly diagnosed with dementia. Like patients with actual dementia (e.g., Alzheimer's disease or vascular dementia), patients with depressive pseudodementia may be unable to follow directions and may experience short-term memory deficits. However, unlike those with organic dementia, they may be more apt to complain of memory loss and difficulty with thinking. Usually people with dementia do not complain about cognitive changes but try instead to minimize or hide deficits (Gurland & Toner, 1983). Importantly, the cognitive deficits of pseudodementia are temporary and associated with the depression. Once the depression clears, the person is able to return to normal cognitive functioning.

Gurland and Toner (1983) described the tragic situation where the individual with a depressive pseudodementia was misdiagnosed as organically impaired. Instead, the patient was experiencing a state of diminished concentration, distractibility, and increased anxiety, often with an awareness of decline in function. Given the grave potential for misdiagnosis (especially with nursing-home residents), OTs need to become familiar with the symptoms of pseudodementia so that this syndrome is recognized and appropriate referrals can be made.

PERSONALITY DISORDERS

Long-standing personality disorders also put older adults at risk for depression (Abrams, Alexopoulus, & Young, 1987). Older adults who lack lifelong coping skills are at an increased risk for the development of depression in late life. Depressed older adults with personality disorders often challenge a therapist's clinical skills, making increased demands for time and attention at this time of crisis. While staff may tend to avoid these patients, that might only intensify the individual's rage and dependency. The personality traits tend to become magnified during a depression. Therefore, it is important to acknowledge some of the behaviors and to formulate initial strategies for creating a therapeutic alliance. Groves (1978) described and categorized three commonly seen personality disorders. Interestingly, Groves suggested methods for intervening that may seem contrary to those usually practiced by therapists.

Patients with dependent personality disorder (or the "dependent clinger") (Groves, 1978) may realize for the first time that all attempts to secure emotional stability have failed, and they can become very frightened, regressed, and ultimately depressed. Their apparent symptoms can be a way of calling out for help (e.g., they can become manipulative and extremely needy). Interestingly, most therapists respond negatively to this type of behavior. When dependency needs increase, therapists may tend to set limits and pull away from the patient. That strategy further fuels the dependency needs, especially during a depressive episode. Instead, perhaps the dependency should be allowed as a transitional experience towards recovery. With guidance, these individuals could learn how to use the dependency as a source of support during a period of change. Here, fears can be expressed and strategies for increasing self-reliance can be introduced, while the person clearly has the support of the occupational therapist.

The "entitled demanders" (Groves, 1978) are the older narcissistic patients, who do not age well without supports.

They tend to be very hostile in treatment, accuse staff of not taking their needs into consideration, and devalue all suggestions. They may also use guilt as a means of threatening or intimidating the therapist. With this group of depressed older adults, the therapeutic relationship should begin with the validation of the patient's past and present strengths before confronting the oppositional behaviors. Usually the depressed older adult is well aware of his or her deficits and failing support system, but the exploration and, importantly, the validation of strengths can be an excellent aid in forming a therapeutic alliance.

The "manipulative help rejecters" (Groves, 1978) need constant emotional supplies in order to sustain involvement in activities. Their pessimism and tenaciousness tends to intensify as the therapist's efforts and enthusiasm increases. They, in fact, do not seek true symptom relief but rather an inexhaustible relationship with a constantly providing caregiver. With this group, extreme sensitivity to the effects of retreating and setting limits is necessary. Commonly, therapists will say, "I have offered you many options and you don't seem ready to act on any of them. When you're ready to discuss these options, please come and find me." Instead, patients should be helped to recognize and identify ways to form long-lasting relationships that can provide support through change. Symptoms seen in the help rejecters tend to continue as long as the symptoms provide the means for ongoing support.

The collection of symptoms mentioned above can be seen in all settings where therapists work with depressed older adults. It is important to be aware of the suggested strategies presented as methods of establishing a therapeutic alliance. It is never too late to develop a new repertoire of coping skills, motivated by a desire for improved relationships and relief from depression.

ASSESSMENTS

It is important for occupational therapists to become familiar with a variety of assessment tools available for measuring depression. By using standardized and validated measures, credible and relevant findings can be established. Four assessment tools, effective for identifying depression in the elderly, are discussed below. These tools are not specific to occupational therapy, but they are highly reliable resources for the recognition of depressive syndromes and can provide the groundwork for sharing findings with other members of the health care team. Additionally, the impact of affect on function can be more readily understood. All tools can be rater or self-administered, with the exception of the SHORT-CARE (Gurland, Golden, Teresi, & Challop, 1984).

The Geriatric Depression Scale (GDS) provides the rater with a reliable and valid measure of depression with 30 Yes or No questions (Yesavage, 1986; Yesavage & Brink, 1983). If a person's response matches the yes or no that corresponds to each item, it is considered a significant finding. This tool also asks questions that are sensitive to the somatic presentation of depression as seen with the elderly (Gallo, Reichel, & Anderson, 1988) (see figure 12–2).

The Beck Depression Inventory (BDI) lists 21 characteristics of depression and asks the individual to choose the best response that most accurately reflects feelings and state of health within the past week (Gallagher, 1986). Here again, the higher score is indicative of a depression. This tool is also

well validated and, like the GDS, is sensitive to the psychosomatic presentation of depression (Gallo et al., 1988).

The SHORT-CARE (Gurland et al., 1984), a multidimensional assessment for use with elderly, is a 45-minute interview assessing depression, dementia, and functional disability. The validity and reliability of this tool are well-established, and it focuses on six areas: subjective memory impairment, sleep disorders, activity limitations, somatic symptoms, dementia, and depression (Gurland & Wilder, 1984). This tool, available through Columbia University, requires training, to assure for inter-rater reliability, and provides tremendous versatility as a screening mechanism in many treatment settings.

If an occupational therapist suspects depression as the underlying reason for unmotivated behavior in any treatment setting, then a well-validated tool could provide support to clinical observations. Case study 2 illustrates the value of using standardized assessments for this purpose.

While the prospect of asking personal and often painful questions of patients may feel uncomfortable, therapists should not shy away from probing and exploring emotional responses. It is often the only opportunity people have to explore and recognize feelings. In addition, it provides an invaluable opportunity to begin the treatment planning process with the depressed older adult's needs in mind.

Treatment Planning and Individual Work

One of the first steps of the treatment planning process is to help the depressed individual to examine the relationship between feelings, perceptions, and their current activities health (Cynkin & Robinson, 1990). Activities health is manifested in the

Figure 12–2. Geriatric Depression Scale

Please answer the following questions.

1. Are you basically satisfied with your life? (N)
2. Have you dropped many of your activities and interests? (Y)
3. Do you feel that your life is empty? (Y)
4. Do you often get bored? (Y)
5. Are you hopeful about the future? (Y)
6. Are you bothered by thoughts that you just cannot get out of your head? (Y)
7. Are you in good spirits most of the time? (Y)
8. Are you afraid that something bad is going to happen to you? (Y)
9. Do you feel happy most of the time? (Y)
10. Do you often feel helpless? (Y)
11. Do you often get restless and fidgety? (Y)
12. Do you prefer to stay in your room rather than go out and do new things? (Y)
13. Do you frequently worry about the future? (Y)
14. Do you feel that you have more problems with memory than most? (Y)
15. Do you think it is wonderful to be alive now? (N)
16. Do you often feel downhearted and blue? (Y)
17. Do you feel pretty worthless the way you are now? (Y)
18. Do you worry a lot about the past? (Y)
19. Do you find life very exciting? (N)
20. Is it hard for you to get started on new projects? (Y)
21. Do you feel full of energy? (N)
22. Do you feel that your situation is hopeless? (Y)
23. Do you think that most people are better off than you? (Y)
24. Do you frequently get upset over little things? (Y)
25. Do you frequently feel like crying? (Y)
26. Do you have trouble concentrating? (Y)
27. Do you enjoy getting up in the morning? (N)
28. Do you prefer to avoid social gatherings? (Y)
29. Is it easy for you to make decisions? (N)
30. Is your mind as clear as it used to be? (N)

ability of the individual to participate in socioculturally delineated and directed activities with satisfaction. An activity that has no meaning to the individual lacks therapeutic value. Activities define not only human existence, but also the means and ends for the development or restoration of function. With this framework, the individual can examine and compare past and present activity patterns and identify the qualities that are most important in determining how one spends time. Asking depressed older adults to complete and critique their activities health assessment (similar to a time configuration) is guided by the following questions:

1. What do you find most striking about your activities health assessment?

2. According to your observations, how would you say your current health impacts on the way you spend your time?

3. What are the major differences that you notice with this configuration compared with the way you would like to spend your time?

4. What do you enjoy in this configuration?

5. What do you do because you feel you must do it?

6. What would you like to change?

This assessment helps to begin the problem-solving process by identifying the ways that the depression has impacted on daily involvement in activities. It also helps to define the goals of treatment and the means for attaining those goals.

Next, a frame of reference is employed to guide intervention and counseling strategies. There are a number of frames of reference available, such as psychodynamic and life review (Miller, 1987). However, one of the most useful techniques for working with the depressed elderly is the cognitive therapy framework. Cognitive therapy (Beck, 1963, 1967; Beck, Rush, Shaw, & Emery, 1979) serves as a natural link to occupational therapy practice, because its basic assumption is that one's thoughts influence behavior. In this model, actions are based on thoughts and perceptions. According to cognitive therapy principles, a "triad" is activated when an individual becomes depressed. For example, an older woman who has suffered a stroke may say, "I'm no good because I can't move my arm any longer." She then sees that there is little activity in her environment that she can perform and says, "I can't do anything around here." That belief then generalizes, offering little hope, and she says, "The future is hopeless; I'll never get better." Once depressed older adults activate this process, it is vitally important to understand the internal sentences that they are telling themselves, since this can influence all behavior.

By knowing how or what someone thinks, their motivation to perform an activity can often be predicted. For example, in geriatric psychiatry units, when staff come into the patients' rooms, they may say, "Come on, everyone out of bed ... time for groups!" While the patients may in fact attend the groups, little was done to help them understand how their negative thoughts affected functional outcomes. With the cognitive therapy strategy, one might say, "What are you thinking when I encourage you to get out of bed? What are you thinking to yourself?" The depressed individual needs help to understand how his or her belief system interacts with and influences the ability to function.

Using this model, the person can begin to learn about the relationship of depression to symptoms. Significantly, therapists must begin by discussing the inactivity cycle. This can be summarized as follows: "The less you do, the less you feel like doing, until you're doing little that you feel good about. This cycle can lead to depression." By stating, "Let's break this inactivity cycle together," a therapeutic alliance or partnership may be formed. It is important that the treatment process begins by a person's engaging in activities that are within his or her abilities. Depressed older adults need therapists to analyze and break down tasks into manageable steps so that they can experience a positive reward for involvement in activities. If the individual refuses, then it is critically important to have him or her explain the reason for refusing. For example, the therapist can say, "I understand that you don't want to take a walk today, but I would like to understand what you are thinking. It would help if you could share your thoughts with me. What are your concerns about taking a walk?" By listening carefully to the responses, a plan can be created in response to these specific concerns. In addition, a positive outcome may be quite powerful, offering a dramatic contrast to the original negative expectations. By engaging in a simple activity with a high probability of a successful outcome, the therapist has the opportunity to show the person how the result contradicted his or her initial expectation. This is how it is possible to begin to shift mind-sets and alter perceptions of what is and is not possible. (See case studies 3 through 6.)

This framework, supported by the Activities Health Assessment process, can provide a well-blended and solid framework for meeting the individualized functional needs of the depressed older adult.

Treatment Planning and Group Work

Through a partnership with the patient, occupational therapists create a safe place to practice the skills necessary for recovery. Groups can provide a powerful mechanism for discovering the universality and commonality of needs among older adults with depression. In group programming, therapists need to continually analyze the individual's goals and to understand how the activity will foster the skills needed to accomplish these goals (see case study 7). Generally, all groups can be classified into areas of occupational performance: self-management, leisure,

work, and family. The activity group interventions, described below, were carried out in two settings. The inpatient groups were developed in collaboration with Colleen Heaney at the New York Hospital, Cornell Medical Center, Westchester Division, Geriatric Psychiatry Division, in White Plains, New York, and the Community Treatment Programs were implemented at the Saint Joseph's Geriatric Day Care Program in Yonkers, New York. Models for group work in each area of occupational performance, for both inpatient and community settings, will be described.

SELF-MANAGEMENT

The continuum of disability varies greatly in self-management. For example, a depressed woman may barely be able to manage personal hygiene or may minimally interact with others, while another older adult may struggle with setting limits on an entitled adult child who insists that the grandparent babysit constantly. The complexity of this area of functioning is obvious, and, therefore, programming can be a challenge (figure 12–3).

LEISURE

The ability to enjoy leisure is a hallmark of healthy functioning. Leisure serves the purpose of aiding reentry into functioning and helps individuals to sustain skills needed for community involvement. Careful programming involves flexibility of staff. For example, some facilities create specific groups in response to the emerging needs of the patients. If a patient with specific talents or interests is hospitalized, then a group can be created that will validate that person's skills through a coleadership experience. For example, when a playwright was hospitalized for

Figure 12–3. Self-Management—Inpatient and Community Treatment

INPATIENT TREATMENT

Delectable Dining: Combats the "regressive" pull of hospitalization, by providing individuals with an opportunity to choose their own dinner (in the staff cafeteria), to assert themselves by asking questions, and to eat with peers.

Intergenerational Cooking: Offers depressed older adults and hospitalized adolescents an opportunity to practice and transfer the interpersonal skills necessary for relationships with family members at home.

Budget and Resources: Provides information on community resources and provides opportunities to practice the higher level skills needed for community reentry (budgeting).

COMMUNITY TREATMENT

Communication: A group targeting older women who consistently alienate themselves (secondary to severe character disturbances). Members of this group need to develop alternative methods of expressing their needs to others and are encouraged to practice these techniques in ongoing interactions with family members and home health aides.

Choices: A group for elderly alcoholics to provide them with an opportunity to explore history of abuse, barriers to sobriety, and activity patterns associated with drinking. (This group was funded through a grant from the Westchester Community Foundation of New York.)

Fit and Fabulous: Grooming, choosing and buying clothing, and establishing an exercise routine are the focus of this intervention program.

---

depression, a play-reading group was created as a means for this man to continue to practice lifelong skills. When these groups are kept flexible, individuals are allowed to validate skills through a co-leadership experience (figure 12–4).

WORK

Work involves paid employment and meaningful volunteer job placements. Here, it is unclear whether the problem begins with a poor match between the person's interests and job chosen, or interpersonal problems exacerbate problems at the employment site. Most impotant, depressed older adults need help in identifying the most appropriate volunteer or paid work opportunities, but they also need help in practicing the skills needed for job retention. This should be a major focus of treatment (figure 12–5).

FAMILY

Finally, practicing the behaviors needed for the maintenance of family roles is an essential component of reentry to family life. Occupational therapists must look at the skills needed for resuming one's role in the family. Programming should reflect these needs as well (figure 12–6).

Summary

In conclusion, occupational therapists can provide an important role in the assessment and treatment of mental

Figure 12–4. Leisure

Inpatient and Community Treatment

INPATIENT TREATMENT

Fitness Walk: Provides opportunity for early morning outdoor walks. Improves the use of exercise as a scheduled part of one's day.

Games: Provides opportunities to practice the skills expected and needed for adapting to senior center activities. Participants are assisted in seeking out peers for activity involvement.

Consumer Determined Leisure Groups: Types and availability of groups can be influenced by the hospitalized population. For example, when a playwright was hospitalized for depression a play-reading group was developed and he assumed coleadership responsibilities.

Leisure Planning: Provides opportunity to explore and identify leisure interests and find resources in the community. Participants contact these resources and plan involvement for increased activity pursuits upon discharge. In addition, participants practice making and carrying out plans for one new activity per week in the community. (Also can be modeled in community settings; here learning ways to access public and specialized transportation services is essential.)

COMMUNITY TREATMENT

T'ai Chi: Provides opportunity for meditative form of exercise. Participants practice relaxation and visualization through an imagery guided exercise experience.

Heart Smart Bakers: Provides opportunity to use lifelong cooking interests to prepare low-fat loaves of sweet breads at bake sales. Combines socialization and cooking interests into an activity intervention.

"Golden Gourmet" Column: An agreement was created with a local newspaper to print a monthly "Golden Gourmet" column for depressed older adults in need of validation of lifelong roles and interests. Participants supply the newspaper with a "family recipe" and a reminiscent story about the significance of the recipe to the individual. Being printed in a newspaper serves as a major force in providing validation and reinforcement of skills.

Remember When ...: Provides opportunity to use life-review techniques and reminiscence to talk about specific life stages and reflect on past strengths and coping styles.

health problems in the elderly. As experts in the evaluation of functional skills, occupational therapists are in a unique position to address the impact of mental illness on everyday activities. When psychiatric symptoms are identified in patients, therapists, as advocates for good care, are in a position to alert physicians and other health providers, so that proper treament can be instituted. Most important, occupational therapists can play an invaluable role in helping to rehabilitate and restore function and quality of life to older individuals with mental health problems.

Figure 12–5. Work

Inpatient and Community Treatment

INPATIENT TREATMENT

Work Choices: Provides opportunity to reflect on interests and past work-related experiences. Members explore options available in the community, and vocational testing is involved.

Video Group: Simulated volunteer or paid employment interviews are videotaped. Group members and leader provide feedback and suggestions.

Boutique: Group members participate in one of three designated production areas (design of products, production, or marketing). All products created in group are sold at a special boutique in the hospital.

Liturgy in Action: Members volunteer at a large community church in a variety of ways (thrift shop, free book store, or serving meals to the homeless).

Volunteer Jobs: Volunteer jobs in the hospital must be tailored to meet the individual's needs. Many older adults volunteer in the gift shop, when, in fact, they have skills in many other areas. We must advocate for creative volunteer job opportunities! Examples include: administrative assistant hospitalized for depression volunteered in the research library at the hospital. A director of maintenance for a college campus was hospitalized and began a volunteer job in the maintenance department of the hospital to assess skills needed for returning to work.

COMMUNITY TREATMENT

Workshop: Contacts were made with local organizations and vendors in order for patients to assist with mailings, sorting of items, and collating materials. This group provides members with meaningful work experience and, in return, most organizations make a donation (used for special outings) or they provide patients with special refreshments.

Bridal Boutique: Members produce bridal sachets filled with birdseed for bridal processions. People from the community purchase these sachets. *Every* program should have a valued item produced by members and recognized by the community.

Volunteer Jobs: Volunteer jobs have been created and adapted for the frail, depressed old adult. Supervising the magazine and book cart at the hospital and delivering supplies to all waiting areas has been a very successful volunteer job.

Intergenerational Program: Readers Digest Foundation funded this intergenerational program. The members were trained in child development and play therapy. They purchased toys and books for this activity program. The program involves three specified activity models:

1. **Grandparent Story Hour**—Older adult chooses and reads books to pre-schoolers at the local library. Prior to the reading, the older adult practices reading and receives feedback from peers.

2. **Adopt-a-Tot**—Older adults plan a one-hour activity group of gross motor activities, crafts and finger plays with three- and four-year-olds at a local daycare center.

3. **Heal-the-Children:**—Older adults attend the Family Health Clinic (upstairs from the Day Program) in order to play with children in the waiting room.

The intergenerational programs allow the older adults to practice and model communicating with young children in order to improve their relationships with their grandchildren.

Figure 12–6. Family

Inpatient and Community Treatment

Family Activity Groups: Parent-adult child or spouse-spouse activity programs provide a valuable opportunity to practice communicating skills. This group also assists families in reengaging in meaningful activities.

Special Events: Families should be included in all special events. They should have opportunities to share positive and empowering experiences with their loved one.

Case Studies

CASE STUDY 1

Mr. L, an 83-year-old married man, was a prominent and well-respected leader in the entertainment field. He was being evaluated at a major teaching hospital for an undiagnosed hematological disorder. The anemia caused by this disorder typically causes symptoms of weakness and fatigue. His family, extremely supportive and worried about his health, were extremely well informed health care consumers. They asked for an occupational therapy evaluation as a means of developing a plan to promote his strength, energy, and endurance for renewed involvement in all of his functional activities. Upon initial evaluation, Mr. L proudly showed the therapist his strength and range of motion (both were within functional limits). However, upon closer examination, his affect and interest in activities were far below the premorbid level of functioning reported by his family. His family described him as a gregarious and extremely generous man who enjoyed supporting artists by collecting and displaying their work. Despite a lifetime commitment to supporting the arts, he currently had no interest in his sculpture garden. He also resisted all social activities. Significantly, his personality and affect had changed. When questioned about whether or not he experienced some of the vegetative signs of depression, he admitted that his appetite and sleep had changed. Following this assessment, the occupational therapist arrived at a functional diagnosis of depression. He exhibited both vegetative (e.g., sleep and appetite changes, concentration deficits) and functional (e.g., decreased interest and activity) signs of depression. When the therapist called his internist to discuss the need for further evaluation and possible consideration of antidepressant medication, the physician's response was, "If you were his age and physically sick, wouldn't you be depressed?" The therapist answered, "Depression is not a natural, automatic accompaniment of old age or sickness. Perhaps I should refer the patient to someone who will evaluate him further?" The physician agreed to formally evaluate him for depression. Mr. L was started on fluoxetine, an antidepressant, and slowly began to revisit his sculpture garden, reengage in meaningful social and philanthropic activities, and enjoyed being with family and friends. Thus, though he had physical reasons for weakness and fatigue (anemia), clearly his depression also strongly contributed to his diminished energy and interest in meaningful activities.

CASE STUDY 2

A 55-year-old woman who had suffered a CVA was inconsistently attending her outpatient occupational and physical therapy sessions. She rarely followed up on recommendations, and she appeared so poorly motivated that the rehabilitation department considered discharging her from treatment. The therapist decided to assess the patient with the Beck Depression Inventory, because she suspected a depressive etiology. The patient scored significantly for depression, and the occupational therapist shared the findings with the patient's neurologist. The physician then referred the patient for psychiatric follow-up and treatment. After a few weeks of medication and therapy, the patient expressed great relief with the fact that there had been a "real" and "diagnosed" reason for her apathy. She was encouraged by her renewed investment and motivation in her rehabilitation plan.

CASE STUDY 3—COGNITIVE THERAPY

Mrs. C is an 82-year-old woman with depression and severe arthritis. When encouraged to help bake cookies for children, she refused, claiming to be in too much pain. The therapist acknowledged how much pain she must be in and discussed how refusing offers her no opportunity to focus on something pleasurable, and that, instead, she is choosing to watch and guard her pain. The therapist, once again, encouraged the patient to join the baking activity. When she refused, she was asked to share her reasons. The patient replied, "It's too hard for me to walk to the kitchen; my legs are killing me." The therapist then said, "Well, let's try something else, because we would really like to have you in the group. Why don't we bring some of the supplies to you, and let's see how you feel while joining us baking for the kids." While preparing the cookies, she reminisced with other group members, and at the end of the group she said, "I'm okay. This was nice." Using the cognitive therapy framework, she was asked to compare the outcome of this activity with what she originally expected or feared (pain). She hesitantly replied, "I enjoyed this. I guess I can do more than I think ... sometimes." The next time she refused involvement in activities, she was reminded of this positive experience and how the outcome had differed from what she had expected. In future activities, she was less resistant to options offered and began to take the initiative in some functional tasks.

CASE STUDY 4—COGNITIVE THERAPY

Mr. J is a 76-year-old man with depression, who suffered a subdural hematoma following a fall. He was left with significant physical findings and had become increasingly frustrated by all activities of daily living. He experienced everything as a failure, and he could not identify any positive aspects of his current functional performance. The occupational therapist encouraged him to list ten positive aspects of his functional performance at the end of each day. At first, he complained about the assignment, but he quickly became increasingly more observant and was able to identify and recognize positive outcomes as they occurred. For example, the occupational therapist recognized that his perception had changed when, during a dressing activity, he said, "Look at that; I just did those buttons completely by myself."

CASE STUDY 5—COGNITIVE THERAPY

Ms. R is a 67-year-old recently widowed woman with an agitated depression. She was hospitalized shortly after her husband's death and complained of increased anxiety during hours spent alone at home. When she was further questioned about her time spent at home, she identified the dinner hour as most anxiety-provoking for her. Eating alone was an activity that she felt she could not tolerate. Using cognitive therapy, the occupational therapist analyzed and broke down the activity of eating alone into incremental, manageable steps. At first, she drank a cup of coffee for 5 minutes, while sitting alone in the cafeteria. She then left the cafeteria and discussed the outcome with her therapist. Gradually, the patient was able to increase the amount of time spent dining alone. By discharge, she was able to eat alone for 30 minutes without significant signs of anxiety. This intervention involved a blending of cognitive therapy and behavioral or systematic desensitization concepts.

CASE STUDY 6—COGNITIVE THERAPY

A 62-year-old woman, who had worked as a schoolteacher, was hospitalized for depression. One weekend, she was encouraged to keep a journal of her thoughts and perceptions. This was intended to heighten her awareness of her negative thought patterns and how they impact on motivation and function. The occupational therapist divided the page into two columns, the Negative Thought and the Positive Thought. Every time she had a negative thought, she was encouraged to note it and then identify the alternative, or positive, perspective. For example, in the Negative Thought column, she listed, "My niece is visiting me only because she pities me and thinks I'm old and lonely." The positive column read, "We have been close for many years and she cares about me." By the end of the weekend, she was able to recognize the shift in her thoughts and was encouraged by her ability to recognize a positive perspective.

CASE STUDY 7—TREATMENT PLANNING WITH A DEPRESSED OLDER ADULT

Mrs. N is a 67-year-old woman who suffered a left hemisphere CVA 8 years ago. Her husband of 40 years died 10 years ago. They had no children, but Mrs. N has an extremely supportive family of sisters, nieces, and nephews living close by. Since her CVA, she has had trouble ambulating (she uses a quad cane) and has experienced residual weakness in her right arm. Although she has full active range of motion in her right upper and lower extremity, she is concerned about the impact of weakness on gait and complains of intermittent dizziness. She is left dominant. She lives alone in a two-bedroom apartment and had worked as an artist for most of her adult life. She prefers to paint on masonite and primarily paints scenery from photographs.

Five years ago, she began attending an adult day-care program to improve her overall functional status and to ameliorate depressive symptoms. Since the stroke, she has not responded favorably to numerous trials of antidepressant medications. Upon initial evaluation at the program, she complained of losing interest in the activities she had once enjoyed and only wanted to discuss how sick she felt. After completing the Activities Health Assessment, she observed that her day was empty and void of anything that makes her feel good. When asked, "What do you feel is missing? If you had the energy, what activities would you like to see in this schedule?" she replied, "My art. But, I don't have the energy for this. I can't do it. I don't have my apartment set up for this."

Clearly, it had been a long time since she had painted, and this activity needed to be slowly reintroduced. By breaking down the task into manageable steps, Mrs. N could have a positive experience that would contrast with her current negative expectations. Importantly, she needed to adjust her expectations, in order to see any movement towards painting as positive. To begin, she chose a small masonite board and asked for specific colors ahead of time. At the day program, all of the supplies were set up and arranged for her (to create as much of a supportive environment as possible). This setting was the natural place to begin painting because it allowed for the greatest amount of support. Despite her initial negative comments, such as, "I can't do this; I'm not going to be any good at this," she was encouraged to explore the truth and to find out what she was still capable of doing with painting. Other patients wandered into the room and provided her with positive feedback. This gave her hope, and after a few sessions of painting, she was encouraged to identify the positive aspects of her work. Although she did comply with this request, she then immediately retorted, "But it's not as good as it used to be."

This process continued for a few weeks, with therapists encouraging her to rephrase negative comments and to identify the "truths" behind negative perceptions. Cognitive therapy had clearly begun to work when she arrived one day at the program saying, "I clipped out some pictures from a National Geographic that I'd like to paint." She eventually recognized this activity as an important part of her life and, more important, she perceived it as something she was able to perform. She began to take the initiative and was responsible for the full set-up of supplies. It was at this point, when she needed minimal support, that the therapist reviewed her Activities Health Assessment with her to identify times of the day that would be appropriate for painting at home. A home evaluation was conducted to help Mrs. N decide the best physical layout and lighting for painting.

She was hopeful and motivated. Within a few weeks, she had a list of acrylic colors she needed, and a visit to the art store followed. As she continued to improve, this dramatic improvement in mood and function left her uncomfortable. She clearly did not trust the change completely and was struggling with the new concept of "wellness." The trip to the art store proved regressive, with comments like, "I'm too sick to do this; maybe we should go back." She was encouraged to discuss how she felt during painting and how those benefits should be the focus of the outing. She also was encouraged to talk about how alien it was for her to feel contentment or happiness since her husband's death and her stroke. This helped her to talk about her ambivalence about getting better and her related fears of failing.

Despite increased involvement in painting, she needed further validation of her skills. NARSAD (National Alliance for Research of Schizophrenia and Affective Disorders) publishes greeting cards of artwork designed by people with a mental illness. Recognizing the potential power of national recognition, the therapist photographed Mrs. N's work, helped her to determine titles for each photograph, and submitted her work for consideration. NARSAD accepted one of her works as a holiday greeting card, and this marked the true cornerstone of change. She was now a nationally recognized artist paid for her work, and this outcome contrasted completely with the image of herself she had developed. With this recognition came increased involvement in groups at the program, renewed involvement in painting at home, and, for the first time in years, a significant change was observed in her affect. The activity provided the means for skill development and ultimately broke the inactivity cycle. She was able to redesign her use of leisure time and chose to become involved in meaningful and gratifying activities.

Review Questions

1. What percentage of people over 60 have some symptoms of depression?
2. What factors account for the failure of older people with depression to seek treatment?
3. List some possible causes of depression in the elderly.
4. What symptoms of depression are often misinterpreted as signs of physical illness?
5. What are the symptoms of depression?
6. What is the symptom of behavior that is a strong indicator for dysphoria?
7. List some medical conditions that have been associated with depression.
8. What is unique about the occupational therapist's contribution to the team treating depression in the elderly?
9. What is meant by "somatization"?
10. What is pseudodementia?
11. What symptoms differentiate the patient with dementia from the one with depressive pseudodementia?
12. Describe an appropriate approach to the patient with dependent personality disorder.
13. How did Groves (1978) recommend that health professionals deal with older narcissistic patients (entitled demanders)?
14. What are the characteristics of the manipulative help rejecters and how are they best handled by the occupational therapist?
15. List four assessments that are useful for measuring depression.
16. What is an important first step in the treatment planning process with the depressed patient?
17. What is the assessment that can identify the ways that depression has impacted daily involvement in activities?
18. What is the basic assumption of cognitive therapy?
19. How can occupational therapists use cognitive therapy in their treatment programs for depressed patients?

References

Abrams, R. C., Alexopoulos, G. S., & Young, R. C. (1987). Geriatric depression and DSM-IIIR personality disorder criteria. *Journal of the American Geriatrics Society, 35*(5), 383–386.

American Psychiatric Association. (1994). *Diagnostic and statistical manual of mental disorders* (4th ed.) (DSM IV). Washington, DC: American Psychiatric Association.

Beck, A. (1963). Thinking and depression. *Archives of General Psychiatry, 10,* 561–571.

Beck, A. (1967). *Depression—clinical, experimental and theoretical aspects.* New York: Harper & Row.

Beck, A. T., Rush, A. J., Shaw, B. F., & Emery, G. C. (1979). Cognitive therapy of depression. New York: Guilford.

Blazer, D., Bachar, J. R., & Hughes, D. C. (1987). Major depression with melancholia: A comparison of middle-aged and elderly adults. *Journal of American Geriatric Society, 35,* 927–932.

Clark, D. C., Cavanaugh, S. V., & Gibbons, R. D. (1983). The core symptoms of depression in medical and psychiatric patients. *Journal of Nervous & Mental Diseases, 171,* 705–713.

Coleman, D. (1995, September 6). Depression in the old can be deadly, but the symptoms are often missed. *New York Times.*

Cynkin, S., & Robinson, A. M. (1990). Occupational therapy and activities health: Toward health through activities. Boston: Little, Brown

Davidson, M., Harvey, P. D., Powchik, P., Parrella, M., White, L., Knobler, H. Y., Losonczy, M. F., Keefe, R. S., Katz, S., & Frecska, E. (1995). Severity of symptoms in chronically institutionalized geriatric schizophrenic patients. *American Journal of Psychiatry, 152*(2), 197–207.

Gallagher, D. (1986). The Beck Depression Inventory and older adults: Review of its development and utility. In T. L. Brink (Ed.). *Clinical gerontology: A guide to assessment and intervention* (pp. 149–163). New York: Haworth Press.

Gallo, J., Reichel, W., & Anderson, L. (1988). Handbook of geriatric assessment. Rockville, MD: Aspen.

Groves, J. F. (1978). Taking care of the hateful patient. *New England Journal of Medicine, 298*(6), 883–887.

Gurland, B., Golden, R., Teresi, J., & Challop, J. (1984). The SHORT-CARE: An efficient instrument for assessment of depression, dementia, and disability. *Journal of Gerontology, 39,* 166–169.

Gurland, B., & Toner, T. (1983). Differentiating dementia from nondementing conditions. In R. Mayeux & W. G. Rosen (Eds.), *The dementias* (pp. 1–17). New York: Raven Press.

Gurland, B., & Wilder, D. (1984). The CARE interview revisited: Development of an efficient systematic clinical assessment. *Journal of Gerontology, 39,* 129–137.

Hendrie, H. C., & Crossett, J. H. W. (1990). An overview of depression in the elderly. *Psychiatric Annals, 20*(2), 64–69.

Katerndahl, D. A., Realini, J. P. (1995). Where do panic attack sufferers seek care? *Journal of Family Practice, 40*(3), 237–243.

Miller, P. (1987). Models for treatment of depression. *Physical and Occupational Therapy in Geriatrics, 5*(1), 3–11.

National Institute of Mental Health (NIMH). (1993). Plain talk about depression (Publication No. 93–5561). Rockville, MD: NIMH.

National Institute of Mental Health (NIMH). (1995). If you're 65 and feeling depressed (Stock No. 017-024–01398–6). Rockville, MD: NIMH.

Nielsen, A. C., & Williams, T. A. (1980). Depression in ambulatory medical patients: Prevalence by self-report questionnaire and recognition by non-psychiatric physicians. *Archives General Psychiatry, 37,* 999–1004.

Popkin, M. K., & MacKenzie, T. B. (1980). Psychiatric presentations of endocrine dysfunction. In R. Hall (Ed.), *Psychiatric presentations of medical illness somatopsychic disorders* (pp. 139–156). New York: SP Medical & Scientific Books.

Robinson, R. G., Starr, L. B., Kubos, K. L., & Price, T. R. (1983). A longitudinal study of post-stroke mood disorders: Findings during the initial evaluation. *Stroke, 14,* 736–741.

Small, G. W. (1991). Recognition and treatment of depression in the elderly. *Journal of Clinical Psychiatry, 52*(6), 11–22.

Smith, S. L., Sherrill, K. A., & Colenda, C. C. (1995). Assessing and treating anxiety in elderly persons. *Psychiatric Services, 46*(1), 36–42.

Sunderland, T., Lawlor, B. A., Molchan, S. E., & Martinez, R. A. (1988). Depressive syndromes in the elderly: Special concerns. *Psychopharmacology Bulletin, 24*(4), 567–576.

Weekes, C. (1990). *Hope and help for your nerves.* New York: Penguin.

Yesavage, J. A. (1986). The use of self-rating depression scales in the elderly. In L. W. Poon (Ed.), *Clinical memory assessment of older adults.* Washington, DC: American Psychological Association.

Yesavage, J. A., & Brink, T. L. (1983). Development and validation of a geriatric depression screening scale: A preliminary report. *Journal of Psychiatric Research, 17,* 37–49.

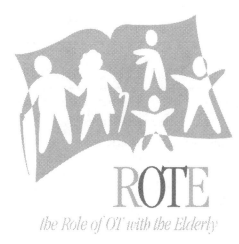

ROTE

the Role of OT with the Elderly

Evaluation and Interventions for the Performance Areas

Section 1.
Evaluation and Interventions for the Performance Area of Self-Maintenance

Diane Foti, MS, OTR

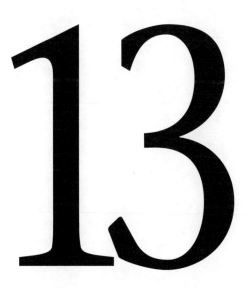

Abstract

One of the occupational therapist's chief contributions to a sense of well-being in elderly people is to help them build independence and competence in self-maintenance.

Introduction

The performance areas consist of activities of daily living (ADLs), work and productive activities, and leisure tasks (table 13–1). Each of these categories can be further divided into more specific tasks that can require assessment and in some cases treatment when working with the elderly.

The ADL performance area includes self-maintenance tasks—hygiene, grooming, dressing, nutrition, eating, food and medication management, sexual function, and personal mobility. The performance areas of work and productive activities and of leisure activities are discussed in subsequent sections of this chapter.

Aging results in many physiological, psychological, and social changes with a potential for declining independence in performing self-maintenance tasks. The aging individual must cope with normal physical

Table 13–1. Performance Areas

Activities of Daily Living	Work & Productive Activities	Play & Leisure Activities
Self-Care dressing eating or nutrition toilet hygiene bathing grooming oral hygiene medication management health maintenance socialization functional mobility functional communication sexual function	**Home Management** shopping meal preparation or clean-up cleaning clothing care household maintenance money management safety procedures	play or leisure exploration play or leisure performance
	Care of Others children parents spouse or partner pets	
	Educational Activities school work-sponsored activities community activities	
	Vocational Activities vocational exploration job acquisition work or job performance retirement planning volunteer participation	
	Safety Management fire safety awareness able to call 911 responds to smoke detector identifies dangerous situations	

Source: Data from AOTA, 1994.

changes, such as declining strength, and visual, hearing, pulmonary, and cardiac changes. The aging individual may also be affected by specific disease processes that create a complex combination of symptoms and functional deficits.

A client may be able to retain independent self-maintenance during the aging process by gradually adapting to progressive changes. However, the sudden onset of disability, such as an exacerbation of rheumatoid arthritis or a sudden paralysis from a stroke, creates a new situation that requires further adaptation and coping with greater disability.

Self-maintenance should be individualized by the occupational therapy practitioner on the basis of treatment setting and care classification of the client, who may require acute care, subacute care, extended care, home care, or health maintenance provided at senior centers and adult day health centers.

The treatment process first involves evaluation to identify deficits, then progresses to a consideration of general treatment principles, and finally consists of treatment interventions specific to each activity.

ADL Evaluation

The occupational therapist's role is to gather baseline data by reviewing the elderly client's medical history, by performing objective assessments (manual muscle test [MMT] and standardized ADL, range of movement [ROM], sensory, coordination, cognitive, and perceptual tests), and by conducting subjective assessments (interview of client, family, and friends; evaluation of the environment). Once the baseline data have been gathered, the elderly client's rehabilitation potential is determined and realistic functional

goals are developed for the client so that he or she may return to an optimal living situation for the maximum level of functioning. The occupational therapist must also consider the client's learning potential and how it will affect rehabilitation potential and the chosen treatment approach.

Medical history is gathered from documents, such as the client's medical records and transfer orders, and from the client, the client's family, and other persons who have a significant relationship with the client. (In this section, significant others and partners are included in the term "family.") A thorough medical history ensures that all potential treatment precautions are considered and assists the occupational therapist to understand how specific disease processes affect the client's activity before beginning the evaluation. The elderly client may have a series of medical problems that complicate performance of an activity. For example, the occupational therapist may be treating a client for a cerebral vascular accident (CVA). The effect of other factors, such as diabetes, coronary artery disease, and aging, however, must also be considered.

The aging individual is typically treated in a continuum of care. Therefore, several occupational therapists may have assessed and treated the client. For example, the client may have entered an acute care hospital, then transferred to a skilled-nursing facility for short-term rehabilitation, and then returned home. It is likely that the client has been treated at each setting by a different occupational therapy practitioner. Because of this continuum, each therapist works on a small component of the treatment plan or short-term treatment objectives to help the client attain the maximum independence possible.

To obtain a perspective on how the client has progressed and the response to occupational therapy, written documentation throughout the course of treatment is needed. Each therapist must be diligent in obtaining and forwarding results of assessments, progress notes, and discharge summaries. With more knowledge about the client's previous treatment, the current occupational therapy practitioner is able to develop a more realistic treatment plan and establish attainable goals. Time lost in redundant treatment and repetitious questions to the family and client in the different treatment settings is minimized and the patient progresses with less disruption.

The interview involves the client and significant others. Inclusion of the elderly individual's partner is important, since there is often an interdependence for certain ADLs or home management tasks and social support. The client's partner may also be elderly and have limitations. The clinician may choose to interview them together or alone, depending on the family dynamics. The interview is pertinent in gathering information about the client's and family's perception of the disability, level of functioning, ability to assist with care, and the home or discharge environment. The caregiver may be pivotal in determining the potential for a client to return or remain home and to prevent institutionalization.

Along with the interview the evaluation should include assessment of specific performance components, such as strength, ROM, sensation, coordination, cognition, and perception. In the evaluation process cognition may be the key performance component in determining the appropriate treatment approach and the client's capacity to learn new methods to perform self-management. If a client has a physical, sensory, or perceptual limitation to overcome but cognition is intact, then

teaching the client is much less complex than when there is also a cognitive impairment. If a cognitive deficit is suspected, then an objective cognitive assessment is needed. The occupational therapist should become familiar with the cognitive assessments available and select the appropriate tool. Chapter 11 discussed assessment tools and chapter 12 addressed cognitive evaluation and treatment.

It is important, though, to combine evaluation of performance components with a performance evaluation to determine the client's actual functional abilities. A performance evaluation will identify what the client is actually capable of doing versus what the family thinks the client is able to do. A family may report that an elderly individual is unable to perform a certain task when actually that person is able to do the task, but has not been allowed to do it or has chosen not to do it. It can also transpire that the family reports that a client is capable of performing a simple ADL but, when observed, the client performs poorly or in an unsafe manner.

Results of a performance evaluation may also clarify how deficits with performance components (cognition, psychological, sensorimotor) actually affect functional activities. The elderly person who has had a general decline in physical and cognitive function may have compensated for these deficits and remains quite functional. For example, when evaluating for performance components, a client demonstrates a lack of shoulder strength. The therapist may then assume that combing hair or reaching for objects on a shelf is impossible. In the actual performance evaluation the client has compensated for the lack of strength by propping elbows on a dresser when combing hair and has rearranged the kitchen so all items are within easy reach. This example demonstrates the need for a combination of approaches to evaluation.

Assessment of the client's present environment and of the environment to which the client may be discharged is needed to make realistic goals and to determine family teaching needs. The environmental evaluation includes the immediate home or institution and the surrounding community. The environment is critical in supporting the individual who has functional limitations. Modifications may be necessary to support greater independence with self-maintenance activities. For the individual with cognitive deficits, a familiar environment that provides many cues may make the difference between needing only supervision for ADLs and needing maximum assistance.

Through use of assessments, interview, and a performance evaluation the occupational therapist determines the client's learning potential and the best teaching style. If the client has limited potential to learn, as with a progressive disease such as Alzheimer's, the focus may be on caregiver education and considering methods to modify the environment to promote independence and safety. If the elderly client has potential to learn, teaching self-maintenance skills is directed to the client and to the family for reinforcement of newly learned skills.

The client's rehabilitation potential, the ability to reach his or her maximum level of independence, must also be taken into account before establishing treatment goals. To determine rehabilitation potential, the following factors about the client should be considered: previous functional level, prognosis for recovery, motivation of the client and family, and the environmental restrictions. The previ-

ous functional level is needed to estimate the client's maximum level of independence. For example, if a client was independent with self-maintenance prior to a stroke and is getting good strength back in the hemiplegic side, has intact cognition, and is motivated, the rehabilitation potential for independence is good. Conversely, if a client has a history of multi-infarct dementia, has required supervision with self-care, and has a new stroke resulting in a dense hemiplegia, the rehabilitation potential for independence is guarded. Goals for the latter client may involve teaching the caregiver how to provide care and proper cuing to elicit maximum functioning from the client. These examples reflect the importance of gathering a history of the client's previous functional level in order to select the most appropriate goals and treatment approach.

Evaluation of the elderly individual is multifaceted, because it involves the client, the family, and the environment. The client's medical and social history may be complex. The investment of performing a thorough evaluation will result in a more individualized treatment plan addressing the specific needs and personal style of the elderly client.

At completion, the evaluation data are analyzed, problems identified, rehabilitation potential determined, and short-term and long-term goals developed. Goals are established jointly with the elderly individual and the family to ensure that treatment is directed to attain their goals and that the scope of the occupational therapy services is understood.

Interventions

Some treatment interventions are applicable to all self-maintenance activities: use of assistive devices, energy conservation and work simplification, posture, and mobility. These factors affect the client's ability to successfully perform self-maintenance tasks and are presented first. Each self-maintenance activity is discussed individually as it applies to working with an aging client. For information on interventions for specific disabilities, the reader is referred to the reference list.

ASSISTIVE DEVICES

There are many assistive devices to compensate for lack of range of motion, limited strength, and incoordination. When working with the elderly the occupational therapy practitioner needs to assess the client's ability to learn to use an assistive device and receptiveness to a device. If the client has a cognitive or perceptual problem, learning to use assistive devices requires much repetition and reinforcement by the occupational therapy practitioner and family and may not be appropriate. Compensatory techniques, rather than using an assistive device, are the treatment of choice whenever possible. The occupational therapy practitioner must also assess what the use of the assistive device will mean to the client. Some clients may see an assistive device as creating independence, while others may see it as evidence of being less capable, or a sign of disability or aging.

Some general concepts regarding assistive devices are as follows:

- Assess client's potential learning to use new tools.
- Use a compensatory technique instead of an assistive device whenever possible.
- Select multipurpose assistive devices to simplify tasks and set-up.
- Make assistive devices easily accessible; for example, if a client uses a

walker, it should be possible to carry it safely.

- Determine whether the family will support and reinforce use of the assistive device.
- Provide the client with resources to maintain or replace an assistive device.
- Consider the cost of an assistive device and the client's ability to purchase, replace, and repair the item.

ENERGY CONSERVATION AND WORK SIMPLIFICATION

The principles of energy conservation and work simplification can be applied to all tasks of ADL, work, play, or leisure. The aging process involves a general decrease in strength, endurance, and cardiac and pulmonary function; therefore, simplifying everyday tasks can help the elderly individual pace activity throughout the day and maintain independence for a longer period.

To apply work simplification principles, the occupational therapist must first analyze the task. Three parts of the job should be analyzed: the preparation; the performance of the task, and the clean-up. Whether the job is essential, when or where it is to be done, the timing of the job, who the most appropriate person is to do the job, and the simplest method to complete the job are considered. Some concepts to apply are as follows:

- Plan ahead and eliminate all unnecessary work.
- Spread out difficult jobs and provide periods of rest.
- Work at a moderate pace.
- Sit to work whenever possible.
- Have needed equipment within easy reach to avoid unnecessary walking.

- Use two hands when possible to perform a job.
- Work in a well-lighted and ventilated room to avoid fatigue (Hittle, Pedretti, & Kasch, 1996).

Examples of applying energy conservation and work simplification techniques to bathing are showering every other day instead of daily, using a shower seat to sit while bathing, using a hand-held shower to eliminate standing and turning to rinse, sitting on the toilet or a chair to dry, donning a robe, and resting afterwards before getting dressed.

The elderly individual may have well-established routines. With demonstration and practice of a new approach to an everyday problem, the client may accept a new method to resolve a troublesome activity of daily living. Application of energy conservation and work simplification may allow more energy to participate in other activities throughout the day.

POSTURE

An important component underlying ADLs in the elderly is posture. In the elderly, poor posture may be caused by osteoporosis, with potential for spinal deformities, generally decreased muscle strength and tone, or neurological deficits. All activities are influenced by posture. Risk of falling is increased with poor standing posture, which also affects gait. Vital capacity; oxygen intake; and mental awareness, alertness, and function decrease with poor sitting posture. When posture is poor, the head drops forward, visual contact is then compromised or may require extreme extension of the neck. With the neck extended, swallowing is difficult and may contribute to aspiration (Wells, Chew, Lang, Campbell, & Chenderlin, 1988). Treatment programs should include daily range of motion, stretching exercises, deep breathing, and exercises to strengthen the diaphragm to improve posture and alertness.

The upper extremities are free to peform activities if there is good posture and trunk stability. An elderly person who needs to hold on to a wheelchair to keep from falling forward will have difficulty eating independently, since it requires releasing the wheelchair. For the ambulatory individual with poor posture, reaching items in a cupboard and carrying things will be difficult (Wells et al., 1988).

If a client must remain in a wheelchair a proper seating evaluation is needed. The evaluation includes physical factors, functional needs, and environmental concerns. The physical factors are ROM, strength, muscle tone, sensation, voluntary and involuntary movements, sitting balance, skeletal deformities, breathing, and circulation. Functional needs are methods of transfer, propulsion, self-maintenance, caregiver needs, and communication. Accessibility to home, work (if appropriate), community, transportation, and safety is included in the environmental needs (ABLEDATA, 1990). The client's financial status must be assessed for covering the cost of any equipment recommendations. Medicare, Medicaid, and private insurance companies have changing policies; therefore, the occupational therapy practitioner needs knowledge of the current guidelines regarding coverage for durable medical equipment.

Wheelchair Posture

The key point of control or stability in the sitting position is almost always the pelvis. A good base of support can enhance the ability to balance, reach, propel, and transfer, and to perform activities of daily living. The postural support provided by a folding wheelchair seat is not adequate for extended periods of time. A seating system begins with a solid seat insert. It distributes pressure over as broad a sitting surface as possible, maximizing the base of support and minimizing pressure. A cushion can then be placed on top of the seat board to provide padding and support (ABLEDATA, 1990). Cushions range from a simple foam to more complex air and gel cushions. Cushions that meet the client's seating, skin-care, functional, and financial needs should be selected. The most expensive cushion is not always needed.

In addition to a firm seat board and cushion, a strap to secure hips in flexion may be required. A wheelchair seat belt is usually placed at waist level and does not secure the hips. It can be repositioned at hip level or behind and below the buttocks so that it is approximately at a 45-degree angle to the seat. This prevents the client from scooting the hips forward and sitting with a kyphotic posture.

A firm back support that provides lumbar support will improve posture and prevent deformities and back pain. If the client has a tendency toward lateral flexion, lateral trunk supports, chest straps, or wheelchair trays may help to prevent this deforming posture. Lateral trunk supports may be contoured into a molded back support or may be a separate attachment.

Armrests should be supportive but not cause excessive shoulder elevation. Specialized arm supports for the individual with hemiplegia can be attached or substituted for the traditional armrest. Wheelchair lap trays can also increase the arm support surface and provide an eating area or area for other ADLs or leisure activities. Wheelchair lap trays come in a variety of materials and styles. Some are full size, reaching from one armrest to the other, and some are hemi-style. The hemi-style is supported by only one armrest and is designed to support a hemiplegic arm. The hemi-style lap tray allows for use of a urinal without removing the tray.

Footrests and legrests should be adjusted to provide support to take pressure off the posterior thigh and prevent foot deformities and injuries. A nonskid surface on the foot pedals, heel loops, calf-pads, and ankle straps are all modifications that will allow for proper foot position and provide foot and leg stability.

Many factors must be considered when evaluating a client's posture in a wheelchair. Modifications may range from simple and inexpensive to more elaborate and very expensive. If a highly technical seating system is needed, the occupational therapy practitioner usually works closely with other team members, such as the physical therapist, physiatrist, rehabilitation engineer, and medical equipment dealer.

MOBILITY AND TRANSFERS

Mobility is particularly critical for the elderly client. Changes in posture, strength, range of motion, endurance, and vision loss due to aging can contribute to difficulties with ambulation. If a client also has sensory and perceptual deficits the risk of falls and difficulty with ambulation may be compounded. Up to 40% of the elderly who live in the community fall each year (Tinnetti, 1987). Caregivers are often willing to help with dressing and bathing, but once an individual has difficulty with ambulation, care becomes much more of a burden.

The physical therapist assesses and treats the client for specific ambulation difficulties, but if the occupational therapy practitioner is developing a comprehensive approach to ADLs, the client's safety and ability to ambulate while performing an ADL and getting to social functions are also considered. Frequently the elderly individual will walk with a caregiver or the physical therapist, then remain in the wheelchair the rest of the day. The occupational therapy practitioner can integrate skills the client has learned in physical therapy into ADLs, for example, ambulating into the bathroom or to the dining room table for meals instead of using the wheelchair. This integration can be accomplished in a long-term care facility or skilled nursing facility so that ambulation is not a separate activity. The client can then sit in a firm standard chair with arms, which generally provides better support than the seat sling of a folding wheelchair.

Functional mobility also involves evaluation and treatment of the client's ability to stand from a seated position and to sit down from a standing position, to properly use mobility aids, to safely manage stairs when performing self-maintenance tasks, to reach for objects on the floor, and to carry personal items when using a mobility device.

Sit to Stand

Extensor musculature weakens before flexors in the elderly. This weakness can be noted when the client plops into a chair or pulls up from a seated position by grabbing a door jamb. Both are signs of hip extensor weakness. Such weakness makes the simple movements of going from sitting to standing or standing to sitting laborsome and a cause of falls. For the client who is wheelchair bound, this weakness will also contribute to difficulties with transfers. Evaluation and treatment may include teaching proper sit-to-stand and stand-to-sit techniques, modifying a chair by raising it, adding grab bars, or discussing a lower-extrem-

ity strengthening program with the physical therapist.

Following are some basic principles for movement from sitting to standing that can be applied to ease mobility for the aging individual. (This technique should not be used with individuals who have had a recent hip arthroplasty.)

The client should

- Sit in a firm chair with arms.
- Select a chair that allows feet to rest on the ground.
- Make sure the ambulation aid is placed nearest the arm used or, if a walker is used, it should be in front of the client.
- Scoot to the edge of the chair.
- Flex knees so that feet are below or slightly posterior to knees.
- Flex hips forward and extend the trunk so that the head is at or just anterior to the knees.
- Place arms on armrests, on knees, or reaching forward.
- Stand and move hands to the ambulation aid.
- Do not use walkers and canes as a support for standing or for returning to a sitting position.

Stair Climbing

The client should lead with the strong leg when going up stairs and lead with the weaker leg when descending. The phrase "Up with the good, down with the bad" has been used to reinforce this approach with clients. A hand rail should be available on the stairs. Some clients will need a hand rail on both sides of the stairs, depending on their limitations and the width of the stairway.

AMBULATION DEVICES

The type of ambulation device is identified in the initial evaluation. The client may use a cane, quad cane, hemi-walker, walker, crutches, or a wheelchair. The client will need to be evaluated for proper use of the device throughout the house or facility. Bathroom doorways may be too narrow to be approached directly with a walker but can be negotiated if approached sideways. Bathrooms generally do not have enough space to turn a wheelchair around, but space may be adequate to turn a walker around tightly. To prevent falls, throw rugs, loose carpets, and long cords should be removed or fastened properly to prevent the mobility aid from catching.

Cane

For the individual with lower extremity involvement but enough hand strength on the same side, the cane is carried on the affected side. For the person with hemiplegia and a nonfunctional hand the cane is carried in the unaffected hand. The length of the cane is measured to the height of the trochanter, so that the elbow is slightly flexed when the cane is grasped.

Walker

Choices include pick-up style walkers and front-wheeled walkers. The pick-up style walker requires better balance to use. A walker is held with both hands. The user never moves it more than one step ahead. The walker is not to be used for balance when sitting down or standing up, since it is unstable and a fall could result.

Manual Wheelchairs

Manual wheelchairs can be ordered with many features. If an individual is to use a wheelchair at all times, it should be custom fitted. The occupational therapist can order a wheelchair in consultation with an equipment vendor. The size and weight of a wheelchair are considered in relation to where it will be stored in the car. If a caregiver must place the wheelchair in a car trunk, his or her strength should also be taken into consideration.

Motorized Scooters and Electric Wheelchairs

A scooter or electric wheelchair can increase an individual's mobility in the home and community. Both require good visual, perceptual, and motor planning skills. Generally, scooters do not provide good trunk stability, because of the design of the seats, but electric wheelchairs can be designed with a supportive seating system. The evaluator should consider how much upper extremity strength and range of motion is required to run the scooter and electric wheelchair. Scooters generally are less expensive than electric wheelchairs.

Carrying Personal Items and Reaching

Use of an ambulation aid frequently results in difficulty carrying objects because the hands are holding a walker or cane or pushing a wheelchair. Walker baskets and bags, wheelchair cupholders, lap trays, and packs will allow for organization of personal items and the potential to do meal preparation independently. Often a small fanny pack or waist pack will be enough to carry a wallet, book, glasses, and cordless phone, while allowing both hands to be used on the walker or cane.

The use of an ambulation aid may indicate that the client will also have difficulty stooping, kneeling, and reaching items on the floor. The evaluation then may include the client's need to reach items in low drawers or cupboards, shoes in the closet, and other self-maintenance activities. The elderly individual may be shown how to kneel safely or may use a reacher to compensate for this inability.

ASSISTING WITH AMBULATION

If assistance is needed for ambulation or transfers a gait or transfer belt will provide a good handhold for the person assisting.

When assisting with ambulation the therapist should

- Use a gait belt.
- Have the mobility aid within reach.
- Walk behind the client and to the weaker side.
- Place hands on the gait belt or client's waist, where they can provide support at the hips, a key point of control.
- Never pull on the arm to lift a person from sitting or to lower to sitting.

Transfers

For the individual who has difficulty with ambulation or is primarily wheelchair bound, transferring to other surfaces is often difficult. Transferring is initiated using sit-to-stand principles described earlier. Instead of standing fully erect the elderly individual may stay in a semi-flexed posture and pivot over to the transfer surface while reaching for the armrest or edge of the chair. To sit, the client again extends the trunk while flexing at the hips, so that the head is over the knees, and continues to flex the hips and knees to control the descent into the chair.

For the elderly individual requiring assistance with transfers, the evaluation should include the caregiver's ability to physically assist with the transfer and to learn safe techniques. The caregiver and occupational therapy practitioner should consistently use proper body mechanics when assisting with transfers so that elderly people are not injured in the process. Transfer style depends on many factors including the client's and caregiver's deficits, strengths, and environmental restrictions. Each transfer must be suited for the individual and the surface being transferred to. Some basic principles for assisting with a transfer follow.

- Secure a gait belt around the client.
- Get as close to the transfer surface as possible and lock the wheelchair.
- Swing away footrests and place client's feet on the floor.
- Remove armrest closest to the transfer surface.
- Position practitioner in front of the client.
- Scoot the client's hips to the edge of the chair.
- Have client flex knees so that feet are below or slightly posterior to knees.
- Have client flex hips so that head is at or just anterior to the knees.
- Have client place arms on armrests, on knees, or reaching forward but preferably not on the person assisting with the transfer.
- Make sure practitioner guards client's balance at all times.
- Have practitioner place hands securely on gait belt, at key points on the trunk, or at the waist and hips to assist with pivot, but not in a way that limits the client's ability to bend forward and not on the client's arms.
- Have practitioner signal the client to pivot and reach for the transfer surface.
- Make sure client is lowered to the transfer surface.
- Make sure client is assisted back into a stable seated position.

Learning transfers or a new style of transfers can cause the client to feel apprehensive and fearful of moving. If a client is able to understand verbal directions, the occupational therapy practitioner informs the client of each step of the procedure. For those with cognitive and perceptual deficits, tactile cues are more effective than verbal directions during a transfer. Transfer training requires not only demonstration with verbal directions but also much practice so that the elderly client and caregiver develop the necessary transfer skills and a sense of competence in handling a potentially difficult situation.

Functional mobility encompasses many small components related to self-maintenance. The physical therapist is primarily responsible for gait evaluation, training, and recommendations for a mobility aid. However, the OT practitioner then determines how the client's functional mobility affects ADLs. For independence the client needs to be able to get up from a variety of surfaces and carry and reach personal items for self-maintenance activities.

Nutrition, Eating, Swallowing, and Managing Food

Some elderly persons are at risk for changes in nutritional status. Some of the factors contributing to inadequate nutrition are inability to eat independently or without great effort, poor appetite, inability to prepare foods or purchase foods at a store, low income, and inadequate knowledge about a balanced diet (Ebert, 1989). Occupational therapy practitioners work with elderly clients on several activities of daily living that apply to adequate nutrition, such as eating, swallowing, shopping, and preparing food.

NUTRITION

Although the specifics of nutrition are addressed by the dietician and nurse, the occupational therapy practitioner should have a basic understanding of the nutritional needs of the elderly and some of the potential problems that can contribute to poor nutrition. Occupational therapy intervention with eating, swallowing, preparing meals, and shopping may prevent or alleviate potential for poor nutrition.

Basic dietary needs are a balanced portion of milk and cheese, vegetables and fruits, bread and cereals, and protein, along with a recommendation for low fat, sodium, sugar, and alcohol consumption. Fluid intake should consist of 1 1/2 to 2 liters daily depending on the client's level of activity and metabolic demands and on the weather (Ebert, 1989).

Occupational therapy practitioners may be evaluating a client's ability to plan a meal. In this case the client can be directed toward selecting nutritional foods, and the therapy situation provides an opportunity for educating the client about a proper diet. If an elderly client has a swallowing problem (dysphagia), liquids and some food consistencies can be difficult; therefore, the occupational therapy practitioner may request that the client or family measure fluid intake to determine the client's intake of fluids and food. This is usually done as a team approach in conjunction with a dietician and nurse.

The elderly individual's cultural background may influence nutritional issues: food preferences may be determined by ethnic background. Residents of long-term care facilities are generally fed the same meal, leaving little choice. These meals are typically a western diet with very little seasoning. The lack of choice, especially for the institutionalized elderly individual, may contribute to a poor appetite and lead to inadequate nutrition. In order to improve nutrition or compliance with changing food consistencies the OT practitioner should be sensitive about the client's ethnic background and related food preferences. Families may be instructed on how to modify the preferred diet and adhere to changes in food consistencies. Recommendations that include the foods the client would typically eat will probably result in improved compliance and nutritional intake.

Certain disease processes require alterations in nutritional intake. Most common in the elderly are diabetes, osteoporosis, hypertension, and cardiovascular diseases. For each of these the occupational therapy practitioner should understand dietary needs and restrictions.

SWALLOWING

Many elderly adults have swallowing problems, which can be due to changes in dentition, a neurological disease process, or cognitive impairment. Changes in dentition—tooth loss, tooth loosening, and use of dentures—may contribute to difficulty with chewing. The aging individual also loses significant muscle strength, which limits ability to chew (Bennett, 1979). Changes occur in the oral mucosa and decreased salivation in the oral stage of the swallow. It may appear that these changes are not significant problems. However, the results of a study by Feinberg and Ekberg (1991) concluded that for 50 elderly subjects with a history of aspiration, 23 of the 50 aspirated because of dysfunction in the oral stage of the swallow. Accordingly, the clinician needs to perform a simple screening of oral and pharyngeal-stage functioning of the elderly client. This check will help determine the need for a more comprehensive dysphagia assessment. Many evaluations are available to the clinician for detailed dysphagia assessment (Logemann, 1983; Nelson, 1996).

Once specific swallow deficits are identified, a treatment program is developed. The treatment program may involve compensatory techniques, specific swallow exercises, or a program combining both. A speech pathologist may be involved in the treatment of dysphagia. Therefore, role delineations are made to provide continuity of treatment and to prevent duplication of services. Because specific compensatory techniques and swallow exercises are very individual, only general guidelines can be outlined:

- Position the individual to sit as upright as possible; provide lateral trunk support with pillows if necessary.
- Ensure that the head is flexed slightly and in midline.
- Select the food consistency that allows for a safe and efficient swallow for the particular client.
- Present small portions of food or small sips of liquid.
- Observe for swallow after each bite of food.
- Check for pocketing of food in cheeks; client may clear this with a finger or the tongue.
- Provide oral hygiene after meals to eliminate food remaining in mouth.
- Have client sit up for at least 30 minutes following a meal.
- If any new difficulties with swallowing occur, such as gurgly voice quality and coughing, complete a thorough dysphagia reassessment. If coughing is involved, note what food consistencies appear to produce the cough and when the cough occurs (Nelson, 1996).

Recommended changes in food consistencies to a ground or pureed diet or to thickened liquids should be discussed with the elderly individual and caregiver. For clients who have many functional impairments, eating is often one of the few enjoyable activities. Therefore, changing food consistencies may result in resistance from the client and family. Also, chopping, pureeing, and thickening foods may increase caregiver stress. The elderly individual and caregiver may need extensive repeated education regarding the necessity for specific food or liquid consistencies.

EATING

Independent eating should be encouraged whenever possible but not at the expense of adequate nutrition. Self-feeding involves determining the appropriate set-up and whether adaptive equipment is needed. Many types of adapted utensils exist to compensate for specific deficits. Therefore, the evaluation should determine why the client is having difficulty with self-feeding, in order to make the appropriate recommendations. Some adaptive equipment that may improve self-feeding are nonskid materials placed under plates or bowls, a plate guard or scoop dish, built-up handles, and cups with spill-proof lids.

The environment to encourage self-feeding should be pleasant and calm. That atmosphere presents a particular problem in the institutional setting where there are many clients and staff. Dining programs with quiet music and tablecloths, where dinnerware is removed from the trays and the staff members sit with the residents, have been found to be helpful. Set-up for the individual involves determining which utensils are needed and whether all of the food is to be set out at once. For the individual with a cognitive deficit, providing one utensil and one food item at a time will decrease distractions and increase focus on that food item. If a client has a visual deficit, food items on the tray should be identified and, if needed, the client's hand guided to each item.

Self-feeding is begun with finger foods or by holding a cup. Using a guiding technique to place the food in the client's hand and then bringing it to the mouth may be needed initially. The guiding technique is particularly helpful when feeding an individual who is tactilely defensive around the face. With this technique the client receives tactile and proprioceptive cues that something is approaching the face and is more likely to open the mouth to eat. A potential problem for the self-feeding individual who is impulsive is eating dessert first or filling up on beverages, which may contribute to inadequate nutrition. In such a situation the caregiver needs to provide one food item at a time.

For clients who need assistance with eating, the following guidelines are suggested:

- Position the client upright.
- Inform the client that it is mealtime and what is to be eaten.
- Provide small bites on a spoon; do not overload the spoon.
- Inform the client when a cup is being placed on the lips.
- Have the person feeding the client sit or stand in view.
- Present the spoon horizontally at the center of the lips and on the mid portion of the tongue. If the client is unable to close the mouth to remove food with the lips, a quick, light pressure on the tongue, with the spoon anchored on the lower incisors, will initiate a reflex closure of the jaw. The spoon is then removed slowly. The client may require manual closing of the lips.
- Do not clean food particles off the chin until the person swallows, for this action may initiate a reflex opening of the mouth and interfere with chewing and swallowing.
- Observe for swallow after each bite of food.

- Check for pocketing of food in cheeks; client may clear this food with a finger or the tongue.
- Provide oral hygiene after meals to eliminate food remaining in mouth.
- Have client sit up for at least 30 minutes following a meal (Nelson, 1996; Wells et al., 1988).

MANAGING FOOD

To maintain adequate nutrition, the aging individual must be able to shop for and prepare food. For the institutionalized individual those needs are filled by the staff. For the person living in the community with mobility impairment, limited endurance, or limited transportation, shopping and meal preparation may be difficult. Shopping may be difficult because of the weight of the grocery bags, limited endurance to walk around the grocery store, or even getting to and from the car. The home management evaluation should reveal the specific difficulties the client is having with shopping so that an individualized treatment approach can be recommended. The principles of energy conservation and work simplification apply to the task of shopping. For individuals who cannot get out to shop, many communities offer a low-cost home delivery of hot meals once a day. Some grocery stores will even deliver food orders.

Evaluation also involves determining the individual's ability to prepare meals. Evaluation should begin from simple, cold-meal preparation to more complex hot-meal preparation. Evaluation and intervention includes retrieving objects from the refrigerator and cupboards, carrying objects, opening and closing containers, stirring, measuring, and cleaning up. Any cognitive, sensory, or perceptual deficits that may require specific training, impair safety, and limit meal preparation should be noted. If an ambulation aid or wheel-chair is used, the client should be assessed while using the needed device. A walker basket or wheelchair tray is helpful for safely carrying items.

Hygiene and Grooming

Ability to maintain proper hygiene and grooming skills is important for the client's health and self-esteem. Hygiene and grooming includes personal care, such as oral hygiene, applying make-up, shaving, toileting, and bathing. Usually all of these tasks are performed in the bathroom, but if the bathroom is inaccessible another room may be selected and set up for hygiene and grooming. Once access has been determined, organization of equipment and tools used for each task can make the difference between being independent or requiring assistance. To simplify tasks, all tools are to be stored within reach and have a counter top on which to place them. Often the elderly client fatigues when performing morning care and should sit while working. Oral hygiene, shaving, make-up application, and washing at the sink can all be completed while seated. Cabinet doors can be removed to make it easier to reach the sink, and mirrors can be lowered and tilted for easy viewing. The ability to open containers, handle faucets, and judge water temperature is included when assessing hygiene and grooming skills. Modified lever handles and lowering the temperature on the water heater may be called for.

The ability to safely handle an electric or manual razor is evaluated. An individual may be unsafe with a manual razor but may be safe with a cordless electric razor. Because draping electric cords across a sink should be avoided, cordless tools are recommended.

Approaches to oral hygiene are determined by whether the client has teeth or wears dentures. Care of dentures is a two-handed task and requires great care to avoid breakage. It is important that the occupational therapy practitioner learn whether the client typically brushes the dentures, soaks them, or does both. If a client wears dentures there may be more steps involved and more packaging, such as denture cleaning tablets, a cleaning machine, and denture adhesives. A denture brush that suctions to the sink allows one-handed brushing for the person with incoordination, weakness, or paralysis. A built-up handle on a standard toothbrush for cleaning teeth or dentures may also be helpful if there is weakness or arthritis.

TOILETING

The treatment approach to toileting depends on whether a client is continent or incontinent. For the continent client the ability to handle clothes when toileting, use toilet tissue, clean adequately, and transfer safely are assessed. Techniques to handle clothes more easily and recommendations for easy-to-handle clothing may be needed. If reaching to clean with toilet tissue is difficult, a pair of kitchen tongs may serve to extend the elderly person's reach, thereby resolving the problem. Several toilet paper holders are available in rehab equipment catalogues. The individual can then wash with a long-handle soft sponge to clean well following toileting.

The standard toilet is often too low for the elderly individual. An elevated toilet seat can be used or a commode chair can be placed over the toilet to provide an elevated seat. The elevated toilet seat or commode seat should be adjusted so the user's feet touch the floor. Grab bars can be installed in the studs in the wall nearby so the client can hold on to them when sitting and standing. A commode chair can also be

used at the bedside with a pan. For the aging person, frequent urination is common, and it may be necessary to get up several times a night to void. The individual who needs assistance, is at risk for falls, or has difficulty with ambulation can use a commode or urinal at the bedside. The use of the bedside commode can provide safety while a client is alone at night and allow the caregiver to have a good night's sleep. Whether the client is able to safely empty the commode pan or the caregiver is willing to empty it also must be considered.

The aging person is at high risk for incontinence. Fourteen to 40% of the elderly are affected by urinary incontinence. Symptoms include dribbling or puddling, urine odors in the home or on clothes, and reluctance to leave home. Incontinence places the individual at risk for skin breakdown, social isolation, and poor self-concept. It can also cause a shrinking of the bladder, which can create an ongoing problem with incontinence. Incontinence can result in overburdening the caregiver and in the placement of the elderly person in an institution (Specht and Cordes, 1979).

The occupational therapy practitioner may help the client avoid incontinence by ensuring that no functional skills or environmental barriers contribute to incontinence. Discussing the client's typical routine and developing a regular schedule of toileting may help eliminate incontinence. A suggested program to begin continence retraining is to make sure the client is taken to the bathroom every 2 hours.

If incontinence is present, the client or caregiver may need instruction on how to use incontinence pads or diapers for greater ease and independence. A client may use a catheter and urinary collection bag, such as a leg or bed bag. The client or caregiver must learn about handling the catheter and leg bag independently, such as how to approach a urinal or toilet to empty a leg bag, or how to open the clamp on the leg bag.

Fecal incontinence is less common and is often associated with severe debilitation, cognitive deficits, or a neurological deficit (Bartol & Heitkemper, 1979). A physician, nurse, and dietician should be involved with the client who has onset of fecal incontinence, because it may indicate a changing medical condition or bowel impaction. The client's diet, medications, and bowel care regimen require review. If environmental barriers or functional skills are contributing factors, occupational therapy intervention is needed.

Toileting is addressed in each ADL evaluation. The elderly individual may be apprehensive about discussing a problem but once it is brought out in the open may be relieved that someone is willing to help. The OT practitioner works closely with other members of the health care team on this interdisciplinary issue.

Toilet Transfers

Because of the small space available in most bathrooms, there is usually little room for maneuvering if the elderly individual uses a wheelchair. Equipment that helps ease the difficulty with toilet transfers are a raised toilet seat with grab bars, toilet safety rails, and a commode chair. A walker can sometimes substitute for grab bars by being placed so the front of the walker is touching the toilet tank. The walker then surrounds the seated person and can be used to push up. Although a walker is not an ideal support because it is usually too high, it can be an adequate substitute for grab bars in some cases.

BATHING

Bathing may be a difficult task for the elderly individual because of the physical barriers in the bathroom, the time required to complete the task, and the risk of falls on wet, slippery surfaces. An initial evaluation should determine whether or not the client is able to enter and exit the shower stall or bathtub and to sit in the tub. The client's ability to stand safely for the entire length of a shower should also be determined. If a caregiver is assisting with bathing, the interviewer needs to listen closely to the difficulties that may arise during bath time to determine whether there are interventions that would be helpful.

If standing is difficult, a number of shower seats are commercially available. If the client is unable to step over the edge of the tub safely, a transfer tub bench reduces this barrier. Shower and tub doors can be removed to increase ease of the transfer. Grab bars installed in strategic locations can prevent falls and allow for greater independence.

When it is impossible or impractical to use the shower or tub, a sponge bath at the sink or at the bedside is an alternative. Given a chair at a sink, the elderly person may be able to wash independently, eliminating the need for the caregiver to carry water to and from the bedside.

Reaching for soap and water faucets and washing and drying feet can be a taxing part of the bathing process. Simple pieces of adaptive equipment that improve reaching are long-handled sponges or brushes and soap holders to prevent the soap from slipping.

For the individual residing in a skilled nursing facility, bathing can be a stressful activity. Staff members should extend the client respect and ensure privacy to maintain the individual's dignity. A client capable of assisting with bathing and walking to and from the shower should be encouraged to do so.

Bathtub and Shower Transfers

The elderly individual with ambulation or endurance limitations will benefit from the use of a shower seat or transfer tub bench. Transfers to these areas require assessment, since the bathroom is an area with a high risk of falls. Assessment should cover the client's ability to transfer safely over the lip of a shower stall; step over the edge of the tub; and, if realistic, sit in the bottom of the tub and get up. Strategically placed grab bars will increase safety. If there are doors on the bathtub, they can be replaced with a rod and shower curtain to increase independence with the transfer. If assistance is needed with bathing, this modification will ease the reach of the caregiver. If a client is unable to safely step over the edge of the tub, a transfer tub bench will provide a safe transfer surface.

DRESSING

Dressing may pose problems for the aging individual because of the need to reach for the feet, pull clothing over the head, or handle small fasteners. Easy-to-handle clothing that eliminates fasteners is recommended. Use of a reacher, a dressing stick, and sock aid decreases the need for reaching. A dressing stick or reacher can be used to push clothing over the head if there is limited upper extremity range of motion. A button hook will help with buttoning. Slip on shoes or elastic laces will eliminate the need for tying shoe laces.

Assessment includes the client's ability to retrieve clothing from closets and drawers. If the client uses a walking aid, a method should be developed for carrying clothing safely. If the client is maneuvering from a wheelchair, it may be necessary to lower closet rods.

Clothing that is most frequently used should be placed in easily reached drawers.

For the more debilitated individual living in a skilled nursing facility, dressing can be quite difficult. Staff should ensure that the client is dressed appropriately and not for the convenience of the staff. Some clothing is designed for wheelchair users and is both attractive and easy to don.

The client should

- Wear stretchable, comfortable pull-up pants and loose shirts or blouses.
- Sit to dress and undress.
- Start dressing the most difficult arm or leg first.
- Wear slip-on shoes or use elastic shoe laces.
- Lay clothes out the night before if getting dressed during the first part of the morning.

Medication Management

Taking medication is a major self-maintenance task for many elderly people. Although medication management is generally the role of other team members, the occupational therapy practitioner may make a contribution by alerting other team members to evaluation findings that may affect self-management of medication or by making specific recommendations for schedules and assistive devices. Some deficits that may affect adequate medication management are poor vision, hearing loss, hand weakness, incoordination, sensory impairment, cognitive deficits, and perceptual deficits.

The elderly person should be given clear, simple instructions to understand the purpose and the proper use of each medication. How to take the medication, for example, with meals or on an empty stomach, should be understood. Side effects should be noted and reported to the physician. A written list of medications to include name of medication, time of day the dose is to be taken, purpose, side effects, and effects if discontinued improperly can help prevent problems. Pill containers for organizing daily and weekly doses and pill splitters are important assistive devices.

When considering an individual's daily routine, taking medications several times a day must also be factored into the schedule. The occupational therapy practitioner should note the client's ability to open pill bottles and handle small pills. If an individual has swallowing deficits, it may be necessary to crush pills and place them in applesauce or to order them in liquid form. A nurse, physician, or pharmacist should be consulted to determine whether crushing a pill will change the effects of that medication.

For the individual with diabetes the occupational therapist can work jointly with a nurse to assess the client's ability to manage insulin and injections. Proper diabetic management requires good organizational skills, decision-making skills, and perceptual and motor-planning skills. Large-print syringes and insulin bottle holders are some of the assistive devices available to improve safety and independence with diabetic management.

Summary

Self-maintenance activities are critical for independent living. The significance of being capable of performing simple self-maintenance activities should not be underrated in building a sense of competence in directing one's life and maintaining a positive self-esteem (Kielhofner, 1985). The occupational therapy practitioner promotes independence with self-maintenance by evaluating the client's skills and needs, the caregiver's ability to assist

with care, and the environment. In cooperation with the aging individual and caregiver a treatment plan is developed to address the most pertinent goals. The client's needs and goals are the primary focus of treatment with the ultimate goal being to maintain the individual's sense of competence and positive self-esteem.

Activities

1. Interview an elderly person to learn about his or her level of independence in all of the performance areas. How has the person's activity level changed with aging? What is the significance of these changes to this individual?

2. Use a walker or a wheelchair for a day. Write a two-page summary to include (a) the feelings evoked during performance of daily activities, (b) a description of the types of social and physical barriers experienced, and (c) how self-maintenance activities were modified so they could be accomplished.

Review Questions

1. How can age-related physical and mental changes affect performance of self-maintenance tasks?

2. What are the subjective and objective elements of activities of daily living evaluation?

3. Why is a performance evaluation critical to accurate assessment when working with an elderly person?

4. Which ambulation devices are typically used by the elderly?

5. What are the factors that place an aging individual at risk for inadequate nutrition?

6. What types of intervention do occupational therapy practitioners provide to prevent or improve inadequate nutrition?

7. What are the common problems of older persons with eating, hygiene, toileting, bathing, and dressing?

8. What are the interventions and types of adaptive equipment that will improve function with eating, hygiene, toileting, bathing, and dressing activities?

9. Give an example of how energy conservation and work simplification techniques can be applied to the task of dressing.

10. How should a client be positioned to ensure safe swallowing?

11. Describe how the environment may be modified to encourage independent feeding.

12. What type of adaptive equipment can be used to improve a client's ability to carry items when using an ambulation device?

13. List the principles for ascending and descending stairs when a person has lower extremity impairment?

14. What types of bathroom equipment can be used to improve independence with toileting and bathing?

Case Studies

CASE STUDY 1

Mrs. R lives with her husband in a single-level home. She is 76 years old and has had chronic obstructive pulmonary disease (COPD) for 10 years. Mr. R is 82 and has had a mild stroke, leaving him with a slight memory impairment but no physical deficits. Mrs. R gets short of breath after 10 minutes of standing activity and then must rest. She has always taken care of the household chores. Mr. R is willing to assist but only helps with the household jobs if asked.

What further information is needed about the social situation?

What self-maintenance tasks may Mrs. R be having difficulty with?

How would the concepts of energy conservation and work simplification be applied to the difficult self-maintenance tasks?

What type of equipment might be used to improve Mrs. R's endurance?

What concerns might Mrs. R have about Mr. R's preparing a meal?

Describe several approaches or situations where Mr. R could be included in the treatment process.

CASE STUDY 2

Mr. D is a resident of a long-term-care facility. He has a history of a cerebral vascular accident (CVA), with a right hemiparesis. He is alert and oriented. He sits in a wheelchair all day, except when the nursing aide walks him once a day. When sitting he leans to the left and is unable to hold himself upright. He also is found at meals with food on his lap after he has eaten. He would like to be able to do more for himself.

Occupational therapy has been requested to evaluate Mr. D's self-feeding skills.

What information is needed from previous occupational therapy practitioners and staff working with Mr. D prior to beginning an evaluation?

List Mr. D's problems.

What is the first intervention to be addressed prior to evaluating self-feeding skills?

What type of adaptive equipment could improve seating and self-feeding?

What other areas of self-maintenance could be assessed?

References

ABLEDATA. (1990, May). Modular seating components (Fact sheet #10). ABLEDATA/NARIC, 8455 Colesville Road, Suite 935, Silver Spring, MD 20910. http://www.ABLEDATA.com

American Occupational Therapy Association (AOTA). (1994). Uniform terminology for occupational therapy (3rd ed.). *American Journal of Occupational Therapy, 48,* 1047–1054.

Bartol, M. A., & Heitkemper, M. (1979). Gastrointestinal problems. In D. Carnevali & M. Patrick (Eds.), *Nursing management for the elderly* (pp. 331–357). Toronto: J. B. Lippincott.

Bennett, J. (1979). Oral health maintenance. In D. Carnevali & M. Patrick (Eds.), *Nursing management for the elderly* (pp. 111–127). Toronto: J. B. Lippincott.

Ebert, N. (1989). Nutrition in the aged and the nursing process. In A. Yurick, B. Spier, S. Robb, & N. Ebert (Eds.), *The aged person and the nursing process* (pp. 563–569). San Mateo, CA: Appleton & Lange.

Feinberg, M., & Ekberg, O. (1991). Videofluoroscopy in elderly patients with aspiration: Importance of evaluating both oral and pharyngeal stages of deglutition. *American Journal of Roentography, 156,* 293–296.

Hittle, J., Pedretti, L. W., & Kasch, M. C. (1996). Rheumatoid arthritis. In L. W. Pedretti (Ed.), *Occupational therapy: Practice skills for physical dysfunction* (4th ed., pp. 639–660). St. Louis: Mosby-Year Book.

Kielhofner, G. (Ed.). (1985). *A model of human occupation.* Baltimore: Williams & Wilkins.

Logemann, J. (1983). *Evaluation and treatment of swallowing disorders.* San Diego, CA: College Hill.

Nelson, K. (1996). Dysphagia: Evaluation and treatment. In L. W. Pedretti (Ed.), *Occupational therapy: Practice skills for physical dysfunction* (4th ed.). St. Louis: Mosby-Year Book.

Specht, J., & Cordes, A. (1979). Incontinence. In D. Carnevali & M. Patrick (Eds.), *Nursing management for the elderly* (pp. 387–398). Toronto: J. B. Lippincott.

Tinnetti, M. (1987). Decreasing the risk of falling. *Clinical Report on Aging* (American Geriatrics Society), *1,* 15–16.

Wells, M., Chew, T., Lang, B., Campbell, B., & Chenderlin, J. (1988). Activities of daily living. In L. Davis & M. Kirkland (Eds.), *Role of occupational therapy with the elderly* (pp. 269–281). Rockville, MD: American Occupational Therapy Association.

Related Readings

Allen, C. K., Earhart, C., & Blue, T. (1992). *Occupational therapy treatment goals for the physically and cognitively disabled.* Rockville, MD: American Occupational Therapy Association.

Hopkins, H., & Smith, H. (Eds.). (1993). *Willard and Spackman's occupational therapy.* Philadelphia: J. B. Lippincott.

Kiernat, J. (1991). *Occupational therapy and the older adult.* Gaithersburg, MD: Aspen.

Lewis, S. (1989). *Elder care in occupational therapy.* Thorofare, NJ: SLACK.

Pedretti, L. W. (Ed.). (1996). *Occupational therapy: Practice skills for physical dysfunction* (4th ed.). St. Louis: Mosby-Year Book.

Section 2.
Prevention of Falls in the Elderly

Amy Cook, MS, OTR
Patricia A. Miller, MEd, OTR, FAOTA

Abstract

Falls are an important health concern for older persons and can lead to disability, fear, activity limitation, depression, loss of independence, and an overall increase in health care expenditures. Occupational therapists can play a vital role in preventing falls among older adults through careful assessment for potential fall risks and in implementing interventions that maintain the ability to perform activities safely and with satisfaction and confidence.

Demographics of Falls

Falls are a common occurrence among the older population, leading to potentially serious injury, reduced functional ability, and emotional distress. This section addresses the multifactoral nature of falls, methods of assessment for fall risks, and the occupational therapist's role in preventing falls and in reducing the negative consequences of a fall.

Approximately 95% of the older adult population in the United States reside in the community (Reinsch, MacRae, Lachenbruch, & Tobis, 1992), and about one third of community-dwelling elderly persons over the age of 65 fall each year (Tinetti, Speechley, & Ginter, 1988). Although only 5% of the elderly population reside in nursing homes, the fall rate among this population is twice that of the community-dwelling elderly (Neufeld et al.,

1991). Accidents are the fifth leading cause of death in older persons in this country (Watzke & Kemp, 1992), with falls being the leading type of accident that causes death in the elderly (Reinsch et al., 1992).

While not all falls result in fatality, the consequences can still be severe. The statistical probability of an older person's suffering a fracture after a fall is 1 in 3, and approximately 200,000 of such fractures occur at the hip (Bear-Lehman, 1995; Deily, 1989; Kiernat, 1991; Tinetti, 1986). Falling can lead to loss of independence, inactivity, decreased mobility, medical complications, depression, and fear of falling (Reinsch et al., 1992; Tideiksaar, 1991). In long-term care institutions, falls may result in increased financial burdens for facilities: the cost of caring for patients with hip fractures, for example, is more than $750 million annually (Parent, 1990).

Causes of Falls

Falls are usually due to a combination of both intrinsic and extrinsic factors, making the nature of falls a complex, multifactorial issue (Tideiksaar, 1991). Intrinsic factors may include sensory loss or changes, syncope, hemiplegia, hypotension, cardiac problems, balance impairment, gait impairment, progressive neurological disorders, decreased range of motion and muscle strength, side effects of medications, cognitive or perceptual impairment, vertigo, or any disease state that may influence mobility (Tideiksaar, 1989; 1991). One study by Tinetti (1986) found several intrinsic factors to be closely related to falls risk, including balance and gait abnormalities, and musculoskeletal difficulties such as decreased knee strength and the presence of imbalance during neck movements. A later study revealed that mental status, use of sedatives, podiatric problems, vision, hearing, and reflexes also strongly contribute to falls risks (National Institute on Aging [U.S. Department of Health and Human Services] [DHHS], 1990). According to Berkman and Miller (1991), the causes and results of falls are cyclical in nature, "whereby the fall leads to restriction of activity, loss of autonomy and self-confidence, depression and anxiety, deconditioning, possible prescription for psychoactive drugs, subsequently placing the individual at increased risk for falling" (p. 34).

Intrinsic emotional factors such as depression, anxiety, and fear can also cause falls, because emotional difficulties can cause a reduction in autonomic nervous system responses or in concentration that may place the person at risk for falling. Frequently, older persons may deny the fact that they are at risk for falls. A consequence of denial is the exhibition of high-risk fall behavior. Extrinsic factors involve the environment surrounding the person, such as placement of furniture, existence of obstacles, use of assistive walking devices, lighting, stairs, presence of pets, or any other object in the person's environment that may put one at risk for falls.

Prevention of Falls

By identifying those at risk for falls and employing methods of prevention, practitioners can curtail the severe physical, emotional, and economic consequences of falls. According to Tideiksaar (1991), "The cornerstone of fall prevention is a thorough clinical evaluation to identify [those] at risk and a careful assessment of the causes" (p. 12). The prevention model consists of the following three levels of prevention:

1. Primary Prevention: Primary prevention of falls involves imparting information to older persons, their families, and caregivers about risk factors and prevention of falls. This is achieved through indirect service, consultation, education, and advocacy (Miller, 1988). Examples of primary prevention are developing a protocol for environmental modification and elimination of fall risks in a senior housing complex.

2. Secondary Prevention: Secondary prevention consists of eliminating factors that may cause a fall. This prevention can be accomplished through a biopsychosocial assessment of clients, making referrals to appropriate services, and beginning direct treatment (Miller, 1988). For example, after a practitioner visits a client's home, recommendations to secure loose carpeting, move cluttered furniture, obtain stronger prescription glasses, use adequate lighting, and other environmental modification to match the individual's needs are secondary preventive measures. A further example is conducting a safety education group at an adult day care center for participants specifically deemed at risk for falls. Many of these participants have experienced a fall without, as yet, sustaining serious consequences.

3. Tertiary Prevention: Unfortunately, many older persons are seen after a fall, when hospitalization occurs for fractures or related complications. Tertiary prevention involves provision of restorative therapy in order to remediate deficits after a fall injury occurs (Miller, 1988). Dealing with a fall after hospitalization is the least cost-effective method of preventing future falls.

Falls and the Role of Occupational Therapy

Because of the multifactorial nature of falls, an occupational therapy frame of reference in assessing and treating problems related to falls should encompass these multiple factors. An activities health (Cynkin & Robinson, 1990) approach takes into account all the activities of a person and how that person's perception of a balance between work, leisure, and self-care activities leads to activities health. The Model of Human Occupation (Keilhofner, 1995) examines the intrinsic and extrinsic factors that guide human occupation. A prevention model (described above) involves detecting potential problems before they occur, when they are just beginning, or when intensive interventions are required that reduce or eliminate fall risks. Application of these frames of reference to occupational therapy interventions related to falling are therapeutic, empowering of older persons, congruent with occupational therapy principles, and cost effective.

While some published writings exist on falling in the occupational therapy literature (Deily, 1989; Walker & Howland, 1991), this topic needs further exploration. No published studies in the occupational therapy literature ascertain whether occupational therapists are actually assessing for falls in their patients. One unpublished exploratory study on falls examined whether health professionals in a metropolitan university hospital (physicians, physical therapists, occupational therapists, nurses) were conducting falls assessments with their patients (Beres, Elmore, & Miller, 1990). The study revealed that out of the 23 subjects only 11 were assessed for falls risks, with only one of those assessments conducted by an occupational therapist. An unpublished document, the "Falls Safety Self Study Packet," was developed by Colmar and Carey (1995). This document provides guidelines for assessing the home environment and risk of falling. Colmar and Carey have made their home health care staff much more aware of fall risks in the elderly (Hettinger, 1995).

Because of further interest in determining whether occupational therapists are considering falls when assessing and treating their patients, a pilot study through a telephone survey was conducted using a sample of convenience. Occupational therapy department heads of health care facilities, which included two rehabilitation hospitals, two long-term care facilities, one acute care setting, one mental health setting, and one home health care service, responded. Out of seven facilities, only one routinely screened for falls risks in all patients as part of an initial occupational therapy assessment. None of the facilities uses formalized fall risk assessments. One long-term care facility provided tertiary falls intervention by assessing and intervening in wheelchair positioning after a reported falling incident. As part of treatment, one facility routinely engaged in primary prevention by educating all of their rehabilitation patients about proper ways to stand, transfer, and get up after a fall. A home health service reported that a specific falls assessment was not included on the occupational therapy evaluation form and that methods for assessing for falls were not standardized. Three facilities reported that other disciplines are more involved in fall prevention, such as nursing or physical therapy, and that occupational therapy is called in only after a fall occurs.

Many falls occur during the performance of daily living activities (DHHS, 1990). Because the fundamental premise of occupational therapy is to assist individuals to achieve optimal functioning in performance of daily living activities, gerontic occupational therapists should consider the need to assess, prevent, and intervene for fall risks routinely.

ASSESSING FOR FALLS

Because falls are multifactorial in nature, assessment for falls should be multifactorial and should include tools that rely on observation of performance, patient self-report, and interview of family or caregivers. Several falls assessment and screening tools exist that are appropriate for use by occupational therapists.

Berkman and Miller (1991) developed a therapist-administered, semistructured Falls Interview Schedule (FIS) (Appendix 1) as part of a larger falls questionnaire, which relies on community-dwelling patients to provide information on their history of falling. While validity and reliability have not been established for this instrument, it has been piloted several times. Modifi-cations were made, and results indicated that subjects were comfortable with the interview and able to provide therapists with crucial information about their fall history. The FIS serves as a screening tool, enabling occupational therapists to determine when further assessment and interventions to reduce or eliminate fall risks are indicated.

Tinetti, Richman, and Powell (1990) developed a valid and reliable self-report tool called the Falls Efficacy Scale (Tinetti, Mendes, Doucette, & Baker, 1994), which was modified by Berkman and Miller (1991) and Cook and Malloy (1991). According to Tinetti et al. (1994), falls efficacy is defined as the subjective level of confidence persons feel they have in performing basic and instrumental activi-ties of daily living without sustaining a fall. The modified Falls Efficacy Scale measures a person's level of confidence in performing 14 activities, on a Likert scale of 1 to 5, 1 meaning no confidence and 5 meaning very confident. Although subjective on the part of the patient, this tool can provide the therapist with information on the person's level of confidence in performing activities and to what extent, if at all, a fear of falling exists. An example is asking the patient whether he or she has stopped taking a bath or shower or has reduced the frequency of either. The therapist next records whether the person has either stopped or reduced participation of this activity or has no problem with this activity. Then the client is asked to rate confidence in bathing or showering, on the 1 to 5 scale. Confidence scale results are also recorded. A low total confidence score denotes low falls efficacy and should alert the therapist that the client may be restricting activities out of a fear of falling. Other examples of activities that are questioned are climbing up or down stairs, doing light housekeeping, answering the door or phone, and getting in and out of bed.

Assessment of movement and neuromuscular performance are other methods of detecting fall risks in the elderly. Tinetti (1986) recommended using a performance-oriented mobility evaluation that looks at gait and balance. (A copy of such a tool may be found in Gallo, Reichel, and Andersen, 1995.) The clinician observes the older person walking and carefully examines the sequences involved in gait. The client is then observed during a series of balance tests, such as rising from a chair, standing balanced with eyes closed, or completing a 360-degree turn while standing. The therapist then rates the client's performance after observation, giving a numerical score for normal, adaptive, or abnormal for each component of gait and balance assessed. The lower the score, the more at risk the person may be for falling.

For example, when observing a client rising from a chair, a normal score would involve the client's rising in a single movement without assistance of arms; an adaptive score would involve the client rising while using the arms to push up; and an abnormal score would involve multiple attempts to rise or being unable to rise without human assistance (Gallo et al., 1995; Tinetti, 1986). The results of this assessment can provide the therapist with an understanding of how gait or balance performance may put the patient at risk for falls. It is important for occupational therapists to apply this information to occupational performance by examining the components of gait and balance a client may be having difficulty with and by relating it to specific activities. For example, persons who demonstrate balance difficulties while standing with their eyes closed may be at risk for falls when pulling a shirt over their heads while standing. By looking at specific components of gait and balance, the practitioner can use the information to educate clients in ways to avoid or modify certain movements or activities.

It is imperative that the environment of the older person be carefully assessed in order to control the extrinsic factors that cause falls. A comprehensive environmental checklist ascertains fall risks in all rooms of the household and includes the environs of the residence, such as outer stairs, sidewalks, or thresholds. Tideiksaar (1986) and Berkman and Miller (1991) developed comprehensive environmental checklists that examine risks in the household. Tideiksaar's (1986) checklist provided information on correcting environmental hazards with a rationale for each correction. Berkman and Miller's checklist (1991) divided the home environment into the categories of exterior, interior, kitchen, bathroom, and bedroom. Each category contains specific questions about potential hazards, with a total of 48 questions making up the tool. Each question requires the therapist to rate whether there is a general fall hazard and whether it poses a hazard for the *specific individual* being assessed.

Making a determination between what is a general hazard and what is a hazard for a particular individual is important to consider when evaluating the environment. For example, persons whose stairs are not outlined with contrasting colored tape may not necessarily be at risk for falling on those stairs unless they have a visual deficit that would necessitate such an intervention (see Appendix B). Because clients are sometimes resistant to preventive environmental changes, this assessment helps the therapist to prioritize recommendations for modifying the environment on the basis of immediate needs. Recommendations are more easily accepted by the client when "felt" and when "real" needs are met.

Tideiksaar (1989, 1991) developed the acronym "SPLAT" to guide assessing and remediating falls risks, which may be used after a fall occurs: S=symptoms; P=previous falls; L=location; A=activity; T=time. Examining these five factors can assist the therapist to determine how persons felt during the fall, whether they had fallen before, where they have fallen, what they were doing, and when they fell. This examination may help establish a pattern surrounding a person's falls so that future falls can be prevented through modification of the environment or activity performance.

Because most falls occur during the performance of activities (U.S. DHHS,

1990), older persons should be observed performing activities of daily living in order to assess for potential risks. Activities that involve bending, reaching, or walking are best observed, for example, while a patient prepares a meal in the kitchen, does laundry, or puts on shoes.

OCCUPATIONAL THERAPY INTERVENTION

Occupational therapists can use a variety of interventions when remediating problems related to falls. Educating caregivers and family about falls risks and falls prevention is imperative, particularly if the older person is dependent on others for certain aspects of care, for example, in a skilled nursing facility or during home care visits. Older persons should explore their daily activity patterns and discuss those they perform and those they avoid. Reasons for avoidance, such as fear of falling, should be explored and remediation should take place if appropriate.

Encouraging the older person to turn on lights, tack down rugs, move objects to arm's reach, or remove extension cords may save that person from an injurious fall. Asking persons to modify their environments takes care and understanding. Many persons are reluctant to change their homes, particularly if they have been set up a certain way for many years. Establishing a level of trust; making recommendations slowly; giving a person choices; and, most important, engaging the person in the problem-solving process are ways to institute this type of change.

Cognitive-behavioral therapy (Beck, Rush, Shaw, & Emery, 1979), in conjunction with traditional occupational therapy, may be a successful mode of changing a person's perceptions about falls when that person has excessive fear of falling or other psychological

consequences (Berkman & Miller, 1991). This method involves using activities that perform the following functions:

- Improve concentration and learning.
- Examine fantasied consequences of feared behavior (e.g., walking outside or transferring to the bathtub).
- Question negative cognitions (e.g., "I'm too old to change").
- Teach relaxation techniques.
- Establish realistic short- and long-term goals in order to instill hope.
- Promote problem solving in order to learn to cope with chronic illness or disability and to develop healthy activity performance (Berkman & Miller, 1991).

An example of changing maladaptive cognitions to positive, adaptive thinking follows. Frail, older, depressed homebound patients may spend a lot of their days napping in a chair or spending time in bed stating, "I have nothing to do and I'm too tired to do anything." When functional activities are suggested by therapists, patients refuse with that or a similar refrain. Inactivity leads to disuse atrophy, a deconditioned state, and an increased risk for falls. This cycle often fosters further depression and fear of falling. Using a cognitive-behavioral approach, therapists need to question the reasoning of patients who are napping and inactive all day. One patient might say, "If I do anything, I'll feel worse." The therapist can gently challenge this by stating, "You feel pretty bad now, don't you? Do you really know that you'll feel worse if we do something together?" Or, "Let's see if you really do feel worse if you get out of bed and we do something together for a little while." If patients agree to try an activity, the negative cognitions can be explicitly stated after completion of the activity and compared to the more positive thoughts from having had a successful experience.

Grading activities to reduce fear of falling and teaching safer activity performance are other important occupational therapy interventions. For example, a client who is reluctant to transfer to a shower chair out of fear of falling on a hard, slippery surface can practice such a transfer in another room of the house (e.g., with a chair placed on a carpeted living room floor next to a wall) until he or she is comfortable with the concept of using such a shower chair. Once simulated activity has helped to establish confidence, the activity can be graded so that the client tries it on a floor without a carpet and, finally, in the bathtub with the presence of a nonslip mat and grab bars.

Summary

Falls can be due to intrinsic or extrinsic factors. Falls can limit mobility as a result of fractures, cause soft tissue injuries, cause atrophy from disuse, limit activity, or promote excessive fear. Some people even deny the risk of falls and carry out potentially hazardous risk-taking behaviors. Occupational therapists, with expertise in activity performance, can play a crucial role in preventing or remediating fall risks. Routinely including a falls assessment in all evaluations of older persons is recommended in order to prevent falls from occurring, and intervenion is recommended when indicated. Because of the holistic philosophy and education of occupational therapy practitioners, they are qualified to recommend environmental and activity modifications and to suggest helping the individual change maladaptive behaviors to adaptive behaviors, thereby preventing or reducing numbers of falls and increasing quality of life for older persons.

Review Questions

1. List four intrinsic factors that may cause falls in older persons.
2. List four extrinsic factors that are potential fall risks.
3. How can an occupational therapy practitioner play a role in preventing older persons from sustaining a first fall?
4. Describe two occupational therapy frames of reference that guide fall assessment and intervention.
5. Name two assessment instruments that can assist in identifying the etiology of falls and guide occupational therapy interventions.
6. Describe a treatment strategy that may be useful with an older person who has discontinued engagement in several activities of daily living because of fear of falling.

Case Study

Mrs. S is a 74-year-old woman who underwent a girdlestone procedure of the left hip, prompted by repeated difficulties with several left hip replacements, beginning at age 51. Significant medical conditions included osteoarthritis and insulin-dependent diabetes mellitus. After being in traction for 4 weeks, followed by a 2-week course of inpatient rehabilitation (both occupational and physical therapy), Mrs. S was discharged home to receive home care therapy. Left hip precautions included weight-bearing precautions of 10–15 pounds. Occupational therapy orders were for ADL evaluation and treatment.

Mrs. S resided in a one-story home with her husband. Prior to the surgery, she was an active member of her local planning board, drove a car, and engaged in all housekeeping tasks. Her roles include that of mother, grandmother, and wife. Much of her day, prior to her illness, involved preparation for planning board meetings, with long hours of attendance at weekly meetings. In the early weeks of home care therapy, she was greatly limited in fulfilling her role as a planning board member, which was a very important role to her.

An occupational therapy evaluation revealed normal bilateral upper-extremity strength and active range of motion. Left hip flexion was limited to 0–20 degrees. She ambulated with a walker and had to wear an elevated shoe on her left foot to compensate for shortness of the left leg. Cognition was normal and the patient was cooperative and motivated for treatment. Visual perceptual functioning was good, except for some minor deficits in visual acuity. The patient's affect was bright, although she did have some complaints about being inactive and homebound. The patient needed minor assistance with basic activities of daily living. She needed moderate to maximum assistance with instrumental activities of daily living, particularly cooking and laundry. A falls assessment included an environmental checklist (Berkman & Miller, 1991) and administration of a performance-oriented gait and balance tool (Tinetti, 1986). Mrs. S was able to compensate well and showed many adaptive behaviors during the balance and gait assessment. Many movements were limited, however, because of the hip precautions and inability to flex her hip beyond 20 degrees. Bending and reaching, by impairing balance and stability, seemed to put her most at risk for falls. Her home was generally safe, except for the placement of throw rugs and small items on the kitchen floor. Moreover, she tended to walk throughout the house with the lights off.

The occupational therapy treatment program involved basic and instrumental ADL retraining and provision of assistive devices, as well as instruction in activity modifications. Recommendations were made to Mrs. S, her husband, and her home health aide regarding minor environmental modifications. One of the most significant modifications was removing throw rugs and moving commonly used items found in the kitchen and laundry to lower areas to increase ease in access. Therapy sessions also involved constant reinforcement to turn on lights, close closet doors, and remove clutter from kitchen floor areas. With repetition, and active participation by the patient in problem solving, instructions for changes were easily followed and accepted.

Mrs. S accomplished the goals of therapy and was independent in all her basic and instrumental daily living activities with compensation and assistive devices after a 4-week course of occupational therapy, twice a week. Toward the end of therapy, she was turning on lights when entering every room and was vigilant about avoiding chair legs and other fall risks. She worked slowly on all activity completion. She attended her first planning board meeting after being home for 4 weeks.

Appendix A.
Falls Interview Schedule (FIS)

Instructions: Circle or fill in the correct response as indicated.

1. Have you fallen in the past year?   Yes   No   DK   NA

2. Have you had any times where you almost fell?   Yes   No   DK   NA

3. How many times have you fallen?   _____times

4. How many times have you almost fallen?   _____times

   Were you tripped, did you slip, or were you shaky
   when you stood up?   Yes   No   DK   NA

5. Tell me about the most recent time you fell.

   a. When did it happen?
      within the past week ____; within 2–4 weeks ____;
      within 1–3 months ____; within 3–6 months ____;
      more than 6 months ____; don't remember ____

   b. How did it happen?
      (What were you doing immediately before the fall?
      What caused the fall?)_____

      _____

      _____

   c. What time of day did the fall occur? __:___ a.m.; ___:___ p.m.

   d. How difficult was it for you to get up after the fall?
      no/almost no difficulty ____; some difficulty ____;
      a lot of difficulty ____; couldn't get up without someone's help ____

   e. How long was it before you got up? ____ minutes; _____ hours

   f. Did you hurt yourself? _____ yes _____ no _____ don't remember

   g. Where exactly did you hurt yourself?
      arm ____; leg ____; hand ____; foot ____;
      hip ____; head ____; other (explain) _____

   h. What kind of injury was it?
      cut ___; bruise ___; muscle strain ___; hip fracture ___; wrist fracture ___
      head injury ___; other (explain)_____

   i. How long did it take your injury (or injuries) to heal?
      less than one week ____; one month ____; 3–6 months ____;
      6–12 months____; more than one year ____; don't remember ____

   j. How much is that fall on your mind?
      never/not much ____; somewhat ____; a great deal ____

   k. Did you tell anyone about the fall?   Yes   No   DK   NA

   l. Whom did you tell? _____

   m. What did this person say or do for you?

      _____

      _____

n. Do you still have problems as a result of the fall, such as pain or limited movement?   Yes   No   DK   NA

o. Are there ways for you to prevent this particular type of fall from happening again?   Yes   No   DK   NA

p. How much do you worry about falling? _____ never; _____ sometimes; _____ frequently; _____ always

6. Comments: _____

_____

_____

_____

(If patient answered 2 or more times to question #3, continue.)

7. "Tell me about another fall you had this year," and then repeat all of the questions in #5 for each fall.

This is an unscored interview. Checks are used for ease of administration and to review findings expeditiously.

Appendix B.
Home Assessment Checklist for Fall Hazards
(Examples from checklist)

	Checklist (Circle one)				Represents Hazards for This Person? (Circle one)		
Exterior							
1. Are step surfaces nonslip?	Yes	No	DK	NA	Yes	No	DK
2. Are step edges visually marked to avoid tripping?	Yes	No	DK	NA	Yes	No	DK
3. Are steps in good repair?	Yes	No	DK	NA	Yes	No	DK
4. Are stairway handrails present?	Yes	No	DK	NA	Yes	No	DK
5. Are stairway handrails securely fastened to fittings?	Yes	No	DK	NA	Yes	No	DK
6. Are walkways covered with a nonslip surface?	Yes	No	DK	NA	Yes	No	DK
7. Are walkways free of objects that could be tripped over?	Yes	No	DK	NA	Yes	No	DK
8. Is there sufficient outdoor lighting to provide safe ambulation at night?	Yes	No	DK	NA	Yes	No	DK
9. Are lights bright enough to compensate for limited vision?	Yes	No	DK	NA	Yes	No	DK
10. Are light switches accessible to the person before entering room?	Yes	No	DK	NA	Yes	No	DK
11. Are lights glare free?	Yes	No	DK	NA	Yes	No	DK
12. Are stairways adequately lighted?	Yes	No	DK	NA	Yes	No	DK
13. Are handrails present on both sides of staircases?	Yes	No	DK	NA	Yes	No	DK
14. Are handrails securely fastened to walls?	Yes	No	DK	NA	Yes	No	DK
15. Are step edges outlined with colored adhesive tape and slip resistant?	Yes	No	DK	NA	Yes	No	DK
16. Are throw rugs secured with nonslip backing?	Yes	No	DK	NA	Yes	No	DK
17. Are carpet edges taped or tacked down?	Yes	No	DK	NA	Yes	No	DK
18. Are rooms uncluttered to permit unobstructed mobility?	Yes	No	DK	NA	Yes	No	DK
19. Are chairs throughout home strong enough to provide support during transfers?	Yes	No	DK	NA	Yes	No	DK

Home Assessment Checklist for Fall Hazards (continued)

	Checklist (Circle one)				Represents Hazards for This Person? (Circle one)		
Interior							
20. Are armrests present on chairs to provide assistance while transferring?	Yes	No	DK	NA	Yes	No	DK
21. Are tables (dining room, kitchen, etc.) secure enough to provide support if leaned on?	Yes	No	DK	NA	Yes	No	DK
22. Is the room free of low-lying objects (coffee table, step stools, etc.)?	Yes	No	DK	NA	Yes	No	DK
23. Are telephones accessible?							
24. Is there an absence of high pile or shag rugs?	Yes	No	DK	NA	Yes	No	DK
25. Is there an absence of electrical cords on or near the floor?	Yes	No	DK	NA	Yes	No	DK
26. Is there an absence of dogs or cats?	Yes	No	DK	NA	Yes	No	DK
Kitchen							
27. Are storage areas easily reached without having to stand on tiptoe or chair?	Yes	No	DK	NA	Yes	No	DK
28. Are linoleum floors nonslip?	Yes	No	DK	NA	Yes	No	DK
29. Is there a nonslip mat in the sink area to soak up spilled water?	Yes	No	DK	NA	Yes	No	DK
30. Are chairs wheelfree, armrest equipped, and of the proper height to allow for safe transfers?	Yes	No	DK	NA	Yes	No	DK
31. Are step stools strong enough to provide support and are treads in good repair and slip resistant?	Yes	No	DK	NA	Yes	No	DK
Bathroom							
32. Are doors wide enough to provide unobstructed entering with or without a device?	Yes	No	DK	NA	Yes	No	DK
33. Are there raised door thresholds?	Yes	No	DK	NA	Yes	No	DK

Home Assessment Checklist for Fall Hazards (continued)

	Checklist (Circle one)				Represents Hazards for This Person? (Circle one)		
34. Are floors not slippery, especially when wet?	Yes	No	DK	NA	Yes	No	DK
35. Are skid-proof strips or mats in place in the tub or shower?	Yes	No	DK	NA	Yes	No	DK
36. Are tub or shower grab bars available?	Yes	No	DK	NA	Yes	No	DK
37. Are tub or shower grab bars securely fastened to the walls?	Yes	No	DK	NA	Yes	No	DK
38. Are toilet grab bars available?	Yes	No	DK	NA	Yes	No	DK
39. Are toilet grab bars securely fastened to the walls?	Yes	No	DK	NA	Yes	No	DK
40. Is an elevated toilet seat available to assist in toilet transfers?	Yes	No	DK	NA	Yes	No	DK
41. Is there sufficient, accesssible, and glare-free light available?	Yes	No	DK	NA	Yes	No	DK
Bedroom							
42. Is there adequate and accessible lighting available?	Yes	No	DK	NA	Yes	No	DK
43. Are nighlights or bedside lamps available for night-time bathroom trips?	Yes	No	DK	NA	Yes	No	DK
44. Is the pathway from the bed to the bathroom free of hazards or obstacles (e.g. objects, loose rugs, thresholds) that might obstruct mobility (especially at night)?	Yes	No	DK	NA	Yes	No	DK
45. Are beds of appropriate height and firmness to allow for safe on and off transfers?	Yes	No	DK	NA	Yes	No	DK
46. Are floors covered with a nonslip surface?	Yes	No	DK	NA	Yes	No	DK
47. Are floors free of objects that could be tripped over?	Yes	No	DK	NA	Yes	No	DK
48. Can a person reach objects from closet shelves without standing on tiptoe or a chair?	Yes	No	DK	NA	Yes	No	DK

Source: From Berkman, C., & Miller, P. A. (1991). Falls interview schedule. Comprehensive falls questionnaire for community-dwelling elders. In P. Miller, *Programs in occupational therapy* (pp. 40–42). New York: Columbia University.

References

Bear-Lehman, J. (1995). Orthopaedic conditions. In C. A. Trombly (Ed.), *Occupational therapy for physical dysfunction* (4th ed., pp. 753–772). Baltimore: Williams & Wilkins.

Beck, A. T., Rush, A. J., Shaw, B. F., & Emery, G. (1979). *Cognitive therapy and depression.* New York: Guilford Press.

Beres, D., Elmore, D. B., & Miller, P. A. (1990). *The circumstances and consequences of falls among the elderly: An exploratory study.* Unpublished master's research project. Columbia University, New York.

Berkman, C., & Miller, P. A. (1991). Falls interview schedule. Comprehensive falls questionnaire for community-dwelling elders. In P. Miller, *Programs in occupational therapy* (pp. 40–42). New York: Columbia University.

Berkman, C., & Miller, P. A. (1991). *Reducing dysfunctional sequelae of falls in the elderly.* Unpublished manuscript, Columbia University, New York.

Colmar, M., & Carey, M. (1995). *Falls safety self study packet.* Unpublished manuscript. Adventist Health Care Mid-Atlantic, Adventist Home Health Services (AHHS), 10800 Lockwood Drive, Silver Spring, MD 20901.

Cook, A. G., & Malloy, L. M. (1991). *Comparison of methods for evaluating fear of falling in older adults: a pilot study.* Unpublished master's research project. Columbia University, New York.

Cynkin, S., & Robinson, A. (1990). *Occupational therapy and activities health: Toward health through activities.* Boston: Little, Brown.

Deily, J. (1989). Home safety program for older adults. *OT in Health Care, 6,* 113–124.

Gallo, J. J., Reichel, W., & Andersen, L. M. (1995). *Handbook of geriatric assessment* (2nd ed.). Gaithersburg, MD: Aspen.

Hettinger, J. (1995, September 14). Falling down. *OT Week,* pp. 18–19.

Kielhofner, G. (1995). *A model of human occupation: Theory and application* (2nd ed.). Baltimore: Williams & Wilkins.

Kiernat, J. M. (1991). Preventing falls in the hospital and home. In. J. M. Kiernat (Ed.), *Occupational therapy and the older adult* (pp. 123–136). Gaithersburg, MD: Aspen.

Miller, P. A. (1988). Preventive treatment approaches. In L. J. Davis & M. Kirkland (Eds.), *The role of occupational therapy with the elderly* (pp. 227–235). Rockville, MD.: American Occupational Therapy Association.

Neufeld, R. R., Tideiksaar, R., Yew, E., Brooks, F., Young, J., Browne, G., & Hsu, M. (1991). A multidisciplinary falls consultation service in a nursing home. *The Gerontologist, 31,* 120–123.

Parent, L. H. (1990). Orthopedic conditions. In C. A. Trombly (Ed.), *Occupational therapy for physical dysfunction* (3rd ed., pp. 531–542). Baltimore: Williams & Wilkins.

Reinsch, S., MacRae, P., Lachenbruch, P. A., & Tobis, J. S. (1992). Attempts to prevent falls and injury: A prospective community study. *The Gerontologist, 32,* 450–456.

Tideiksaar, R. (1986). Preventing falls: Home hazard checklists to help older patients protect themselves. *Geriatrics, 41.*

Tideiksaar, R. (1989). Geriatric falls: Assessing the cause, preventing recurrence. *Geriatrics, 44,* 57–61.

Tideiksaar, R. (1991). Falls in nursing home residents. *Long-Term Care Forum, Fall,* 12–14.

Tinetti, M.E. (1986). Performance-oriented assessment of mobility problems in elderly patients. *Journal of the American Geriatrics Society, 34,* 119–126.

Tinetti, M. E., Mendes, C. F., Doucette, J. T., & Baker, D. I. (1994). Fear of falling and fall-related efficacy in relationship to functioning among community-living elders. *Journal of Gerontology: Medical Sciences, 49,* 140–147.

Tinetti, M. E., Richman, D., & Powell, L. (1990). Falls efficacy as a measure of fear of falling. *Journal of Gerontology, 45,* 239–243.

Tinetti, M. E., Speechley, M., & Ginter, S. F. (1988). Risk factors for falls among elderly pesons living in the community. *New England Journal of Medicine, 319,* 1701–1707.

U.S. Department of Health and Human Services (DHSS), Public Health Service, National Institutes of Health. (1990). *National institute on aging special report on aging 1990.* Washington, DC: Author.

Walker, J. E., & Howland, J. (1991). Falls and fear of falling among elderly persons living in the community: Occupational therapy interventions. *The American Journal of Occupational Therapy, 45,* 119–122.

Watzke J. R., & Kemp, B. (1992). Safety for older adults: The role of technology and the home environment. *Topics in Geriatric Rehabilitation, 7,* 9–21.

Section 3. Transportation

Susan Pierce, OTR, CDRS

Abstract

Driving is important to older persons because it enables them to be independent, but many age-related impairments can affect driving ability. Occupational therapists who specialize in driver rehabilitation services can provide interventions to help older drivers keep their mobility.

Demographics

In 1900, 4% of the population was 65 or older. By the late 1980s, 12% of the population was in this age group. Of 165 million licensed drivers in the 1990s, more than 22 million are age 65 or older (Retchin & Anapolle, 1993). It is projected that by the year 2000, licensed drivers over 55 years of age will account for more than 25% of the total driving population (Malfetti, 1985). More than 50 million older persons will be eligible to drive, and almost half of these drivers will be 75 or older (Transportation Research Board, 1988).

On the one hand, the Transportation Research Board stated that 80% of trips by those 65 and over are made in automobiles, and this percentage is continuing to increase (Transportation Research Board, 1988). On the other hand, the emphasis that American society puts on mobility places those who are not as mobile at a severe disadvantage. The lack of accessible or effective public transportation can hinder an older person's lifestyle and survival greatly.

Driving as an Activity of Daily Living

Activities of daily living (ADLs) in the older adult take on a different perspective than in the younger adult still working at a full-time job and years from retirement. Despite the different priorities for road travel, mobility in the community remains important and imperative for the old and young alike. Without a mode of transportation, a person has no access to medical treatment, food, medications, and other necessary services for survival. Bonnie Kantor, director of Ohio State University's Office of Geriatrics and Gerontology stated that "older people's number one fear isn't death—it's losing their independence and becoming burdens to their loved ones" (Blum, 1993). Driving in this country is equated with independence; therefore, when older persons have to give up their driver's license, they know in reality they are giving up their independence. According to Kantor, when older adults stop driving, their ability to function goes down, with a corresponding increase in depression and isolation, and even nutritional problems, because many older people regularly eat out (Blum, 1993).

Driving is one of the most complex activities of daily living that persons of any age perform in their daily routine. It is an activity that is performed on a daily basis for many miles with no thought of the skills involved in moving and handling a vehicle in an ever-changing traffic environment. Driving is an overlearned task that involves areas and skills that can be significantly affected by the aging process. It entails the use of skills in many performance components including the sensorimotor (vision, visual processing, visual perception, and physical capacities); cognitive; and psychosocial. Driving is a decision-making process that is dependent on perceptions and judgments. Because 85 to 90% of the perceptions in driving are visual, driving and visual perception are closely related. Drivers must not only see objects in the path of travel but also understand their implications for safety in order to adjust their driving accordingly (Milone, 1985).

Age-Related Impairments Affect Driving

Driving abilities can be impaired as a result of adverse drug effects or many age-related factors such as physiologic changes and age-associated diseases such as arthritis, cataracts, memory loss, and hearing loss. As visual functioning declines in the elderly person, that person must understand how this visual decline can affect driving performance. For example, a person who suffers a CVA and has resulting homonymous hemianopsia does not have the 120 degrees of total peripheral field of vision required in most states to drive. A person with cataracts or glaucoma may not have adequate vision to drive at night or may have poor glare recovery.

A slowing of physical functioning can affect reaction time in responding to something in the environment. The loss of strength or range of motion can prevent the person from operating the vehicle's primary or secondary controls safely. A decline in cognitive functioning can significantly alter a person's performance in traffic so that decision-making capabilities are slow and inadequate concentration and poor judgment exist. Poor insight into the diagnosis or problem areas can be very dangerous as the driver may not be aware of the serious mistakes he or she makes while driving.

Driver Assessment

Some decreases in physical function can be accommodated with various kinds of adaptive equipment or driving aids, such as a left foot gas pedal or hand controls. Loss of neck range of motion can be accommodated by special panoramic mirrors. What is misunderstood by many is that compensatory techniques with special equipment for driving only assist with the task of controlling a vehicle and do not resolve the older driver's declining functional skills. A comprehensive driver assessment conducted by an occupational therapist specializing in driver rehabilitation services can consider all performance components that can be affected by the person's age, diagnosis, or disability. Occupational therapists can explain how limitations in any of these areas are affecting the driver's abilities to control a vehicle and to react appropriately and safely in traffic. They have the background and understanding to interpret the driving behavior observed in traffic and to judge exactly what is needed so the older driver can remain on the road safely. If the person requires special equipment, instruction and training on the devices in a dual-controlled vehicle is crucial to prevent any accidents while the person is becoming familiar with the devices and before he or she begins to drive alone. The older driver generally requires a longer period of training as adaptation involves breaking old habits, for example, using hand controls instead of the feet for pedal operation.

In the past 20 years court precedent has been established that makes physicians responsible for protecting the public health, even when it may conflict with the patient's right to privacy and confidentiality. This duty to warn has been increasingly recognized by the courts and has consequently extended the physician's liability to third parties. As America's passion for lawsuits continues to rise, the medical doctor and other professionals treating older drivers should take careful consideration of the necessity of having them appropriately evaluated for safe driving skills if there is any question about their skill level.

As driving is an activity of daily living, the occupational therapist is the most logical team member to make sure this issue is addressed, whether the therapist works in a rehabilitation or temporary residential care facility or through a home health agency. If the older person is not being seen for rehabilitation, the primary care physician will often be the first professional to identify deficits in skills that may affect driving performance. The Department of Motor Vehicles may demand an evaluation if the older driver is involved in a collision, receives a ticket, or is reported for unsafe driving behavior. In any case, the physician or Department of Motor Vehicles should know the community resources that offer driver rehabilitation services. The social and ethical dilemma faced by the medical profession and the Department of Motor Vehicles and Driver Licensing is to attempt a balance between protecting the older adult's privilege to drive and the safety of other road users, including pedestrians, other drivers, and vehicle passengers.

Preventing Accident and Injury

Another area of concern is the susceptibility of older adults to more serious injury than younger adults in motor vehicle accidents. Current statistics from the Transportation Research Board show that drivers 75 and over are more at risk of crash involvement than the average driver.

Older occupants in vehicles are much more likely to be severely injured or killed than middle-aged occupants in crashes of equal severity. Specifically, their data show that people 65 and older are more than three times more likely to die than a 20-year-old occupant from injuries of equal severity (Transportation Research Board, 1988). Motor vehicle injuries are the leading cause of injury-related fatalities among 65- to 74-year-old persons and are the second leading cause (after falls) in persons 75 years old and over (Waller, 1985). In 1987, 7,600 fatalities among older adults resulted from motor vehicle collisions. Except for drivers under 25 years of age, elderly vehicle occupants sustain the highest rate of fatalities (per 100,000 drivers and per mile driven) of any age group, even though they are known to curtail their driving miles and avoid driving during the busiest times of day (National Center for Health Statistics, 1987).

The Driving Environment

Aside from special training or the use of special devices, the Department of Transportation has researched the driving environment for areas that may warrant changes or improvement to accommodate the needs of older drivers. The Transportation Research Board recognizes that when automobiles and highways were originally designed in the 1940s, the design characteristics were aimed at a younger population. For example, research in the 1940s, when only 7% of the population was 65 or older, formed the basis for the current sign letter height standards that correspond to visual acuity of 20/25. This is not satisfactory today when the visual acuity of about 40% of licensed drivers who are 65 to 74 years old is below this standard (Transportation Research Board, 1988). Clearly, an improvement in sign visibility, intersection design, road markings, and vehicle crash-worthiness are a few areas to which state and national agencies can contribute for the improved safety of older drivers and vehicle occupants.

Assistance for Older Drivers

Community services and educational classes are available for older adults to assist them in keeping a driver's license as long as possible. For example, the American Automobile Association (AAA) Foundation for Traffic Safety offers a booklet entitled *Drivers 55 Plus: Test Your Own Performance* (Malfetti & Winter, 1986). The self-rating package helps mature drivers to recognize their limitations and unsafe practices, as well as making them aware of remedial actions such as planning a trip to avoid busy intersections, to use these intersections at less congested times, or to plan an alternate route to avoid left turns at busy intersections. The American Association of Retired Persons (AARP) offers a similar exercise and questionnaire booklet titled *Older Driver Skill Assessment and Resource Guide* (AARP, 1992). Since 1979, AARP has sponsored driver refresher courses called 55 ALIVE/MATURE DRIVING that are offered in most states. Many states' Departments of Motor Vehicles have special departments that evaluate individual driving abilities and offer special licensing programs where deemed appropriate. A driver assessment from a local driver rehabilitation program could be very helpful to determine exactly what the limitations are by providing an actual behind-the-wheel assessment in traffic similar to that in which the older driver travels. The Association of Driver Educators for the Disabled (ADED) can be contacted for state and local resources for driver rehabilitation services (see the Appendix of resources at the end of this section). The Association of Driver Educators for the Disabled is the primary resource for occupational therapists who wish to become driver rehabilitation specialists.

The Handicapped Driver's Mobility Guide by AAA provides a listing for driver evaluation and training resources as well as Mobility Equipment Dealers (AAA, 1995).

Surrendering the Driver's License

When the time comes for the driver's license to be taken away, then transportation alternatives must be explored and confirmed in order to assist the person in surviving. Before a family member, physician, or other medical professional decides it is time to "take away the keys" of the older driver, the following steps are recommended to make the reality easier to accept:

1. The person closest to the driver should have a frank discussion with him or her about why it is unsafe to continue driving. A discussion of observed driving behaviors is helpful.

2. The driver should be encouraged to have his or her driving skills evaluated. The doctor can judge reflexes, medication levels, and eyesight, and the driver rehabilitation specialist or occupational therapist can offer a more complete and practical assessment of overall driving abilities. This objective assessment may be the most helpful in convincing the older person to refrain from driving.

3. Available counseling should be sought to make the transition easier. Many senior centers offer counseling services that help elderly individuals to cope with many changes in their lives.

4. Transportation problems may be solved by enlisting an assistant (family member, volunteer) to drive the person to appointments and on errands. Information should be provided about senior transportation services available in the community and about the nearest bus routes that may offer viable transportation alternatives.

The Occupational Therapist as Driver Rehabilitation Specialist

For the therapist interested in getting involved in driver rehabilitation services, the Association of Driver Educators for the Disabled offers a certification examination and an annual conference with educational opportunities for the beginner and experienced driver rehabilitation specialist. A few other organizations, such as AAA; Adaptive Mobility Services, Inc.; and Louisiana Tech University offer yearly educational workshops and seminars related to various levels of driver rehabilitation services. (See list of resources at the end of this section.) AOTA offers networking opportunities through presentations and meetings at their annual conference. Driver rehabilitation services is a unique area that requires specialized training for the medical professional who is interested in providing this service. As population ages, with greater numbers over 65, the demand for driver rehabilitation services will increase as referrals are generated from family members, physicians, and driver licensing authorities.

Summary

By the year 2000, more than 25% of drivers will be over 55 years of age.

Mobility is important to older persons because it enables them to keep their independence and facilitates their performance of many activities. When older persons must stop driving, they usually experience decreased function and increased depression and isolation.

Driving is one of the most complex ADLs. It engages the integration of all of the performance components. Age-related impairments can affect driving performance and necessitate evaluation and intervention. A comprehensive driver assessment conducted by an occupational therapist specializing in driver rehabilitation services can consider all performance components that can be affected by the person's age, diagnosis, or disability. Special devices, instruction, and training may make driving possible. Changes in the driving environment, such as improved sign visibility, intersection design, road markings, and vehicle crash-worthiness would be valuable for the improved safety of older drivers and passengers.

Resources to assist older drivers to maintain independence in driving for as long as possible are available from agencies such as AAA and AARP. The difficulty of surrendering a driver's license can be eased through evaluation, discussion of limitations, counseling, and provision of alternative transportation.

Case Study ━━━━━━━━━━━━━━━━━━━━━━━━━━━

DATE SEEN: JUNE 17, 1995

REPORT: DRIVER EVALUATION SUMMARY

The client is a 70-year-old woman with a diagnosis of bilateral BK amputations. She was referred to Adaptive Mobility Services for a driving evaluation by her vocational rehabilitation counselor. She received medical approval for the evaluation from her doctor who has followed this client since 1994.

The client gives the following medical history: In 1992, she was bitten on the left ankle by a brown recluse spider. She subsequently developed an infection in the foot and leg that finally led to a below-the-knee amputation in October 1993. Apparently because of some carryover of the infection, she had similar symptoms develop in her right leg that required a below-knee amputation in November 1994. The client states that she has had her left prosthesis since December 1992 and her right prosthesis since December 1993. She states that her gait training has been slowed by infections that developed in both of her stumps. She underwent surgery to the right leg in April 1995 for an apparent bone chip in the leg.

She states that she is presently able to walk approximately 200 feet using her walker and her prostheses. She is presently receiving physical therapy for gait training at Sunbelt Living Center three times a week. She still requires a refitting of the prostheses as she is still not comfortable with their fitting.

The client denies having any other medical problems except for arthritis in her hands that required PIP joint replacements in her right hand in 1991. She denied having any arthritic problems in her elbow and shoulder joints although she later admitted to having bursitis type symptoms in her right shoulder.

The client presently lives alone, although her son, who is a truck driver, occasionally comes to be with her in between jobs. She is presently attending vocational training for typing with computers. She states that she had 32 years of office work in a public affairs office in the government in Washington, D.C., before moving to Florida. Prior to 1992, she was working in the food and beverage department at Walt Disney World. She is presently interested in returning to employment at Disney, although in some type of office work. She hopes to be back on the job by August.

The client was able to drive until April 1993 when she lost her right leg. She presently owns two vehicles. She has a 1972 Mercury Comet that she considers to be in the classic stage, and she does not want to drive this vehicle but would rather sell it as a classic. She has a 1983 Chevrolet Camero that has over 200,000 miles on the odometer. She is interested in purchasing a new car, states she has the finances to do so, and is eager to have recommendations given for vehicle selection.

The client is on the following medications: daily vitamins, a medicine for minor high blood pressure problems, Visteril for sleep, and Darvocet that she takes once or twice at night and as needed for pain.

The client holds a valid Florida driver's license that was issued 6-8-89 and expires 12-2-95. Only the restriction of glasses is noted.

CLINICAL ASSESSMENT

Physical evaluation of the upper extremities reveals normal active range of motion in the shoulder and elbow joints. She does exhibit some limitations in the extreme ranges of wrist flexion and extension, although it does not appear to limit the function of her hand. She demonstrates normal MCP movement, although she also demonstrates severe arthritic deformities in the PIP and DIP joints of her fingers. Little movement is noted in the joints, and she is unable to make a full composite flexed hand. She feels her left hand is more mobile but that her right hand has greater strength, as was noted on the dynamometer. Her grip strength is very weak at 16 pounds on the right hand and 8 pounds on the left hand. The client denies having any pain in her hands. She does not use any splints or cuffs or any other orthotic devices for her hands in functional activities.

The client appears to have good use of her hips and knees bilaterally. She is able to come to a standing position if she has guarded standby assistance. She does use a manual wheelchair that she has had since her first amputation. It is noted to be a heavy manual wheelchair with elevating foot rests. She states that she does not use the foot rests or arm rests at home, and she is able to use her legs to help push the chair in her house.

The client denies having any visual problems. She has not been diagnosed with glaucoma or cataracts. She saw her doctor just recently who stated that her vision remains 20/20 to 20/30. She presently has progressive lenses in her glasses that she uses for near and far distance. She states that she has worn glasses since her 20s.

Functional evaluation reveals the client to be independent in all activities of daily living, although she requires some assistance with heavy cooking and house-keeping activities. She depends on public transportation at the present time as she lives alone and is able to use her son only occasionally.

VEHICLE AND EQUIPMENT ASSESSMENT

Because the client has bilateral prostheses, she does require hand controls for operation of the gas and brake pedals. Because of the arthritis in her hand, I would also recommend the push right-angle type in addition to a quad handle to provide her hand and wrist more support. She will need the remote horn and high beam switches, but could use them similar to the para handle controls.

For steering, the client will require some type of steering device to assist in one-handed steering. A moving assessment revealed the client to have difficulty using a spinner knob. It was finally decided after some time of training that the single post steering device was best for her. Initially, she did have some difficulty turning the steering wheel between the 8 and 11 o'clock position on the steering wheel. After watching the client carefully, I repositioned the driver power seat three or four times to place her in the most up position with a slight tilt forward to give her greater advantage on the steering wheel. This did appear to help her, and with the additional driving practice, she was able to demonstrate better steering control by the end of her lesson today.

Depending on the type of vehicle that the client chooses, she may or may not require some other adaptations on the accessory and secondary controls. This need would have to be assessed in the vehicle that she purchases. Because she needs hand controls and the arthritic condition of her hands, she requires a vehicle with automatic transmission, power steering, and power brakes. She requires the easiest type of power steering. Although she is interested in a Ford Probe, I explained to her that the steering would be too stiff in this vehicle. I will discuss this matter with her son so that he will understand the exact car she needs. I have encouraged them both not to purchase a vehicle until she has approved it through me.

As a result of her mobility in a manual wheelchair, the client requires some means of loading and storing her wheelchair. Again, because of the arthritis in her hands, I would not recommend that she load the vehicle into the back seat area of the car. Neither could she load it into the trunk of a vehicle. She could use either a chair topper, which would load the chair effortlessly on the top of her car, or a wheelchair loader, such as a Bruno Backsaver, which would be on the rear bumper of the vehicle. To use the Backsaver, the client would have to walk from the rear of the vehicle to the driver's seat. My best recommendation is for the client to use the Braun chair topper as this would eliminate her having to do any ambulation. In addition, her wheelchair would be stored out of the weather. It is important that she purchase a vehicle that will accommodate the installation of the chair topper.

IN-VEHICLE ASSESSMENT

The client was introduced to the push right-angle hand controls with a single-post steering device. She was initially taken into a neighborhood and given practice and instruction in the use of the equipment. She was given approximately 1 hour and 45 minutes of practice in a neighborhood environment. She demonstrated a lot of anxiety and nervousness about driving. However, with cuing, directions, and instructions, she was able to become more comfortable in driving after the first hour. She did occasionally confuse the gas and brake motions and, as stated above, occasionally had difficulty on turns. By the end of the first hour, I was able to train her in the use of the turn signals so that she was able to reach quickly and efficiently using her left hand from the hand control handle.

SUMMARY AND RECOMMENDATIONS

A comprehensive driver assessment reveals that this client has excellent potential to be an independent driver. She does require a new vehicle and is able and willing to purchase an appropriate vehicle to be adapted for her driving needs. She will require a vehicle with the easiest power steering that is allowed.

For adaptive equipment, the client will require a set of hand controls, a special steering device, and a Braun chair topper. The prescription will not be written until the client has an appropriate vehicle to adapt.

The client does require additional driver training so that she can progress into traffic and become a safer operator of the vehicle with the controls recommended. On June 28, 1995, I contacted the VR counselor by telephone who verbally authorized 10 additional hours of driver training, although she stated that the authorization could not be cut until approximately July 10.

I will continue to counsel the client on vehicle selection and write the prescription at the appropriate time when we are assured she has a proper vehicle.

I was in touch with World of Independence, a local vendor and was given a price of $3,560.00 for the car topper, hand controls, and steering device. I do not feel that a bidding conference is needed on this prescription, although I would recommend a final vehicle inspection following installation to ensure proper installation, proper fitting, and adjustments of the hand control and steering device for her safe use.

PLAN

Send report to VR counselor and referring physician. Schedule client for additional 10 hours of driver training. Follow-up services for a final vehicle inspection can be done as requested.

Write prescription for driving needs when client has an appropriate car.

Susan Pierce, OTR, CDRS
Driver Rehabilitation Specialist

NOTE: July 7, 1995: The client went car shopping over the weekend. She found a 1994 Cutlass Ciera and asked me to look at it to approve it for her driving needs. During one of her lessons, our instructor was able to drive this car to me to look at. It is properly equipped with AT, power brakes, and the easy power steering that she needs. It is an appropriate size for the chair topper. After a few more successful training sessions, I will finalize Rx. S. Pierce, OTR.

Review Questions

1. What is the projected percentage of drivers who will be over 55 years of age by the year 2000?
2. About how many of those drivers will be over 75 years of age?
3. What are the limitations an older person confronts when independent mobility is no longer possible?
4. Which performance components are involved in driving?
5. List at least three general factors and three specific diagnoses that can have an effect on driving performance?
6. Why is an appropriately trained occupational therapist well suited to conduct driver assessment?
7. What are some environmental changes that would contribute to improved safety for older drivers and vehicle occupants?
8. List two agencies that provide education and information for the older driver.
9. If an occupational therapy practitioner wishes to become a driver evaluator, what agency should he or she contact?

Appendix.
Resources

Seniors

AAA Seniors
Box 78
1000 AAA Drive
Heathrow, FL 32746-5080
Phone: (407) 444-4000

ADED
109 West Street
Edgerton, WI 53534
Phone: (608) 884-8833

AARP
601 E Street, NW
Washington, DC 20049
Phone: (202) 434-2277

Therapists

Adaptive Mobility Services, Inc.
116 East Gatlin Avenue
Orlando, FL 32806
Phone: (407) 855-8050

Louisiana Tech University
Department of Biomedical Engineering
711 S. Vienna, Room 200
Ruston, LA 71270
Phone: (318) 257-4562

References

American Association of Retired Persons. (1992). *Older driver skill assessment and resource guide.* Washington, DC: AARP & ITT Hartford Insurance Group.

American Automobile Association. (1995). *The handicapped driver's mobility guide.* Heathrow, FL: Author.

Blum, J. (Ed.). (1993, August). Keeping seniors on the move. *Columbus Monthly,* 72.

Malfetti, J. L. (1985). *Drivers 55+: Needs and problems of older drivers.* Falls Church, VA: American Automobile Association.

Malfetti, J. L., & Winter, D. J. (1986). *Drivers 55 plus: Test your own performance.* Heathrow, FL: American Automobile Association.

Milone, A. M. (1985). Training and re-training the older driver. In J. L. Malfetti, *Needs and problems of older drivers: Survey results and recommendations* (p. 38). Heathrow, FL: American Automobile Association.

National Center for Health Statistics. (1987). Advance report of final mortality statistics. *Monthly Vital Statistics Report, 38* (suppl. to no. 5) 16.

Retchin, S. M., & Anapolle, J. (1993). An overview of the older driver. *Clinics of Geriatric Medicine, 9*(2), 279.

Transportation Research Board. (1988). *Special report 218: Transportation in an aging society: Improving mobility and safety for older persons* (Vol. 1, pp.1–5). Washington, DC: Author.

Waller, P.F. (1985). Preventing injury to the elderly. *Aging and public health, 3,* 103–146.

Section 4.
Sexual Expression in Later Life

Patricia A. Miller, MEd, OTR, FAOTA
Nikki D. Couloumbis, MS, OTR

The authors gratefully acknowledge Donna Adams, MS, OTR/L; Elise Henry, MS, OTR/L; and Ira Silverman, MS, OTR/L, for their contributions in conducting the first pilot study of the knowledge, attitudes, and interventions of rehabilitation professionals regarding sexuality in the older adult.

Abstract

Sexual expression is an important domain of practice for occupational therapists. The authors discuss physical, psychological, and social obstacles to sexual expression often experienced by older adults. Approaches to guide occupational therapists' interventions are provided to help older clients mitigate or eliminate sexual limitations.

Introduction: Defining the Issue

Despite cultural stereotypes that depict elderly individuals as uninterested and uninvolved in sexual relationships, recent data clearly suggest otherwise (Brecher, 1984; Cross, 1993; Starr & Weiner, 1981). Incorrect perceptions of older people as nonsexual are shared by health professionals as well as the public at large, so that relatively little research on late-life sexuality has been conducted. With inadequate information and little training, many practicing health professionals may be unprepared to address the sexual topics that are regarded as important for older age groups (Cross, 1993; Kaplan, 1991). Therefore, even conscientious occupational therapy practitioners may be failing to meet the full spectrum of health needs in elderly persons (Couloumbis & Miller, 1994).

Recent studies have contributed to a more accurate profile of sexual behavior in late adulthood (Cross, 1993). Data gathered from thousands of men and women show that over 50% of the healthy elderly population remains sexually active on a weekly or more frequent basis (Brecher, 1984; Starr & Weiner, 1981). In a national survey of 3,260 adults over 65, 53% of men and 41% of women reported that they had a reasonably active sex life, enjoying greater spousal intimacy than when they were younger (Sherman, 1993). Research results support assessment of the need for sexuality interventions with elderly patients (Cross, 1993).

Sexuality is formally recognized as part of the occupational therapy domain; "sexual expression" is included in the activities of daily living of occupational performance in the second edition of "Uniform Terminology for Occupational Therapy" (AOTA, 1989) and is defined as "engaging in desired sexual and intimate activities" in the third edition (AOTA, 1994, p. 1052). In this section, sexuality is defined as the conscious use of the body, including caress and gesture, to share or provide pleasure for oneself or another with or without sexual intercourse (Miller, Adams, Henry, & Silverman, 1993). Occupational therapy practitioners who wish to address sexuality with elders may first prepare by examining their individual knowledge of and attitudes toward the topic, as these will guide clinical practice.

Conceptual Framework

Two concepts that guide practice have been chosen to ground this analysis. First, because of the roles played by biology, society, and psychology in the determination of sexuality, the consideration of issues in late-life sexuality has been based upon a biopsychosocial approach. The dynamic and interactive forces of biology, social context, and personal psychology are interdependent in shaping an individual's sexual function, behavior, and expression (Ferrini & Ferrini, 1993; Whitbourne, 1992), and one's sexual behavior and expression become major components of self-concept and social identity (Ferrini & Ferrini, 1993; Neistadt, 1993).

The second concept is informed by the paradigms of Havighurst, Neugarten, and Tobin (1968); Cynkin (1979); and Cynkin and Mazur-Robinson (1990), which state that a positive relationship exists between activity level and patterns and overall life satisfaction (Croft, 1982). It follows that maintaining satisfying sexual activity for as long as possible would be expected to contribute to an individual's sense of independent function and personal well-being if sex is a valued activity (Atchley, 1989; Miller et al., 1993). Because occupational therapy pursues restoration, adaptation, and maintenance of a patient's physical and psychosocial function (with preservation or establishment of meaningful roles and activities), it is within the domain of the profession to assess the need for interventions and provide them as necessary to enable sexual expression, regardless of age.

Aging: Real and Imagined Obstacles to Sexual Expression

Some physiological changes due to the aging process are normal and require adaptive techniques but do not mean the end of sexual functioning (Ferrini & Ferrini, 1993; Fry, 1986;

National Institute on Aging [NIA], 1992; Whitbourne, 1992). Simple methods of accommodating physical changes can be used by partners who wish to continue sexual enjoyment (Cross, 1993).

For men, age-related changes include decreased levels of testosterone and penile sensitivity that can make erection slower or require more stimulation (Ferrini & Ferrini, 1993; NIA, 1992). However, changes in hormone levels may not be solely related to aging, as pathology and medication can alter endocrinal function (Whitbourne, 1992). Although erections in older men may not be as firm and an increased refractory period may mean fewer erections are possible physiologically (NIA, 1992), function and sensation during orgasm remain unimpaired.

For postmenopausal women, lowered levels of estrogen lead to some changes in the shape, flexibility, and lubrication of the vagina (Fry, 1986; NIA, 1992). However, these don't change sexual capacity if properly addressed through the use of water-soluble lubricant (NIA, 1992), extended stimulation by the partner, or appropriate hormonal supplementation selected from the wide range of traditional estrogen therapies (Fry, 1986) or alternative natural progesterone therapies (Kamen, 1993) now available. Kegel exercises can improve vaginal tone for women who experience laxity from previous pregnancies (Kaplan, 1991). Clitoral and nipple responsiveness and capacity for orgasm is undiminished in the healthy older woman (Ferrini & Ferrini, 1993).

Actual changes in the human genital system caused by aging are minimal and do not necessarily decrease desired sexual expression and enjoyment. In fact, appropriate intervention by a proactive therapist can go a long way; elders reporting higher levels of sexual activity experience fewer of the age-related sexual changes than those who report lower levels (Ferrini & Ferrini, 1993). However, four obstacles to sexual expression do exist for older adults:

1. Demographic factors that affect partner availability
2. Social attitudes that affect sexual behavior
3. Affective and cognitive changes caused by psychological conditions
4. Pathophysiological changes caused by the onset of disease (Croft, 1982; Ferrini & Ferrini, 1993; Fry, 1986; NIA, 1992).

DEMOGRAPHIC FACTORS

Partner availability is the single most important factor found to determine sexual activity in later life. Having a healthy spouse, or being able to find an accessible partner, is the major predictor of sexual activity in older adults. Certain demographic factors make partners less available for older women than for older men. First, because of their longer life expectancy, elderly women outnumber men by at least 1.5 to 1; single elderly women outnumber single men by 4 to 1 (Cross, 1993). Furthermore, women tend to marry men who are older than they are, making the probability of widowhood even greater. Older men are more than twice as likely to be married as older women (Knopf, 1975), and older widowers (who are 8.6 times more likely than older widows to remarry due to the noted sex differential) usually remarry younger women (Anderson, 1979). The result is that maintenance of a sexual relationship in late life is much more difficult for women than for men, unless they are bisexual or lesbian (Knopf, 1975).

SOCIOCULTURAL ATTITUDES

Attitudes about aging and elderly individuals have been shown to strongly influence sexual activity in later life. Conflicting stereotypes depict the elderly as either uninterested in sex or inappropriately interested in sex ("dirty old man") (Steinke, 1988). Some elderly people internalize ageist stereotypes, changing their behavior to conform to sociocultural expectations. Croft (1982) referred to a generalized process of sociogenic aging that occurs with no physical basis as a result of negative social attitudes and stereotypes.

Clinicians are influenced by stereotypes and may not recognize or feel comfortable addressing sexual issues that exist for older patients (Fry, 1986). Unfortunately, within a biopsychosocial framework, the social inputs received influence volition, affective responses, and behavioral outputs (Kielhofner, 1988, 1995). Widespread negative social inputs can prevent help-seeking behavior by patients, compounding the trouble caused by misinformation about sexual decline during aging and often contributing to the development of secondary non-physiological impotence or dysfunction (Whitbourne, 1992).

PSYCHOLOGICAL CONDITIONS

Psychological conditions that may affect sexual function include depression and dementia. Depression leads many elderly individuals to withdraw from their partners, or it may be precipitated by the loss of a significant other. Decreased libido is one symptom of depressive disorders, and many of the drugs used to treat depression have side effects that also negatively impact libido or sexual potency.

Organic brain diseases and dementias can cause sexual acting out, resulting in the need for special medical management of the patient and counseling of the spouse or family. Yet, dementia may not rule out satisfying sexual relations (Walz & Blum, 1987). In the early stages, the caregiver and affected partner may still share satisfying experiences. However, as the disease progresses, cognitive losses and personality changes can reduce the viability of sexual involvement.

PHYSICAL CONDITIONS

Arthritic conditions may limit sexual activity by causing joint pain and stiffness, and drugs prescribed for relief can decrease libido. However, compensatory strategies including rest, warm baths before and after sex, and changes in intercourse position or timing can help control arthritis pain (Ferrini & Ferrini, 1993).

Hypertension-related sexual problems, usually induced by antihypertensive medications, are more frequently documented in men because they are more observable (Walz & Blum, 1987). These drugs can cause erectile dysfunction in men even at normal therapeutic doses and may reduce vaginal lubrication and orgasm in women (Ferrini & Ferrini, 1993). Using lubricants and extra stimulation may be helpful to some women, and new medications may offer hope for men who can take them (Walz & Blum, 1987).

Diabetes can cause erectile dysfunction in men as nerves controlling the dilation of penile arteries are damaged (Ferrini & Ferrini, 1993). However, sensation and orgasm are unaffected, so that implants can be used in treatments. In women, diabetes does not affect function but appears to reduce orgasmic capacity (Ferrini & Ferrini, 1993).

Cardiac conditions often lead older people to relinquish sexual activity out of fear. However, the risk of death during intercourse is extremely low. With medical advice, an active sexual life can be resumed within 12 to 16 weeks after a heart attack (NIA, 1992) and sometimes as early as 8 weeks later (Walz & Blum, 1987).

Strokes may more seriously impact sexual activity, causing tone-related limitations of movement (NIA, 1992) that may require adapted sexual positioning. Cancer's effects on sexuality can be direct, as in breast or prostate cancer, or indirect, as treatment side effects reduce desire and function (Ferrini & Ferrini, 1993).

An empathetic physician and the patient's partner should be involved in therapeutic interventions. Proper medical management as well as compassionate support are necessary to help a patient overcome sexual problems associated with any primary diagnosis.

Primary, Secondary, and Tertiary Care Options

To select an approach to sexuality intervention requires self-assessment of personal knowledge and attitudes. Clinicians will not be able to provide effective and responsible interventions if they are misinformed. After appropriate education, clinicians can address their own perceptions of the myths that can complicate treatment of late-life sexual dysfunction and better understand how their zone of personal comfort may affect professional behavior.

Well-informed therapists may play an important role in primary prevention of geriatric sexual problems by developing educational programs, becoming involved in policy planning at an institutional level, or by providing information to primary caregivers. When therapists are educated enough, direct and indirect services in secondary prevention can be provided by conducting thorough assessments of existing needs and following up with early recommendations for adaptive techniques or referrals to specialists.

Therapists who are prepared and comfortable should incorporate sexuality intervention into individual treatment plans when providing tertiary care. In determining the type of intervention to be used at this level, therapists should be aware of the range of intervention choices that exist, from specific suggestions for exercises and positioning to simple grooming activities. For patients who don't participate in actual intercourse, some level of sexual expression is still possible, and maintaining established makeup and grooming habits can be a very practical way of enhancing feelings of attractiveness—in effect, helping to preserve some aspects of sexual identity and expression.

The primary, secondary, and tertiary prevention model described here (Miller, 1988) can be combined with the PLISSIT Model developed by Annon (1976). PLISSIT provides guidelines for therapists to grade their approach using cues from the patient through the use of a multi-stage assessment and intervention process: P—giving permission to raise sexual concerns, LI—provision of limited information, SS—specific suggestions, and IT—intensive therapy. Specialized training is necessary to intervene on the IT level of the model; professional judgment may require a referral to a sex therapist or other specialist in order to ensure the best care for the patient. An example of a patient in need of IT is the patient experiencing impotence after prostate surgery (Smedley, 1991).

Research Findings

A 2-year pilot study was conducted to examine the knowledge level and attitudes of occupational and physical therapists working in gerontology toward the sexuality and sexual behavior of older adults. The impact of knowledge and attitudes on clinical practice was also examined. A demographic questionnaire and two instruments, the Adult Sexuality and Knowledge Test developed by Walz and Blum (1987) and a Clinical Practice Intervention Scale developed by Miller et al. (1993), were used to survey 150 occupational and 150 physical therapists. Results from 177 respondents (1993: n = 88, 1994: n = 89) showed that despite overall positive attitudes, knowledge levels were insufficient to ensure competent intervention, and that intervention levels were generally low. Although not statistically significant, a stronger correlation was found to exist between attitude toward sexuality and the level of clinical intervention than between knowledge about sexuality and the level of clinical intervention. The most striking finding in 1993 was that therapists did not consistently respond to patients' initiation of sexual concerns (Miller et al., 1993). The most striking finding in 1994 (Couloumbis & Miller, 1994) was that therapists who had received information on the sexuality of older adults during their education or clinical practice reported intervention levels 27.8% higher than therapists unexposed to this information. Study findings support research that shows the elderly population's needs for intervention in the area of sexuality may be underserved by clinicians, and that specific education in this area may improve levels of clinical intervention and competence.

Summary

Considering the facts about late-life sexuality and the social attitudes that can obscure them, the question that confronts occupational therapists is whether the full range of needs of the geriatric population is being adequately addressed. The prevention and PLISSIT models provide the responsibly informed therapist with guidelines to address sexual expression, an area of occupational performance that is often overlooked, at the level of their expertise in a manner that meets the needs of the patient through direct intervention or referral.

Occupational therapy practitioners are uniquely trained to maintain the functional performance of patients in their chosen activities. This is understood to be the central treatment objective. Failure to address potential sexual dysfunction as a result of professional bias, low level of knowledge, or personal discomfort undermines clinical competence and discredits what occupational therapy values philosophically. These authors hope that this introduction and related self-study materials will serve as an impetus to occupational therapy practitioners to serve older clients more comprehensively.

Review Questions

1. What percentage of healthy older adults remains sexually active?
2. Why is sexual expression in the domain of occupational therapy?
3. Define sexuality according to the authors of this section.
4. What important step must occupational therapy practitioners take before addressing sexuality issues with elders?
5. Why does sexual activity contribute to an individual's sense of independent function and sense of well-being?
6. List four possible causes of sexual dysfunction in older men.
7. How can the effects of lowered estrogen levels be addressed in the older woman who wishes to remain sexually active?
8. List four obstacles to sexual expression for older adults.
9. What are two common stereotypical beliefs about sex and older persons?
10. Which psychological conditions of age may affect sexual function?
11. What are some of the physical conditions and medications that can affect sexual function?
12. Briefly define the three-stage prevention model for intervention.
13. The PLISSIT Model developed by Annon (1976) provides guidelines for therapists to grade their approach based on cues from the patient.
14. What important research findings underscore the need for more knowledge and greater intervention by occupational therapists?

Appendix.
Case Application of PLISSIT and Prevention Models

The following is an excerpt of a discussion held during a therapy session to prepare a female patient and her husband for the transition to home after a total hip replacement. In this example, the therapist responds to cues from the patient's spouse with a permissive attitude, limited information, and a written form of primary prevention. For confidentiality, the names have been changed.

Background Information: At 83, Ruth Myers's medical history was uncomplicated. During her stay at the rehabilitation hospital, she had returned to her prior level of independent ADL performance and was ambulating safely with a walker. She and her 79-year-old husband had both been trained for transfers and equipment use.

OT: Let's review the equipment we've ordered for the bathroom. One elevated toilet seat, one shower chair. You have a very large shower, 6' × 8', so the chair can be placed beneath the showerhead or you can use the hand-held nozzle.

Mrs. Myers: I'll probably use the hand-held. We also got those grab bars you told us about, one near the toilet and two in the shower according to the diagram.

OT: Good. You can plan to take your long-handled sponge home with you, because you won't be able to bend at the hip freely for the rest of the three-month healing period. Now, would you like to go over the transfer again? You've been doing quite well getting over the practice ledge with your walker.

Mrs. Myers: Actually, I feel good about it. The shower's so big I can take the walker right in with me and put it near the chair. I don't feel anxious about it.

OT: Okay. But be sure to dry off the walker if you do take it in with you, before getting up.

Mr. Myers: I can also help Ruthie getting in and out, and stay in there with her while she bathes if she needs me to.

OT: Hmmm ... that's not a bad idea. There's definitely room for two in that shower.

Mr. Myers: Sometimes we like to take our showers together.

OT: Well, it certainly makes me feel that Mrs. Myers will be quite safe. Just be sure you don't slip if you bend down to try to help her with her feet.

Mrs. Myers: No, I'll use the sponge for that, but Jim can help me with my back. Besides, we have that nonslip stuff on the floor.

OT: Good. I think that's a special way to be able to express your affection for one another while you're recovering completely. You shouldn't feel as if you can't enjoy yourselves physically. Will that bathing arrangement satisfy both of you for the time being?

Mrs. Myers: I've always liked it in the past, so I don't see why not. There won't be anything more now, not until I feel up to it.

Mr. Myers: There's no reason to rush anything. Besides, we both have a little back trouble these days, and that can act up if we aren't careful.

OT: Do you mean that you have back pain during or after sex?

Mr. Myers: Sometimes I do; sometimes Ruth does.

OT: I have a specific booklet on back pain and sexual activity. If you'd like, I can copy it for you. I'll put a line through all the positions or suggestions that Ruth should not try due to her hip precautions, and I'll bring it to you this afternoon. That way, the two of you can look at it over the next couple of days and ask any questions before you leave. The booklet also has some information on using hot showers and massage to relieve back pain, so you might find it helpful.

Mrs. Myers: It sounds good. We've been wondering what to do for a while.

OT: Okay, so I'll take care of that. Do you have any other intimate concerns? No? All right, then, let's talk about your home exercise program.

References

American Occupational Therapy Association. (1989). Uniform terminology for occupational therapy (2nd ed.). In H. Hopkins & H. Smith (Eds.), *Willard and Spackman's occupational therapy* (8th ed.). Philadelphia: J. B. Lippincott.

American Occupational Therapy Association. (1994). Uniform terminology for occupational therapy (3rd ed.). *American Journal of Occupational Therapy, 48*(11), 1052.

Anderson, B. G. (1979). *The aging game: Success, sanity, and sex after 60.* New York: McGraw-Hill.

Annon, J. S. (1976). The PLISSIT Model: A proposed conceptual scheme for behavioral treatment of sexual problems. *Journal of Sex Education Therapy, 2*(2), 1–15.

Atchley, R. (1989). A continuity theory of normal aging. *Gerontologist, 2*(2), 183–190.

Brecher, E. M. (1984). *Love, sex, and aging: A Consumers' Union report.* Boston: Little, Brown.

Couloumbis, N., & Miller, P. (1994). *Knowledge, attitudes, and interventions of rehabilitation professionals regarding late-life sexuality: A survey.* Unpublished manuscript, Programs in Occupational Therapy, Columbia University, New York.

Croft, L. H. (1982). *Sexuality in later life: A counseling guide for physicians.* Boston: PSG.

Cross, R. J. (1993). What doctors and others need to know: Six facts on human sexuality and aging. *Sex Information and Education Council of the U.S. [SIECUS] Report, 21*(5), 7–9.

Cynkin, S. (1979). *Occupational therapy: Toward health through activities.* Boston: Little, Brown.

Cynkin, S., & Mazur-Robinson, A. (1990). *Occupational therapy and activities: Toward health through activities.* Boston: Little, Brown.

Ferrini, A. F., & Ferrini, R. L. (1993). *Health in the later years.* Dubuque, IA: Brown & Benchmark.

Fry, P. (1986). *Depression, stress, and adaption in the elderly.* Rockville, MD: Aspen Publishers.

Havighurst, R. J., Neugarten, B. L., & Tobin, S. S. (1968). Disengagement and patterns of aging. In B. L. Neugarten (Ed.), *Middle age and aging* (pp. 161–172). Chicago: University of Chicago Press.

Kaplan, H. S. (1991). Sex therapy with older patients. In W. A. Myers (Ed.), *New techniques in the psychotherapy of older patients* (pp. 21–37). Washington, DC: American Psychiatric Press.

Kamen, B. (1993). *Hormone replacement therapy: Yes or no?* Novato, CA: Nutrition Encounter.

Kielhofner, G. (1988). Occupational therapy—Base in occupation. In H. Hopkins & H. Smith (Eds.), *Willard and Spackman's occupational therapy* (7th ed., pp. 84–92). Philadelphia: J. B. Lippincott.

Kielhofner, G. (1995). *A model of human occupation: Therapy and application* (2nd ed.). Baltimore, MD: William & Wilkins.

Knopf, O. (1975). *Successful aging.* New York: Viking Press.

Miller, P. (1988). Preventive treatment approaches. In L. J. Davis & M. Kirkland (Eds.), *The role of occupational therapy with the elderly* (pp. 227–235). Rockville, MD: AOTA.

Miller, P., Adams, D., Henry, E., & Silverman, I. (1993). *Knowledge, attitudes, and interventions of rehabilitation professionals regarding sexuality in the older adult: A survey.* Unpublished manuscript, Programs in Occupational Therapy, Columbia University, New York.

Neistadt, M. (1993). Human sexuality and counseling. In H. L. Hopkins & H. D. Smith (Eds.), *Willard and Spackman's occupational therapy* (8th ed., pp. 148–154). Philadelphia: J. B. Lippincott.

National Institute on Aging. (1992). *Age page: Sexuality in later life.* Washington, DC: U.S. Department of Health and Human Services, National Institute of Health.

Sherman, B. (1993, April 24). Senior sex. *New York Newsday*, Part 2, pp. 17–19.

Smedley, G. (1991). Addressing sexuality in the elderly. *Rehabilitation Nursing, 16*(1), 9–11.

Starr, B., & Weiner, M. B. (1981). *The Starr and Weiner report on sex and sexuality in the mature years.* New York: Stein & Day.

Steinke, E. (1988). Older adults' knowledge and attitudes about sexuality and aging. *IMAGE: Journal of Nursing Scholarship, 20*(2), 93–95.

Walz, T., & Blum, N. (1987). *Sexual health in later life.* Lexington, MA: Lexington Books.

Whitbourne, S. K. (1992). Sexuality in the aging male. In L. Glasse & J. Hendricks (Eds.), *Gender and aging* (pp. 49–52). Amityville, NY: Baywood.

Section 5. Transition to Home After Hospitalization or Rehabilitation Program

Nancy Richman, OTR/L, FAOTA
Coralie H. Glantz, OTR/L, FAOTA

Abstract

Occupational therapists can smooth the transition from a hospital or rehabilitation facility to home by careful planning and attention to the continuum of care. Educating caregivers, becoming familiar with community resources, and recommending appropriate environmental adaptations and assistive devices all play a part in enhancing the older person's independence and safety.

Introduction

The increase in the number of elderly individuals in relationship to younger persons in this country is having an influence on the delivery of occupational therapy services to older persons. With Diagnosis Related Groups (DRGs) and insurance company restrictions on lengths of stay, the occupational therapist is involved with discharge planning from the outset of treatment. The therapist accumulates data relative to the client, the client's support system, caregiver involvement, and the physical environment at the time of evaluation. This is necessary to support the establishment of appropriate treatment goals that are relative to discharge plans. If occupational therapy personnel employed in hospitals, rehabilitation centers, long-term-care facilities, and private practice know what services are offered in their communities and where an elderly individual can go to gain entry into systems (Benzing, 1988), they can ease the transition barriers for their clients.

Health care systems have grown so complex that many clients and their families find it difficult to obtain appropriate care in a suitable setting. It is often a difficult process for them and they may be unable to obtain proper information and sort out their options. They may need an advocate to help them define their treatment goals and ensure that clients, families, and the treatment team keep those goals in mind during the discharge process (Barone, Costante, & Ennis, 1989).

Delivery Systems

Transition involves an understanding of the continuum of care and how it relates to the clients whom occupational therapists serve. One definition of a continuum of care from Evashwick (1989) states that it is "an integrated system of care that guides and tracks patients over time through a comprehensive array of health, mental health, and social services spanning all levels of intensity of care. It [comprises] both services and integrating mechanisms" (Evashwick, 1989, p. 36). When an efficient continuum of care exists, the transitions may be easier.

One model for continuum of care is a continuing care retirement center (CCRC). In this system, the focus is on keeping older adults healthy and allowing them to age in place in their homes. A variety of options is available in a CCRC, such as independent living units, congregate housing with meals and housekeeping, assistive living with the ability to buy services as needed, and possibly a nursing unit. The focus of these living arrangements is often on instrumental activities of daily living (IADLs). The medical model continuum, however, is more focused on treating illness, as it is associated with a health care entity with hospital beds, skilled-nursing beds, home health care agency links, or a tie to durable medical equipment and supplies. A Preferred Provider Organization (PPO) component may offer care coordination (Evashwick, 1989). An OT practitioner involved in the CCRC type of model or the medical model continuum works with different aspects of transition and has a different set of options than an OT practitioner who is working to discharge a client to home without connected resources and well-defined systems in place.

The involvement of occupational therapy practitioners in a care management system must also be addressed as they look toward appropriate transition models. "Care management refers to the care planning and organization of services and resources needed to meet needs and maintain independence" (Fanale, Keenan, Hepburn, & Von Sternberg, 1991). Discrete systems of acute, institutional, and home-bound care exist, and the goal of care management is to bridge these systems. All of the anticipated benefits from innovative approaches to community-based long-term care projects have not been achieved through these care management systems. Quality of life and levels of independence may have improved, but rates of institutionalization and overall health care costs have not been positively affected (Fanale et al., 1991; Kane & Kane, 1987). These are important issues for occupational therapy practitioners. Could more therapist involvement influence these outcomes? Some examples of care man-

agement projects are the National Long-Term Care Demonstration (channeling); the On-Loc Senior Health Services Community Care Organization; the South Carolina Long-Term Demonstration Project; the Social/Health Maintenance Organization; and the ACCESS long-term program in Monroe County, New York (Fanale et al., 1991; Kane & Kane, 1987).

The government is trying to restructure resources and entitlement programs that are now available for older adults to ease transition to the community. This approach may trigger significant changes. Budgetary concerns are driving political interest in shifting from an age-based policy to a need-based policy. These need-based criteria may require wealthier older persons to pay greater taxes or pay a larger share for services than those older persons who have less income (Binstock, 1994).

To be effective, the occupational therapy practitioner must understand the systems involved as the client leaves the hospital or rehabilitation program, which resources will be available for that individual, and whether the move to a home setting involves relocation for the client. The home situation can then be analyzed from many aspects: intrapersonal-cultural biases, support people, community resources, client preparation for termination of treatment and follow-up care, caregiver availability, environmental modifications, and adaptive equipment. Occupational therapists are prepared to promote independence, but as the older adult's need for help is identified, his or her readiness to accept help must be identified (Benzing, 1988). Many things must be taken into consideration. The client and caregiver self-image, lifestyle, and culture are all relevant. Occupational therapists may design appropriate interventions with excellent team collaboration, but clients will decide what they will do and when and how they will do it (Yerxa, 1991). Caregivers define, approach, and react to their caregiving role in distinct ways and occupational therapy practitioners need to consider these unique situations as they offer caregivers support in their roles. A framework should be developed from which to evaluate the specific and individualized needs of caregivers. A health care system that is community- and home-based will demand it.

Social Dimensions

Social dimensions (such as the availability, attitude, and capabilities of caregivers); environmental dimensions (such as architectural barriers); and qualities of deprivation versus enrichment (Rogers, 1988) can promote or hinder functional improvement. Recipients of care need to have trust, opportunities for socialization and support, and increased security from knowing that someone is available to respond to needs and problems. Those needs can often be ignored when care is being given by a homecare worker and timeliness, task performance, and unit costs take precedence over interpersonal relationships (Capitman, Abrahams, & Ritter, 1994). Occupational therapists must remember that when care is being provided by a spouse, he or she may be as infirm as the client and is probably experiencing the problems associated with aging. With environmental barriers to leaving the home and lacking available transportation or somewhere appropriate to go for leisure, the motivation for improvement or even maintenance of skills previously gained diminishes.

Intrapersonal Aspects

To understand the intrapersonal aspects involved in transition, the OT practitioner must "attend to each individual's unique personal history. The personal history includes one's skills and abilities (performance components), the past performance of specific life tasks (performance areas), and experience within particular environments (performance contexts)" (American Occupational Therapy Association [AOTA], 1994, p. 1049). An understanding of the family dynamics, financial ramifications, and the community is essential preparation for transition. Pollock (1993) stated that occupational "performance is predicated on the interaction of the person's mental, physical, socio-cultural, and spiritual performance components. It is also related to roles, role expectations and developmental stages." These performance contexts, such as support available from other persons and adaptation of structure and objects within the environment, must be considered (AOTA, 1994) as part of the parameters of concern.

Different cultural patterns influence readiness to accept care. It may be appropriate for a daughter to provide care but not a daughter-in-law. If there are no female family members to provide care, it may be thought inappropriate for an available male family member to make the sacrifice. Formal sources of care (such as homemaker services, adult day care, and home health care) account for only 15% of care for disabled older persons. Informal caregivers are usually women who often sacrifice employment and other family obligations to provide the care to a relative (Katz & Karuza, 1992). Roles that family members may undertake include more than physical caregiving. Cultural aspects may include financial support, emotional support, decision making, and crisis intervention, which will influence family roles. Older people frequently have a long history of experience with health care providers that influences their beliefs about the meaning of health and how they interpret treatment, and they may have habits and idiosyncrasies that are firmly entrenched. Older peoples' life-long experiences in work, family, problem solving, religion, culture, aesthetics, and social arenas influence their reactions to illness and accepting care (Hasselkus, 1988a).

Culture

Culture encompasses ethnic and religious orientation, behaviors, ideas, and values. Occupational therapy practitioners must put aside their own cultural orientation to work with and accept the culture of the family. Burgess & Ragland (1983) gave some guidelines to follow:

1. Speak the right language. In order to make sure the client understands all terms, use interpreters.

2. Talk to the appropriate person. Who is making the decisions? Is the person receiving the care instructions actually going to give the care?

3. Be aware of cultural taboos that may relate to privacy or modesty.

The therapist should make some observations as to how health and illness are perceived. Is there denial of the problem or do the client and family seek and follow advice? Is the client being hidden because the cultural biases of the family characterize disability as upsetting, embarrassing, ugly, or even contagious? Has the client followed instructions given by other health care professionals in the past? Does the client always say "yes" because it would be impolite to disagree? Does the client have personal

beliefs about what will restore health? It may be necessary to incorporate folk medicine into the treatment plan for optimum success. Does the client's culture feel that attempts to make an older person independent are disrespectful and that the person should be cared for in bed? Habits concerning food, hygiene, dress, and leisure time must be taken into consideration. How does the family function? Their sex and age roles and caregiving practices are important. How do they establish patterns of communication and how do they make decisions (Groves, Glasser, & Kelsey, 1988)? What is the meaning of home and how does the occupational therapy practitioner determine which aspects of the home are important to the client (Thiers, 1993)? All of these factors are significant issues in planning transition.

Ethnographic Perspective

Gitlin, Corcoran, and Leinmiller-Eckhardt (1995) suggested that an ethnographic perspective be used to develop a framework for occupational therapy practitioners. An ethnographic perspective is "to understand another way of life as it is viewed and given meaning by participants. The ethnographer is interested in the values, meanings, and viewpoints of persons and how persons make sense of or perceive their own context" (Gitlin et al., 1995, p. 802). Occupational therapists can function in a way that is similar to ethnographers by trying to elicit the client's perspective and use this information about the client's value and meaning structure to develop treatment protocols (Gitlin et al., 1995).

Hasselkus (1990) described a system using ethnographic interviewing techniques with family caregivers and Gitlin et al. (1995) designed a framework for occupational therapists to use for evaluating the needs of family caregivers. They suggest the use of four key terms—informant, emic, reflexivity, and interpretation—"to derive an understanding of the perspective of the family member, the personal meaning of providing care, how care is provided in the home, and specific aspects that are perceived to be problematic" (Gitlin et al., 1995, p. 803).

IDENTIFY AN INFORMANT

Informants are a key source for the therapist to learn about daily practices and behaviors and to gain insight about the meaning of an activity or routine. They have knowledge of the cultural system and Hasselkus (1988b) viewed informants as lay practitioners because of their primary role in managing, coordinating, and providing hands-on care. By viewing family members as practitioners, the OT practitioner is encouraged to view the therapist's role as that of an enabler rather than that of a prescriber.

THE EMIC APPROACH

The *emic* approach is to obtain "an insider perspective or the point of view of an informant as to how things are and why.... The occupational therapist interviews and observes the lay practitioner(s) to identify their perspective of the meaning that shapes their act of caregiving" (Gitlin et al., 1995, p. 804). Observation of the home goes beyond traditional evaluation of accessibility and safety and the therapist uses a more inclusive observation method. This observation includes how "caregivers set up objects for daily routines, the presence of photographs and other objects of meaning, and the extent to which caregivers have rearranged the home to accommodate the level of competence of the family member who is impaired" (Gitlin et al., 1995, p. 804).

SELF-REFLECTION

In *self-reflection,* self-questioning is used by therapists to put their values and beliefs in perspective relative to those values and beliefs that exist in the cultural setting of the home. Questions for the therapist to ask are "(a) What do I see happening in this home? (b) Do I understand the perspective of the family members? and (c) Is my vision of the family members' needs the same or different from those of the lay practitioner(s)?" (Gitlin et al., 1995, p. 804).

FRAMEWORK FOR INTERPRETING INFORMATION

On the "basis of interviews, observation, active listening and reflexivity," the occupational therapist "derives an interpretation or analysis of the emic perspective, or how things work and what is important for the lay practitioner" (Gitlin et al., 1995, p. 804). This interpretation is continually changing and evolving on the basis of incoming information. It involves clinical reasoning in interpreting meanings and adapting treatment strategies to fit the individuality of the family unit. The occupational therapy practitioner observing the family members' behavior constantly asks these questions: "(a) What does the disability or impairment mean to the care receiver and the family member? (b) How do the family member and care receiver experience the caregiving activity? and (c) On the basis of the underlying meaning that informs care, what is an appropriate treatment strategy to support the efforts of the family unit?" (Gitlin et al., 1995, p. 805).

"The ethnographic framework for evaluating the family members' perspective ... can serve as a helpful structure for integrating the client's psychosocial, physical and emotional dimensions in treatment planning" (Gitlin et al., 1995, p. 807).

Caregiver Education

The family is involved with planning for discharge early in the treatment process. Most clients desire to return home if at all possible. The therapist must communicate with the practitioners in the other disciplines involved in the patient's care to ensure that all aspects of the client's functional needs are being addressed. Some of the following points should be reviewed to develop an understanding of the formal and informal support systems available at home and to develop a self-care plan prior to discharge. The goals that are most important to the client and family must be addressed quickly, because clients are being discharged at lower functioning levels and time is at a premium now and is anticipated to be more of a premium later. This enables the client to have a head-start on adjusting to the home environment and have a successful transition period. The Omnibus Budget Reconciliation Act (OBRA), the federal law governing long-term care facilities, mandates that a post-discharge plan contain the following points:

- Preferences for care
- How services are to be accessed and paid for
- How care is to be coordinated
- Identification of specific needs
- Personal care issues
- Sterile dressings
- Therapy
- Client or caregiver educational needs.

The occupational therapy practitioner is involved in making and researching some of these issues as well as incorporating appropriate parts into their treatment plans (Glantz & Richman, 1991).

The following questions further guide transition issues:

1. What is the status of the patient's or client's independence in essential activities of daily living?
2. Is the home adaptable for safety?
3. Are social contacts available for regular interaction?
4. Does the patient or client have projects that provide a sense of achievement?
5. Is transportation available?
6. Is the patient or client aware of resources available in the community? Is he or she willing to use them?
7. Will loneliness and activity planning become a problem? (Wells, 1988, p. 136)

Appropriate assistance for the client depends on the family's and friends' understanding the client's abilities and losses. Instruction and observation with the OT practitioner will help them to be an essential and integral part of the rehabilitation process (Wells, 1988). As the therapist and the client are working toward increased functional independence, the family may insist on providing unnecessary assistance. This adds to the family's burden, undermines the client's results from the established treatment plan, and jeopardizes the client's ultimate independence (Hunt, Baum, & Lottes, 1988). Occupational therapy personnel should not use their own value judgments about what the client should do and the role the family should play. The family may like cooking for the client, and the client may like to have his wife bathe him even though he can do more for himself. The therapist does need to emphasize how important realizing potential in each activity is to the client's recovery (Groves et al., 1988).

Transition for the person experiencing problems with dementia brings additional consideration for occupational therapy practitioners. Physical assistance is only one component to consider, but coping with constant care adds considerably more stress to the situation. Day care or other forms of respite and support groups may ease the burden for the caregiver (Wells, 1988) in such situations. It is appropriate for the occupational therapy practitioner to consider these options for the caregiver when planning discharge.

Follow-Up

Continuity of newly acquired self-care skills is often a problem when clients are discharged after a short hospital stay and they attempt to function with new methods of adaptation in their old environment. Follow-up efforts by telephone, in person, or through a community agency providing continuity of care is likely to contribute to more appropriate patterns of care and prevent dysfunctional patterns from emerging. The following points should be addressed during follow-up contacts:

1. Is the patient or client using the adaptive skills that were learned in the treatment setting?

2. Is the patient or client maintaining an interest and activity level that is as independent and creative as possible?

3. Have the caregivers established realistic expectations of the patient's or client's involvement in self-care? Is the patient or client demanding more assistance than is necessary?

4. Has the environment been adapted appropriately to maximize function, independence, and safety?

5. Does the caregiver interact with the patient or client with exercises and activities designed to maintain and improve strength and abilities?

6. Are the patient or client and the family involved in a support group? (Wells, 1988, p. 137).

Availability of Services

Independence is important to most people. At any age, persons strive for independence. Two important symbols of independence are a car and a home. Both are symbols of control over our lives. Being forced to move away from one's home can be demoralizing to an older adult. Poor health, financial hardship, or a deteriorating neighborhood can all contribute to the need for relocation. Having no choice about the decision to move increases the sense of alienation, loss of control, and dependence (Averyt, Furst, & Hummel, 1987). Relocation diminishes knowledge of resources and in some cases changes available support people or reduces their number. Understanding the intensity of the need for control and how it affects transition from hospital or rehabilitation program to home is important for the occupational therapy practitioner in the establishment of treatment goals.

Transition is aided by the full awareness of support services designed to keep older adults living at home. Such services include meal programs, home health aides, friendly visitors, homemaker aides, and Lifeline services. Subsidized community housing, shared housing, foster homes, halfway houses, caregiver arrangements, and "granny flats" all postpone the need for institutionalization (Averyt et al., 1987).

Gaps in the continuum of services can be created when existing services are not appropriate or available for an older adult returning to the community after hospitalization. Having available resources is necessary for the older adult to return to the community with an acceptable quality of life. Availability, accessibility, and acceptability should be part of the community long-term care system. Availability determines whether a service is provided; accessibility means the service is accessible to the population that needs it; and acceptability means the service is culturally appropriate for the population (Wallace, 1990).

It may be difficult for older adults with declining health, disability, and lack of financial resources to stay in their own homes because of a lack of knowledge about how to find support services.

Area agencies on aging have resources to help the older adult or caregivers find essential services such as the following:

- Homemakers' aides
- Home-health aides
- Chore services
- Support groups
- Adult day care
- Hotline numbers
- Medical equipment suppliers
- Hospice services
- Available senior discounts
- Meal services
- Help with Medicare paperwork
- Legal help for writing a will or a living will
- Friendly visitors.

Senior services directories have information about organizations available for help and can describe services available. (Information on these directories often are available from area agencies on aging and senior centers.)

Neighborhood churches and synagogues may offer or have information about the following services:

- Food banks
- Emergency shelters
- Volunteers to help with repairs and chores
- Persons to be a live-in companion
- Persons to do light housekeeping.

Financial Assistance

Utility Assistance Programs are available in most areas to help low-income older persons with their heating bills.

Many communities have *free weatherization* programs to make older homes more energy efficient and less costly to heat. These programs may be sponsored by local utilities, state public service departments, or state and county extension services. Information may be obtained from area agencies on aging, public service departments, state energy offices, or local social and welfare offices.

For telephone service, Lifeline services are available. The high cost of telephone service has meant that one in five older persons has had to curtail telephone service. The American Association of Retired Persons (AARP) and other public-interest organizations fear that more older adults will have to give up this necessity. For the older adult, the phone is not a convenience; it is a vital link to family, friends, social services, and emergency assistance. Its loss will mean greater isolation. Many states have passed "lifeline" legislation that is directed at keeping telephone service available for the elderly. For information about reduced-cost telephone service in a given area, call the area agency on aging, the local phone company, or the state public-service commission (Averyt et al., 1987).

Environmental Modification and Adaptive Equipment

Home modifications for comfort, ease, and safety are important and the occupational therapy practitioner can match specific needs with the appropriate modifications for the client to promote independence and successful aging in place (AOTA, 1995). The most appropriate way to determine which adaptations are needed to compensate for the person's inability to perform certain tasks is through a home visit. Without a home visit, the client's true needs may not be identified. Even with home visits, Christensen (1995) suggested that it is difficult for occupational therapy practitioners to be aware of all the assistive services and products available. Recommendations must be made in a timely fashion and therapists may make decisions about suggesting equipment that more appropriately should be made by the client and family. A thorough evaluation of the client's capabilities and the status of the living environment must be completed to allow the therapist to identify appropriate solutions to alleviate some of the identified problems. Enhancements Adapting Senior Environments (EASE), developed by Lifease, Inc.,* is one tool that may be used for this purpose.

Environmental adaptations for safety may be difficult for the client and family to make. They may be unwilling to remove clutter, area rugs, or cords crisscrossing the apartment or house. Furniture rearranging may require strength or balance that the client or caregiver does not possess. Do the support persons understand the reasons behind changes so that they can comply with the adaptations necessary (Wells, 1988)? Does the client's home have the physical layout to support his or her needs? There are many obvious considerations such as stairs, size of bathroom, size of doorways, types of floor surfaces, and distances between areas of the home. It is important to know whether the client owns the home or rents, whether modifications can be made, and to what extent they are practical and feasible. Another consideration is accessibility to the areas of the home that have meaning to the client. The decision to turn the dining room into a bedroom for the client may be appropriate from a functional perspective but not acceptable from the perspective of the client who has been spending a lot of leisure time in an upstairs den surrounded by the memorabilia of career days. Moving the memorabilia into the dining room may be unacceptable to a wife, for example, who has always maintained a "company" downstairs area. Is leisure for this client associated with the garage or basement work area and how important is using these areas safely to the client?

Other environmental issues that the therapist must consider when preparing a client for transition into the community is where grocery stores, laundry, and bus stops are located and the characteristics of the locale, such as curb cuts, hilly terrain, and safety. The occupational therapy practitioner should observe proximity of neighbors, condition of the home and surrounding environment, mobility barriers, and indications of the client's feelings of safety (bars, locks, dogs, etc.) (Groves et al., 1988).

Assistive devices can enable an individual with a disability to live life to its fullest potential. Obtaining funding for equipment has become increas-

---

*Stoney Lake Office Park, 2451 75th St., NW, Suite D, New Brighton, MN 55112.

ingly more difficult in this era of cost containment, particularly when devices are considered high-tech and expensive. Many managed care and insurance companies supply only one wheelchair for a person's entire lifetime and have stopped paying for repairs. Therapists and equipment suppliers need to provide objective documentation as to need and they must justify every piece of equipment. Strong, clear language must be used and denials must be appealed. If funding is denied through Medicare, Medicaid, and private insurance, more creative sources should be approached, such as Lions, Elks, Variety Club, and health associations (Daus, 1995).

Adaptive equipment issued in a hospital setting may often be inappropriate for the client at home. Bath benches that don't fit the client's space gather dust and may place the client in an unsafe situation when a task is attempted without the necessary equipment. The valuable resources of the elderly and the systems that provide the required equipment cannot be wasted or abused. Care must be taken in ordering equipment, and adequate training is essential for its appropriate use. The occupational therapy practitioner must assess the caregiver's ability to understand information given on safe, appropriate use of equipment. Even when the equipment has been issued in the hospital or rehabilitation setting, appropriate transition requires that the client is retrained for proper and safe procedures in his or her unique environment (Steinhauer et al., 1995).

The same factors for acceptance of new technology apply to all consumers regardless of age. These factors are motivation, knowledge, and affordability. Some seniors resist using products that are difficult to use or of inferior quality. Such resistance is positive and benefits the consumer. Some resistance is detrimental to consumers: for example, the consumer would benefit from technology but does not want to use it. The therapist needs to take resistance factors into consideration, as well as the following characteristics of products or environmental modification, to help understand the client's acceptance or opposition to technology:

1. Relative advantage—Is this idea, modification, or product much better than what it supersedes?
2. Compatibility—Is it consistent with existing values, past experiences, and current needs?
3. Complexity—Is there a perception that it is difficult to understand and use?
4. Trialability—Can it be tried without a large investment (Brink, 1995)?

Preparation for Emergencies

SAFETY

Safety as it relates to the client's discharge is a priority issue. The occupational therapy practitioner must use a holistic approach to this issue, involving assessment of cognitive and physical abilities. Safety in relation to medication management is an important area to evaluate from a cognitive and motoric standpoint. The treatment plan should include teaching medication management and how to recognize and cope with emergencies in this domain (Steinhauer et al., 1995).

COMMUNITY RESOURCES

Telephone reassurance programs are meaningful in assuring older persons that someone cares about them and will be checking on them regularly to ensure their safety. Volunteers for telephone reassurance programs ideally have training in referral and know the person through regular telephone visits. They give the isolated older person a point of contact (Benzing, 1988).

The client needs to have a plan for emergencies. The plan should be posted near the phone. Numbers to include are as follows:

- Police
- Fire department
- Poison control
- Doctor
- Family member
- Friend or neighbor conveniently located.

Has the treatment plan included training in telephone skills, adaptive equipment if needed, and safety issues of placement and accessibility of the phone? Technology now gives us portable phones for increased safety in the bathroom, phones that can be programmed for one-step or one-number dialing, and portable doorbell systems that can be placed in distant or most-used rooms.

Carrier alert, which is operated by the U.S. Postal Service and its workers' union in conjunction with a local sponsoring agency, checks on older citizens who might be isolated or in need of medical attention. A special decal is available to place on the mailbox to alert the letter carrier to be attentive to any potential problems.

The "Lifeline Emergency Response System" provides individuals with immediate access to emergency medical care. Families and older persons who live alone can have peace of mind about getting immediate help in case of an accident or other medical problem, even if they cannot get to their telephone. The system works by activating a unit attached to the telephone that automatically dials the emergency response center at a local hospital pro-

viding Lifeline service. It is triggered by a cordless "help" button worn on a necklace or bracelet. The hospital then attempts to reach the person by phone or sends a predesignated individual to the person's home. Information about Lifeline systems in a specific area can be obtained by calling 1-800-451-0525.

"Link to Life" is another system that reaches designated people to check on the subscriber, or if no one is available, it alerts the community emergency system. Information can be obtained by calling 1-800-338-4176.

"Medic Alert" is an identification system for medical information to be easily accessible in an emergency situation. The client wears a bracelet or neck chain with vital information engraved on it and there is a phone back-up hot line. Information can be obtained from 1-800-ID-ALERT.

HOME SAFETY

In preparing for the client's transition to the home, the OT practitioner must address all aspects of safety. Safety concerns exist for elderly persons experiencing normal changes of aging, for those individuals with more extensive impairment, and for caregivers of individuals with dementia. Education and training are essential for the client and the caregivers.

General Principles for Home Safety

The following conditions should exist in the home:

- Adequate lighting
- Uncluttered, uncrowded rooms with clear pathways
- No loose scatter rugs
- No cords in exposed areas
- Carpets or rugs that do not impede wheelchairs, walkers, or canes

- Water temperature controlled-heater set below 140 degrees.*

Kitchen Safety
- Check appliance cords for wear
- Remove objects from high shelves or cupboards
- Remove stove and oven knobs*
- Install cut-off systems for stoves*
- Lock up sharp knives*
- Put away appliances.*

Bathroom Safety
- Shower control gauge
- No-slip decals or mats in the tub and shower
- Installation of grab bars to eliminate reliance on less secure places to grab
- Nonskid rugs or mats to prevent slipping on a wet floor
- Bathtub or shower bench; hand-held shower
- Raised toilet seat
- Medication locked up.*

Bedroom Safety
- Stable furniture at bed height next to bed for support.

Specific Safety Issues for Persons With Dementia

The caregivers need to use specific precautions if the client wanders. Clients require an ID bracelet or some other form of identification that will always be with them. Recent photos should be kept handy to assist police in case the person wanders off. Local health departments or police departments may have a wandering program. Environmental changes should be made to prevent wandering, such as putting latches and locks higher or lower than eye level or using systems designed with two or more parts need-ed to unlock doors. Electronic technology should be used, if possible.

Education and Training

Education and training for potential emergencies should involve the client and caregivers in preparing written instructions. That enhances cooperation and helps to secure the success of the interventions. Carefully written instructions may help to avoid some emergencies. Included should be instructions on positioning, transfer procedures, appropriate cuing, and reasonable expectations for functional independence in feasible time constraints. The therapist needs to ensure that all verbal and written instructions can be understood and used by the client and family in emergency situations. Clients and their families should understand the functional, mental, and emotional changes that the client may experience.

Summary

The transition from the hospital or rehabilitation facility to home or a community living situation is complex. It begins at the outset of the treatment program and involves knowledge of the continuum of care and community resources. Good planning, preparation, and client and caregiver education will all ease the transition. The occupational therapist has a critical role to play in the process by recommending environmental adaptations, providing assistive devices that enable greater independence and safety, and ensuring that the client and caregiver are prepared to function in the discharge environment.

---

* For clients with dementia.

Activities

1. Do an initial interview with a client, using the ethnographic approach described in this section. What did you learn about the client's unique values, meanings, and viewpoints? Were you able to see the situation from the client's perspective? How did this form of interview differ from previous initial interviews you have conducted? Do you think the information was more helpful to you in formulating a treatment plan for the client in the home or community living situation?

Review Questions

1. Define "continuum of care."
2. Compare the medical model continuum with the CCRC model.
3. What is "care management"?
4. What are the intrapersonal aspects involved in transition?
5. What is meant by "ethnographic perspective"?
6. Why is follow-up care important?
7. What points should be addressed during follow-up contacts?
8. How can the occupational therapy practitioner address safety issues in the home?
9. Why is the ethnographic perspective important to occupational therapy practitioners?
10. What are some specific safety issues for people with dementia?

References

American Occupational Therapy Association (AOTA). (1994). Uniform terminology for occupational therapy (3rd ed.). *American Journal of Occupational Therapy, 48,* 1047–1054.

American Occupational Therapy Association (AOTA). (1995). *Growing older in your home.* Bethesda, MD: Author.

Averyt, A. C., Furst, E., & Hummel, D. D. (1987). *Successful aging: A source book for older people and their families.* New York: Ballantine Books.

Barone, W., Costante, P. A., & Ennis, R. S. (1989, June). The challenge to adapt. *Health Progress, 70,* pp. 50–52.

Benzing, P. (1988). Community networking. In L. J. Davis & M. Kirkland (Eds.), *Role of occupational therapy with the elderly* (pp. 393–404). Rockville, MD: American Occupational Therapy Association.

Binstock, R. H. (1994). Changing criteria in old-age programs: The introduction of economic status and need for services. *Gerontologist, 34,* 726–730.

Brink, S. (1995). Are there problems of technology adoption among seniors? *Aging, Disability, and Rehabilitation Network of the American Society on Aging, 3,* 1–2.

Burgess, W., & Ragland, E. C. (1983). *Community health nursing: Philosophy, process, and practice.* Norwalk, CT: Appleton-Century-Crofts.

Capitman, J. A., Abrahams, R., & Ritter, G. (1994). Measuring the adequacy of home care for frail elders *(HCFA Home Care Quality Report).* Waltham, MA: Institute for Health Policy, Brandeis University.

Christensen, M. A. (1995). Assessing an elder's need for assistance: One technological tool. *Generations, 19,* 54–55.

Daus, C. (1995, June/July). Reimbursement for assistive technology. *Rehab Management, 8,* 54–57.

Evashwick., C. J. (1989, June). Creating a continuum. *Health Progress, 70,* pp. 6–39.

Fanale, J. E., Keenan, J. M., Hepburn, K. W., & Von Sternberg, T. (1991). Care management. *Journal American Geriatrics Society, 39,* 431–436.

Gitlin, L., Corcoran, M., & Leinmiller-Eckhardt, S. (1995). Understanding the family perspective: An ethnographic framework for providing occupational therapy in the home. *American Journal of Occupational Therapy, 49,* 802–809.

Glantz, C. H., & Richman, N. (1991). *Occupational therapy: A vital link to the implementation of OBRA.* Rockville, MD: American Occupational Therapy Association.

Groves, J. K., Glasser, C., & Kelsey, T. T. (1988). Home health. In L. J. Davis & M. Kirkland (Eds.), *Role of occupational therapy with the elderly* (pp. 153–170). Rockville, MD: American Occupational Therapy Association.

Hasselkus, B. R. (1988a). Assessment. In L. J. Davis & M. Kirkland (Eds.), *Role of occupational therapy with the elderly* (pp. 123–127). Rockville, MD: American Occupational Therapy Association.

Hasselkus, B. R. (1988b). Meaning in family caregiving: Perspectives on caregiver/professional relationships. *Gerontologist, 28,* 686–691.

Hasselkus, B. R. (1990). Ethnographic interviewing: A tool for practice with family caregivers for the elderly. *OT Practice, 2,* 9–16.

Hunt, L. F., Baum, C. M., & Lottes, E. M. (1988). Institutional settings for gerontic occupational therapy practice, the acute hospital. In L. J. Davis & M. Kirkland (Eds.), *Role of occupational therapy with the elderly* (pp. 139–152). Rockville, MD: American Occupational Therapy Association.

Kane, R. A., & Kane, R. L. (1987). *Long-term care principles, programs and policies.* New York: Springer.

Katz, P. R., & Karuza, J. (1992). Service delivery in an aging population: Implications for the future. *Generations, 16,* 49–54.

Pollock, N. (1993). Client-centered assessment. *American Journal of Occupational Therapy, 47,* 298–301.

Rogers, J. C., (1988). Roles and functions of occupational therapy in gerontic practice. In L. J. Davis & M. Kirkland (Eds.), *Role of occupational therapy with the elderly* (pp. 117–121). Rockville, MD: American Occupational Therapy Association.

Steinhauer, M., Austill-Clausen, R., Menosky, J., Young, J., Youngstrom, M. J., & Hertfelder, S. (Commission on Practice Home Health Task Force). (1995). *Guidelines for occupational therapy practice in home health.* Bethesda, MD: American Occupational Therapy Association.

Thiers, N. (1993, September 23). Home sweet home: Recognizing the importance of place. *OT Week, 7,* pp. 14–15

Wallace, S. P. (1990). The no-care zone: Availability, accessibility, and acceptability in community-based long-term care. *Gerontologist, 30,* 254–261.

Wells, M. A. (1988). Continuity of care. In L. J. Davis & M. Kirkland (Eds.), *Role of occupational therapy with the elderly* (pp. 133–138). Rockville, MD: American Occupational Therapy Association.

Yerxa, E. J. (1991). Nationally speaking: Seeking a relevant, ethical, and realistic way of knowing for occupational therapy. *American Journal of Occupational Therapy, 45,* 199–204.

Section 6.
Evaluation and Intervention for Work and Productive Activities

Ferol Menks Ludwig, PhD, OTR/L, FAOTA, GC, and Barbara L. Kornblau, JD, OTR, DAAPM, CIRS, CCM

Abstract

Work and productive activities have served as central themes in occupational therapy, reflecting the core philosophy, values, and commitment dating back to the founding of the profession. Historically, work and other productive activities have been used to build skills and habits that were considered to be essential requisites for the development and maintenance of good character and well-being (Meyer, 1922/1977; Slagle, 1922).

Occupational therapy developed from the functional pragmatic philosophical base, which valued the productive use of time and ascribed a strong moral tone to one's engagement in occupation. Occupational therapy was based on the proposition that there was both health-maintaining and health-generating potential in the purposeful use of one's time if it was balanced among work, rest, and play. When this deteriorated, individuals lost their ability to lead a balanced life and to satisfy and adapt to daily needs and demands (Meyer, 1922/1977; Slagle, 1922). Hall (1910, p. 12) spoke of the "work cure." Reilly (1966) built on this foundation and added an important emphasis on the work-play continuum and the need for competence.

Many of the current cohort of older adults in the United States were born and raised during the era of occupational therapy's founding and development. Older adults and occupational therapists continue to find themselves heavily influenced by the work ethic and they highly value work and productive activities.

Continuity Theory

Continuity theory provides a useful framework from which to examine performance areas in older adulthood. This section discusses continuity theory as it relates to evaluations and interventions concerned with the meaning of work and productive activities in late adulthood.

Continuity theory contends that people will pursue occupational patterns consistent with their life experiences that have meaning to them and are an essential part of their sense of self and personal narrative (Atchley, 1989). For example, events such as retirement have been found to have less effect on inner continuity than role theorists hypothesized (Atchley, 1982). To predict the effect of a specific change such as retirement, one must know how that change in occupation is interpreted by the individual and how it is linked to his or her identity and themes of meaning.

Kaufman (1986) emphasized the importance of subjective interpretations of continuity and change over time for each individual. She found that her informants dealt with specific changes, problems, and events as they had been doing throughout their lives and that they interpreted these in reference to themes they formed earlier. Meaning in old age was derived from being oneself, which relied on a sense of continuity of self over time and is "a critical resource for remaining healthy" (p. 6).

People come to know and explain themselves through the development of themes, which they create to interpret and evaluate their life experiences (Kaufman, 1986). Themes provide continuity and occupations that serve to reflect themes are meaningful. Themes are socially constructed from historical, geographical, and social circumstances such as the values of American society and the cultural expectations of how a life should be lived. Productivity, achievement, work, progress, and usefulness have been found to constitute major themes of meaning in older adults that reflect the ideals, values, and norms of their sociocultural heritage (Kaufman, 1986; Ludwig, 1995).

Older adults interpret their own development with cultural ideals, and their age and cohort values are the standards by which they measure whether they became and are continuing to be the type of person that they value. Erikson (1963) referred to this as achieving a sense of integrity versus despair. Older adults assess their success in meeting these culturally based ideals through what they have done and what they are doing. Thus, through engagement in work and productive activities, they integrate and evaluate themselves and their lives.

Following is a discussion of relevant literature and evaluation and intervention strategies for work and productive activities. The specific areas are work, retirement, caregiving and care receiving, home management, and financial affairs.

WORK

Occupational therapy has always recognized work as a significant need in one's life. The role of worker fills many basic human needs and many older adults are choosing to work longer than others have in the past. Instead of contemplating retirement, many older employees might be thinking of new challenges and ways to contribute at work. They want to use their experience and continue in the workplace where they derive satisfaction. Workers also might need to remain in the labor force because they cannot financially afford to retire.

Most of the elderly have much potential for making continued productive contributions. Stereotypes of declining physical capacity, although partially correct, must be monitored on an individual basis. Although the incidence of health problems does increase with age, in many cases work abilities of older employees show no significant impairment. Furthermore, they often have much better attendance and safety records than their younger counterparts (Rosen & Jerdee, 1985).

Older employees need help developing strategies that will keep them employable if they desire to continue working. Rosen and Jerdee (1985) described the challenges of managing older employees:

1. Increasing economic pressure to delay retirement
2. Preventing employee obsolescence
3. Expanding legal protection for older workers, which requires positive steps from management
4. Creating a major push for extending work lives.

The primary reasons older workers currently find themselves out of work include the following:

1. Voluntary or mandatory retirement
2. Layoff or discouragement
3. Infirmity or disability
4. Technological changes

5. Problems of reentry

6. Career switches

7. Poor qualifications (Bass, 1988).

The nature of work is changing, requiring workers to deal with new kinds of information, people, and machines. These changes are more threatening to older employees who have limited skills but are more challenging to older more adaptable workers. Job displacement remains a serious problem for all workers, especially older ones who are more likely to be unemployed for longer periods of time and who often suffer greater salary reductions when they do find new employment. Their previous specialized skills may no longer be needed and their seniority may not be useful in new situations. Realistic counseling needs to be provided for these people who have to change not only their positions but also their status and compensation. Older workers who are eligible for training and who want it should be given equitable access to regular Job Training Partnership Act training programs under Title II and access for displaced workers under Title III (Shapiro & Sandell, 1987).

MacRae (1991) stated that as the supply of younger workers decreases and the aging population expands, more employers will court older workers and that occupational therapists can act as advocates for aging workers to provide linkages between them and employers. As the population continues to age, many of the available occupational activities will become more varied. The role of occupational therapy will expand in the areas of health promotion and functional assessments of aging people who are capable and motivated to work. "One of occupational therapy's most important contributions to the future might be advocacy—promoting the well-being of an aging society via wellness programs, developing adaptive and compensatory techniques, and ensuring the right and the means to pursue work activities throughout life" (MacRae, p. 364).

Work assessment and intervention programs can be used with older clients, but the programs should incorporate several factors. People should have an accurate understanding of the normal age-related processes, as distinguished from the disease and disuse processes. The incidence of chronic disease increases with age and older workers are more likely to have several chronic diseases such as arthritis and high blood pressure. Occupational therapists can assess the work or home environment to determine what adaptations are necessary to promote continued productive employment.

A strong need might occur for occupational therapy practitioners to carefully assess the performance of older employees. Current and complete job descriptions, with special emphasis on delineating the physical and psychological demands associated with each job, play an important role. Both employee capacities and limitations need to be noted. Experimenting with job redesign facilitates the effectiveness and employability of the older worker.

Traditionally, OT practitioners have viewed the onset of a stroke or other disability in an older adult as the end of the individual's working days. The onset of a stroke or other potentially work-interrupting disability, however, need not mean the end of a person's working life or career. The Americans with Disabilities Act (ADA, 1990) gives older workers with disabilities the tools they need to be able to return to the workplace or workforce. These tools include a mandate requiring employers to make reasonable accommodations for individuals with disabilities to enable them to perform their jobs.

Under the ADA (1990), if an older individual has an impairment that substantially limits a major life activity, but the individual still is able to perform the essential functions of his or her job, the employer must make reasonable accommodations. These reasonable accommodations might include, for example, allowing the worker to sit instead of stand or providing the worker with adaptive equipment (called auxiliary aids under the ADA) such as an adjustable book stand to hold work equipment. Reasonable accommodations include making the workplace accessible by putting in ramps or grab bars to allow the worker access.

The reasonable accommodations requirement adds a whole new dimension to the provision of occupational therapy services for the elderly worker. Traditionally, in the rehabilitation setting, occupational therapists have performed home assessments of individuals before discharge following an accident or illness, to enable performance of the person's activities of daily living at home. Now, with the ADA firmly in place, in assessing the older adult, the occupational therapy practitioner needs to look at doing a work visit and assessment as part of the rehabilitation package.

Like the home visit, the work visit will enable performance of activities of daily living but will be specifically focused on the performance of work. The work visit allows the occupational therapy practitioner to observe the work and get a feel for the job. This assessment gives the occupational therapy practitioner information about the type of work the worker performs and how the work is performed—basically a task analysis of the job.

Job analysis is an essential component in the development of a specific worker's qualifications and reasonable accommodations. The skillful occupational therapy practitioner will carefully look at the work, the worker, and the workplace to create a match between the worker, any accommodations that might be needed for the way the work is performed, and any ergonomic changes in the workplace that might be needed. Job analysis should include a sequential list of essential job functions the worker must perform. The job analysis includes the physical requirements of the job as well as the cognitive, psychological, environmental, and physiological considerations of the job (Reynolds-Lynch, 1985).

The skillful occupational therapy practitioner will look at specific measurements, tools, and equipment used on the job, as well as the frequency with which the worker performs specific work tasks, including repetitive motions. Furthermore, both the number of employees performing the work task and the percentage of time the individual tasks are performed will be important factors in the job analysis (Ellexson & Kornblau, 1992).

The occupational therapy practitioner then can compare the work with the worker's functional abilities and determine areas of difficulty that will need reasonable accommodations. With this information, the occupational therapy practitioner can provide reasonable accommodations information to the employer so that he or she can modify the job, or provide information to the elderly worker to advocate for his or her reasonable accommodations needs in the workplace.

A typical workplace accommodation might include redesigning the worker's work station, pertaining not only to the actual elements of the job task but also to all of the job processes and the worker's interactions with the job components and the workplace environment. Workers vary considerably, yet most work stations currently lack the features required to accommodate individual workers' needs and promote optimal comfort, efficiency, and performance (Smith, 1989). Specific features of the work environment must readily be adjusted to meet the needs of all workers, not just the older worker. These features can involve adapted seating, job station design, injury prevention, and the use of ergonomic principles to accomplish the work.

In spite of these workplace accommodations, some older workers might find that they no longer are able to work on a full-time basis but still wish to remain active players in the work force. Part-time work provides a viable alternative. With the shortage of younger workers, many companies such as McDonald's have sought out older workers from among the retired set. Additionally, under the ADA (1990), allowing a worker to work part-time instead of full-time can be considered a reasonable accommodation. Thus, OT practitioners should consider this option for older workers who wish to continue working in their previous occupations. If this is not possible, the older worker could explore other positions with accommodations.

Many older adults wish to continue with productive employment but also want adjustments in their work situation. They may desire primarily to free themselves from the rigid 5-day-a-week work schedule and may seek more flexibility and discretion in their work, not wanting the daily hassles they had to tolerate in the past.

Flexible work schedules are gaining in popularity as an option for the older worker. Many older adults want to work but want to work part-time, a desire that increases with age. Part-time work provides a natural transition from full-time work to retirement, yet sudden retirement is the norm. Reality tells us that part-time work usually is poorly compensated and can result in diminished Social Security benefits, depending on the age of the worker (Jondrow, Brechling, & Marcus, 1987).

RETIREMENT

Retirement is regarded by some older adults as the reward for work they have accomplished over many years, whereas for others it is viewed as a roleless role and as forced idleness (Atchley, 1982). Two primary factors that determine retirement are wealth and health, not age (Rosen & Jerdee, 1985). Until recently, people worked until they perceived that they could afford to retire or were too infirmed to continue working. With the increases in Social Security, pension plans, and savings, larger numbers of people find themselves able to retire and are living longer as retired persons.

The trend toward early retirement continues, but it is being offset by economic forces such as the increase in age eligibility for Social Security and other factors that erode funds and create pressure for maintaining more older persons in the labor force. Their increased longevity creates the need for more resources to support themselves and their families for a longer period of time in the postretirement years. Many older workers are being steered to delay retirement by the macroeconomic forces that keep them working longer. Healthy individuals who retire early tend to get more satisfaction from their leisure activities than they did from their work, whereas motivated older employees tend to find more satisfaction from their jobs (Rosen & Jerdee, 1985).

Planning

Both late career stages and retirement require special planning and flexibility. It is hoped that the older worker has effectively planned for retirement much earlier in life. One must understand the individual's career and retirement aspirations and how these contribute to his or her sense of continuity and themes of meaning.

Transition to Retirement

For some people, work is very much tied into their identity and, for these people, retirement is seen as a discontinuity that is hard to reconcile. Self-imposed routines that provide structure can be helpful in such cases to provide the discipline that work once provided in organizing one's day. Work frequently serves to structure time, give purpose to living, and provide self-esteem (Olmstead, 1975). Work and productive activities also could be needed to create a time structure for leisure because freedom from obligations can only exist in relation to obligation (Berman, 1994). Retirement necessitates a renegotiation of the balance of work and play/leisure, which could take 1 to 2 years for many older adults.

Psychosocial Aspects of Retirement

Retirement has serious consequences for older persons and clearly affects the way they spend their time and income, who they interact with, and their physical and mental health and well-being. The discussion continues about whether and how retirement affects attitudes and life satisfaction (Palmore, Burchett, Fillenbaum,

George, & Wallman, 1985). One needs to assess this on an individual basis by asking the person how he or she feels about being retired. For example, people who were forced to retire for poor health likely will find themselves having more difficulty adjusting to retirement than those who chose and planned for retirement. Poor health in many workers preceded retirement and may have caused unhappiness with retirement rather than vice versa.

Palmore et al. (1985) found that retirement at the socially expected age of 62 to 65 has little or no adverse effect on health. Some people become more dissatisfied, whereas others become more satisfied. More negative effects were noted among those retirees who were forced to retire early because of health reasons, age discrimination, or other involuntary reasons. Thus, evidence indicates that public policy and occupational therapy practitioners need to focus on reducing unemployment for those who wish to continue to work. Those who retire as a result of poor health are the most vulnerable and most negatively affected group (Palmore et al., 1985).

Health status seems to be much more related to life satisfaction than labor force status. The primary factors of better adjustment are better health, income, education, more activities, and being married (Palmore et al., 1985). Social activities become increasingly more important after retirement and occupational therapy practitioners need to help older persons maintain or increase opportunities for social activities. Loneliness was found to be a serious problem that was more common among retirees over age 65 than for those persons over age 65 who continued to work (Sheppard, 1988).

The effect of retirement on the marital relationship depends on what that relationship was like to begin with.

Division of labor often is renegotiated. Olmstead (1975, p. 35) wrote in his retirement journal: "Since I no longer go out and drudge all day in an office in order to bring home the bacon, perhaps it has now come time for me to lighten the work load C has been carrying at home all these years." More time exists for shared activities, and individual time has new dynamics.

Many older adults experience a sense of relief from having decreased obligations and responsibilities that permit them more time to do things they value and enjoy. Some report enjoying the freedom from the rushing and frenetic activity that characterized their earlier years when they worked and had children at home (Ludwig, 1995; Olmstead, 1975).

Work Substitutes

Economically developed nations consider that productive work and gainful employment is paid work usually performed in the employ of others. The payment one receives for work outside of the home is a widely used measure of productivity in modern Western nations. Today, however, infinite varieties of work or participation in productive activities exist that fit one's skills and abilities and contribute to the welfare of others or society at large.

Volunteer Work

Productive work includes work for the community or unpaid work for the family. Volunteer work often substitutes for paid employment and can help to satisfy one's need to feel useful and to contribute to the common good. Some older adults, however, do not find work that is unpaid, or work below prevailing rates of pay, to be an acceptable alternative.

Some older adults who are financially secure chose the flexibility of volunteer work rather than paid employment. The reasonable accommodation provisions of the ADA (1990) apply to volunteer work under the public accommodations provisions. These provisions require that places of public accommodation that offer programs to the public make their programs accessible and usable by individuals with disabilities. For example, if a woman wished to be a "pink lady" volunteer in the local hospital, and she required certain accommodations to participate in the volunteer program, such as a volume-controlled telephone, the hospital would have to provide the accommodation. The occupational therapy practitioner should consider reasonable accommodations wherever possible to enable older persons to participate in volunteer programs.

Advisory Roles

Older adults might serve in paid or unpaid advisory roles to businesses, institutions, organizations, and persons. Retired Senior Volunteer Services, or RSVS, is one example of a voluntary advisory organization.

Education

Colleges and universities have developed numerous programs to serve the needs of older people. Few, however, concern themselves with career education and training for older adults. The most common programs are tuition-waiver programs within the regular college or university. Most of these enable the older person to enroll on a space-available basis. Few supportive services are offered specifically for the older adult, but such services legally must be provided and older adults also can tap into existing services for special students.

Continuing education programs, which primarily are targeted at leisure or personal-enrichment programs, account for the largest enrollments of older adults. Institutes for retired professionals often are designed with university resources that enable older people to plan, administer, and teach their own educational programs that serve both intellectual and social functions.

Elder Hostel is another extensive program that uses a wide variety of settings to provide in-residence learning experiences in an ever-widening catalog of courses taught all over the world.

CAREGIVING OR RECEIVING

Caregiving and care receiving are common productive activities of older adults. At various times, they may find themselves both caring for others as well as receiving care themselves. Older persons can function as viable resources in either the primary or the secondary labor market. They can assume productive work roles that serve others as paid or unpaid workers.

WHO ARE THE CAREGIVERS?

Meeting the needs of older family members has become "a normative family crisis" (Brody, 1985, p. 19). When parents become old and frail, their adult daughters or spouses most likely will provide caregiving. Sixty-two percent of all medical and personal care to elderly in the community comes from family members (Cicirelli, 1992).

Caregivers are quite heterogeneous. Their age varies and their caregiving obligations often recur throughout their life span for adult children, grandchildren, parents, and spouses. Unfortunately, the traditional option of choosing to assist in family responsibilities, such as caring for grandchildren, has changed for many older adults. This responsibility has changed from an option to a requirement as the structure of the family has changed.

The emergence of a plethora of single-parent households, as well as single working parents and drug-addicted mothers, forces many older adults into the primary caregiver role for their grandchildren. For example, some 80-year-old women provide care for adult children and grandchildren. This care can involve having adult children move in or providing financial help and babysitting (Ludwig, 1995).

Among caregivers 70% are female, with an average age of 46. Interestingly, 15% of caregivers are over 65 years of age. One-third are caregivers because of their proximity to the older person. A full 54% have children under 17 years of age living at home. Half of the caregivers work for pay full-time, a number that continues to increase. The average age of care receivers is 77. The typical caregiver is a female who is juggling job, family, and elder dependent. The majority of caregivers provide personal services with instrumental and personal activities of daily living (Zimmer, 1991). Most family caregivers indicate that a sense of family responsibility and love motivates them to engage in caregiving.

Demographic trends indicate a growing likelihood that midlife and older workers will be expected to serve as caregivers. Thus, the need arises to design and implement services to facilitate and support caregivers and to help ease their burden. For example, a 49-year-old working caregiver can easily have an elderly parent, age 67, who will survive another 16 years or more; the caregiver also may have a grandparent age 85 years or older. She could be caring for them as well as for relatives of her husband (Gibeau, 1988). Many women function as the sole support for dependent children and as caregivers for their frail elderly. Decreases in family size lead to a beanpole family structure that provides fewer available children to care for family members.

Caring for a dependent older family member is often a long-term obligation and the choice to become caregiver has serious implications for one who so chooses, especially for his or her later years (Gibeau, 1988). Some sacrifices may be loss of benefits and economic contributions.

STRESSES

One must distinguish between subjective and objective feelings of burden. Studies have found that perceived burden is more related to caregiver burden and stress than the tangible load (Montgomery, Gonyea, & Hooymana, 1985).

Caregiving is physically and psychologically demanding. Caregiving and paid work embraces two full-time jobs. Time pressures and conflicts often ensue as the caregiver tries to juggle roles. Generally, the major loss is in personal time, particularly leisure. The caregiver frequently experiences social isolation, decreased physical well-being, emotional exhaustion, depression, fatigue, and stress-related illnesses. Caregiver burden can lead to abuse and neglect of the patient and depression and substance abuse in the caregiver.

Financial stress can cause conflict and pressure. Caregivers struggle with setting priorities, ethical dilemmas, intergenerational conflicts, and knowing how much is reasonable for them to do. Often caregiving duties arise when one expects to be free of obligation and responsibility for the daily care of others. Old family conflicts can arise after decades of independence and distance (Ludwig, 1987). Role reversal also can occur.

The demands of caregiving generally continue over an extended period and the stressors of caregiving can change. This is particularly true for caregivers of persons with Alzheimer's disease.

Many caregivers are in their 70s and may have some diminutions in their physical or mental status while at the same time caring for parents in their 90s or a spouse. Adult children also may need their parents for financial, emotional, and physical support.

NEEDS

Occupational therapy practitioners evaluate the needs of the patient and the caregiver's ability to provide care. The goal is to both maximize the independence of the care receiver and to minimize the burden of care on the caregiver. Treatment should help the caregiver and the family to provide support (Baum & LaVesser, 1994). This involves doing informed discharge planning; giving caregiver training in specific needed skills; facilitating the development of caregivers' confidence in their ability to provide quality care and handle situations as they arise; helping caregivers to recognize and protect their own mental and physical health needs, to receive positive feedback, and to establish or maintain a positive relationship with the care receiver.

Caregivers must to be able to recognize when and how to help. They need training in the skills related to how to care for the older person; how to manage the disease and learn difficult concepts, such as the difference between lying and confabulation; how to use emergency measures; and how to access resources, such as respite care and home health services. They need to learn how to manage and recognize problems and deficits as necessary for safe and effective management of the care receiver. Emotional support serves to help caregivers learn how to handle stress and resolve the dilemmas of their demanding situation.

Hasselkus (1994) viewed the family caregiver as a lay practitioner with whom the health professional must establish a "therapeutic alliance" (p. 340). Each party holds his or her own perspectives and beliefs. As occupational therapy practitioners work with each caregiver, they transfer responsibility for the care to the caregiver so that the caregiver can take over. According to Hasselkus, this very complicated process should be delicately and sensitively handled. Issues, such as beliefs about illness and causation, cultural differences, and power, play strong roles in this process. She advocated discussing these issues in an effort to form an alliance. Discrepancies between views should be addressed. Ethnographic interviewing has been suggested as a way to understand the caregiver's orientation that influences his or her caregiving actions. The process is both reflective and reflexive.

Likewise, information should be presented to caregivers in ways that are most conducive to their learning styles. For older caregivers, written instructions should be printed in a size of at least 12-point type and should be sharp, standing out on the printed page. For caregivers over age 75, information might need to be presented more slowly, with only a few major ideas and details at a time. Building on previous knowledge and skills is particularly effective. Handouts and written instructions are important memory aids. Pictures are particularly helpful. Audiotapes or videotapes also can be useful for older adults.

PERSONAL AUTONOMY

One must keep in mind the ethical principle of autonomy whenever decisions have to be made about the care of older adults. Autonomy can be enhanced or diminished through the actions of caregivers (Cicirelli, 1992). Older individuals have a right to maximum self-determination and dignity. The practitioners must examine autonomy issues in the caregiving of older adults, especially by family members, as the practitioners weigh the care receiver's wishes against the caregiver's concern for safety (which often is paternalistic).

Caregiving for older adults involves extensive decision making, especially in relation to the type and amount of help one should provide to an aged person. It is important that the OT practitioner determine who actually makes the decisions in the caregiving decision-making system. Many times who makes the decisions is influenced by cultural factors as well as by the beliefs and attitudes of each of those involved toward elderly adults. Occupational therapy practitioners must be sensitive to differences in autonomy, attitudes, and paternalistic beliefs between decision makers, to be more sensitive to areas of conflict and congruence.

Occupational therapy practitioners must try to avoid premature and unnecessary paternalism. Intervention should empower older adults by teaching them safe ways to do things and ways to compensate for deficits and limitations. It is important that caregivers be able to express their concerns, yet see the older person engaging in functional performance as independently and safely as he or she chooses or is able to. Caregivers, as well as the care receivers, can benefit from information and further education about a disease or disability and its management. In many cases, autonomy is shared and negotiated by members of the decision-making system and is based on trust and confidence between family members (Cicirelli, 1992).

Independence in some areas of occupational performance might not be desired by the caregiver or care receiver family system. The occupational therapy practitioner will need to negotiate realistic options and describe to those parties the consequences.

HOME MANAGEMENT

Home management refers to "obtaining and maintaining personal and household possessions and environment" (AOTA, 1994, p. 1052). Clothing care, house cleaning, meal preparation and cleanup, shopping, money management, household maintenance, and safety procedures all are activities needed to remain independent in the community. Home management, independent living skills, and instrumental activities of daily living (IADL) are used to refer to these types of activities. Home management activities are more complex than those for self-care and require higher cognitive processing and neuromuscular function and endurance.

Assessment

The Instrumental Activities of Daily Living Scale and the Activities of Home Management Form, adapted from the Occupational Therapy Department, University Hospital, Ohio State University, Columbus, Ohio (Foti, Pedretti, & Lillie, 1996, p. 468), can be used to evaluate many home management activities. If possible, all evaluations should be done by having individuals actually perform in their natural setting. Home evaluations, such as the checklist adapted from the Ralph K. Davies Medical Center and Alta Bates Hospital cited by Foti, Pedretti, and Lillie (1996, p. 470), are useful for evaluating the older adult's ability to function in his or her home environment.

Enhancements Adapting Senior Environments (EASE) is a comprehensive software program that was designed for occupational therapy practitioners to use to help older adults live at home longer and more safely (Christenson, 1995). It identifies potential problems by measuring the functional abilities of the individual with the functional requirements of the home environment. EASE then identifies specific solutions for each problem and identifies resources. (Refer to Module II, chapter 8, for more detail on this software application.)

Other assessment tools that use interviews could be helpful. These are mainly screening devices, however, and do not observe actual performance in context. The IADL Screener was created to identify older community dwelling residents who are at risk for dependency by screening a person's ability to do housework, travel, shop, prepare meals, and manage personal finances (Fillenbaum, 1985). The Functional Activities Questionnaire (FAQ) screens normal older adults and those with mild dementia who function in the community (Fillenbaum, 1988). Its advantage is that it includes specific aspects of financial management, such as writing checks and ability to track and manage forms needed for such things as Social Security and taxes. Someone close to the person being evaluated, such as a spouse or close friend of the patient, completes the FAQ, which has its own special advantages and disadvantages.

The Safety Assessment of Function in the Environment for Rehabilitation, or SAFER, is a Canadian evaluation that focuses on physical and cognitive safety in home management and community activities. Its reliability and validity currently is being studied by Letts (1995).

It is essential to determine which tasks the person needs to be able to perform as well as those that he or she would like to perform or delegate to others. The occupational therapy practitioner needs to consider:

1. Consistency

2. Time

3. Level of independence or assistance needed

4. Quality of the performance.

Safety, in particular, needs to be noted for the older adult. The OT practitioner frequently evaluates the potential for the person's remaining at home by using the home management evaluation.

It is important to keep in mind that the functional status of older adults fluctuates with exacerbations and remissions of chronic conditions, such as arthritis, and periods of inactivity secondary to hospitalization. Return to independent function is realistic in many cases for older adults who exhibit functional losses in home management skills. Optimally, the home evaluation is multidisciplinary and health professionals and family are present to contribute to a comprehensive performance-based assessment. It is important to assess the family's expectations and resources for the patient.

Occupational therapy practitioners assess how the environment limits or fosters performance. From these data, the OT practitioner delineates the problems and suggests additional safety equipment, modifications, assistive devices, and home rearrangement. For example, the kitchen storage areas frequently should be rearranged to allow for energy conservation, work simplification, limited range of motion, and prevention of falls (Foti, et al., 1996). The recommendations, costs, and resources are discussed with the patient and his or her family, if the patient permits the therapist to discuss this information with them. The therapeutic relationship is confidential and therapists working with older adults must have their permission to discuss this with family members unless the family member is legally designated to be in charge. (See *Conservator and Guardianship* later in this chapter.)

Today many adult children live in other communities away from their aging parents. The extended family has dwindled in importance in mainstream American culture, leaving many aging adults alone in the world with few support systems outside of friends or church or synagogue. As aging friends pass on, older adults might find themselves completely alone in the world, with absent children—who can provide no day-to-day assistance—in some faraway place.

How do the elderly manage? There are some alternatives. Many communities have Meals on Wheels or congregate lunch-type programs to ensure that older adults get at least one nutritious meal per day. Area Aging Offices provide some community services and other grants-in-aid provide an aide to come into the home to help bathe the older adult and do some simple household chores such as laundry. Unfortunately, the current climate of budget cuts to social services is taking its toll on many of these programs. Social health maintenance organizations could become more predominant and help to fill needs for social support.

Another alternative exists for older adults who can afford to pay for these same types of services. Many communities with large elderly populations have private companies that provide assistance to older adults. This assistance can include taking the older adult to the bank or grocery shopping, or helping the client balance a checkbook. Sometimes the service includes making a friendly visit or calling on a daily basis to make sure the client is safe. Private companies providing these services often market their services to the adult children by advertising, in newspapers in major cities, to provide services to the older parents in some of the popular retirement areas such as those found in Florida and Arizona.

Environmental Adaptations and Modification

Having elderly people remain at home will often entail finding ways to simplify home management. This can mean using adaptive equipment, assistive devices, and auxiliary aides that promote the elderly staying in their homes as long as possible. To determine deficit areas, the occupational therapy practitioner can simulate various home maintenance activities in the clinic and may make a home visit. By analyzing these tasks, the occupational therapy practitioner can zero in on the specific deficits in performance. After deficit areas are identified, the occupational therapy practitioner will problem solve to see how the deficits can be overcome. Many assistive devices are available from occupational therapy equipment sources to make just about any home maintenance activity easier to perform.

Sometimes required adaptations in the home can mean changing physical features in or around the dwelling. For example, the use of a walker or wheelchair may necessitate the addition of a ramp on the premises. If an individual lives in a condominium or apartment building, the landlord or condominium board could disapprove of the addition of the ramp, disabled parking space, or other accommodation.

Although the ADA (1990) does not provide any help to the older adult in this sort of situation, another law exists under which older adults can seek assistance. The Fair Housing Act Amendments (1988) requires that reasonable accommodations be allowed in multiple dwelling housing to accommodate individuals with disabilities. Under the Fair Housing Act Amendments, unlike the ADA, however, the individual in need of the accommodations must pay for those accommodations. The landlord or condominium board is required under the law to allow the individual to make the accommodations. Thus, the need for accommodations in an apartment or condominium should not stand in the way of the older adult remaining in an independent living situation.

The Fair Housing Act Amendments (1988) has some caveats. The landlord can require that the modifications be undone when the person vacates the premises, if those changes can be made. In fact, the landlord can require the individual to deposit funds in an account in advance to make sure that the premises will eventually be restored to their original state.

If the occupational therapy practitioner should find that an older adult has been denied these reasonable accommodations, he or she should recommend that the person call the U.S. Department of Housing and Urban Development to file a complaint. The administrative process includes a conciliation process to try and facilitate settlement.

FINANCIAL AFFAIRS

Planning for one's financial affairs at retirement is a long process that spans adulthood. At the time an individual begins his or her first job, planning for retirement begins in the form of payment for Social Security. This payment continues throughout adulthood with the addition of other forms of retirement benefits, such as individual retirement accounts, investments, or other types of retirement plans. If one waits for late adulthood to begin financially preparing for retirement, it probably will be too late to amass the amount of money one should have to live comfortably through retirement. Social Security does not provide enough money for the majority of retirees to maintain their preretirement standard of living.

Most retirees experience a sharp decrease in income when they retire, to an average of three-fourths of preretirement income (Palmore, et al., 1985). It is important to examine other types of income or resources such as dividends, food stamps, and home equity.

Olmstead (1975, p. 64) questioned in his retirement journal, "Is Social Security manly?" Even though he contributed to Social Security for 40 years and believed that he deserved it, he felt diminished as a man by taking it. Older adults vary widely in their beliefs and attitudes regarding receiving and spending money.

Saving money becomes incorporated into purposeful activities that organize parts of an older person's days. They may cut coupons and shop carefully for specific cost savings.

Conservator and Guardianship

When older adults are no longer able to care for themselves, they can reach a point where the state (usually in the form of the state's Health and Rehabilitative Services [HRS] agency) steps in, has the person declared incompetent, and appoints a guardian or a conservator. These terms may vary by state but are essentially the same. This situation often happens when an individual is too confused to take care of his or her own affairs. A bank often will initiate this process, calling HRS

when it detects irregularities in the accounts or transactions of an older person whom it may suspect has been swindled out of money. Hospitals may call HRS when they are unable to contact relatives before discharging an older patient.

To effectuate the conservator or guardianship process, the state usually proceeds to court to prove the individual needs supervision because he or she is unable to take care of his or her needs. The individual deemed incompetent becomes a ward of the state. Some states such as Florida have a limited guardianship, which means the state appoints a guardian to act for the ward only in specific, limited situations. For example, the court might decide that the individual cannot manage finances and appoint a guardian to handle the funds and make all decisions about how and when money will be expended.

In some states, occupational therapy practitioners may participate in the guardianship or conservator process by providing the courts with information about the person's current status in relationship to his or her ability to take care of himself or herself, funds, and other related matters. This arrangement would involve the occupational therapy practitioner's performing an activities-of-daily-living assessment, focusing extensively on community living skills such as balancing a checkbook and other money-handling tasks, and making informed decisions about selecting medical care and a place of residence on par with the amount of care one requires. The occupational therapist might be asked to give information about the individual's ability to make appropriate decisions regarding his or her own care and needs.

Depending on the laws of the particular state, and the person's condition, when he or she is found to be incompetent and a guardian or conservator is appointed, the person will lose all or some of his or her rights. These lost rights can include, among others, the right to choose one's place of residence, the right to select a medical care provider, the right to vote, the right to handle one's financial affairs, and the right to contract for goods and services.

After appointment, the guardian or conservator acts in place of the individual. The person is no longer permitted by law to act on his or her own behalf. So, for example, if a ward has a stroke and is in need of occupational therapy services, under the law, the ward cannot sign consent for treatment. Only the guardian or conservator can give consent for occupational therapy services. This situation can be complicated further by out-of-state guardians or conservators, which some states permit, or guardians who are appointed from social service agencies solely devoted to providing guardians or conservators. In both cases, these guardians often are difficult to reach.

Dealing with guardians might present the occupational therapy practitioner with an ethical problem. Most states will make every effort to appoint a family member as the guardian or conservator. A family member who is serving as a guardian or conservator often is listed in the ward's will and therefore has a personal interest in the ward's financial situation. The less the guardian or conservator spends on the ward during the ward's lifetime, the more money will remain for the family member-guardian or conservator to inherit.

Suppose, for example, that the guardian or conservator refuses to give consent for occupational therapy services and the occupational therapy practitioner feels the services are necessary. What can the occupational therapy practitioner do? Under the law, when a guardian or conservator is appointed, he or she has a duty to act in the best interest of the ward. The guardian or conservator in most states is obligated to make an annual report to the court and thus performs his or her services under the ultimate supervision of the court. Depending on the law of the particular state involved, the occupational therapy practitioner might be able to petition the court for permission to treat the patient.

This guardianship situation can be totally avoided with a little advance planning before the individual becomes incompetent. Older adults and even younger adults might want to consider the *durable power of attorney* as an alternative or preventative measure to avoid finding themselves as wards of the state. Although all 50 states provide for durable powers of attorney, these laws vary by state so it is best to tell clients and patients to seek advice from an attorney who specializes in elder law in the appropriate state. Attorneys who specialize in elder law can be found by contacting the National Association of Elder Law Attorneys.

The durable power of attorney is a legal document in which the person signing the document gives to another person the power to act in his or her place. On the one hand, the difference between a regular power of attorney and a durable power of attorney is the regular power of attorney ceases to be in effect when the individual becomes incompetent. The durable power of attorney, on the other hand, survives incompetency, remaining in place in spite of the individual's incompetency. Durable powers can be general or special, depending on the scope of the powers given. In other words, the power can be limited to business or banking purposes, for example, or general enough to cover all legal decisions that need to be made (Buchanan, Kaplan, & Gilfix, 1991).

The durable power of attorney must be given with extreme care because it takes effect at the moment it is signed. If the power is given to an unscrupulous individual, he or she could potentially empty all of the person's bank accounts the same day the papers are signed. Thus, although power of attorney forms can be found readily in stationary and office supply stores, the older adult should consult a knowledgeable attorney for advice to ensure that he or she will be protected as much as possible.

If done properly, the durable power of attorney may in some states effectively prevent a guardianship or conservatorship procedure. With the durable power of attorney in place, the guardianship or conservatorship may not be necessary, because under the durable power of attorney, someone already is legally appointed to care for the older person.

Additionally, in the rare case in which the court might find it necessary to appoint a guardian in spite of the existence of a durable power of attorney, many courts will consider the older person's wishes about who to appoint as the guardian or conservator. If the person already is named in the older adult's durable power of attorney, the court usually will follow that wish and appoint the named person as the guardian or conservator.

In practical, day-to-day application, the person appointed by the durable power of attorney can assist the older individual by doing the banking, signing Medicare or Social Security documents and forms, and signing almost anything else that requires a signature, including selling property or stocks

and bonds. This can be very helpful to an older adult whose mobility may be limited or to a healthy elderly individual who is taking precautions for the future.

Protection from Con Games and Theft

Every day older adults, especially older women, are conned out of money by slick telemarketing schemes, mailings, and door-to-door sales pitches for all sorts of overpriced services or goods. Some of these predators wedge themselves into the lives of their victims and take everything that they have. Fraud is a major problem for the elderly and it is believed that the crimes are underreported because the people affected are embarrassed and fear being judged incompetent. The National Center on Elder Abuse in Washington, D.C., reported more than 29,000 cases of exploitation for 1994 (Harris, 1995).

After an older person falls prey to one of these scams, he or she is identified as an easy mark because con artists sell names of these persons to one another. Thus, he or she will be contacted repeatedly with various schemes. Instead of believing that they have been taken, many justify their actions by believing that they will win this time (Harris, 1995).

Four factors put current seniors at greater risk than ever before: more leisure time, isolation, anxiety, and richer assets. For many older adults, participating in contests and telemarketing schemes provides them with contact with others and engages them in activity. The need for human contact and activity is the hook of such schemes. Computer-generated letters even use recipient's names and seem to personalize the approach. Someone seems to care and is willing to do something for them, which in turn obligates them to do something in return.

Other scams involve relatives, repairmen, and caregivers. These persons gain entry and become familiar with the senior's financial life and start taking money or valued items. This usually starts out small but quickly escalates, especially as the older person becomes more frail. Minor impairments play nicely into the scam artist's plans. For example, minor visual impairments can cause an older adult to sign documents that he or she has not read or understood and that do not say what he or she has been told they say.

Law enforcement agencies in Florida, California, New Jersey, and a few other states have special units that investigate elder scams. Harris (1995) has stated that the main burden of safeguarding the elderly from fraud belongs to their families. It is important to encourage adult children to stay involved with their parents and become as familiar with their assets and spending as the parent is comfortable. Those working with older adults should look for potential indications of fraud—for example, numerous shoddy products and offers lying about and arriving in the mail. Adult children might check telephone bills for 900 number calls to sources that promise big prizes or merchandise.

Above all, an older person should not be judged as incompetent solely because he or she has been conned. Many competent younger adults have been victims of such schemes. If, however, the person has not learned from the experience and does not recognize the situation, then the earlier discussion about guardianship and conservatorship might be indicated, or some less severe limitation of access to funds, such as a joint signature with a trusted family member.

Summary

This section discussed evaluation and interventions for work and productive activities for older adults. Both occupational therapists and the current cohort of older adults continue to find themselves heavily influenced by the work ethic and highly value work and productive activities. Meaning in old age is derived from a sense of continuity of self over time and is an important adaptive resource. Some older employees wish to continue to work for pay and seek to remain as productive as they can. Occupational therapy practitioners can provide valuable services to help them remain in the work force through work assessment, job analysis, and design of an ergonomic work station.

Older adults view retirement in a wide variety of ways. Planning for retirement must begin early in life and be continuous. Retirement reconstitutes a whole new negotiation of relationships and time allocation among one's occupations. Those persons in poor health seem most at risk for poorer adjustment to retirement. Volunteer work, consultancy, and education can substitute for work.

Caregiving and care receiving are other productive activities that make up a substantial part of middle-aged and older adults' lives. Occupational therapy practitioners evaluate the needs of the patient and the caregiver's ability to provide care. The goal is to both maximize the independence of the care receiver and minimize the load on the caregiver. Therapists need to form a therapeutic alliance with caregivers (Hasselkus, 1994).

Home management assessments and interventions play crucial roles in determining whether an older adult can safely remain at home and with what environmental modifications.

Conservatorship or guardianship might be necessary for those older adults who cannot independently and safely take care of themselves. Occupational therapy practitioners have an essential role in helping older adults function at their maximal independent and productive manner for as long as the older adult wishes. Skillful use of occupational therapy assessment and intervention very likely will enable the older adult to remain engaged in meaningful occupations that significantly contribute to his or her own continuous sense of self, integrity, and mental and physical well-being.

Activities

1. Think of the reasons that you engage in work and productive activities. How do they relate or not relate to your identity and themes of meaning?

2. How would you spend your time if you were retired? What major adjustments would this entail? In what ways would retirement alter your life?

3. Describe how older adults might be involved as caregivers. How might that impact their physical and mental well-being?

4. You are an occupational therapy practitioner working in home health with an older adult who has sustained a hip fracture and who has severe rheumatoid arthritis as well. The family believes that older persons should be pampered and taken care of instead of being taught to do things independently. How would you form a therapeutic alliance with the caregivers and how would this affect your treatment?

5. Look back in your life to a volunteer position or job you have held. Imagine you are 68 years old and trying to perform the same job:
   - Following total hip replacement surgery
   - With severe osteoarthritis in your hands
   - With macular degeneration.

   Describe the volunteer position in detail. For each condition, describe the types of reasonable accommodations you would need to perform the tasks required.

6. Make a list of how much money you would need to meet your expenses if you were to retire now. What changes would you have to make in your lifestyle in order to retire? What is the minimum amount you need at this time to retire? Suppose you are 65 and need to plan for the next 25 years of retirement. How much money is necessary?

7. A patient has been referred for occupational therapy and the physician demands that you begin treatment immediately. The conservator refuses to authorize occupational therapy. You believe that therapy is in the patient's best interests and without it, the patient will have a significant loss of function due to contractures, decreased strength, etc. What is the ethical and legal dilemma? What are the options?

Review Questions

1. How can the ADA help older workers in their efforts to return to work?

2. What are the implications of continuity theory for the meaning of work and productive activities for older adults?

3. How can work provide a person with a sense of identity and continuity?

4. How can retirement provide a person with a sense of identity and continuity?

5. Why do some older persons prefer not to participate in volunteer work?

6. What are some educational opportunities that have been specially designed for older adults?

7. What are the responsibilities of a guardian and conservator? What does this mean in terms of the patient's or client's personal autonomy?

8. How can the occupational therapist assess whether a patient or client is at risk for being conned or has been conned or is a victim of theft?

Case Studies

CASE STUDY 1

Mort is a 62-year-old man who has recently had a right CVA. He owns a large print shop with approximately 25 employees. Mort has been in business for 30 years and never gave a thought to retiring, thinking he would die with ink on his hands.

Mort is attending occupational therapy as an outpatient. He walks, with the aid of a quad cane, at a fairly steady gait. He is independent in ADL. His left-hand grip strength is 20 pounds and his right-hand grip strength is 65 pounds. (He is right-handed.)

Mort confides in you, the occupational therapy practitioner, that he wants to return to work but his wife is against it because she fears he will not be able to do the work and it will be unsafe to try. What do you do?

Case Study Analysis

Because Mort wants to return to work, the occupational therapy practitioner must look carefully at Mort's current level of functioning, the work he must perform, and the environment in which he must perform the work. To begin this task, the occupational therapy practitioner should ask Mort's physician whether he or she has placed any work restrictions on Mort, such as limitations on carrying and lifting. Next, the occupational therapy practitioner will want to perform a job analysis, preferably at the job site. Many readers may think they know what a printer does on the job, but in reality the job turns out to be very different when seen on-site as part of a job analysis.

During the job analysis, the occupational therapy practitioner will look at the tasks performed, the physical requirements of the tasks themselves, and the physical layout of the work site. Keeping in mind Mort's current level of function and restrictions, the occupational therapy practitioner will look at ways to simplify the tasks, decrease the amount of physical labor required, and lower energy expenditures. Fortunately, because he is the boss, Mort can make additional accommodations that an entry-level worker may not find at his disposal, as Mort ultimately pays for his own accommodations.

After carefully comparing the job analysis with Mort's physical capacities, the occupational therapy practitioner might find, for example, that Mort can return to work if he reduces the amount of carrying or lifting he requires of himself. Conversely, one might find that Mort spends a great deal of his time sitting at the computer, a task that is not so physically challenging.

Mort's fears about returning to work might be lessened by simulating some of his work tasks in the occupational therapy clinic as part of his therapy and gradually increasing the amount of time he spends performing the work tasks. On the basis of his experience in the occupational therapy clinic, Mort could find that returning to work on a part-time basis meets his early return-to-work needs. He might want to stay at the part-time level and may want to gradually increase to full time. Working with Mort, the occupational therapy practitioner can give him guidance about how to lower various stress factors at work, allowing him to make a smooth transition from client to worker.

CASE STUDY 2

Jeanne is an 82-year-old divorced woman who works as a volunteer 3 mornings a week at the botanical gardens and has an active social life with friends. Two months ago her daughter and two grandchildren, ages 6 and 8, moved in with her. Since that time, Jeanne's routines often have been altered by those of her family. For example, Jeanne has to drive the children to school when her daughter, a student, has early classes; she also has to pick them up after school. She is trying to adjust her new family obligations with those that she has been enjoying since she retired 12 years ago. She sadly comments that she frequently has to miss her volunteer work and outings with her friends because "something always comes up and my daughter needs help with the grandchildren."

Jeanne fell and sustained a Colles fracture of her dominant right hand. She explained her duties to the occupational therapy practitioner and started to cry because she does not know how she is going to manage now that she will be almost one-handed for several months. The occupational therapist determines with Jeanne and the orthopedic surgeon what her functional limitations are. Jeanne is quite adept with her left hand and is taught to adapt many of her activities. Adaptive equipment and techniques are suggested to aid her with her home management, self-care, and volunteer activities. For example, she is taught to use suction cups and similar equipment and compensatory techniques to stabilize items when cooking or repotting plants. Jeanne and the occupational therapy practitioner agree that the grandchildren can help her with kitchen and other household activities, which would be a useful occupation for all of them. The occupational therapy practitioner and Jeanne plan how they can use her home management and volunteer work activities as therapeutic activities for her wrist rehabilitation.

The occupational therapist, Jeanne, and her daughter work on solving additional problematic areas and decide that a car pool would be a good way to cover taking the children to school on days their mother cannot drive. This car pool would relieve Jeanne of those duties. Jeanne expresses considerable relief at now being able to meet her family obligations and being able to continue with the other meaningful occupations in her life.

References

American Occupational Therapy Association. (1994). Uniform terminology for occupational therapy (3rd ed.). *American Journal of Occupational Therapy, 48,* 1047–1054.

Americans with Disabilities Act of 1990, P.L. No. 101–336, 42, U.S.C.A. §12101 (1990).

Atchley, R. C. (1982). The process of retirement: Comparing women and men. In M. Szinovacz (Ed.), *Women's retirement.* Beverly Hills, CA: Sage.

Atchley, R. C. (1989). A continuity theory of normal aging. *Gerontologist, 29,* 183–190.

Bass, S. A. (1988). The role of higher education in creating economic roles. In R. Morris & S. A. Bass (Eds.), *Retirement reconsidered: Economic and social roles for older people* (pp. 222–231). New York: Springer.

Baum, C. M., & LaVesser, P. (1994). Caregiver assistance: Using family members and attendants. In C. Christiansen (Ed.), *Ways of living: Self-care strategies for special needs* (pp. 453–482). Rockville, MD: American Occupational Therapy Association.

Berman, H. J. (1994). *Interpreting the aging self: Personal journals of later life.* New York: Springer.

Brody, E. M. (1985). The Donald P. Kent memorial lecture: Parent care as a normative family stress. *Gerontologist, 25,* 19–25.

Buchanan, S., Kaplan, N., & Gilfix, M. (1991). Advanced directions in advanced directives. Proceedings of the National Association of Elder Legal Attorneys Third Annual Symposium on Elder Law. Orlando, FL: NAELA.

Christenson, M. A. (1995). Assessing an elder's need for assistance: One technological tool. *Generations, 19,* (Spring), 54–55.

Cicirelli, V. G. (1992). *Family caregiving: Autonomous and paternalistic decision making.* Newbury Park, CA: Sage.

Ellexson & Kornblau, 1992 [more info to come?]

Erikson, E. H. (1963). *Childhood and society.* New York: Norton.

Fair Housing Act Amendments of 1988, P.L. No. 100–420.

Fillenbaum, G. G. (1985). Screening the elderly: A brief instrumental activities of daily living measure. *Journal of the American Geriatrics Society, 33,* 698–706.

Fillenbaum, G. G. (1988). *Multidimensional functional assessment of older adults.* Hillsdale, NJ: Erlbaum.

Foti, D., Pedretti, L. W., & Lillie, S. (1996). Activities of daily living. In L. W. Pedretti (Ed.), *Occupational therapy: practice skills for physical dysfunction* (4th ed.). St. Louis: Mosby-Year Book.

Gibeau, J. (1988). Working caregivers: Family conflicts and adaptations of older workers. In R. Morris & S. A. Bass (Eds.), *Retirement reconsidered* (pp. 185–204). New York: Springer.

Hall, H. J. (1910). Work cure, a report of five years experience at an institution devoted to the therapeutic application of manual work. *Journal of the American Medical Association, 54,* 12.

Harris, M. J. (1995, November). Elder fraud: Con artists steal billions from seniors each year—or worse. *Money,* 145–154.

Hasselkus, B. R. (1994). Professionals and informal caregivers: The therapeutic alliance. In B. R. Bonder & M. B. Wagner (Eds.), *Functional performance in older adults* (pp. 339–351). Philadelphia: F. A. Davis.

Jondrow, J., Brechling, F., & Marcus, A. (1987). Older workers in the market for part-time employment. In S. H. Sandell (Ed.), *The problem isn't age:*

Work and older Americans (pp. 84–99). New York: Praeger.

Kaufman, S. R. (1986). *The ageless self: Sources of meaning in late life.* Madison, WI: University of Wisconsin Press.

Letts, L. (1995, October). SAFER. [On-line]. Occupational Therapy List Serve available from <lettsl@fhs.csu.McMaster.ca.>

Ludwig, F. M. (1987). Caregiving and developmental issues of mid life. *Gerontology Special Interest Section Newsletter, 10*(4), 2, 6.

Ludwig, F. M. (1995). *The use and meaning of routine in women over seventy years of age.* Unpublished doctoral dissertation, University of Southern California, Los Angeles.

MacRae, N. (1991). The older worker. In K. Jacobs (Ed.), *Occupational therapy: Work-related programs and assessments* (2nd ed., pp. 358–364).

Meyer, A. (1977). The philosophy of occupational therapy. *American Journal of Occupational Therapy, 31,* 639–642. (Original work published 1922).

Montgomery, R. J. V., Gonyea, J. G., & Hooymana, N. R. (1985). Caregiving and the experience of subjective and objective burden. *Family Relations, 34,* 1–8.

Olmstead, A. H. (1975). *Threshold: The first days of retirement.* New York: Harper & Row.

Palmore, E. B., Burchett, B. M., Fillenbaum, G. G., George, L. K., & Wallman, L. M. (1985). *Retirement: Causes and consequences.* New York: Springer.

Reilly, M. A. (1966). A psychiatric occupational therapy program as a teaching model. *American Journal of Occupational Therapy, 20,* 61–67.

Reynolds-Lynch, K. (1985). Job analysis. In M. Kirkland & S. C. Robertson (Eds.), *Planning and implementing vocational readiness in occupational therapy* ([PIVOT] pp. 155–157). Rockville, MD: American Occupational Therapy Association.

Rosen, B., & Jerdee, T. H. (1985). *Older employees: New roles for valued resources.* Homewood, IL: Dow Jones-Irwin.

Shapiro, D., & Sandell, S. H. (1987). The reduced pay of older job losers: Age discrimination. In S. H. Sandell (Ed.), *The problem isn't age: Work and older Americans* (pp. 37–51). New York: Praeger.

Slagle, E. C. (1922). Training aids for mental patients. *Archives of Occupational Therapy, 1,* 11–17.

Smith, E. R. (1989). Ergonomics and the occupational therapist. In S. Hertfelder & C. Gwin (Eds.), *Work in progress: Occupational therapy in work programs.* Rockville, MD: American Occupational Therapy Association.

Zimmer, A. H. (1991). More than a nine-to-five job: Issues of the employed caregiver. *Work, 2,* 61–66.

Section 7. Evaluation and Intervention for Leisure Activities

Coralie H. Glantz, OTR/L, FAOTA

Nancy Richman, OTR/L, FAOTA

Grow old along with me!
The best is yet to be,
The last of life, for which
  the first was made.
Our times are in his hand
Who saith, "A whole I planned;
Youth shows but half. Trust God;
  see all, nor be afraid!"

— "Rabbi Ben Ezra"
    by Robert Browning, 1864
    (Averyt, Furst, & Hummel,
    1987, p. 441)

Abstract

Our older years can represent nearly one quarter of our entire lives. These years can be some of our most rewarding years. Like Rabbi Ben Ezra, we must focus on and remember our successes and not dwell on our past failures. Our later years must be infused with meaningful activity and expectation, not with self-pity. "The secret of successful aging is more than the ability to tap the resources in our community but we must able to tap the resiliency of our own spirit" (Averyt, Furst, & Hummel, 1987, p. 442).

Dane Davis, when he was an 84-year-old former governor of Vermont, put the same thoughts in modern vernacular: "There's a vast difference between aging and growing old. There's not much you can do about aging … but there's a whole lot you can do about growing old." Davis knew a man who was so ready to die that he never bought green bananas. "That's not the way to live. Go out and buy green bananas. Make sure every single day is full of life, full of adventure, and full of function. Life is acting, thinking, doing, being, and growing" (Averyt et al., p. 442).

Recreation and Leisure in Adult Life

Adult play is classified as recreation and leisure. Recreation regenerates energy to support the worker role (Kimmel, 1974). Leisure can be defined as freely selected activity pursued simply for the pleasure of it. The social role obligation is minimal and there is freedom from constraint, along with a pleasant recollection and recall. (Crepeau, 1986). However, some activities are not clearly classified as either work or leisure. These are called coordinated and complementary leisure (Kimmel, 1974). Coordinated leisure is work-related activity that has the element of being freely chosen; learning computer skills by playing computer games is an example of coordinated leisure. Complementary leisure is a role-related activity. For example, professional association involvement relates to the work role and being a Scout leader relates to community and family roles (Crepeau, 1986).

A homeostatic alliance exists between work and play. Everyone has a unique pattern of activity that provides for structure and routine in daily life. Because this offers a secure base of need fulfillment and support in many social roles (Kielhofner, 1977), it enables people to use their time effectively and adapt to life changes as they arise (Bell, 1976). Leisure skills can be cultivated and assimilated into the changing pattern of daily activity (Bell, 1976; Kielhofner, 1980).

Daily activities maintain health by providing mental and physical challenges to keep body and mind adequately stimulated (Yerxa, 1980). Normal aging affects activity levels and activity choices. A process of time expansion can be seen in some retired adults. Activities previously rushed through are pursued at a slower pace (Keiber & Thompson, 1980). More enjoyment can be achieved in carrying out the activity because more time is available. People are moving from active mastery of the environment to more passive approaches. Reminiscence and the use of fantasy increase as declines in mobility and other resources limits physical movement (Gubrium, 1973; Rowles, 1978). The home environment increases in importance, and distant places that are visited infrequently but that have strong emotional ties are thought about more often (Rowles, 1978).

The Role of Occupational Therapy in the Development of Leisure Skills

Because occupational therapy is aimed at an older adult's competence to function independently in all facets of daily living, be they work, self-care, play, or leisure, the therapist should be involved in the evaluation of the client's lifelong interests; priorities in pursuit of those interests; and physical, psychosocial, and cognitive ability to pursue those interests.

Successful performance promotes feelings of personal competence and provides opportunities for individuals to achieve mastery of their environment (Fidler & Fidler, 1979). To experience successful outcomes in the pursuit of leisure activities requires coordination between the individual's sensory motor, cognitive, and psychosocial systems in the context of interpersonal, cultural, and environmental conditions (American Occupational Therapy

Assocation [AOTA], 1993). Occupational therapy education addresses activity analysis and synthesis that enable the therapist, in collaboration with the individual, to design occupational experiences that offer opportunities for effective action. These experiences are considered purposeful in that they assist and build on the individual's abilities and lead to the achievement of personal goals (AOTA, 1993; Hinojosa, Sabari, & Pedretti, 1992).

An occupational therapy practitioner analyzes from several perspectives. First, the activity is examined to identify its component parts to determine which skills and abilities are necessary to complete the task. Second, it is examined in terms of the context in which it will be performed. Third, the practitioner considers the person's age, occupational roles, cultural background, gender, interests, and preferences that can influence the meaningfulness of the activity for the individual. All this information is considered to assist the occupational therapy practitioner in synthesizing (i.e., adapting, grading, and combining) activities for therapeutic purposes for a particular individual (AOTA, 1993, p. 1081; Hinojosa et al., 1992).

Such activity analysis is applied to leisure activities to ensure that clients can succeed in their performance.

Activity analysis reflects a sociocultural and idiosyncratic patterning of the activity for each individual. If the occupational therapy practitioner can discover and understand past activity patterning, present and future activity planning can be more effective. Activity organization, time allotment, categorization, priorities, expectations, accepted variations, consistencies, and irregularities (Cynkin, 1979) all are part of the activity patterning and can play a role in choosing the activities that have the highest probability for success.

Occupational therapy practitioners teach skills relative to performance components and occupational performance areas; they adapt tasks and the environment to facilitate performance. Throughout a purposeful activity, the occupational therapy practitioner modifies the setting, the method of personal interaction, and the physical handling to achieve the success (AOTA, 1993; Hinojosa et al., 1992).

Supportive or assistive devices or techniques frequently are used by the occupational therapy practitioner to ensure success. Such techniques or devices are considered to facilitate or prepare for performance of purposeful activity and are used to enhance the effectiveness of an activity or facilitate performance (Henderson et al., 1991; Pedretti, 1996).

Leisure routines are an important aspect in all settings in which an elderly person may be living. Occupational therapy practitioners can sometimes be reimbursed by Medicare for one to two visits for leisure evaluation and program planning in the home health setting (Health Care Financing Administration, 1986), although it is recommended that developing a leisure-based program be combined with other activities, particularly ones involving activities of daily living (ADL) skills or physical components that occur during a treatment session focusing on leisure routines. The occupational therapy practitioner should document both the physical and leisure components of the activity (Steinhauer et al., 1995).

Leisure activities such as card playing, arts and crafts, puzzles, work games, video or computer games, reading, talking on the telephone, social gathering, and watching television all can be very beneficial in helping to stimulate an individual's cognitive awareness and perceptual processing abilities. As part of the initial evalua-

tion, a history of leisure-time pursuits should be obtained from the client and the family or friends. It should be determined if these activities currently are of interest to the person. The occupational therapy practitioner can then adapt the leisure routine to fit the needs of the individual receiving service. A creative occupational therapy practitioner will find ways to incorporate components of the patient's preferred leisure-time activities into the occupational therapy program (Steinhauer et al., 1995).

Leisure time can include driving. The act of driving may in itself be a leisure interest or it can enable the person to gain access to leisure pursuits in the community. Thus, another area to be addressed by the occupational therapy practitioner is the ability to transfer into a car. Predriving assessment tests can help the occupational therapy practitioner focus on the skills most relevant to facilitate predriving training. The occupational therapy practitioner needs to document very carefully the reason car-transfer training and predriving activities are incorporated into treatment, as such activities could indicate the patient is no longer homebound. (Steinhauer et al., 1995).

For most older persons, the major source of socialization is the family, although in the American culture most socializing takes place among people of the same age, with couples being the "normal" unit for social activity. When aged persons are single, they often are excluded from many social activities. This situation has led to the creation of programs designed to promote socializing, such as senior citizen centers, congregate meal sites, and social clubs in senior housing (Edinberg, 1987). The staff members in these sites may recognize a problem or need and be a referral source for therapy evaluation and services. The occupational therapy practitioner may become involved in these community-based settings through development of support groups for elderly persons who are experiencing some stress because of the normal aging process, with changes in mobility, memory, and sensory abilities, as well as changes in family relationships. The occupational therapy practitioner can help these individuals increase their independence and feeling of self-worth and to use problem-solving skills in making new adjustments (Petty, Moeller, & Campbell, 1976).

Treatment Settings for Leisure Activities

The occupational therapy practitioner can assist with socialization and leisure-time fulfillment for the elderly person in a variety of settings. Whether in the client's home, a retirement home, an assistive living situation, a day care setting, or a nursing facility, the therapist can do a complete evaluation that could include safety issues, ADL skills, client interests and priorities, current available resources, and possible adaptations or modifications needed to improve function and quality of life. These evaluations can occur when there has been a change in function, such as when the person is moving into the retirement home, assistive living center, or nursing facility. Thus, the fee may be covered under home health Medicare A, rehabilitation agency Medicare B, private insurance, private pay, or Medicare A or B in the nursing facility. In some of these settings, the occupational therapy practitioner can serve as a consultant to activity staff, helping them develop programs and tasks appropriate to the abilities and interests of the individual residents. Their skills can be used to promote meaningful activities for all

residents, activities that offer choice, make use of clients' strengths and capabilities, and reflect individual interests. The therapist can work with staff members to develop appropriate empowerment, maintenance, and supportive activities to enhance their programs, community involvement, work programs, and small group programs to meet psychosocial needs and problems (Glantz & Richman, 1991). Disease-induced reduction of activity can lead to progressive decline through disuse and can cause further decrease in activity levels. As the pathological changes occur in any aspect of the resident's competence, the pleasurable challenge of activities may narrow. This pattern can, however, be broken: many activities can be continued if they are adapted to require less exertion or if the resident is helped to adapt to specific deficits. In some cases, compensatory strategies, such as task segmentation, may be helpful (Cornelius, Perschbacher, Reublinger, Cook, & Sinclair, 1991). Training in activity analysis and occupational performance concepts enables the occupational therapy practitioner to provide an important perspective for the activity coordinator. In earlier times, this role might actually have been filled by an occupational therapist, but in today's marketplace it is often assumed by individuals of varying background and education. Therefore, a consultant is needed to provide expert guidance and training for activity coordinators working in these settings (Jaffe & Epstein, 1992). With her or his ability to use adaptive or compensatory techniques to ensure that the resident experiences success, the certified occupational therapy assistant often is an ideal person to conduct or coordinate activities in a nursing facility or assisted-living facility.

Dementia Care and Leisure Skills

In the area of dementia care, the occupational therapy practitioner can help the person with dementia experience some meaningful leisure-time activity and thereby improve the current quality of life. In this situation, very often the past interests may need to be changed to allow for successful, satisfying experiences.

When dealing with persons with Alzheimer's disease and related disorders, the occupational therapy practitioner's focus is to maintain, restore, or improve functional capacity and to promote participation in activities that optimize physical and mental health. This focus should include leisure skills, which are such a vital component in the quality of life. Leisure activities are appraised to determine interest, skill, and level of participation. The assessment considers the person's ability to initiate, sustain, and complete tasks. It yields a description of the tasks that the person can do independently, easily, and safely. A continuous modification of tasks and the physical and social environments in which these tasks are performed can help persons with dementia maintain their abilities, retain some control over their lives, and maintain a sense of personal dignity. Leisure activities such as exercise, games, and crafts can be used to maintain joint mobility, muscle strength, mental alertness, social skills, and self-esteem. Each task must be analyzed for its component parts, and each part is then evaluated in terms of the person's ability to continue to perform it. Even though the person might not complete all steps of the task, he or she is not deprived of using the abilities that remain (AOTA, 1994). Cultural issues should be considered when conducting needs assessments and structuring leisure activities as part of the initial planning and outreach efforts (Goldberg, Carroll, & Dobrof, 1991). To assist in the development of positive leisure-time experiences, the occupational therapy practitioner may utilize the following skills:

1. Modification—Use task simplification and task segmentation to adapt for success and limit the chance of failure as abilities decline.
2. Repetitiveness—Use familiar and routine activities.
3. Safety—Make sure that the activity does not present a hazard to the resident, other residents, staff, or family.
4. Adaptability—Make participation be individual, small group, or large group and seated, standing, or lying down; having activity being spontaneous or planned.
5. Dignity—Use approach and involvement to ensure the resident's self-respect and sense of worth.
6. Fun—Ensure pleasure from the activity by using past interests and skills, and not requiring a perfect end-product.

Anything residents do or are involved with is their activity at that moment. If we can shift the focus from doing an activity for the resident to one of doing an activity with the resident or allowing independent involvement, we can help stimulate wellness (Hellen, 1992). Like all people, people with dementia need to have a purpose and a feeling of usefulness. They are capable of achieving success if the task, the environment, and the technique are appropriate. The use of task simplification, task segmentation, strict routine, cuing and coaching, removal of extraneous and distracting environmental stimulation, and a calm atmosphere without time constraints all can facilitate and enhance successful performance. Communication must be respectful and specifically directed to the individual, using short simple phrases, and it must allow time for the information to be understood. Leisure pursuits enable individuals to feel useful and a part of the family and community. It gives them an opportunity to call on their life experiences and enables them to successfully use the skills they still possess (Morris & Hunt, 1994).

In addition to providing direct services to persons with dementia, an occupational therapy practitioner can act as a director of a special unit in a living center. He or she can provide consultation and educational services to facilities and programs serving people with dementia. Typically, these services involve the following:

1. Designing environments that support function, provide optimal sensory stimulation, and promote safety

2. Teaching strategies and techniques for managing task performance deficits and disruptive behaviors

3. Recommending activity programs that maintain physical, cognitive, and social abilities

4. Suggesting alternatives through programming for physical and chemical restraints (AOTA, 1986, 1994).

Summary

Old age should be an enjoyable time in life. Leisure time plays a vital role in determining a person's quality of life. Occupational therapy practitioners possess many skills that can help elderly persons experience enjoyable times and attain the quality of life they seek. Practitioners can modify or adapt elderly persons' lifelong interests to allow for their continued participation, and practitioners can explore and assist in the initiation of new interests in which the person can experience success, enjoyment, and satisfaction. By working to establish priorities and set objectives, the occupational therapy practitioner can help older persons achieve their life goals and dreams.

Activities

1. List three things you like to do in your leisure time. Now consider that you are 86 years old and have suffered a CVA resulting in left hemiplegia, homonymous hemianopsia, and a body-image deficit. Develop an occupational therapy plan that would help you to attain your life goals and dreams for successful and enjoyable leisure pursuits.

2. Analyze three of the following activities and adapt them so that they are appropriate for a person with middle-stage Alzheimer's disease: card playing, sewing, Rosary, bingo, checkers, woodworking, baking, reading the newspaper, handicrafts, drawing, plant care, and exercising.

3. Describe four functions you could provide in consultation to a living center for people with dementia.

Review Questions

1. Give some examples of coordinated and complementary leisure activities in your own life or the life of an elderly person whom you know.

2. Why do you think an occupational therapy practitioner would be a good consultant to activity-program development and activity-staff effectiveness?

3. When working with persons with dementia, how can you focus on and stimulate wellness?

4. What are the two major perspectives from which an occupational therapy practitioner analyzes an activity?

5. What feelings does success in leisure-time pursuits promote for an individual?

6. What are three modifications that an occupational therapy practitioner can make to enable a client's successful participation in purposeful activity?

7. What are the five areas the occupational therapy practitioner should evaluate in order to assist in the development of successful leisure time activities?

8. What compensatory strategy can be used to help a client adapt to a deficit such as a decline in memory?

Case Studies

CASE STUDY 1

An 83-year-old woman was admitted July 25, 1995, with a diagnosis of right CVA (July 10, 1995), diabetes mellitus, osteoarthritis, and organic brain syndrome. Within 48 hours of admission, the resident was seen by an occupational therapy practitioner for evaluation. At that time, the resident was observed in a wheelchair with a vest restraint, leaning severely to her left. The therapist's evaluation indicated that the resident had a left hemiplegia, homonymous hemianopia, unilateral neglect, and deficits in postural balance, visual-motor integration, and problem solving. On speaking with the family, the therapist learned that they intended to have her and her 86-year-old husband live with the daughter. Therefore, she needed to be safe in her wheelchair, be able to transfer with her daughter's help, and be as independent as possible in her ADL. The daughter was concerned about what her mother would do all day, especially because her mother had always been active and could no longer pursue her walking, exercising, her handiwork (quilting club and knitting), or her cooking and baking. The therapist's plans included working on all of the foregoing items, with the daughter present whenever possible.

Although the resident made progress during her first few weeks of therapy, it became apparent that the daughter, who had medical problems herself, would not be able to transfer her mother to their home. The decision was made to move the resident and her husband into an assistive living facility. At the time of the transfer, the therapist had fabricated a seating and positioning device that allowed the resident to sit safely in her wheelchair without using the safety vest. The resident had learned to move and direct her chair by using her right arm and leg, and to always check the position of her arm to make sure it was properly placed in the arm trough before moving the chair. The therapist was able to evaluate and modify the resident's apartment in the assistive living facility before she moved in, to compensate for her homonymous hemianopia, her wheelchair mobility and access, and her transfer needs. The therapist continued working with the resident, her husband, and the caregivers in the assistive living facility. The caregivers learned to safely transfer the resident and to assist her with bathing. The husband was taught to assist with dressing while the resident was still in bed, and he was able to do any necessary problem solving for the resident.

Development of new leisure activities that met her interest was a real challenge. Before her discharge from therapy, the resident was provided with adaptive cooking and baking devices that she practiced with during her therapy sessions. The therapist worked with a frame for quilting, but it proved to be frustrating and unsuccessful and the resident was unable to continue her needlework. New potential interests were explored, and the resident chose painting. After learning compensatory techniques for the hemiopsia, the resident was able to paint quite well; in fact, a hidden talent was discovered. The therapist spoke with the activity director at the assistive living facility and found that cooking, baking, and painting were activities the resident could pursue in her new setting. The activity director welcomed the suggestions for such interests the resident could pursue and welcomed the guidance of the therapist in developing a wheelchair fitness trail that the resident could use either alone or with her husband.

CASE STUDY 2

An 86-year-old man returned to his apartment in the retirement home after a 4-day stay in the hospital following a mild CVA. His son telephoned the occupational therapy practitioner and was irate that the administration of the retirement home refused to turn his father's stove on, fearing that it would be an unsafe situation because of his loss of coordination. The son stated that it was very important to his father to cook because this was something that he had done as a hobby for many years.

The occupational therapist did a thorough functional, safety, and cognitive assessment of the resident and also evaluated his environment. She found three problem areas that could make it unsafe for him to use the stove, two of which were present before the CVA: Before the CVA, the man had a hearing deficit, which prevented him from hearing the buzzer on the stove; he was also unable to recognize the smell of smoke. Since the CVA, the resident had an attention and a memory deficit. His motor skills, including his coordination, were within normal limits. The therapist was able to put an alarm on the stove that the resident could hear over the sound of the television, a light indicator on the smoke detector, and an automatically timed shut-off capability on the stove. With these adaptations, the resident was able to safely use his stove and pursue his hobby of cooking. To celebrate, he made a special soup luncheon for his son, the therapist, and the facility administrator.

Appendix.

RESOURCE ORGANIZATIONS

Following is more information about organizations mentioned in this chapter:

Retired Senior Volunteer Services (RSVS)
Corporation for National Community Services
1201 New York Avenue
Washington, DC 20524

Elder Hostel
Department JD
75 Federal Street
Boston, MA 02110
To request a catalog, specify domestic, international, or service programs.

Lifease, Inc.
Stoney Lake Office Park
2451 75th Street, NW, Suite D
New Brighton, MN 55112

National Association of Elder Law Attorneys
1604 North Country Club Road
Tucson, AZ 85716

References

American Occupational Therapy Association. (1986). Occupational therapy services for persons with Alzheimer's disease and other dementias: A position paper. *American Journal of Occupational Therapy, 40,* 822–824.

American Occupational Therapy Association. (1993). Purposeful activity: A position paper. *American Journal of Occupational Therapy, 47,* 1081–1082.

American Occupational Therapy Association. (1994). Occupational therapy services for persons with Alzheimer's disease and other dementias (Statement). *American Journal of Occupational Therapy, 48,* 1029–1031.

Averyt, A. C., Furst, E., & Hummel, D. D. (1987). *Successful aging: A source book for older people and their families.* New York: Ballantine Books.

Bell, B. (1976). Role set orientations and life satisfaction. In J. F. Gubrium (Ed.), *Times, roles, and self in old age,* (pp. 148–164). New York: Human Sciences Press.

Cornelius, E., Perschbacher, R., Reublinger, V., Cook, J., & Sinclair, S. (1991). Resident assessment protocol: Activities (pp. F43–F46). In *Resident assessment instrument training manual and resource guide.* Nantick, MA: Elliot Press.

Crepeau, E. L. (1986). Treatment approaches: Activity programming; Module III: In *Role of occupational therapy with the elderly.* Rockville, MD: American Occupational Therapy Association.

Cynkin, S. (1979). *Occupational therapy: Toward health through activities.* Boston: Little, Brown.

Edinberg, M. A. (1987). *Talking with your aging parents*. Boston, MA: Shambhala Publications.

Fidler, G. S., & Fidler, J. W. (1979). Doing and becoming: Purposeful action and self-actualization. *American Journal of Occupational Therapy, 32,* 305–310.

Glantz, C. H., & Richman, N. (1991). *Occupational therapy: A vital link to the implementation of OBRA*. Bethesda, MD: American Occupational Therapy Association.

Goldberg, A., Carrol, D., & Dobrof, R. (1991). *How to start and manage a group activities and respite program for people with Alzheimer's disease and their families: A guide for community-based organizations*. New York: Brookdale Foundation Group, The Brookdale Center on Aging of Hunter College.

Gubrium, J. F. (1973). *The myth of the golden years: A socio-environmental theory of aging*. Springfield, IL: Thomas.

Health Care Financing Administration. (1986). *Home health agency manual* (Pub. No. 11). Washington, DC: U.S. Government Printing Office.

Hellen, C. (1992). *Alzheimer's disease activity-focused care*. Newton, MA: Andover Medical Publishers.

Henderson, A., Cermak, S., Costner, W., Murray, E., Trombly, C., & Tickle-Gegnen, L. (1991). The issue is: Occupational science is multidimensional. *American Journal of Occupational Therapy, 45,* 370–372.

Hinojosa, J., Sabari, J., & Pedretti, L. (1992). *Purposeful activity: A position paper*. Rockville, MD: American Occupational Therapy Association.

Jaffee, E. G., & Epstein, C. (1992). *Occupational therapy consultation: Theory, principles and practice*. St. Louis: Mosby-Year Book.

Keiber, D. A., & Thompson, S. R. (1980). Leisure behavior and adjustment to retirement: Implications for post retirement education. *Therapeutic Recreation Journal, 14*(2), 5–17.

Kielhofner, G. (1977). Temporal adaptations. *American Journal of Occupational Therapy, 31,* 235–242.

Kielhofner, G. (1980). A model of human occupation, part 3: Benign and vicious cycles. *American Journal of Occupational Therapy, 34,* 572–581.

Kimmel, D. (1974). *Adulthood and aging*. New York: Wiley.

Morris, A., & Hunt, G. (1994). *A part of daily life: Alzheimer's caregivers simplify activities and the home* (Videotape and resource book). Bethesda, MD: American Occupational Therapy Foundation and American Occupational Therapy Association.

Pedretti, L. W. (1996). Occupational performance: A model for practice in physical dysfunction. In L. W. Pedretti (Ed.), *Occupational therapy: practice skills for physical dysfunction*, (4th ed., pp. 3–11). St. Louis: Mosby-Year Book.

Petty, B. J., Moeller, T. P., & Campbell, R. Z. (1976). Support groups for elderly persons in the community. *Gerontologist, 15*(6), p. 522.

Rowles, G. D. (1978), *Prisoners of space? Exploring the geographical experience of older people*. Boulder, CO: Westview Press.

Steinhauer, M., Austill-Clausen, R., Menosky, J., Young, J., Youngstrom, M. J., & Hertfelder, S. (1995). *Guidelines for occupational therapy practice in home health*. Bethesda, MD: American Occupational Therapy Association.

Yerxa, E. (1980). Occupational therapy's role in creating a future climate of caring. *American Journal of Occupational Therapy, 34,* 529–534.

Related Resources

Allen, C. K. (1987). Activity, occupational therapy treatment method. *American Journal of Occupational Therapy, 41,* 563–575.

Alzheimer's Association. (1992). *Guidelines for dignity: Goals of specialized Alzheimer's/dementia care in residential settings.* Chicago: Author.

Alzheimer's Association, Conference Proceedings. (1993). *Alzheimer care strategies: Partners in quality care.* Chicago: Author.

American Occupational Therapy Association. (1994). Occupational therapy and long-term-care position paper. *American Journal of Occupational Therapy, 48,* 1035–1036.

Borg, R. M., Kennedy, S., & Smith, B. (1994). *Bringing out the best—dementia programming and activities.* Winston-Salem, NC: Bowman Gray School of Medicine of Wake Forest University, Department of Psychiatry and Behavioral Medicine. Partners in Caregiving: The Dementia Services Program.

Born, B. (1993). *Occupational therapy and long term care position paper.* Rockville, MD: American Occupational Therapy Association.

Davis, N. B., & Teaff, J. D. (1980). Facilitative role continuity of the elderly through leisure programming. *Therapeutic Recreation Journal, 14*(2), 32–36.

Fuller, E. (1992). The biology of aging. *Generations, Journal of the American Society of Aging, 16*(4).

Fuller, K. (1994). Frontline workers in long-term care. *Generations, Journal of the American Society of Aging, 16*(4).

Fuller, K. (1994). Current ethical issues in aging. *Generations, Journal of the American Society of Aging, 18*(4).

Fuller, K. (1995). Technology and aging: Developing and marketing new products for older people. *Generations, Journal of the American Society of Aging, 19*(1).

Glantz, C., & Richman, N. (1992). *Empowerment through wellness.* Riverwoods, IL: Glantz/Richman Rehabilitation Associates, Ltd.

Glantz, C., & Richman, N. (1993). The wellness model in long-term care facilities. *Quest, The Journal of the Illinois Health Care Association,* 7–11.

Glantz, C., & Richman, N. (1994). *Enhancing rehabilitation services for older people.* Seventh Annual Continuing Education Program on Issues in Aging, Wayne State Institute of Gerontology, Detroit, MI.

Jenny, S., & Oropeza, M. (1993). *Memories in the making—A program of creative art expression for Alzheimer's patients.* City, CA: Alzheimer's Association.

Kleemeir, R. W. (1964). Leisure and disengagement in retirement. *Gerontologists, 4,* 180–184.

Parker, R. A., & Downe, G. R. (1981). Recreation Therapy: A model for consideration. *Therapeutic Recreation Journal, 15*(3), 22–26.

Rathbone-McCuan, S., & Levenson, J. (1975). The impact of socialization therapy in a geriatric day care setting. *Gerontologists, 15,* 338–342.

Risberg, G., & McCullough, V. E. (1987). *Tough: A personal workbook.* Oak Park, IL: Open Arms Press.

Sheridan, C. (1987). *Failure-free activities for the Alzheimer's patient,* Oakland, CA: Cottage Books.

Thews, T., Reaves, A. M., & Henry, R. S. (1993). *Now what? A handbook of activities for adult day programs.* Winston Salem, NC: Bowman Gray School of Medicine of Wake Forest University.

Tickle, L. S., & Yerxa, E. J. (1981). Need satisfaction of older persons living in the community and in institutions, part 1: The environment. *American Journal of Occupational Therapy, 35,* 644–649.

Zogola, J. (1987). *Doing things: A guide to programming activities for persons with Alzheimer's disease and related disorders.* Baltimore, MD: Johns Hopkins University Press.

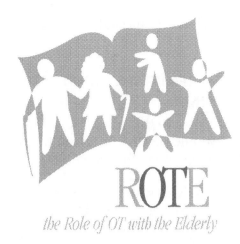

ROTE

the Role of OT with the Elderly

Palliative Medicine and Rehabilitation: Assessment and Treatment in Hospice Care

Kent N. Tigges, MS, OTR, FAOTA, FHIH
William M. Marcil, MS, OTR, FAOTA

Issues of Life and Death

For many generations the American public has had a peculiar relationship with life and death issues. Up until the mid-20th century, people were born, grew up, worked hard, grew old, and died. Many died in childbirth or from early childhood diseases. They were laid out in the family parlor and were buried simply and discreetly with family and friends standing around. Life went on. Grief existed, but it was worked through by returning to life's responsibilities. Little time could be lost in a community of farmers, laborers, shopkeepers, and housewives. People died and life went on.

In the second half of this century modern medicine broke the "death barrier." Elaborate surgical procedures, the harvesting and transplanting of major body organs (Kilner, 1990), medications, and life-sustaining machinery have substantially affected the way people perceive their relationship with life. Life can be prolonged and death can be postponed.

In the meantime, the value system of the American public has changed. Along with these changes, many delicate and highly charged issues are being debated.

- When does life begin?
- When does death occur?

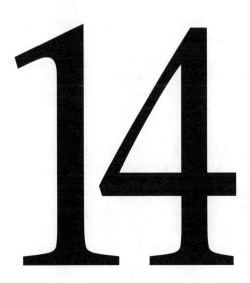

- Should life be sustained at all cost?
- Who should rightfully receive an organ transplant?
- Should one be permitted to end one's life in private or in concert with others?

Only three of these issues will be discussed:

1. When does death occur?
2. Should life be sustained at all cost?
3. Should one be permitted to end one's life?

WHEN DOES DEATH OCCUR?

Curiously, death does not occur in much of today's society—people "pass," "pass away," or have "passed on."

The terms *death* and *died* have somehow become either too uncomfortable to use or are considered insensitive or incorrect. Some people suggest that the use of these euphemisms helps people avoid the blunt reality of death.

The American obsession with extending life has altered the concept of when death occurs. In times past, death occurred when one stopped breathing and an ear to the chest could not hear a heartbeat. Today's medicine can fool life's normal functions. When breathing and the heartbeat cease, they can be, and often are, artificially restarted and maintained, unless one has a current and validated "do not resuscitate" (DNR) document on file. The aggressiveness of medical personnel to save a person's physical life, regardless of the outcome to the comprehensive integrity of the victim, is well known to viewers of the television program *ER*.

The time that death occurs has many definitions, medically, ethically, religiously, personally, and professionally. Other factors in determining when death has occurred are whether one is young to middle-aged or is elderly. Socioeconomic status may also be a factor.

SHOULD LIFE BE SUSTAINED AT ALL COSTS?

The answer to this question is relative and should be left entirely in the hands of the competent individual, with or without the knowledge or input of family or significant others. A growing sector of the public voluntarily refuses to have its lives saved or sustained. These people's decision to save themselves or their family members the burden of the painful indignity that is often associated with artificially prolonging life. A variety of documents, such as DNR documents, living wills, and health care proxies, activate such decisions. Legal documentation, appropriate authorization, and who should hold the documents vary from state to state. The well-informed occupational therapist should be knowledgeable about these legal issues, for it is not infrequent that a patient or family members may make inquiries of the therapist.

A sector of the public will attempt to sustain life at any cost, personal or financial. In either instance the individual's decision must be sincerely respected.

Hospice policy recognizes that people who initially choose palliative measures over curative measures, or vice versa, may be admitted and discharged upon request. This policy allows for people to change their minds at any time without jeopardy.

SHOULD ONE BE PERMITTED TO END ONE'S LIFE IN PRIVATE OR IN CONCERT WITH OTHERS?

This question carries strong personal, religious, ethnic, ethical, and legal implications. From the legal point of view, suicide or attempted suicide is not against the law. However, physically helping another person to die is against the law and constitutes a crime with ensuing penalties.

In these days when medicine and rehabilitation can save and often "resurrect" a person's body from many severe physical injuries or provide palliative care for those who have a terminal illness, it is ironic that the public is growingly interested in self-deliverance (Humphry, 1991), commonly known as euthanasia. The most notorious figure in this arena is Jack Kevorkian, M.D., a retired pathologist who invented the controversial "suicide machine" (Kevorkian, 1991). Since 1990, Kevorkian has personally provided the machinery through which at least 25 individuals have ended their lives by their own hand.

Two established organizations advocate euthanasia. The British euthanasia organization known as EXIT[1] and the American counterpart known as the Hemlock Society.[2] Both of these organizations hold and advocate that quality of life is imminently personal and can be evaluated and judged to be worthy only by the individual who is suffering, whether physically, emotionally, or both. It is that individual alone, with or without the consent or passive assistance of others, who has the right to engage in the planning and execution of a plan to achieve death rather than to live with suffering.

It is interesting to note that the established medical community is openly and publicly discussing physician-assisted suicide (Byock, 1993; Drane, 1995; Gates, 1993a, 1993b; Olson, 1995; Piper, 1994).

---

1. EXIT, also known as Voluntary Euthanasia Society of England and Wales, 13 Prince of Wales Terrace, London W5PG, England.

2. Hemlock Society, USA, P.O. Box 11830, Eugene, OR 97440-3900.

Hospice—The Movement and the Need: The First 15 Years

Hospice is a medieval term meaning a place for shelter, refreshment, and care for religious pilgrims and travelers on a long journey. In the early days, crusaders used hospices on their way to the Holy Land. When the Irish Sisters of Charity opened hospices in Dublin in 1846 and in London in 1905, they included many long-stay patients, but because the dying became their special concern, the term hospice came to be equated with their work.

The hospice in the 20th century has emerged out of the very real and substantially different needs of people with advanced metastatic disease (terminal cancer) for whom there is no hope for a cure. Dame Cicely Saunders, M.D. (personal communication, London, 1976) led the development of the 20th century hospice movement. While working in a large London hospital, Saunders, formerly a nurse, later a social worker, and finally a physician, recognized that patients who had terminal cancer with a short life expectancy were inappropriately treated. They were regarded by staff members as curable and treated with aggressive medical methods. Although aggressive medicine is appropriate for those who can be cured or whose life can be prolonged, she thought it inappropriate for those who are dying.

Saunders advocated a model of palliation, care that would provide pain and symptom control, diagnostic honesty, attention to the patient's quality of life, caregiver's support, and bereavement services for the survivors. The model fosters the notion that death is a normal and natural developmental milestone in life and need not be violent, frightening, or feared.

St. Christopher's, the first modern hospice to serve the needs of the terminally ill, opened in 1969 in a suburb of London. Under the medical direction of Dr. Saunders, it gained an international reputation and has become the model for hospices throughout the world.

Two years later, in 1971, St. Luke's Hospice opened in Sheffield, England, under the medical direction of Eric Wilkes, M.D. Whereas St. Christopher's offered only inpatient care for the terminally ill, St. Luke's added home and day care services. First in the United States was the Connecticut Hospice in New Haven, Connecticut. It was established in 1971 as a free-standing unit offering inpatient and home care services. The first hospice in Canada began operating in 1973 at the Royal Victoria Hospital in Montreal, under the medical direction of Balfour Mount, M.D. This hospice is associated with a large research and training hospital. These two hospices have provided the model for hospices in North America (E. Wilkes, M.D., personal communication, London, 1980).

The National Hospice Organization (NHO), developed through meetings of representatives of the early hospice programs in the 1970s, was incorporated in April 1978. Hospice programs now exist in every state of the union. An estimated 2,500 hospice programs in the United States offer varying degrees of services. Regulations for certification of Medicare providers became effective November 1, 1983. The first hospice to provide coverage under Medicare regulations was in Schenectady, New York. The majority of the nation's major insurance carriers now offer hospice care coverage or are developing a benefits package to include such coverage. Studies show that hospice care is less costly than traditional hospital or nursing home care

and in most instances is much more appropriate.

Philosophies and Models of Practice of Traditional and Hospice Occupational Therapy

Traditional occupational therapy in the United States and England focuses on treatment and rehabilitation. The aim is to return the injured or the disabled person to the mainstream of living. Although the paradigms currently used vary in concepts and focus, the patient's pathology has traditionally been the focus and the springboard for occupational therapy assessment and treatment planning. The majority of patients referred to occupational therapy have suffered a temporarily or permanently diminished physical or emotional function or capacity.

Although some would adamantly disagree, quality of life and the total person are not of primary or even secondary importance in treatment. Not one of the health professions can, or does, treat the total person; economics and education do not permit it. Health professionals treat only that aspect of the individual that their professional education has prepared them to address. People do not usually go to hospitals to improve the quality of their lives. They go into hospitals for specific health reasons, and they expect or demand to receive the most expeditious treatment that is available. People assume that their treatment will improve, or at least maintain, their quality of life and that they will be able to resume their chosen and familiar life patterns (occupational roles) and expectations.

Wilkes (personal communication, 1980) claims that the health care professional's greatest liability in dealing with patients is his or her "professional blinkers." The health care professional has been taught how to preside technically over what goes wrong physically with a person but not how to commune with a person when a serious or catastrophic event occurs. Medical management of pain and symptoms cannot be equated with quality of life. Neither can improving a person's occupational roles if other social systems and resources are not in place. If health professionals are truly in the business of preserving the integrity of a person's life, they must look beyond their professional blinkers and examine what services, and in what proportion, are necessary for the quality-of-life concept being advocated. Life without self-direction, independence, interdependence, dependency, self-esteem, purpose, and the ability to interact with and influence other people has little value, purpose, or meaning.

Advocates of the hospice movement have admirably stated that quality of life will be of paramount importance. A. Holland (personal communication, 1995) stressed that the problem with traditional inpatient (hospital, institution, nursing home) care is that patients are immediately put into a passive and dependent role, causing them to lose their sense of personhood and corresponding occupational roles and responsibilities. It is little wonder then that patients have difficulty adjusting from inpatient care to their homes, which are integrated within a community. Although greatly preferable, home care can pose problems similar to the hospital. Well-meaning family or friends may unintentionally place the ill or disabled person in a passive and dependent role. When there are no family or friends, isolation, loneliness, and inactivity can be more devastating than being in a busy hospital.

Given occupational therapy's goals of restoring or maintaining occupational roles, one would think that these goals would remain constant in an acute care hospital, rehabilitation center, institution, nursing home, or hospice facility. Unfortunately that constancy is not necessarily true. In the true sense of hospice, terminal care providers, whether physicians, occupational therapists, nurses, or social workers, have few norms to guide their practice. Hospice care is not, and cannot be, medical or nursing care only. It cannot be rehabilitation or social services care only. Hospice is not an agency or an extension of traditional hospital or nursing home care. Professional care providers do not, and cannot, speak of traditional roles. For occupational therapy personnel, substantial changes and adjustments in therapeutic approaches, goals, and personal perceptions must be made. The notion that tomorrow will bring the opportunity for an altered but nonetheless bright and productive future is completely inappropriate. Many hospice patients literally have no tomorrow; for others, some tomorrows will come, but no shallow reassurances of a predictable future can be offered. What exists, exists now.

The Tenets of Hospice Care

There are five basic tenets of hospice care: pain and symptom control, diagnostic honesty, quality of life, around-the-clock care, and bereavement care.

PAIN AND SYMPTOM CONTROL

Depending on the nature of their disease, patients experience four types of pain:

1. The pain of the disease itself
2. The side effects of chemotherapy, radiotherapy, and medication
3. The pain associated with the effects of long-term inactivity (bed rest)
4. The pain of loss of role.

Taken together or separately, pain can become all-consuming and frequently incapacitates the patient emotionally and physically. In such situations, not only does the patient suffer but also caring family or friends suffer. The first two types of pain patients experience are the single greatest reason that they seek, or are referred for, hospice care. As a result of the hospice movement, substantial pharmacological research has produced established protocols to successfully manage almost all levels of advanced cancer pain—in the majority of cases without adverse side effects or chemical dependency (addiction). This achievement is perhaps the greatest single contribution that medicine has made in the treatment of advanced metastatic disease. With relief from pain, patients can then turn their attention to living and enjoying the time they have. It is tragic, indeed, that many physicians in general hospitals, who treat patients with advanced cancer or other diseases and illnesses, either do not follow the established pain management protocols or have to seek consultation from a hospice physician to secure information to comfort their patient's sufferings.

The third type of pain that the patient with advanced metastatic disease experiences is the pain associated with inactivity and bed rest. This is one of the two areas of pain control that the occupational therapist is the most capable of assessing and treating. It is most generally associated with poor bed or wheelchair positioning, resulting in back, neck, shoulder, hip, or knee discomfort and pain. Poor positioning frequently leads to contractures that result in significant pain and discomfort in bathing, toileting, dressing, and transfers. The result is that patients resist being moved and withdraw from normal and routine activities.

Very frequently the nurse, the primary person who assesses pain and makes medication suggestions to the physician, will assume that the pain results from disease progression, and the physician alters the medication, which does not provide positive results. The occupational therapist can provide substantial intervention that significantly reduces the contractures, while at the same time recommending and teaching proper positioning and transfer techniques that will result in the patient's looking forward to resuming routine activities (Tigges, 1989).

The fourth type of pain, and the second type of pain that the occupational therapist is best skilled to treat, is the pain of loss of role. Once the physical concerns of the patient are under good medical management, the patient's attention turns to the realities of everyday life. Typically, patients feel they no longer have a purpose in life. They experience the pain of loss of role. Panic can ensue: "Time is running out; health is fading. I am dependent; I am helpless and useless." It is during this period in the patient's illness that the occupational therapist, approaching practice from an occupational behavior perspective, can diminish the pain the patient is experiencing. The occupational behaviorist believes that quality of life extends substantially beyond the state of mere survival. Quality of life rests with internalized feelings of positive self-esteem. By making a contribution, people gain respect for themselves and the admiration of others. This respect and admiration lead to feelings of worth and positive self-esteem. Thus competency is realized and a purpose for living is recognized. The occupational therapist can assist the terminally ill person who feels no particular reason to live to realize his or her potential through examining and supporting strategies for achieving self-care, work, and leisure (Tigges, Sherman, & Sherwin, 1984).

DIAGNOSTIC HONESTY

When one is ill and goes to a physician with a physical or emotional complaint, one assumes that, following appropriate examinations and tests, the physician will explain what is wrong and what the course of treatment will be. That is the usual procedure when recovery and rehabilitation are possible. When medical personnel encounter someone whose life cannot be saved, prolonged, or rehabilitated, they often are caught off guard. They may hide behind an attitude of professional detachment, avoiding or overlooking the necessity of taking time to explain to the person what is happening, or in some cases they will lie. These courses of action are referred to as diagnostic evasion or diagnostic dishonesty.

The hospice philosophy recognizes that life is made up of many and varied experiences ranging from successful to unsuccessful, happy to sad, productive to unproductive, and loving to lonely; and that as surely as one is born, one will die. Hospice requires people to be honest and straightforward with one another during the happy as well as the sad times, for by sharing life experiences, one grows in understanding of what living is all about.

Diagnostic honesty is the practice of answering patients' and families' questions openly and honestly. Hospice personnel believe that when direct or indirect questions are asked about the diagnosis and the prognosis, an honest and direct answer will always be given. When and how these answers are given depend on a good understanding and perception of how much the patient actually wants to know and a great sensitivity on the part of the health care team member who is replying to the patient or family members.

QUALITY OF LIFE

Many people diagnosed with cancer have experienced years of knowing that they have cancer and have undergone numerous medical procedures. Their illness and subsequent treatments have either slowly or rapidly eroded their ability to maintain their familiar and preferred life roles in self-care, work, and leisure. People are creatures of habit and therefore have expectations that they will be capable of providing for their basic needs, and of making a significant and valued contribution during their lifetime for many years to come. "Not to be able to carry on with life as a capable, productive, valued and respected person" (Tigges, 1993, pp. 535–536) can, and does, cause an immense erosion in one's perception and realization of quality of life and thus, one's self-esteem. This, perhaps, is the greatest insult to personal integrity.

When a patient is given a final prognosis of less than six months to live, health professionals should not be surprised to see their patients, no matter what their premorbid locus of control profile may have been, express feelings of helplessness, hopelessness, or uselessness. Helplessness is the inability to satisfy basic needs, the loss of control. Hopelessness is the inability to see any purpose in living, a loss of personal safety and security, and a loss of choices. Uselessness is having no perceived personal worth or value, the loss of options (Tigges, 1993).

These very real and justifiable feelings are a result of progressive or rapid loss of physical strength and endurance, and discomfort and pain. Typically, advanced cancer patients come to the painful realization that they will no longer be able to do the things they could in the past, and that they will not be able to achieve all their life goals. Hospice advocates believe that they must deal with the devastating effects and grim prognosis of advanced terminal disease so that the fabric of a patient's life can be rewoven and he or she may live the remainder of life with a sense of accomplishment and purpose. In this reweaving and living, occupational therapy can perhaps make its single most significant contribution.

AROUND-THE-CLOCK CARE

In traditional medical facilities, patients expect that doctors and nurses will be in attendance around-the-clock and that occupational and physical therapists will be available from nine to five Monday through Friday. To fulfill the tenets of hospice care, all disciplines are expected to be on call 24 hours a day. When a patient expresses a need or a concern, the appropriate staff member should be there to address it. This represents a very different model of care for occupational therapists.

For a patient with a life expectancy of 6 months or less, a weekend without occupational therapy represents a significant percentage of life. The likelihood of a need for an occupational therapist in the evening and on weekends is very high, for that is when patients and family members have activities and events that they want to participate in.

BEREAVEMENT CARE

After the death of a patient, life is generally very difficult for those who survive. Families cope with and adjust to death in vastly different ways, depending on their previous roles, their relationships with the deceased, and the practices of their particular religion. Two behaviors seen in the majority of survivors are depression and withdrawal from social activities.

Grief is normal and natural and should be treated as such. On the death and the burial of a patient, the hospice treatment team closes its case and transfers the family to a separate bereavement team. Although not all families participate, a large majority request bereavement services, for both individuals and support groups. Most hospice programs provide such services for one year.

Attitudes and Approaches in Treating the Terminally Ill

In the hospice model of care, a reality that must be considered and accommodated is that all patients will die. Coming to terms with the inevitability of death can pose very real personal and professional problems for occupational therapy personnel because they are accustomed to working with patients who are going to survive. In general, people in American society have difficulty in talking about and facing death. Occupational therapy personnel, like others who work with the terminally ill, must explore and learn to cope with both their professional and their personal feelings and thoughts about dying and death. An open and honest consideration of their own feelings and thoughts is essential to effectiveness in hospice work. Only after such consideration are professionals likely to feel comfortable when patients and families express a need to talk about and question their own feelings about the impending death.

Occupational therapy personnel need to consider the patient's and family's religious values and practices. Religion often provides a structure for a patient and a family to view death, and helps them understand how and why tragedies occur—why bad things happen to good people. In traditional occupational therapy, becoming involved in a patient's religion is considered professionally inappropriate because religion is a personal and private matter and irrelevant in treatment. In hospice care, however, religious issues and concerns invariably become a prominent part of therapeutic intervention. Thus, the occupational therapist must not only be trained to respond appropriately to these concerns but also be knowledgeable about various religious beliefs and practices (Tigges & Marcil, 1988).

Still another matter to understand is the strong humanitarian aspect of hospice philosophy. All efforts are made to comfort, listen to, encourage, and guide the patient in meeting personal needs and wishes. No request is too small to consider. No matter how long a patient wants to talk, or how much he or she wants to be reassured, time is given. Although this is admirable, it can cause problems for the patient and the therapist, so precautions must be taken to preserve the integrity of both.

Because so much caring and time are given, and frequently many intimate feelings and concerns are revealed, it is not uncommon for a patient or a family member to see the occupational therapist as a friend first and a therapist second. This is particularly true because occupational therapists help people recognize their needs and goals in living their last weeks or months as independently and as productively as their disease permits.

In hospice work, going the extra mile and being honest with feelings cause families and patients to want to show their appreciation. They may offer a cup of coffee, a drink, or a meal. Although accepting these expressions of gratitude is an important part of intervention, caution must be exercised. Particularly in a home-care situation, it is not uncommon for patients and family members to regard the therapist as a member of the extended family. After all, the therapist has been there on numerous occasions to assist the patient get out of bed, ambulate to the bathroom, groom, dress, make plans, get out of the house, and experience normal life events. It should come as no surprise, then, when the patient or family members extend the hand of friendship to the therapist. Nevertheless, the occupational therapist must remain friendly without becoming a friend. Should friendship occur, the relationship with the patient will become compromised and fail.

Ending a relationship with a family must also be examined. Occupational therapy personnel are with a family during one of the most significant milestones in life. Families sometimes grow to feel that staff members will continue as a part of the family fabric after the death of the patient. Invitations may be extended to come to the family home for a visit or meal. At the death and during the wake, funeral, or shiva, it is necessary to say good-bye to the family gently, sincerely, and clearly.

It may seem paradoxical to advocate going the extra mile to care for, comfort, share with, and help a patient and a family, and at the same time to keep a professional distance and objectivity. Appropriate balance and perspective in professional and personal relationships with patients and their families are essential, but they are not easy to accomplish. Each situation is unique.

Another attitude to examine in working with the terminally ill is one's criteria for success. In traditional treatment and rehabilitation settings, success is achieved when the patient has recovered or has reached a higher level of independence and productivity. With such achievements the therapist feels a sense of satisfaction, which brings a renewed vigor to the next day's cases. Such a standard of success is obviously not appropriate in treating the terminally ill person. It is a recognized fact that the patient will die. Therefore, it should come as no surprise when the patient begins to deteriorate and ultimately dies. No matter how well educated or experienced occupational therapists may be, they are likely to experience feelings of loss when a patients dies. These very real feelings can be comforted by reviewing these criteria for success.

1. The patient's functional ability was increased and directed towards competence and achievement in occupational roles.

2. Family and primary caregivers were given instruction and guidance in providing the necessary assistance and support to the patient.

3. The patient was given the opportunity to set and accomplish personal goals.

4. The patient lived well, free from pain and symptoms, and even though life was not as long as hoped for, it was completed with a sense of strength, purpose, and dignity, which would not have been possible without the skills and abilities of each and every member of the palliative care team. In the eyes of all, there was hope without a future, a future without time (Tigges, 1993).

HOSPICE: THE PAST 10 YEARS

As with any new idea, concept, philosophy, or model of care, changes occur over time. Hospice is no exception. Initially, hospices admitted only patients with advanced metastatic disease with a life expectancy of 6 months or less. Eventually, with some reluctance, individuals with AIDS were admitted and cared for (Pollatsek, 1987). Today, the population in most hospices includes patients with advanced cancer, AIDS, Alzheimer's, and other life-threatening illnesses.

Although the diversity of the hospice population has changed impressively, many people feel that some of the original tenets of hospice have been dismissed or significantly compromised, particularly in the area of quality of life. Where once every effort was made to facilitate the patient's life ambitions and goals, now the effort is limited to biological pain and symptom management, family support, and bereavement care. Reasons given for this change are reimbursement issues, increased patient loads, the need to cut costs, and changes in administrative philosophy (Silverman, 1984; Sherman, 1987; Ufema, 1989; Williams, 1989).

Despite the numerous changes and adjustments in the hospice movement, it still provides an essential service to patients who otherwise would have little or no alternative but to suffer at home or seek aggressive care in a hospital.

The Role of Occupational Therapy in Assessment

Each health care team member needs to be more than casually knowledgeable about other team members' roles and contributions so that team interventions can be as effective as possible in the limited time available to set and accomplish goals. Ensuring the patient's quality of life is the major consideration for the team.

The patient's or family's first contact is usually with a physician who must ascertain the following:

- Whether the diagnosis and the prognosis are appropriate for admission to hospice care

- Whether the patient and the family (or the primary caregiver) understand the philosophy and the model of care advocated by hospice

- Whether the family has, or can develop, the personal and emotional resources to care for the patient

- What the immediate and future needs of the patient and the family in regard to the physical condition of the patient are, and what the needs of the patient are for enhancing quality of life.

Apart from the appropriateness of the diagnosis, the prognosis, and the medical concerns of pain and symptom control, the physician must have knowledge and understanding of occupational therapy. It is the responsibility of the occupational therapist to orient physicians thoroughly as to the specific contributions that occupational therapy can make and to provide them with key questions from the occupational history to pose to patients and family members on the initial intake visit.

IDENTIFICATION OF PATIENT AND FAMILY CHARACTERISTICS AND NEEDS

The following questions are appropriate for the physician to ask to elicit the information needed to determine whether a full occupational therapy assessment is indicated:

Questions for the Family or the Primary Caregiver

1. *What are you most concerned about in caring for the patient (excluding pain and symptom control)?*

Generally, answers include such concerns as lifting, bathing, toileting, dressing, ambulation (use of walkers and wheelchairs), and getting the patient in and out of bed.

2. *What are you allowing the patient to do for himself or herself? Are you doing everything for him or her?*

This question frequently elicits the information that caregivers are doing everything for the patient. This renders the patient dependent and facilitates feelings of helplessness and hopelessness.

Questions for the Patient

1. *What are the most important things that your illness has prevented you from doing?*

The answer is usually "Everything."

2. *At the present time, what brings you the most pleasure?*

The answer is frequently, "Very little or nothing. I feel so bad that I am such a burden to my family."

3. *What would you like to do tomorrow, if you could?*

Reponses usually take two extremes. On the one hand, patients express the desire to be more independent in self-care: "If only I could take a bath and wash my hair," or "If I could just get out of bed and sit in my favorite chair"; work: "I'd like to do something to help my family out," or "I want to be more useful in some way"; and leisure: "I would love to get out of the house and go visit my friends, but I know that is impossible," or "I used to have so many hobbies, but I can't do them in bed." On the other hand, patients respond with "Nothing!" This response is generally a loud and clear statement that if they cannot do what they did before, independently, they are not interested in doing anything at all, and no amount of persuading is effective.

After asking these questions, the physician is in a good position to determine the appropriateness of an OT assessment.

ANALYSIS OF THE APPROPRIATENESS OF PATIENT NEEDS AND GOALS

What would the patient like to accomplish? What physical limitations interfere with the performance of these roles? For the answer to these questions the occupational therapist administers an occupational history, a temporal adaptation assessment, and a performance assessment (see appendix).

An occupational history is an assessment that looks historically at how the patient's roles in self-care, work, and play have been developed, achieved, and maintained. The occupational history also reveals what roles in the patient's life have been important and have brought a sense of independence and accomplishment.

The assessment of temporal adaptation seeks information to compare past and present routines of daily living. It inquires how the patient has adjusted the routine to accommodate present circumstances.

The administration of the occupational history and the temporal assessment can be stressful for the patient. Recounting one's past occupational talents, abilities, and accomplishments, and one's hopes for the future can bring the futility of the present situation into focus. However, if sensitively handled by the therapist, the patient's review of past accomplishments and setting of immediate goals for continued accomplishment can bring him or her a sense of well-being.

The performance assessment is used to determine the patient's ability to do what he or she would like to achieve before death. The choice of physical assessments is strictly determined by the patient's goals. The therapist must constantly remember that the purpose of the intervention is to restore the desired roles, as quickly and efficiently as possible in the time the patient has left to live.

Occupational therapists must be keenly alert to the feasibility of a patient's accomplishing his or her goals with respect to the disease and its projected course. Just as the physician must be informed about the services that occupational therapy can offer a particular patient, so must OT personnel be knowledgeable about that patient's condition and the patient's progression of the illness so that both on the initial visit, and in the assessment of the patient, realistic goals can be set.

IMPLEMENTATION OF OCCUPATIONAL THERAPY

Work and leisure goals should be intertwined with the facilitation of a higher level of self-care abilities. Should the patient specify certain leisure goals, they should be combined with the self-care goals. Goals are set through assessment and discussions with patients. As patients become more independent, their feelings of isolation and abandonment significantly decrease, because they no longer feel so dependent and useless. In the authors' experience in treating the terminally ill, fewer than one percent of patients have been unable to achieve a significant increase in independence and ability in self-care, work, and leisure.

When a patient's level of independence improves significantly, diagnostic honesty becomes a problem. It is not uncommon to have to deal with newfound independence in relation to the nature of the disease process. This is a paradox. A person who has been told that he or she has a terminal illness for which there is no cure, and that the prognosis is 6 months or less, is referred for occupational therapy.

Therapy, in the eyes of many lay people, means hope for remediation. When the terminally ill are helped to make a significant improvement in their level of independence, some equate increased physical function with survival.

The occupational therapist should directly, yet sensitively, answer questions about the terminal nature of the disease despite an increase in function. No prepared responses exist. The response will depend on the individual circumstance.

Diagnostic honesty, a basic tenet of hospice care, enables the patient and members of the health care team to plan and achieve realistic goals. Being honest in these circumstances is not easy, but it provides a measure of hope that patients can realistically carry out their life ambitions with a sense of integrity in weeks instead of years.

Occupational therapists encounter many difficult and varied problems in working with the terminally ill. An occupational therapist may be at the bedside of a dying patient, because the patient or the family want him or her to be present. However, when it becomes obvious that the patient has fewer than 24 hours to live, the hospice team determines which members are most appropriate to be with the family, and a vigil is arranged.

At such times, a precise order of action is required:

1. Directing all efforts to make the dying person comfortable. This may include bathing him or her, changing the bed linens, or providing ice chips to soothe the patient's thirst.
2. Reassuring the family that the patient is comfortable and pain free.
3. Reassuring family members that they have done everything possible and could not have done anything more.
4. Determining that the person is dead.

Initially, that may be difficult because it is outside the traditional role of the occupational therapist.

Once the person has died, a standard procedure is followed:

1. The primary nurse is notified.
2. The body is laid out, with or without the assistance of family members, in preparation for the arrival of additional family members or the funeral director.
3. Assistance is given to family members in selecting the clothes in which the deceased will be buried.

All of these roles are normal and natural. They have been performed for centuries. However, occupational therapists are not usually trained to act in such situations.

It would be foolish to say that the hospice professional's task of caring for the terminally ill—that is, seeing the patient through death and the family through a wake, a funeral, or a shiva—is easy or becomes so customary as to be done with personal detachment. If that were true, the professional's effectiveness in a hospice program would be seriously questioned. Being a professional in a hospice program requires not only excellent professional skills but also exceptional personal maturity and sensitivity. Although patients die daily, weekly, or monthly, people always have a feeling of great loss. To repress such emotions is to deny that feelings are shared and exchanged with the patient. Hospice personnel recognize the importance of having a time when team members can share and bring closure to a case. If such opportunities are not planned for, staff burnout is inevitable.

Hospice care is a challenge beyond traditional education and experience. It calls for working with people who know they are going to die and who want professionals to support them in fulfilling their last desires. Occupational therapy personnel who practice from an occupational behavior perspective can provide much to the terminally ill by helping them to realize life to its fullest.

Summary

This final chapter of Module 3 examined the role of occupational therapy in the care of the terminally ill. Important questions exist about life and death issues such as when life begins, when death occurs, and whether life should be sustained at any cost. Such questions require the consideration of all health care providers.

The history of the hospice movement evolved from medieval times, when hospice meant a place of shelter and refreshment, to the 20th century, when it became a movement to meet the needs of the terminally ill.

The philosophy of traditional occupational therapy focuses on treatment and rehabilitation, while in hospice care the focus is on quality of life and working within the five tenets of hospice care. The attitudes of health care providers and their coming to terms with the inevitability of death are critical issues in effective hospice practice. Occupational therapy has an important role to play in assessment and treatment of the terminally ill in all phases of hospice care.

Review Questions

1. What are the principal factors that changed attitudes toward death in America from the first half to the second half of the 20th century?

2. What determines whether life should be sustained at all costs?

3. What was the definition of "hospice" in medieval times?

4. When and by whom did dying become a concern in the hospices?

5. How did hospice emerge in the 20th century?

6. Where and when was the first hospice established in the United States?

7. How does the philosophy of traditional occupational therapy practice differ from practice in hospice care?

8. List some attitudes and approaches the occupational therapist must examine if treating the terminally ill.

9. What are the components of the occupational therapy assessment with the hospice patient?

10. How are OT goals determined?

11. How can an increase in function affect the patient's perception of the terminal illness?

12. What personal skills are essential for work in hospice?

13. How do hospice personnel deal with feelings of loss?

Case Study

The following case study uses the occupational history developed for the terminally ill (Tigges, 1993) and is based on the occupational behavior model. All treatment plans are developed from this and related assessments. Because the hospice program described in this case study is a home-based agency, all treatment occurs in the patient's home.

BACKGROUND INFORMATION

Jeffery is a 65-year-old, married man who was diagnosed with amyotrophic lateral sclerosis (ALS) 9 months ago. He recently began hospice services after receiving a prognosis of 6 months. He lives with his wife in a ranch house with a ramped entryway in the rear of the house. His wife is a nurse and, because of recent financial difficulties incurred by his illness, she continues to work every day. Jeffery is Catholic and his wife is Jewish, but they do not actively practice their respective religions. They have four adult children, all of whom live in the area and visit frequently.

OCCUPATIONAL HISTORY

Work history. Jeffery has worked for the past 25 years as a certified public accountant. He has a master's degree in accounting. He worked until 3 months ago, when he developed bilateral upper extremity weakness and was unable to operate his computer. He states that he has always worked since he was a teenager and that the hardest part of his illness is being dependent on others to assist him. Jeffery is aware that it is not feasible for him to return to work. However, he would like to help his family and friends prepare their tax returns. Jeffery states that he never had any hobbies or interest in sports. He enjoys using America Online to communicate with people around the country.

Performance assessment. Jeffery is dependent in all activities of daily living, owing to the rapid onset of his ALS and great weakness of all extremities. Owing to dysphagia, he is unable to eat solid foods and is fed by means of a gastric tube. He is able to drink fluids but is unable to hold and manipulate a cup. Although the therapist is able to transfer Jeffery using a stand-pivot method, his wife is unable to transfer him without a hydraulic lift. He spends most of his day in a recliner although he does have an electric wheelchair for mobility. He has enough finger movement to use the television remote control although this is extremely difficult.

Locus of control assessment. Results of the Reid Assessment (Reid, 1981) reveal that premorbidly, Jeffery was a strong origin personality. Although he continues to demonstrate some origin traits, he also demonstrates an increase in pawn characteristics as evidenced by his growing feelings of being controlled by his environment and other people, with little self-direction.

Self-esteem assessment. According to the therapist's subjective observations and interpretations, Jeffery is experiencing feelings of helplessness and hopelessness as evidenced by his excessive demands on his wife, strained interpersonal relations with his wife and children, and an inability to control his emotions.

Physical assessment. Jeffery is nonambulatory and he is able to bear only partial weight on his legs. He has poor-plus strength in both arms and has no grip strength. Both hands are moderately edematous and very painful to touch and movement. He exhibits marked atrophy of the first dorsal interossei of both hands (a hallmark of ALS). His upper extremity passive range of motion is limited by pain and muscle tightness. He exhibits good head, neck, and trunk control. All sensation is intact and he has no visual-perceptual impairments.

Primary caregiver assessment. Jeffery's wife is concerned that he is alone for a large part of the day because she must continue to work. Although she stops home every day at lunchtime and he has a personal care aide and a hospice volunteer for two hours each day, she is concerned that he will be unable to meet his needs or summon help. She would like to be able to shower him in the tub (she has purchased a bathtub transfer bench), but she is unable to transfer him. She would like to have some personal time on the weekends to go shopping and get her hair done.

PROBLEMS

1. Jeffery is unable to use his computer owing to bilateral upper extremity weakness and bimanual edema with pain.
2. He is unable to perform object manipulation tasks.
3. He is unable to transfer into or out of the bathtub.

NEEDS

Because of his generalized weakness and steady decompensation, Jeffery will require assistance with all ADL. To operate his computer independently, he will require environmental adaptations and assistive devices to foster and facilitate greater independence. It is extremely important to Jeffery that he be able to use his computer. All other goals are secondary.

ASSETS

Jeffery has some voluntary use of both arms and hands. He has good cognitive, perceptual, and visual skills. He has good head and neck control, which will allow him to use a mouth stick even if he loses total use of his arms and hands. Although he is depressed and emotionally labile, he appears to be motivated to maximize his independence. He is aware of the progression of his disease and he holds no false hope for recovery.

GOALS AND METHODS

Goal 1. Patient will independently operate his computer with adaptations and assistive devices.

Methods. Patient will be provided with bilateral mobile arm supports to allow him to utilize the minimal active movement of his arms.

Patient's computer table will be raised 4 inches to allow total wheelchair access.

Patient's work area will be ergonomically arranged to allow ease of access to all equipment.

Patient will be supplied with and trained in the use of a mouth stick to allow him to depress keys on keyboard.

Computer mouse will be replaced with a track ball to allow him to move cursor with less movement of arms and hands.

Goal 2. Patient will be transferred into and out of the bathtub using the stand-pivot transfer method and a bathtub transfer bench.

Methods. Patient's sons will be instructed in the stand-pivot transfer technique, including proper placement of wheelchair. All transfers will be supervised by occupational therapist registered until they can be performed safely.

Goal 3. Decrease bimanual edema or pain.

Methods. Patient will be provided with bimanual pressure gloves and instruct patient's wife in application and removal (with physician's order).

Retrograde massage will be provided to both hands.

Patient and family will be educated in proper positioning of arms and hands to decrease edema.

Patient's family and hospice volunteer will be educated in bilateral upper extremity passive range of motion exercises to maintain joint mobility and decrease pain on movement.

Goal 4. Patient will independently drink water as needed.

Methods. Patient's recliner chair will be adapted to stabilize a large, insulated cup, which will be filled with ice water by family or hospice personnel throughout the day as needed. A long drinking straw will be secured to the cup to allow him to sip water as he desires.

Goal 5. Patient will independently operate the television remote control with relative ease.

Methods. Patient's recliner will be adapted with a bean bag lap tray and Velcro put on television remote and tray to secure remote.

Patient will be educated in the use of the mouth stick to operate the buttons.

The OTR will perform the initial evaluation with a certified occupational therapy assistant present. Following completion of the evaluation, the OTR and COTA will discuss the findings with Jeffery and his wife, presenting what can realistically be accomplished based on Jeffery's desires and his physical abilities. Initially, visits will be made 5 times a week for the first 2 weeks, and 3 times a week for the next 4 weeks. The OTR and COTA will work together for the first week. Following that, the COTA will be responsible for executing the OT plan with supervisory visits every five visits. It is estimated that all of the original goals can be accomplished in this 6-week period.

The OTR will also instruct the hospice volunteers in the OT program to ensure greater coverage of goals. The OTR will report patient's progress to the entire hospice team at the weekly patient review conferences. A meeting with the volunteer coordinator resulted in Jeffery's having a volunteer on Saturday and Sunday to allow his wife some personal time.

Appendix.
Occupational History

Patient's name:

Date of history:

Time of history:

Occupational Inquiries

A. WORK HISTORY (EMPLOYMENT)

1. I understand that before you became ill you were a _____. What an interesting job. How did you get started or interested in that line of work?
2. What sort of training or education was involved?
3. Where did you get your training?
4. What was the first job you had (and subsequent jobs)?
5. What was the last job you had before you became ill?
6. Did you work up until you became sick?
7. (If retired) How long have you been retired?

B. WORK HISTORY (HOMEMAKER)

1. I understand that you have been a housewife or mother for many years. That is more than a full-time job, isn't it?
2. What was the most challenging part of being a housewife, wife, mother?
3. What was the most frustrating part of being a housewife, wife, mother?
4. Apart from being a full-time housewife, were you ever interested or involved in community or religious activities?
5. Were you still active in these activities up until the time you became sick?
6. Since you became ill, what jobs have been the most difficult to give up?
7. What bothers you the most about the jobs you have had to give up?
8. What type of work is/was your husband involved in?

C. FAMILY HISTORY

1. Have you always lived in _____ (city)? If no, where did you live before you moved here?
2. What did your parents do for a living?
3. Do you have brothers and sisters? Where do they live? Do you see/talk to them often?
4. I understand that you have children or grandchildren. Where do they live? Are they married? Do you see or talk to them frequently?
5. (Husband as patient) Before you got sick, what were your duties or responsibilities around the house?

6. Before you got sick, which did you do with your spouse, children, grandchildren?

7. What are the most important things that your illness has prevented you from doing?

8. At the present time, what brings you the greatest pleasure?

9. What are the things that you would like to do now?

D. LEISURE, SPORT, AND RECREATION

1. When you were finished with your day's work, what did you do for relaxation or fun?

2. How often did you engage in these activities?

3. Who did you do them with?

4. When was the last time you enjoyed these activities?

5. If you could, would you like to do them again?

E. TEMPORAL ADAPTATION

1. Before you got sick was it important for you to have a daily schedule? (In what way was it or was it not important to you?)

2. How did you organize your day? Start from the time you got up each morning and tell me everything you did before you went to bed.

3. What is your daily schedule like now?

4. If you had your choice, how would you like to spend tomorrow?

Therapist's Comments:

FUNCTIONAL EVALUATION

Ask patient to demonstrate or describe problems in the following areas:

1. Bathing or toileting, dressing
2. Ambulation
3. Object manipulation
4. Homemaking or home management
5. Child care, parenting or grandparenting
6. Leisure, sport, or recreation.

Source: Occupational therapy by K. N. Tigges (1993), in D. Doyle et al. (Eds.), *Occupational textbook of palliative medicine* [pp. 535-543], Oxford: Oxford University Press. Reprinted with author's permission.

References

Byock, I. (1993). The euthanasia/assisted suicide debate matures. *American Journal of Hospice and Palliative Care, 10*(2), 8–11.

Drane, J. F. (1995). Physician assisted suicide & voluntary active euthanasia: Social ethics and the role of hospice. *American Journal of Hospice and Palliative Care, 12*(6), 3–10.

Gates, R. P. (1993a). Readers say: Don't throw "hospice" out the window. *American Journal of Hospice and Palliative Care, 10*(5), 2.

Gates, R. P. (1993b). Throw "hospice" out the window. *American Journal of Hospice and Palliative Care,10*(2), 4–5.

Humphry, D. (1991). *Final exit: The practicalities of self-deliverance and assisted suicide for the dying.* Eugene, OR: Hemlock Society.

Kevorkian, J. (1991). *Prescription: Medicine.* Buffalo, NY: Prometheus Press.

Kilner, J. K. (1990). *Who lives? Who dies?* New Haven, CT: Yale University Press.

Olson, P. (1995). Physician assisted suicide. *American Journal of Hospice and Palliative Care, 12*(1), 9–12.

Piper, G. (1994). Hospice vs. suicide: The wrong debate. *American Journal of Hospice and Palliative Care, 11*(6), 5.

Pollatsek, M. A. (1987). Hospice for AIDS patients. *American Journal of Hospice Care, 4*(6), 9–10.

Reid, D. W., & Ziegler, M. (1981) The desired control measure and adjustment among the elderly. In H. Lefcourt (Ed.), *Research with the locus of construct* (Vol. 1, pp. 127–159). New York: Academic Press.

Sherman, L. M. (1987). Hospice at the crossroads. *American Journal of Hospice Care, 4*(3), 18–21.

Silverman, H. D. (1984). Hospice is hospice; or is it? *American Journal of Hospice Care,1*(3), 8–10.

Tigges, K. N. (1989). Pain assessment: An interdisciplinary perspective. *Home Health Care Nurse, 7*(6), 18–23.

Tigges, K. N. (1993). Occupational therapy. In D. Doyle, G. Hanks, & N. MacDonald (Eds.), *Oxford textbook of palliative medicine* (pp. 535–543). Oxford: Oxford University Press.

Tigges, K. N., & Marcil, W. M. (1988). Religious practices and funeral rites. In K. N. Tigges & W. M. Marcil (Eds.). *Terminal and life-threatening illness: An occupational behavior perspective* (pp. 185–203). Thorofare, NJ: SLACK.

Tigges, K. N., Sherman, L. M., Sherwin, F. (1984). Perspectives on the pain of the hospice patient: The roles of the occupational therapist and physician. *Occupational Therapy in Health Care, 3,* 55–66.

Ufema, J. K. (1989). Is this hospice? *American Journal of Hospice Care, 6*(1), 7–8.

Williams, R. (1989). Another look at hospice in America. *American Journal of Hospice Care, 6*(5), 15–16.

Module IV

Jeffrey L. Crabtree, MS, OTR/L, FAOTA
Editor

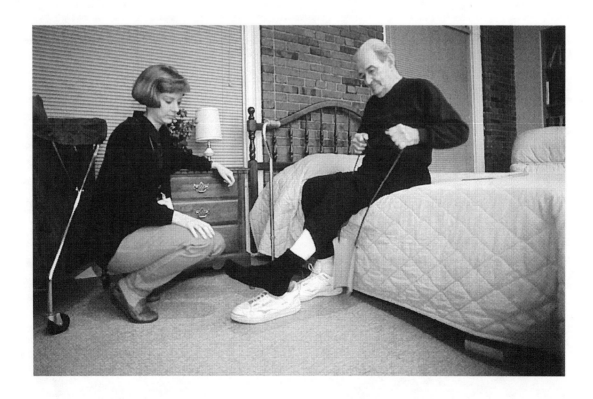

Author Biographies

Jeffrey L. Crabtree, MS, OTR/L, FAOTA, is an assistant professor in the Occupational Therapy Program, Department of Rehabilitation Sciences, at Texas Tech University Health Sciences Center, Lubbock, Texas. He earned his bachelor's degree in occupational therapy from the University of Washington and his master's degree in health sciences from San Francisco State University. Currently he is a member of the AOTA Roster of Accreditation Evaluators. Mr. Crabtree is past editor of the *Gerontology Special Interest Section Newsletter* and has served on the editorial board of the *American Journal of Occupational Therapy* and on several national and local boards. He has published many articles and chapters and is the coauthor of *Home Caregiver's Guide: Articles for Adult Daily Living and In-Home Assessment of the Elderly: An Interdisciplinary Approach.*

Elizabeth Walker Peterson, MPH, OTR/L, is a clinical instructor in the Department of Occupational Therapy at the University of Illinois at Chicago, where she also serves as the Illinois Geriatric Education Center Network Disciplinary Director for Occupational Therapy, with responsibility for developing educational programs for occupational therapists working with older adults. She received her bachelor's degree in occupational therapy from the University of Florida, and her master's degree from Boston University School of Public Health. She has been involved in several research projects dealing with the fear of falling: She is a coinvestigator of a study funded by the National Institute on Aging, entitled *Changing Attitudes and Self-Conceptions to Reduce Fear of Falling,* and also a coinvestigator of a study entitled *Fear of Falling Among Minority Community Dwelling Elderly,* which is supported by the Center for Health Interventions with Minority Elderly.

Timothy A. Reistetter, MS, OT, is a staff therapist at Transitional Hospital of Tampa, a long-term acute care hospital. He works primarily with older adults and was a case manager for Jubilee Associates of Maryland, Inc.

Laurie Rockwell-Dylla, MS, OTR/L, is a clinical associate at the University of Illinois at Chicago, where she earned both a master's degree and postprofessional master's degree in occupational therapy. She has clinical experience in working with the geriatric population in hospitals, long-term care facilities, and home settings. Her teaching experience includes guest lectures on the role of occupational therapy in home health. Ms. Rockwell-Dylla's research experience has been in using qualitative methods to explore older adults' meaning of home.

Matin Royeen, PhD, is an assistant professor in the Department of Occupational Therapy, School of Pharmacy and Health Professions at Creighton University in Omaha, Nebraska. He holds a doctorate in psychology, counseling, and multicultural and international education. Dr. Royeen has worked in a variety of settings, including education, business, and government, focusing on multicultural and international education.

Deborah Walens, MHPE, OTR/L, FAOTA, is a clinical assistant professor and field coordinator at the University of Illinois in Chicago, where she earned both her bachelor's degree in occupational therapy and master's degree in health profession education. Ms. Walens has developed clinical education models throughout the continuum of care. She was the principal investigator on a Federal Allied Health Projects Grant that focused on the training of occupational therapy students in home health.

Learning Outline

Chapter 16
Health Education in Occupational Therapy 805

Elizabeth Walker Peterson, MPH, OTR/L

Chapter 17
Client- and Family-Practitioner Relationships:
Collaboration as an Effective Approach to Treatment 833

Deborah Walens, MHPE, OTR/L, FAOTA, and Laurie Rockwell-Dylla, MS, OTR/L

Chapter 18
Keeping Current with Laws and Public Policy Issues That Influence Practice

Jeffrey L. Crabtree, MS, OTR/L, FAOTA

SECTION 1.

Keeping Current with Legislation

SECTION 2.

Keeping Current with Government Programs

Introduction to Module IV

As the demand for services to an aging and culturally diverse population increases, and as efforts to lower the costs of those services become greater, the demand for occupational therapists to work in interdisciplinary teams and to collaborate with older clients and their families will become more evident. The interdisciplinary issues considered in Module IV can be categorized as teamwork. More and more, occupational therapists are working in teams with other professionals to provide the best type of care for elderly patients, whether in hospitals or nursing facilities or through community-based providers.

Chapter 15 addresses the general concept of teams and how they operate, describing the theoretical stages of teamwork and the different types of teams that may be encountered by occupational therapists.

Chapter 16 discusses theories underlying adult education and the best ways to teach geriatrics new methods of performing tasks. It includes a discussion of different ways to involve adults in their own education.

Chapter 17 discusses teamwork as it applies to the client, the client's family, and the occupational therapist. This team is critical to the success of the occupational therapy.

Chapter 18 presents myriad sources of information on different state and federal laws that have an impact on the provision of services to the elderly, including the Americans with Disabilities Act, Medicare, Medicaid, and the Social Security Act. A comprehensive list of sources on information on aging in general is also provided.

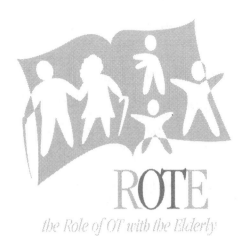

ROTE

the Role of OT with the Elderly

Theories and Models of Teams and Groups

Matin Royeen, PhD
Timothy A. Reistetter, MS, OT

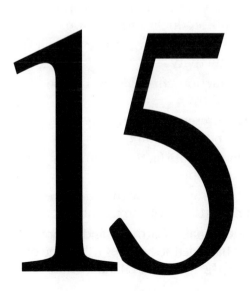

15

Abstract

This unit is divided into three sections: section 1 deals with group theories and models, section 2 with how the models apply to occupational therapy, and section 3 with occupational therapy in different cultural settings.

Section 1 focuses on essentials of group tasks, maintenance, leadership, roles, functions, and different approaches to the study of groups. Other topics covered include formation of small groups, stages of group development, group conflict, and communication. This broad overview is intended to give a general understanding of the theories and principles of group dynamics. Additionally, this section focuses on models of group treatment in occupational therapy followed by a discussion of educational groups with geriatric populations.

Section 2 discusses group models and structures as they apply to occupational therapy services. Specifically, it focuses on the team approach used with the geriatric population. This section covers the interdisciplinary team, multidisciplinary team, and the occupational therapist (OTR) and occupational therapy assistant (COTA) team. Other topics covered include case management and consultancy in occupational therapy.

Section 3 deals with the ethnic and cross-cultural implications of occupational therapy practice in different settings, including the geriatric population. It provides a bicultural approach (i.e., American versus non-American) to working with individuals in different settings. Some specific recommendations are made for working with people whose cultural-ethnic background differs from the mainstream American culture. The section also provides a cross-cultural view of aging.

Section 1. Groups, Theories, and Models

Group life has been an integral part of human existence throughout history. From prehistoric periods to the contemporary era, human beings have been living in groups. People depend on each other not only for survival, but also for accomplishing their collective goals. The basic group is the family whose members share certain responsibilities and perform specific tasks to fulfill their needs. To meet their total goals, families expand their social circles to include playmates, schoolmates, and social, religious, and recreational organizations. As social beings, people need to interact with others and receive satisfaction from their experiences.

Since World War II, the interest in group work has dramatically increased (Mills, 1967). Social scientists, researchers, and educators have researched and taught courses on group behavior. Much of the research focused on individuals and their patterns of interaction as they met in small groups.

According to Mills, the study of small groups is important for a number of reasons. First, the study of small groups is important for practical reasons. Individuals in groups make decisions that could affect the fate of people, communities, and nations.

Second, studying small groups helps us understand the psychosocial pressures faced when individuals meet

in a group. Learning more about the impact of psycho-social pressure on individuals and the way they interact with group members is important.

Third, studying the sociology of understanding small groups may provide empirically based theories about the dynamics of interacting forces in the group.

Fourth, small groups are the microsystems of larger societies. Because the study of large groups is difficult, small groups may serve as models to construct and test theories before applying them to less accessible societies. According to Mills, "Small group research is thus a means of developing effective ways of thinking about social systems in general."

Definition of Small Groups

Cartheart and Samovar (1970) defined a small group as a face-to-face assemblage of individuals whose numbers should not exceed 12 to 15 people. Furthermore, they have identified measurements for task and interaction effectiveness. Group task effectiveness can be measured by the following:

1. The speed with which group members reach their goals

2. The amount of satisfaction expressed by members regarding group products and decisions

3. The quality and quantity of their productivity.

Interaction effectiveness can be measured by

1. The presence of harmony and absence of conflict

2. Member satisfaction with their interaction

3. The congruency with the desired relationships of the members.

Additionally, Cartheart and Samovar (1970) have defined groups using one or more of the following characteristics:

1. **Perceptions:** Each group member should be aware of his or her relationships with other group members and possess a perception of unity.

2. **Organization:** Groups are organized systems of two or more individuals with certain standards and roles to perform within the group.

3. **Goals and motivation:** Individuals join groups to satisfy their needs and meet their goals.

4. **Interdependency:** While pursuing common tasks and shared responsibilities, group members are interdependent on each other.

5. **Interaction:** Group members influence each other through constant communication and interaction.

Howe and Schwartzberg (1986) discuss the following group characteristics. The characteristics have a great impact on the patterns of interactions and decision making in the group. The characteristics are listed below:

1. **Group structure:** the organization and procedures within the group

2. **Group context:** the context, originating outside the environment of the group, in which the group is created

3. **Group climate:** the physical and social environment inside the group

4. **Group size:** the number of members in the group

5. **Closed-group membership:** the number of group members stays the same throughout the life of the group

6. **Open-group membership:** the number of group members changes throughout the life of the group

7. **Voluntary membership:** the member joins the group by his or her own choice

8. **Group and individual goals:** the group and individual members have

goals, and these goals are the shared responsibility of all members.

The Impact of Leadership Styles on Groups

Researchers on group dynamics have identified three different group leadership styles. The democratic leader encourages group participation; the autocratic leader dictates; and the laissez-faire leader leaves power to other individuals within the group. In his study of leadership in different experimental group atmospheres, Lippitt (1940) found the following:

1. Democratic groups were more original than the autocratic and laissez-faire groups.

2. Autocracy was not more efficient than democracy.

3. Members of autocratic groups displayed more dependence and less individuality.

4. More friendliness and group-mindedness was noticeable under democratic leaders.

5. Autocratic leaders led to increased hostility and aggression.

Authority and power are considered to be vital ingredients of leadership and social organizations. Any abuse of power and authority can seriously disturb interpersonal relations within a group. Luft (1970) discussed some symptoms of the corrosive effect of authority on interpersonal relations. Authority figures do the following:

1. **Set up barriers:** They unnecessarily isolate themselves from others.

2. **Use people as tools:** They are impersonal and dehumanizing and do not hesitate to use others for their own personal agenda.

3. **Think they are perfect:** They see no need to evaluate their behavior or seek feedback from others since they believe they can do no wrong.

4. **Stick to their own level:** They relate to others in terms of their positions in the hierarchy. They glorify the elite while condescending to their subordinates.

5. **Eliminate opposition:** They cannot tolerate serious disagreements and deal harshly with dissenters.

6. **Display pseudohumility:** They are patronizing and caring at one time and indifferent at other times.

7. **Stress rules and conformity:** They insist on rules and regulations and emphasize conventional ways and conformity.

8. **Dichotomize:** They view things in terms of good or bad or right or wrong without any tolerance for ambiguity.

9. **Be anti-introspective:** They deny their feelings and do not acknowledge the feelings of others.

Roles

Role refers to the pattern of behavior individuals assume within the group. Bene and Sheats (1978) have identified the following three categories of individual roles in groups: task roles, maintenance roles, and individual roles.

Group task roles reflect the responsibility of individuals toward group goals, especially while the group is forming. The following task roles are assumed by the group leader as well as various members while performing task roles:

1. The *initiator-contributor* introduces new ideas and suggests changes regarding group goals, procedures, and so forth.

2. The *information seeker* asks questions and seeks clarification of ideas and facts discussed in the group.

3. The *opinion seeker* asks for clarification of values related to what the group is doing.

4. The *information giver* provides authoritative facts and generalizations or relates his or her own experiences to the group problem.

5. The *coordinator* clarifies the relationship among various ideas and suggestions, pulls them together, and coordinates various activities of the members.

6. The *orienter* defines the position of the group with respect to its goals.

7. The *evaluator-critic* subjects the group's accomplishments to a standard of group functioning in the context of the group task.

8. The *energizer* drives the group to action or decision and attempts to elevate the group to a higher level of activity.

9. The *procedural technician* facilitates the group movement by performing routine tasks.

10. The *recorder* writes a list of suggestions and decisions and serves as the "group memory."

Group maintenance roles focus on how individuals achieve the group's goals and how different personalities, views, feelings, and relationships are processed by the group:

1. The *encourager* praises, agrees with, and accepts the contribution of other members. He or she displays a very warm and positive attitude toward the opinions of others.

2. The *harmonizer* mediates the differences between other members, attempts to reconcile disagreement, and diffuses tension in conflict situations.

3. The *compromiser* operates within a conflict in which no idea or position is involved. In order to maintain group harmony, he or she is willing to compromise by adjusting his or her stance.

4. The *gatekeeper and expediter* maintains open communication and

actively facilities participation by all members.

5. The *standard setter* establishes standards for the group functioning or for the quality of group processes.

6. The *group observer* and commentator maintains a record of group processes and provides feedback to help the group evaluate its procedures.

7. The *follower* goes along with the movement of the group, serving as an audience in group discussion.

Individual roles are assumed by members to satisfy personal needs that may not be relevant to the group task and maintenance functions. If a group becomes too highly individual centered (as opposed to group centered), the group has problems and should reevaluate its functioning:

1. The *aggressor* lowers the status of others, attacks the whole group and does not care for values and feelings of other group members.

2. The *blocker* seems to be negative, stubborn, and unreasonable with others.

3. The *self-confessor* uses the group audience for expression of his or her own feelings, insights, ideology.

4. The *recognition seeker* attempts to draw everybody's attention by boasting and exaggerating personal achievement.

5. The *playboy* does not display any active involvement in group's process.

6. The *dominator* attempts to assert personal authority or superiority by manipulating group members.

7. The *help seeker* collects sympathy responses from other group members by expressions of insecurity, personal confusion, or self-depreciation.

8. The *special-interest pleader* speaks for special interest groups, usually as a mask for his or her own prejudices and biases.

Effective group functioning is a paradox in which all individuals become one and yet retain their individuality.

The Sociology of Small Groups

Mills (1967) discusses six different approaches to the study of small group models: the quasi-mechanical model, the organismic model, the conflict model, the equilibrium model, the structural-functional model, and the cybernetic-growth model. These models are related to both the task and the maintenance of group needs, as well as how the individuals contribute to the group's work.

THE QUASI-MECHANICAL MODEL

According to this model, the group is like an "interaction machine" in which members can predict each other's behaviors. Group behavior is considered a game in which individuals know both the games and players well enough to predict the outcome. In other words, this model assumes an individual will know who will speak and what type of behavior will be displayed from the beginning to the end. The quasi-mechanical model usually does not deal with emotions, norms, and beliefs within the group.

THE ORGANISMIC MODEL

This model views the group as a biological organism. The group forms, passes through various developmental and growth stages, and reaches maturity. The different individuals within the group assume different roles and responsibilities and display different types of behaviors and emotions as the "organism" matures. This model assumes a group is composed of different individuals with distinct personalities and beliefs in a very complex and dynamic system characterized by change, growth, and development.

THE CONFLICT MODEL

This model states that the individual members' varying needs in a group come in conflict over the limited amount of freedom and available resources. Some individuals have more freedom, while others have more prestige, leading to a sense of inequity within the group. Sometimes, individuals may blame other members for their own problems.

THE EQUILIBRIUM MODEL

This model assumes the group is usually in a state of equilibrium. Often, opposing forces within the group counteract each other, resulting in equilibrium. At times the group attempts to achieve group goals by disrupting solidarity and creating tension among members. However, this state of disruption is followed by establishing a sense of balance between the external demands and the internal needs of the group.

THE STRUCTURAL-FUNCTIONAL MODEL

This model assumes a group faces personal, social, and environmental challenges in pursuit of its goals. To meet these demands and prevent disintegration, the group must not only maximize its resources, but must also be willing to make the necessary changes both in structure and function.

THE CYBERNETIC-GROWTH MODEL

This model hypothesizes that group systems process information to enhance their capabilities. When a group successfully meets both external and internal demands, it develops a degree of self-determination and subsequently achieves self-growth. Every group depends on individual members' capability and degree of commitment to group development. Thus, the individuals play integral roles in the capability of the collective body.

The Primary Group

According to Dunphy (1972), the term "primary group" was first introduced by Charles H. Cooley in 1909. According to Cooley, primary groups have a tremendous impact on the formation of the personalities of their members. Cooley distinguished five characteristics of primary groups:

1. Face-to-face association
2. The unspecialized character of the association
3. Relative permanence
4. The small number of persons involved
5. The relative intimacy among the participants.

Similarly, Dunphy defined the primary group "as a small group which persists long enough to develop strong emotional attachments between members; at least a set of rudimentary, functionally differentiated roles; and a subculture of its own which includes both an image of the group as an entity and an informal normative system which controls group-relevant actions of members."

Dunphy expanded the general classes of primary groups to include the following:

1. Families
2. Peer groups in childhood, adolescence, and adulthood
3. Informal groups such as classroom groups, factory work groups, small military units

4. Resocialized groups such as therapy, rehabilitation, and self-analytic groups.

Primary groups play a critical role during all stages of socialization. The socialization process begins with the family and is carried to the classroom and recreation peer group and completed within the adult organizational work group. Since primary group structures are constantly changing, new groups are continually forming.

Formation of Small Groups

Small groups are formed by individuals with a specific goal or purpose in mind. There are many different types of groups. Barker et al. (1979) cites different reasons for formation of small groups:

1. To search for solutions to common problems

2. To develop new products and programs or deal with existing problems

3. To deal with specific legislation and decision making in government and other settings

4. To deal with problems on a regular basis

5. To implement plans that already have been approved by others.

Status of Group Development

Groups, like individuals, go through several stages of development. As a group forms, each member needs to get to know the others and to develop a sense of ease and comfort. In the process of working together, members experience a diversity of opinion that causes stress, anxiety, and tension in the group.

Tuckerman (1985) outlined four stages of group development:

1. **Forming.** Members deal with the issues of coming together to form groups and learn about each other's talents and resources.

2. **Storming.** Members experience varying degrees of conflict with leadership, tasks, and task management.

3. **Norming.** Individual members resolve conflicts, and the group begins to develop a sense of cohesiveness, norms, and procedures to carry out its activities.

4. **Performing.** The group has established control and works effectively together in pursuit of tasks.

Emotional Patterns of Group Life

Group members experience varying degrees of emotional and psychological swings during the course of group development, all of which affect their productivity and interaction within the group.

Bion (1948), a British psychiatrist, refers to the underlying emotional patterns of group life as "modalities." Among these are the following:

1. Fight-fight modality describes the ways in which group members fight instead of work because of their emotional needs.

2. Flight refers to the ways in which a member runs away or avoids a task.

3. Pairing results when one member joins another to cope with a problem or to increase personal satisfaction.

4. Dependency occurs when individuals seek support from a person they see as stronger than themselves.

The emotional makeup of individual members determines their success in the group. Any unmet need increases the potential for conflicts within the group.

Group Conflicts

Groups often face conflicts as members struggle to deal with varying needs and competing demands and priorities. Thelen (1954) believes that conflicts are inevitable in groups because the larger culture is continually struggling with issues, such as competition versus cooperation, individuality versus conformity, and freedom of expression versus inhibition of feelings. Eubank (1992) identified five ways in which groups deal with conflicts:

1. Eliminating the opposition
2. Subjugating the opposition
3. Forming an alliance to overpower opposition
4. Reaching a compromise with opposition
5. Integrating opposing ideas toward new solutions.

Group Communication

Communication is one of the most important components of group life. Communication takes the form of both verbal and nonverbal articulation of words, thoughts, and feelings. Verbal communication consists of words used to express thoughts or ideas. Nonverbal communications include hand placement, body position, facial expressions, voice tone, touch, and clothes. All communicate something to others. Similarly, the shape of the room; the color of the walls; the type, size, and arrangement of the chairs; and the temperature also communicate and have an impact on behavior in small groups. The patterns of nonverbal communication are deeply rooted in the evolution of human beings. Communication difficulties may result from real or imaginary threats to members of a group and are related to the questions of power and influence.

Models of Group Treatment in Occupational Therapy

Howe and Schwartzberg (1986) have divided treatment groups into the following four categories, some of which may overlap each other:

1. Activity groups are small primary groups in which members perform common activities to learn and maintain occupational performance. The philosophy of activity groups is based on purposeful activity where individual skills are enhanced and positive behavior changes are encouraged. The leader facilitates group interaction by engaging members in structured activities that maximize task performance and foster positive group climate. In selection of activity groups, the leader needs to consider the individual's cognitive, social, emotional, and perceptual-sensory skills.

2. The intrapsychic group's goal is to address the unconscious thoughts and motivations that cause maladaptive behavioral patterns. Intrapsychic groups include therapy groups; projective occupational therapy groups; art therapy groups; and psychodrama groups. The leader helps the members explore and interpret their feelings, beliefs, values, and thoughts.

3. Social system groups help members learn about themselves while participating in common tasks. The members learn about their interpersonal relationships, patterns of communication, and decision making in a group context. The leader helps create a climate that promotes the process. T-groups, laboratory methods groups, and other educational group laboratories are included in social system groups.

4. Growth groups enhance personal growth through the power of the group. The growth group focuses on the needs and inherent potential in every individual. The leader facilitates interaction and learning among members by modeling openness, spontaneity, expression of feelings, and mutual regard.

Contemporary Groups in Occupational Therapy Practice

Duncombe and Howe (1985) surveyed occupational therapists to investigate the scope and nature of group work in their practices. They found the following ten types of groups:

1. **Exercise groups:** Members of the groups engage in physical exercise, such as volleyball, bowling, and ping-pong. These groups are mainly found in rehabilitative centers and schools for the developmentally delayed. The goals of exercise groups are to increase physical ability and facilitate interaction.

2. **Cooking groups:** Individuals in these groups plan, shop, cook, and eat meals. Cooking groups are found primarily in psychiatric and rehabilitative programs.

3. **Activities of daily living groups:** These groups prepare individual members for independent living in the community, as well as teach necessary self-care skills.

4. **Arts and crafts groups:** Group members use arts and crafts for evaluation and treatment of psychosocial disabilities. These groups improve task skills and promote interaction skills.

5. **Task groups:** These groups perform tasks such as planning a picnic, publishing a newspaper, and so forth. They engage in social, recre-ational, and educational activities to facilitate socialization and communication.

6. **Self-expression groups:** These groups engage in activities such as art, music, and self-awareness exercises. The groups' goals are to increase interaction among members and promote individual insight.

7. **Reality-orientation discussion groups:** These groups use topics such as current events, as well as transactional analysis, assertiveness training, and role playing to improve communication and socialization skills.

8. **Sensorimotor and sensory integration groups:** These groups work with children with a wide range of problems, such as learning disabilities, cerebral palsy, developmental disabilities, auditory and visual difficulties, and sensory-integrative disorders. Development of physical abilities and improved sensory integration are the groups' primary goals.

9. **Feeling-oriented discussion groups:** Group members use role playing, poetry, and fantasy for discussion.

10. **Education groups:** These groups provide services that include individuals and their families. The groups provide information on and discussion about issues such as medication and family planning.

In 1993, Duncomb and Howe repeated their survey. The 1993 research revealed an increase in the number of therapists using groups in school systems and nursing homes, while fewer therapists were working in psychiatric facilities. This change from medical-based practice to community-based services potentially redefines the role and scope of occupational therapy.

Focusing on the curative aspects of group therapy, Yalom's (1975) research has identified the following factors that could be applied to occupational therapy:

1. **Instilling hope:** Members with shared problems and health-related concerns do not feel alone. The sense of sharing and interacting instills a sense of hope in members.

2. **Universality:** People who seek help in the group learn that their fears, concerns, and experiences are not necessarily unique to them, but are common to other members as well.

3. **Imparting information:** As a result of group interaction, members have the opportunity to share information about their problems and learn about treatment of specific diseases and dysfunctions.

4. **Altruism:** Membership in therapy groups provides the opportunity to help others. This, in turn, enhances the individual's self-worth and self-esteem.

5. **Corrective recapitulation of the family group:** As a primary group, the therapy group resembles a family group providing a safe environment where members can become aware of and correct their maladaptive behaviors.

6. **Development of socializing techniques:** Therapy groups assist individuals in learning or enhancing their social skills by applying methods such as role playing.

7. **Imitative behavior:** Group members often learn new behaviors from watching each other, especially those who have shared similar experiences with them.

8. **Catharsis:** The expression of feelings and release of tension is a vital part of the healing process.

9. **Existential factors:** Personal concerns regarding isolation, loneliness, helplessness, death, and dying can be shared with the group.

Talking about these issues not only helps members define their attitudes, but also helps them assume responsibility by making some realistic and practical choices.

10. **Cohesiveness:** Group members belong and share their experiences and limitations with others.

11. **Interpersonal learning:** Members of the therapy group learn from their interactions with other members.

Education Groups with Older Adults

Occupational therapy professionals are involved with group and individual education. Education can take the form of teaching about an illness or developing specific techniques, such as energy conservation, joint protection, and independent living skills. Some of the skills that can be addressed with a group approach are assertiveness, problem solving, activity planning, community networking, basic communication, self-esteem, stress management, time management, community networking, and leisure skills. When facilitating education groups, the therapist must keep in mind both educational planning and group dynamics.

Educational planning for older people is frequently overlooked in occupational therapy education programs. Teaching is the final step of the program. The therapist must develop and adjust the topic and the environment to meet the needs of the elderly individuals. Adaptations may include: lighting, noise, the physical layout of the room, the use of visual aids, the number of individuals in the group, time, and so forth. The therapist should be able to break down each step of the skill being taught into the simplest components. For example, a lesson on problem solving may be broken down into the following steps: identifying the problem, generating alternative solutions, hypothesizing the alternative's success, selecting an alternative, executing the problem-solving strategy, and evaluating effectiveness. By breaking each skill down into its specific steps, the therapist is able to assess and facilitate group communication to meet the needs of a specific individual.

Developing a lesson also requires that therapists construct an outline with the strategies they will employ to meet the goal. Generally, the outline includes an introduction of individuals, an introduction of the purpose of the group, a brief description of the topic being discussed, examples of how the topic applies to everyday life, the step-by-step application of the skill (i.e., problem solving using activity analysis), practice with the various skills of the task, and a review of the topic.

Section 2. Team Approach, Case Management, and Consultancy in Geriatric Occupational Therapy

Health care trends have led hospitals and other service agencies to use a team approach to patient care. Occupational therapists have shifted their focus from the patient only, to the patient and the financial stability of institutions (Burke & Cassidy, 1991).

A team approach balances patient-centered care with pressures of diagnostic-related groups and shortening in a patent's allowed length of stay (Erikson & Perkins, 1994). Studies have shown that by using teams, patients decrease their length of stay and, therefore, cost. Erickson & Perkins's (1994) study of the interdisciplinary team approach with hip-and-knee rehabilitation showed that team use resulted in earlier, increased daily living activities, bed mobility, and transfers. In turn, a decrease in patient's overall length of stay was noted.

Nystrom & Evans (1988) identified several advantages to a team approach for both individuals and professionals as follows:

1. Easier access to varied professionals
2. Decrease in duplicated services
3. Easier management of interrelated issues or problems
4. Additional insight into issues
5. Decreased burden on the individual to integrate services
6. Assistance with the decision-making process
7. Increased continuity or carryover between disciplinary interventions.

Conversely, Nystrom and Evans (1988) identified the potential disadvantages to a team approach as follows:

1. Roles can overlap.
2. Team goals may not mesh with individual disciplinary goals.
3. Power struggles may develop within the team.
4. The balance between meeting the geriatric individual's needs versus the institutional needs could give rise to ethical dilemmas.
5. The team approach may interfere with one-to-one relationship.
6. Difficulty may arise over responsibility and decision making among members.
7. The professional may be isolated from disciplinary peers, which could limit his or her professional growth and any needed supervision.

An interdisciplinary team approach can be viewed as having two distinct advantages. First, it provides the individual with easier access to many health care professionals and service providers. Second, it increases the team members' opportunities to develop holistic, cohesive services that foster growth and education. Implementation of a team-care plan will have positive effects on the patient (Crepeau, 1994a). Many of the disadvantages of a team approach revolve around poor interpersonal and group interaction skills that lead to frustration. Occupational therapy professionals' contributions to the team depend on effective communication, cooperation, and collaboration of team members.

Occupational therapy professionals bring a wealth of information regarding the activities of daily living, including self-maintenance tasks; work and productive activities, including purposeful activities for self-development, social contribution, and livelihood;

and play-and-leisure activities, including intrinsically motivating activities for amusement, recreation, spontaneous enjoyment or self-expression (AOTA, 1994c). This holistic view of how an individual's illness is affecting his or her quality of life allows for better understanding and decision making by all members of the team.

The first section of this chapter provided a framework of group models and group dynamics. This section presents (a) the definition of multidisciplinary teams, (b) the definition of the interdisciplinary teams, (c) the occupational therapy assistant and the occupational therapist (COTA-OTR) partnership, and (d) a case study to provide a practical example of a team approach.

Multidisciplinary Teams

A multidisciplinary team is a group of individuals who come from various educational backgrounds and expertise levels. The multidisciplinary team encompasses individuals from different fields, as well as professionals within the same field from different settings. As a result, the multidisciplinary team can be a mix of individuals working within one practice setting (i.e., hospital) to various settings (i.e., hospital versus community agency). Multidisciplinary team members have different goals that focus on their respective disciplines. The purpose of the team is to share information regarding the development and implementation of an individual's comprehensive treatment plan. When executing the plan, each team member works independently of the other professionals. On occasion team members may cotreat; however, during these times, the practitioners' focus remains on their respective goals. Hence, the individual team members are the primary service-delivery agents, not the multidisciplinary team. The multidisciplinary team is often led by the highest ranking individual among all disciplines (Snow, 1988).

An example of multidisciplinary goals for a 75-year-old, right-handed man with left hemiparesis may be to improve left upper-extremity function, strength, and range, through the use of self-care activities (occupational therapy); to improve ambulation abilities through the use of progressive resistive exercises (physical therapy); to monitor vital signs and regulate medication (nursing).

Interdisciplinary Teams

An interdisciplinary team is a group of individuals from different disciplines, who generally work in the same setting. Often within this team are professionals who bring expertise from various areas within their respective fields. Therefore, the team is interested in developing and providing comprehensive services that transcend disciplinary boundaries. An interdisciplinary team could include social workers, occupational therapy professionals, physical therapy professionals, speech-and-language pathologists, doctors, nurses, and a case manager. Even though individuals come from various theoretical and disciplinary backgrounds, they have a collective identity that supersedes each individual disciplinary background (Nystrom & Evans, 1988).

The interdisciplinary team seeks agreement and understanding in working toward a common goal. For example, the goal may be to increase independent living skills at home. Because of the common goal, the team often experiences a cohesive approach to assessment, problem identification, problem solving, and treatment. Generally, the leader of the interdisciplinary team, like the multidisciplinary team, is the highest ranking professional on the team.

In Crepeau's (1994a) study of the team approach, three aspects of a cohesive interdisciplinary team were identified. The three aspects of the interdisciplinary team were called the constructive, ritualistic, and professional images. According to Crepeau, the constructive approach occurs when the team members challenge their knowledge of an illness to come to a consensus regarding a patient's problem. For example, a 62-year-old woman who recently underwent coronary bypass surgery is expected to have difficulties only with upper extremity range and endurance. At the initial assessment, however, the occupational therapist notes that the individual is oriented only to person and is extremely confused. Thus, the team must reexamine its notion of the patient's problem.

The ritualistic component of the team refers to those traditions, procedures, and formats of the team meeting and the hospital. Consistent with Crepeau's (1994b) concept of ritualization, these traditions and customs provide the framework to bind the interdisciplinary team together behind a common goal. Some examples of the ritual component of team meetings might include always beginning the meeting at 3 p.m., followed by discussion of individuals who were recently admitted, discussion of nursing issues, progress in occupational therapy, and so forth.

Finally, the professional image of the team refers to the specific disciplinary knowledge and expertise that each member brings to discussions and treatment planning (Crepeau, 1994a). Collectively, the constructive, ritualistic, and professional aspects of the interdisciplinary team affect goal setting, the development of care plans, and the communication between all professionals and the older adult. The cohesive nature of the team carries over to the interactions between the occupational therapy assistant (COTA) and occupational therapist (OTR).

COTA-OTR Partnership

Much like the interdisciplinary team, the COTA and OTR must act as a cohesive unit. In response to the ever-changing roles between the OTR and the COTA, the American Occupational Therapy Association established a task force to examine how the COTA-OTR relationship is taught in education (Hettinger, 1995). Young and Youngstrom (1995) view the COTA-OTR team as a means to expand available service within the geriatric population. A push to increase the effective and interactive use of the COTA-OTR team exists in the field.

According to the *Guide for Supervision of Occupational Therapy Personnel,* supervision is suggested or required for all occupational therapy personnel, depending on their training and experience level (AOTA, 1994b). The method of supervision is critical to team development. Level of supervision needed should be determined prior to an occupational therapy professional's entry into a system. Much like Crepeau's (1994) professional image component of the interdisciplinary team, the COTA-OTR partnership is based on a reciprocal exchange of ideas, feelings, and perceptions regarding the treatment of elderly individuals. Ultimately, the OTR is responsible for the provision of services (AOTA, 1994a). Standards of Practice for occupational therapy charge the OTR with the responsibility of conducting the initial assessment and developing the appropriate goals and treatment plan. A COTA with experience has valuable information to aid the therapist in developing goals and treatment plans. Following development, a treatment plan is implemented. The delivery of the older adult's individualized treatment plan is conducted either by the COTA or the OTR. Again, varying levels of supervision are necessary depending of the practitioner's level of skill and expertise. Hirama (1994) stated, "one of the strengths of a competent certified occupational therapy assistant is that they can function independently in certain aspects of the occupational therapy intervention process." Similar to the assessment process, the implementation process can be enhanced by keeping communication between the COTA and the OTR open.

The dynamic, interactive process of the COTA-OTR team is an integral part of working with the geriatric population. The team approach transcends the mere use of two sets of hands to become a partnership based on mutual ideas, experiences, feelings, and skills. The case study at the end of this chapter provides the reader with an opportunity to visualize the use of interdisciplinary, multidisciplinary, and COTA-OTR team approaches.

Case Management

Case management has become an integral part of geriatric health care services (Hennessy, 1993). The goal of case management is to increase patient satisfaction with health services while decreasing lengths of stay and cost. This section provides (a) some definitions of case management, (b) an overview of the characteristics of case management, (c) an introduction to a geriatric case management model, (d) a brief review of the types of case management, and (e) a discussion of the relevance of case management to occupational therapy.

DEFINITIONS

Case management can be defined in numerous ways, depending on the

professional's background (Lumadon, 1994) and practice environment. To the hospital, case management involves the connection of inpatient to outpatient services. Social services professionals view case management as incorporating a variety of hospital- and community-based programs. Insurers see case management as a form of cost containment. Hennessy (1993) defines case management as "a mechanism to coordinate the delivery of services intended to prevent or forestall nursing home placement." In Kemper's 1990 study of case-management services, case management is referred to as "the process of assessing needs, acting as an advocate, planning, monitoring, and coordinating services" (Kemper, 1990). In reference to psychiatry and mental health services, Richert & Gibson (1993) state that case management includes advocacy, monitoring of services, analysis of benefits, and individual or family counseling or advice. Young & Youngstrom (1988) define case management in the home-health setting as liaison services that advocate, coordinate, and assist with the acquisition of benefits. Austin & O'Connor (1989) state that case management for the elderly encompasses the coordination of long-term care plans to ensure the most comprehensive set of services to meet the individual's specific needs. Hence, the term case management includes assessment, planning, coordination, advocacy, and monitoring.

Originally, case management referred to the documentation and monitoring of treatment. The term was later adopted by the social services field to signify the coordination of an array of services provided to an individual (Snow, 1988). Traditionally, occupational therapists have not acted as case managers for individuals who are elderly. Often, the role of case manager falls under the auspices of social work or nursing.

ROLES OF THE CASE MANAGER WITH THE OLDER INDIVIDUAL

For the elderly individual, complex health care systems and governmental policy make managing services extremely difficult without the assistance of an effective advocate, family member, or case manager (Snow, 1988). The case manager must be able to negotiate medical and community services concerning reimbursement, eligibility, and availability, while responding in a coordinated and timely fashion. The role of case manager can be too complex for a family member and is often assumed by someone in health or medical services.

Case management includes the following activities (Del Togno-Armanasco, Hopkin, & Harter, 1994; Snow, 1988):

1. Assessing the elderly individual's medical, psychological, and community needs

2. Identifying potential community and medical agencies that would meet the elderly individual's specific needs

3. Negotiating and completing the necessary paperwork in a timely fashion to ensure acceptance into identified programs and agencies

4. Ensuring the implementation of holistic, individualized service that meets the elderly person's needs

5. Reevaluating and reassessing the elderly individual's needs periodically and ensuring they are being met

6. Monitoring and following up with the necessary documentation to maintain service delivery

7. Educating the individual and his or her family about expected community and medical care providers.

The older adult's needs define which roles and characteristics of case management are implemented. For one individual family, education may be the critical part of the service plan, while to another, integration into community programs may be the key to independence. Case management is more than the sum of components; it is the application of a process. With older adults, this process is referred to as the geriatric case management model.

Geriatric Case Management Model

Greenberg, Doth and Austin (1981) identified six stages of geriatric case management models, including the following:

1. Screening

2. Assessment

3. Planning

4. Acquisition

5. Monitoring

6. Reassessment.

The screening phase includes a brief assessment to determine if the individual is eligible and would benefit from case management.

If the individual is deemed eligible, assessment of specific needs is conducted by various professionals. This assessment stage may include nursing, occupational therapy, physical therapy, speech therapy, and so forth.

During the planning stage, the group of professionals, including the case manager, determines the most appropriate and beneficial approach to service delivery for the older individual.

In the acquisition stage the case manager is charged with the responsibility of coordinating and acquiring the services identified by the team. This acquisition often includes establishing formal and informal contracts with various service providers (Austin

& O'Connor, 1989). During the acquisition phase, occupational therapists and other professionals are frequently asked to share their assessments and expertise with potential service providers to ensure effective implementation of services.

After the service plan is in place, case managers are required to maintain communication with providers and the individual to make sure that the services denoted in the team's plan are being carried out (Austin & O'Connor, 1989). This is referred to as the monitoring stage.

The reassessment stage includes follow-up assessments and evaluations to identify the individual's status and to ensure that his or her needs are being met. Reassessments are conducted periodically in accordance with the dates established in the initial service plan.

The geriatric case management model can be conceptualized as a cycle. The reassessments conducted in the final stage can lead to the identification of new needs, requiring the case manager to reenter the screening stage.

The amount of time a case manager or team spends in each area of the geriatric case management model depends on the setting and type of case management being employed. A case manager in a hospital setting is expected to spend less time in the planning and acquisition stages than a case manager in a community-based program. The following section provides a basic framework of the types of case management as they apply to group dynamics and the team approach.

Types of Case Management

Case management can be either an internal or external process. *External case management* refers to situations where the case manager is not em-

ployed by the hospital or service provider. On the one hand, a case manager working for an insurance company would be considered an external case manager. *Internal case management,* on the other hand, denotes that the case manager is an employee of the hospital or service provider. Since occupational therapists deal more with internal case management in the health care system, the remainder of this chapter will be devoted to the internal case management process.

Internal case management is generally divided into four categories. However, to use services with the geriatric population, fluid movement between all four forms of case management is needed (Snow, 1988):

1. *Intradisciplinary intraagency* refers to services provided in one setting by professionals within the same discipline. This is the simplest form of case management because it entails a continuum of service provided by one department or discipline within a single agency. For example, within an acute care facility, a patient is generally assigned to one occupational therapist who is in charge of ensuring that the patient receives all the necessary occupational therapy services. This occupational therapist may work alone or supervise a COTA. However, the occupational therapist assumes responsibility for the occupational therapy provided.

2. *Interdisciplinary intraagency* case management is the coordination of services from various disciplines that are all part of the same agency. Like the previous type, this form of case management occurs within the same setting. However, the responsibility of the case manager is to coordinate services from different disciplines. For example, the case management role of ensuring

appropriate scheduling and the delivery of services within a rehabilitation hospital may be the responsibility of a nurse. This nurse would coordinate the occupational, physical, and speech therapy services. Coordination could take the form of a written schedule posted at the nurses' station or in the chart that allows the therapists involved to see when their sessions are scheduled.

3. *Intradisciplinary interagency* is defined as case management services provided by one discipline in various settings. For example, an occupational therapist providing case management may work primarily with inpatient rehabilitation. Because of the patient's upcoming discharge, however, the occupational therapist or case manager would be involved in the transfer of documentation, referrals, and the initial coordination of outpatient and home therapy.

4. *Interdisciplinary interagency* case management involves services provided by various disciplines in numerous settings. Interdisciplinary interagency case management is most consistent with the previously stated stages and components of case management. Within health care delivery systems, the interdisciplinary interagency type is generally synonymous with case management. In this form, the case manager draws on a variety of interpersonal, group, and management skills to coordinate services for the individual. Like the previous types, the manager must be extremely knowledgeable of the service systems, networks, and community programs that are available to the individual. For example, a social worker at the community geriatric day hospital may act as the case manager and be responsible for ensuring that the patient acquires financial and housing benefits. The case manager would also be interested in making appropriate referrals and coordinating contacts with an outpatient psychiatrist or therapist. While at the day hospital, the case manager would be responsible for completing the appropriate scheduling to ensure the continuity of occupational therapy and nursing. The social worker may encourage involvement in a support group or senior citizens' center, as well as assume the responsibility for reimbursement.

Relevance of Case Management to Occupational Therapy

Because of the occupational therapy professional's focus on a holistic individualized approach, he or she is particularly well suited for the role of case manager. Occupational therapists frequently find themselves filling the role of case manager. Many hospitals have begun providing internal case management in response to increasing demands to contain costs. The current political climate has prompted many hospital administrators and case managers to focus on controlling costs to ensure financial stability. Even if occupational therapists are not acting as case managers, the role has an impact on the team approach as well as the use of occupational therapy services.

As providers of geriatric care, occupational therapists must keep in mind the role of the case manager. Oftentimes, the case manager is the "gatekeeper" to the services the older individual needs. The type of case management used at a facility can affect patient care. As a member of the team or case manager, the occupational therapist is equally responsible for creating a positive team environment based on open communication. By keeping in mind the stages, roles, and types of case management, the occupational therapist has the potential to be the catalyst for the independence of the older adult.

Consultancy

Occupational therapists may find themselves acting as individual, programmatic, or departmental consultants to service providers working with elderly persons. This tendency was first reported by West (1967). According to West, the increase in occupational therapy consultancy was driven by the shift toward preventive services, wellness programs, and the focus on a holistic approach to an individual's illness experience. Consultancy is the process of providing expertise and assistance to individuals to aid in problem solving (Epstein, 1992). Consultancy will continue to escalate with the increase in the number of the nation's elderly and the shortages of occupational therapy practitioners.

Consultants can be found in hospitals, rehabilitation centers, long-term care facilities, skilled nursing facilities, private practice, community programs, outpatient programs, and community mental health facilities (Epstein, 1993). As consultants and team members in diverse settings, therapists may find themselves filling some or all of the following roles (Epstein, 1992; Lewis, 1989):

1. Adviser or facilitator with occupational therapy expertise

2. Evaluator or diagnostician, to identify problems or concerns

3. Trainer, to provide opportunities for others to learn skills

4. Assistant, to help persons developing goals for treatment

5. Educator, to teach the individual, family, and staff about the issues the elderly person is confronting

6. Advocate, to push for benefits in both the health care system and the community

7. Developer, to plan therapeutic programs to be carried out in various settings

8. Collaborator and team member, to work with others in providing geriatric care

9. Informer, to keep various service provider systems informed about appropriate care for the individual

10. Adaptor, to ease the patient into the environment where he or she is currently functioning.

Occupational therapy consultants bring a wealth of information and expertise to the team approach, which is extremely helpful when working with elderly individuals. Crucial to the success of the consultant's interactions is adherence to the general principle of group dynamics and teams. Consultants must keep in mind that they are outsiders to the team and that their information may be viewed as threatening or intrusive by some members. Effective occupational therapy consultants are able to assess team dynamics and assert themselves in a manner that ensures a cohesive team approach. As a result, consultants are afforded the opportunity to impact the lives of elderly individuals positively.

Summary

Occupational therapy professionals rely on a variety of group skills to improve the functional independence and quality of life for older adults. Multidisciplinary and interdisciplinary team approaches provide challenges and opportunities for therapists to apply their knowledge of group dynamics. Consideration of the disciplinary backgrounds, settings, and goals of various professionals is critical to success within a team environment. The constructive, ritualistic, and professional images Crepeau (1994a) lists have implications for understanding and developing a cohesive team. The cohesive team transcends the interdisciplinary and multidisciplinary team to the COTA-OTR partnership. A successful COTA-OTR partnership is based on open communication, feedback, and self-assessment.

On multidisciplinary and interdisciplinary teams, occupational therapy professionals communicate with or fill the roles of case manager or consultant. Working with or as a case manager necessitates an understanding of the roles, types, and stages of case management. The roles of a case manager include assessment, identification of agencies, negotiation of the admission to programs, review, monitoring, documentation, and education. Case management can be either internal or external processes with internal case management placing the highest demands on the occupational therapist's interpersonal and group skills. The types of case management include intradisciplinary intraagency, interdisciplinary intraagency, intradisciplinary interagency, and interdisciplinary interagency. Finally, the stages of case management encompass screening, assessment, acquisition, monitoring, and reassessment.

Consultants bring expertise for program evaluation and development, and advice, training, assistance, and education to the team. Because of limited contact between the consultant and the team, an understanding of the dynamics of positive interaction is essential.

The next section provides an understanding of the potential ethnic and cultural dilemmas that arise when using teams.

Section 3. Cross-Cultural Considerations in Occupational Therapy

The United States is known as the land of racial and ethnic diversity. Millions of people from many different cultures and nationalities have settled here. Some observers have characterized the United States as a "melting pot," meaning that people of various backgrounds adopt the dominant American culture as their own. Immigrants who were committed to becoming "real Americans" assimilated as they accepted the United States as their new home.

Other immigrants chose to confine themselves to their own cultural enclaves and interacted mainly with their own cultural groups. These groups did not assimilate as well into the American mainstream. As these racial and ethnic enclaves grew stronger, "cultural pluralism" emerged. This term implies mutual respect and understanding between majority and minority groups. It means creating an awareness of, and developing appreciation for, this diversity and the issues and problems associated with diversity.

Occupational therapists often work with people of different cultural backgrounds. While this may be challenging, the rewards are great. An awareness of mainstream American characteristics may provide some helpful insights. Consider the following norms:

1. **Scientific orientation:** People in the United States have accepted scientific methods and scientific reasoning as the way to understand the physical world. Everything in the physical world has a logical, understandable basis. Many other cultures to not accept scientific explanations and are likely to be guided in their behavior by mysticism, tradition, or other nonanalytical approaches.

2. **Control of nature and the environment:** Americans think of nature as something that can be altered, conquered, and controlled for their comfort and use. In contrast, many cultures accept nature as a force greater than people and something to which people must adapt rather than something they can change or control.

3. **Progress and change:** Most people accept change as an inevitable part of life. Some cultures tend to look to their traditions as a guide to the future. Americans are more likely to make decisions based on the anticipated future and view change and material progress as good and desirable. Achievement, positive change, and progress are all seen as the result of effort, hard work, and the control of self and nature.

4. **Materialism:** Americans look for measurable results to determine if they are making progress. They often stress material comfort and convenience. Other cultures emphasize spiritual and aesthetic values and inner experience rather than any material result. Americans tend to judge other cultures by their material progress—how many telephones, how many cars—and neglect other values.

5. **Individualism:** American culture emphasizes the individual as the one responsible for making the decisions that affect his or her life. In other cultures, decisions may be made by family, clan, group, or recognized authority figure. Americans

think that individuals should take control of their own lives, develop their own potentialities, use their own initiative to move ahead. Less emphasis is on consultation within the family. Americans desire personal success, to progress socially and economically, and they are not likely to consider social and cultural factors as barriers to their ability to get ahead. As a result, American life is very competitive. Achievement is a dominant motivation in life. Royeen (1979) found that non-American students in U.S. universities viewed individualism as an extension of materialism. American individualism may be synonymous with "selfishness" in non-Western cultures.

6. **Moralistic orientation:** Americans want to win other people over to their way of thinking and, like other cultures, are likely to judge other societies in terms of their own. Because the United States has had great economic and technological progress, Americans often think that others should follow their example and adopt their ways of doing things.

7. **Time orientation:** Americans generally are very time conscious, treating time as a resource to be used to best advantage. People who do not make good use of their time are considered lazy and unmotivated. Americans often have difficulty with people from cultures where time is less important and people are not expected to arrive at a set hour.

8. **Doing rather than being:** Because Americans are motivated by a desire to achieve, they tend to distinguish between work and play. As a result, Americans may have difficulty functioning in cultures where a social relationship must be cultivated before business is transacted. When Americans play, they are more relaxed, time is less important, and there is more emphasis on social relationships. Even at play, however, Americans may strive to improve their ability, take courses or classes to develop their skills and interests, or otherwise "make good use" of their time.

9. **Egalitarianism:** Although many social economies and educational differences exist in the United States, a theme of equality runs through social relationships. Americans tend not to recognize social differences in dealing with other people. As a result, they do not often show deference to people of greater wealth, greater age, or higher social status. Visitors from other cultures who hold high positions sometimes feel that Americans do not treat them with proper respect and deference, and Americans find it very confusing to shift from high to low status as the situation requires. Americans call each other by their first names much sooner and more often than people in most other cultures. People in American society are seen as having equal rights, equal social obligations, and equal opportunities to develop their own potentials.

10. **Prejudice:** People in all societies have rigid, preconceived ideas and feelings about people, customs, religions, and values.

11. **Role of women:** Although women have not yet achieved full societal equality, they play a much more public and visible role in the United States and have much more responsibility and authority than in many other countries. What other cultures may consider the "proper" role for women is considered by American standards to reflect sexism.

12. **Problem solving:** Because Americans feel that they can control their own environment, problems are to be analyzed, discussed, and solved in the short term. In other societies, people can think of a national problem in terms of a hundred or more years. Americans may have difficulty accepting that some problems may not have solutions. This direct approach to problems sometimes leads to confrontations that are shocking to people from other cultures. When faced with a problem, Americans like to get the facts, talk to the necessary people, and make some plan of action. If the problem is interpersonal, Americans are likely to talk directly to the other person to discuss the issue, to confront the situation as directly as possible. If the two people involved cannot solve the problem, they may turn to a third person, such as a counselor or advisor or mutual friend, but they still try to confront the situation directly. This direct approach may insult or offend people from other cultures, because they have a more indirect approach to interpersonal relationships.

13. **Friendliness and openness:** To Americans, a friend can be anyone from a mere acquaintance to a lifelong intimate, and the friend's company may depend on a particular activity. Americans have friendships that revolve around work, political activities, volunteer activities, special interests, and so forth, and those friends rarely if ever meet each other. An American may have many friendships on a casual, occasional basis but only a very few deep, meaningful friendships that last a lifetime. People from other cultures sometimes see these casual relationships as a reluctance to become deeply involved with others. When a person in another culture would turn to a friend for help or support, an American may turn to a professional. Americans live in a mobile society and tend to move frequently in their lifetime. They therefore can form friendships much more easily and with less stress than people in many other cultures.

14. **Hygiene:** Americans are generally obsessed with personal hygiene, and it is not unusual for them to bathe every day, change their clothes every day, and wash their hair several times a week. Americans tend to find natural body odors unpleasant; and, in addition to frequent bathing, they use perfume, cologne, and underarm deodorant on a regular basis. In contrast, people of other cultural backgrounds may not have the same level of personal hygiene.

The aforementioned mainstream American values are based on Royeen's (1979) research as well as personal experiences with many internationals in the past two decades.

Cross-Cultural Suggestions for Occupational Therapists

Occupational therapists often have the opportunity to work with groups from different cultural backgrounds. The following suggestions may help in developing a better understanding and sensitivity toward clients:

1. **Listen and observe:** Remember that culturally different clients operate with different rules, norms, and cues. Listening and observing carefully will help put communications in the proper context. Americans are very frank and direct in their communication, while others tend to be more indirect, especially

when confronted with negative or sensitive information. Also, the client may not show his or her disagreement because he or she does not want to cause loss of "face."

2. **Ask questions:** Don't assume knowledge or understanding of a client's communication. Clients are happy to explain specifics of cultural features that may interfere with effective working relationships. Before entering a working relationship, occupational therapists should ask patients to educate them about the patient's cultural background. By doing so, occupational therapists not only learn something valuable about the patient, but they also establish a positive interpersonal relationship. However, remember not to invade a patient's privacy.

3. **Be nonjudgmental:** Keep in mind that as occupational therapists learn about different cultures, they should be careful not to judge or compare value systems.

4. **Try to empathize:** Remember that as helping professionals, occupational therapists should put themselves in their patient's place and look at the situation from his or her perspective. The same situation may have different cultural interpretations.

5. **Keep a sense or humor:** Know that occupational therapists may make mistakes as they explore and learn more about a patient. Maintain a sense of humor about mistakes. Often, the client will respond with friendliness as they see the human side of their therapist.

6. **Anticipate some anxiety and frustration:** Know that learning the intricacies of the client's cultural background can cause anxiety and frustration for both the client and the occupational therapist. Anxiety and frustration are a normal part of the experience.

7. **Do not stereotype patients:** Treat patients as unique human beings. Don't lose sight of the patient as an individual with a distinct personality.

Ethical Considerations

According to Fletcher (1991), "the ethical foundations of respect for personal choice is grounded [sic] in the principle of autonomy." Occupational therapists are constantly confronted with the personal choices of the older adult, the family, or other health professionals. These choices can give rise to ethical dilemmas. Crabtree (1994) states that choices become ethical dilemmas when there are equal levels of moral support for two or more options. The *Occupational Therapy Code of Ethics* refers to the profession's respect for personal choice (AOTA, 1994c). Principle two of the code of ethics states that "Occupational therapy personnel shall respect the rights of the recipients of their services.... Occupational therapy personnel shall respect the individual's right to refuse professional services." The core concepts for occupational therapy are altruism, equality, freedom, justice, dignity, and truth (AOTA, 1994a).

When working with patients, occupational therapists must respect personal choice. Every individual brings different cultural and personal experiences to the therapeutic relationship. Even though occupational therapists are the "experts" in the use of everyday occupations to promote health and wellness, the choice of whether to use the therapists' assistance should rest solely on the patient.

In Clark, Corcoran, & Gitlin's (1995) study on therapeutic relationships with family caregivers, the need

A Personal View of Aging

Matin Royeen

About 25 years ago, as I was preparing to leave Afghanistan in pursuit of higher education in the United States, a friend of the family, an older man in his 50s, gave me the following advice: "Go to the United States and enjoy your life as a young man, because youth is very much valued and admired in the American culture. But when you get old, come back to this primitive land where your age is respected, your wisdom sought, and your family and friends will take care of you."

This personal note echoes the feelings and sentiments of many people in other cultures toward their elderly. The following points will provide some understanding of how other cultural groups view their elderly:

1. A great number of people of various cultural backgrounds live in extended families. Thus, grandparents, children, and grandchildren live together in the same household. The elderly are treated with respect, and every member of the family feels an obligation to take care of them.

2. The elderly have made their contribution to society by raising their children, who in turn are making their own contributions. Children are expected to take care of their parents during old age. It brings a great deal of shame to their families if they do not take care of the aged.

3. Aging is viewed with respect. The elderly are the source of knowledge and wisdom, and the younger generation treasures their guidance and advice. At a gathering, the elderly have the best seats, are listened to when they talk, and are served first.

4. The elderly enjoy a very positive self-image and self-esteem. Furthermore, their sense of security and confidence is always enhanced when they feel that there is always somebody in the family who will care for them.

to "empower care givers so that they can shape occupational therapy recommendations to match life-styles, values, and goals ranked high." The need to empower family caregivers also applies to older individuals. The occupational therapist is obligated to provide choices that match an individual's cultural experiences. Understanding of the cultural background of the individual not only reduces the ethical dilemmas but also enables the therapist to make sound decisions toward a meaningful and comprehensive treatment plan for the older adult.

Case Study

TEAM APPROACH AT A LONG-TERM-CARE FACILITY

S is an occupational therapist working at a long-term-care facility in a small southern city. Her facility provides occupational therapy, physical therapy, respiratory therapy, speech therapy, social work, nursing, physician services, and recreational therapy. The "rehabilitation team" provides speech therapy, occupational therapy, and physical therapy and meets regularly. The facility also has weekly "medical team" meetings. The medical team provides physician services, nursing, rehabilitation team services, social work, recreational therapy, and administration. S is often asked to participate in meetings with various members of the medical team. All of the occupational therapists meet biweekly to discuss issues. Finally, S works with K, a COTA. S and K together have 26 years of experience and have seen that each brings valuable experiences to team meetings.

Upon admission of an individual, the rehabilitation team conducts an initial screening to determine what services to provide. They begin by examining and reviewing the information already gathered from prior medical history. After the initial screening, S speaks with the person, his or her family, and any other professionals working with the patient to determine the patient's strengths, needs, and goals. Subsequently, S and K, along with other professionals meet with the medical team. During the team meeting, S educates other professionals about the potential benefits of occupational therapy services, advocating for the individual to receive services to improve function and independence. Given a referral from the physician, S begins an assessment of the person's strengths and needs. From her findings, and working with the client and family, S develops a treatment plan for occupational therapy. K and S provide occupational therapy to the individual. At other medical team meetings, the professionals gather to review individualized care plans for each patient. Oftentimes, the overall goal of the care plan is to improve someone's independence with activities of daily living (ADL). In speech therapy, this often translates to goals for eating. Physical therapy's focus may be on ambulation and standing tolerance. Increasing ADL independence for occupational therapy may become goals for dressing and transfers.

Over the years, S and K have gotten used to overlap between members of the rehabilitation team. For example, with one patient, upper-extremity dressing may encompass measures of sitting tolerance; for another, treatment for sitting tolerance may be specifically conducted and billed for by physical therapy. With the pressure of managed care, the administration is drilling the message "two services can't bill for the same thing." This can be a point of frustration for K and S. However, a collaborative care plan or patient-focused care plan would eliminate frustration or confusion. Each team member would know what others were doing based on the specific needs of the client.

S and K rely on their interpersonal and group skills. K and S often remind each other that every person on the team is there to help the patient. The knowledge of each person and the respective disciplines are valuable and needed. Although the differing roles and dynamics within each team can create ethical dilemmas for S and K, they have seen how the team approach has positive impacts on the older patient's quality of life.

Within health care systems, the use of case managers is having an impact on team work. Hospital case managers—whether social workers, nurses, or occupational therapists—are being asked to facilitate the acquisition and delivery of services to older adults. Considering this case study, a case manager would have an impact on the rehabilitation team, medical team, and the COTA-OTR partnership. Hence, an understanding of the case manager's role is essential for the development of a cohesive team approach.

Appendix.
Sample Outline for an Educational Group on Time Management

I. Outline the purpose of the group (i.e., to practice or develop skills for daily living) and the topic of the day (i.e., time management).

II. Discuss the necessity of talking about daily activities?

III. Define wellness as adequate life balance. What areas are we balancing with time management? (Some ideas that might come up in discussion: leisure, play, self-care, eating, sleeping, crafts or hobbies, work, volunteering, senior center activities, medication or doctors, family or friends, household cleaning or maintenance.)

IV. Describe how time management helps balance life, feeling good about self, stress, etc.

V. Outline how to use the calendars to complete weekly activities.

VI. Invite individuals to discuss their use of time and balance of activities.

VII. Identify one enjoyable activity that could be added to a weekly calendar.

VIII. Identify one thing to do today or tonight to better manage time.

IX. Relate the importance of time management to feeling better and encourage everyone to complete the activities they identified.

References

American Occupational Therapy Association. (1994a). Standards of practice for occupational therapy. *American Journal of Occupational Therapy, 48*(11), 1039–1043.

American Occupational Therapy Association. (1994b). Guide for supervision of occupational therapy personnel. *American Journal of Occupational Therapy, 48*(11), 1045–1046.

American Occupational Therapy Association. (1994c). Occupational therapy code of ethics. *American Journal of Occupational Therapy, 48*(11), 1037–1038.

American Occupational Therapy Association. (1994d). Uniform terminology for occupational therapy (3rd ed.). *American Journal of Occupational Therapy, 48*(11), 1047–1054.

American Occupational Therapy Association. (1993). Occupational therapy roles. *American Journal of Occupational Therapy, 47(12)*, 1087–1099.

Austin, C. D., & O'Connor, K. (1989). Case management: Components and program contexts. In M. D. Peterson & D. L. White (Eds.), *Health Care of the Elderly: An Information Sourcebook.* Newbury Park, CA: Sage Publications.

Barker, L., & Cegula, D., Kibler, R., & Wahlers, K. (1979). *Group process: An introduction to small group communication.* Princeton, NJ: Prentice Hall.

Bene, K. D., & Sheats, P. (1978). Functional roles of group members. In L. P. Bradford (Ed.), *Group Development* (2nd ed.). La Jolla, CA: University Associates.

Bion, W. R. (1948). Experiences in group. *Human Relations, 1,* 314–329, 487–496.

Burke, J. P., & Cassidy, J. C. (1991). Disparity between reimbursement-driven practice and humanistic values of occupational therapy. *American Journal of Occupational Therapy, 45*(2), 173–176.

Cartheart, R. S., & Samosar, L. A. (1970). *Small group communication: A reader* (3rd ed.). Dubuque, IA: W. M. C. Brown.

Clark, C. A., Corcoran, M., & Gitlin. (1995). An exploratory study of how occupational therapists develop therapeutic relationships with family caregivers. *American Journal of Occupational Therapy, 49*(7), 587–594.

Crabtree, J. L. (1991). Ethical dilemmas and the older adults. In J. M. Kiernat (Ed.), *Occupational Therapy and the Older Adult.* Gaithersburg, MD: Aspen.

Crepeau, E. B. (1994a). Three images of interdisciplinary team. *American Journal of Occupational Therapy, 48*(8), 717–722.

Crepeau, E. B. (1994b). Rituals. In C. B. Royeen (Ed.), *The Practice of the Future: Putting Occupation Back Into Therapy.* Bethesda, MD: American Occupational Therapy Association.

Del Togno-Armanasco, V., Hopkin, L. A., Harter, S. (1995). How case management really works. *American Journal of Nursing, 95*(5), 24I–24K.

Duncomb, L., & Howe, M. C. (1994). Group treatment, goals, tasks, and economic implications. Manuscript submitted for publication.

Duncomb, L., & Howe, M. C. (1985). Group work in occupational therapy: A survey of practice. *American Journal of Occupational Therapy. 39*(3), 163–170.

Epstein, C. F. (1992). Consultation: Communicating and facilitation. In J. Bair, & M. Gray (Eds.), *The occupational therapy manager* (Rev. ed.). Rockville, MD: American Occupational Therapy Association.

Erickson, B., & Perkins, M. (1994). Interdisciplinary team approach in the rehabilitation of hip and knee arthroplasties. *American Journal of Occupational Therapy, 48*(5). 439–441.

Eubank, K. B. (1972). Study of some factors that affect communication in natural groups. Unpublished doctoral dissertation. U. of Oklahoma.

Fletcher, J. C. (1991). When the patient refuses treatment. In J. C. Fletcher (Ed.), *Introduction to clinical ethics.* Charlottesville, VA: Center for Biomedical Ethics.

Hasselkus, B. R., & Kiernat, J. M. (1991). Education for Empowerment, In J. J. Kiernat (Ed.), *Occupational therapy and the older adult.* Gaithersburg, MD: Aspen.

Hennessy, H. C. (1993). Modeling case management decision-making in a consolidated long-term-care program. *Gerontologist, 33*(3), 333–341.

Hettinger, J. (1995) A question of roles. *OT Week, 9*(39), 18–19.

Hirama, H. (1994). Should certified occupational therapy assistants provide occupational therapy services independently? *American Journal of Occupational Therapy, 48*(9), 840–843.

Howe, M. C., & Schwartzberg, L. A. (1986). *A Functional Approach to Group Work in Occupational Therapy.* Philadelphia: J. B. Lippincott.

Kemper, K. (1990). Case management agency systems of administering long-term care: Evidence from the channeling demonstration. *Gerontologist, 30*(6), 817–824.

Lewis, S. C. (1989). Occupational therapy and the elderly. *Elder care in* occupational therapy. (pp. 223–338). Thorofare, NJ: SLACK.

Lippitt, R. (1940). An experimental study of the effect of democratic and authoritarian group atmospheres. *University of Iowa Studies, 16*(3), 43–198.

Luft, J. (1970). *Group process: An introduction to group dynamics.* Palo Alto, CA: National Press Books.

Lumsdon, K. (1995). Beyond four walls: Case management evolves into management of a continuum of care. *Hospital & Health Networks, 68*(5), 44–46.

Mills, T. M. (1967). *The Sociology of Small Groups.* Princeton, NJ: Prentice-Hall.

Nystrom, E. P., & Evans, L. S. (1988) The interdisciplinary team approach. In L. J. Davis, & M. Kirkland (Eds.), *The role of occupational therapy with the elderly* (pp. 351–357). Rockville, MD: American Occupational Therapy Association.

Richert, G. Z., & Bigson, D. (1993). Practice settings. In H. L. Hopkins & H. D. Smith (Eds.), *Willard and Spackman's occupational therapy* (8th ed.) (pp. 546–551). Rockville, MD: American Occupational Therapy Association.

Rosenfeld, L. D. (1973). *Human Interaction in the Small Group Setting.* Columbus, OH: Charles E. Merrill.

Royeen, M. A. (1979). *Perceptions and attitudes of Taiwanese and Indian students towards the United States and the American people.* Unpublished doctoral dissertation. University of Cincinnati.

Snow, T. L. (1988), Case management. In L. J. Davis & M. Kirkland (Eds.). *The role of occupational therapy with the elderly* (pp. 359–365). Rockville, MD: American Occupational Therapy Association.

Thelen, H. (1954). *Dynamics of groups at work.* Chicago: University of Chicago Press.

Tuckerman, B. W. (1965). Developmental sequencing in small groups, *Psychological Bulletin, 63,* 384–399.

West, W. L. (1967). The occupational therapist's changing responsibility to the community. *American Journal of Occupational Therapy, 21,* 312–316.

Yalom, I. D. (1975) *The theory and practice of group psychotherapy.* New York, NY: Basic Books.

Young, J. A., & Youngstrom, M. J. (1995). Teamwork, personal issues, and supervision in the home health setting. *Guidelines for occupational therapy practice in home health* (pp. 15–20). Bethesda, MD: American Occupational Therapy Association.

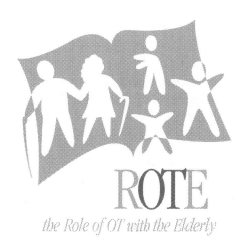

ROTE

the Role of OT with the Elderly

Health Education in Occupational Therapy

Elizabeth Walker Peterson, MPH, OTR/L

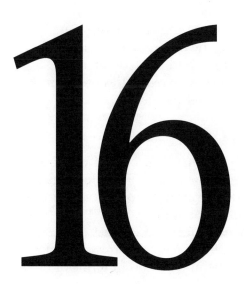

Abstract

No two individuals age in exactly the same way. The quality of life for older adults is influenced by a myriad factors. As health care professionals, occupational therapy practitioners focus on well-being rather than on physical health alone (Bonder, 1994). Health education provides a context in which the biological, social, and psychological influences on wellness are appreciated and incorporated into treatment planning.

Health education is defined as "any combination of learning experiences designed to facilitate voluntary adaptations of behavior conducive to health" (Green, Krueter, Deeds, & Partridge, 1980). Behavioral change, with the intention of promoting health and achieving functional outcomes, is often the goal of occupational therapy interventions. Such change, however, is a complex phenomenon. Behavior includes activities, as well as psychological, physiologic, and social responses (Padilla & Bulcavage, 1991).

Health education philosophy is compatible with general principles of occupational therapy intervention because the client is recognized as the agent for change. With regard to the role of the patient in health education, "the defining characteristic of health education ... is the voluntary participation of the consumer in determining his or her own health practices" (Green et al., 1980). This perspective appropriately acknowledges that occupational performance is heavily influenced by internal motivation. Health education principles also embrace the view that individuals must be understood as a part of the larger system that includes family, society, and culture. Health education principles described later in this chapter will reflect intervention efforts directed broadly to include not only the family, but also other external influences that impact on adjustment to disability.

This chapter provides an overview of health education principles and builds a case for the practicality of using concepts, which were borrowed from health education literature, in clinical practice. Toward that end, this chapter reviews five learning theories from which health education principles are drawn. Just as occupational therapy practitioners use activities that are meaningful and relevant to their clients, they design educational experiences with their clients' unique learning needs in mind. Therefore, the second component of this chapter examines factors that influence learning. These factors are described in the context of the PRECEDE model (Predisposing, Reinforcing, and Enabling Causes in Education Diagnosis and Evaluation) (Green, 1980). The PRECEDE model incorporates learning theories to provide a framework for health education planning. Two models that complement the PRECEDE framework, the Diffusion of Innovations Model (Rogers, 1983), and the Health Belief Model (Rosenstock, 1990), will be described in the second component of this chapter.

The third component of this chapter describes the steps involved in program planning for health education. These steps include development of learning objectives and learning experiences, and evaluation. Special attention to educational strategies that facilitate development of cognitive, affective, and psychomotor skills are presented. The chapter concludes with two case studies describing occupational therapy interventions with an older adult who is experiencing physical disability. The occupational therapy interventions presented incorporate a variety of teaching strategies drawn from the principles emphasized in this chapter.

Learning Theories

Learning theories provide a conceptual framework for the learning process. In the context of learning, such frameworks provide "the source of decisions relative to the selection of learning objectives, choice of learning experiences and teaching strategies, and determination of expectations in the performance of students and teachers" (Reilly & Oerman, 1992). Occupational therapy practitioners use a variety of elements from several theories when developing learning experiences, depending upon the client's preferences and the phase and objectives of the learning experience. In fact, the National Cancer Institute recommends integrating theoretical frameworks in health education programs for behavior change (Office of Cancer Communications: National Cancer Institute).

Inherent in any learning theory are assumptions about human behavior. The assumptions underlying theoretical approaches should be recognized to determine the best possible match between the different approaches to teaching and desired outcomes. Overviews of five theories of learning will be presented next.

HUMANISM

The humanist theory of learning is concerned with individual feelings and experiences leading to personal growth and fulfillment (McKenna, 1995). The humanist theory recognizes that individual differences and stressors can and should be understood in terms of how individuals view themselves and the world around them—the phenomenological approach. The phenomenological theory of Carl Rogers, with its emphasis on human experience, is highly compatible with occupational therapy philosophy. Rogers emphasized that humans are inherently positive beings whose personal growth naturally moves toward a healthy self-actualizing personality.

Because individuals react to the environment as they perceive it, a humanistic health care practitioner strives to understand his or her client and to communicate that understanding. The therapeutic process, in which clients share their feelings and are unconditionally cared for, is highly important in humanist theory. Being empathetic and demonstrating unconditional positive regard creates a climate in which the patient lowers his or her defenses and becomes open to new ideas. (Jourard, 1961). The role of a therapist as an educator becomes one of facilitating a client's personal growth. However, the client is ultimately responsible for his or her own behavior.

Rogers (1983) believes that significant, meaningful, experiential learning has five qualities:

1. It involves the whole person—both feelings and cognitive processes.

2. It is self-initiated with a sense of discovery coming from within.

3. It is pervasive and makes a difference in the behavior, attitudes, and perhaps the personality of the learner.

4. It is evaluated by the learner, who knows if his or her needs have been met or not.

5. The essence of it has meaning.

Occupational therapy practitioners and clients involved in humanistic learning experiences may find the process frustrating at times. On the occupational therapy practitioner's part, consideration of treatment options must be postponed until the patient's perspective is appreciated. Clients who are given the responsibility for learning may be frustrated at not being given "answers" or "prescriptions." Health education interventions that operationalize humanistic principles take time. The benefits of health education programs that embrace patients' world views and emotional responses to given situations, or both, are frequently cited in the medical literature. (McCord & Brandenburg, 1995; Abraham & Sheeran, 1994; Anderson, 1986; Ferrell, Ferrell, Abril, & Tran, 1994).

McCord and Brandenberg's use of open-ended interviews with patients who had diabetes is an excellent example of how humanistic principles can be used to understand and facilitate adaptive behavior change (McCord & Brandenberg, 1995). In those interviews, patients discussed their experiences with diabetes and explored the effect that diabetes had on their lives. Information gleaned from those discussions suggests that the concept of "compliance" may need to be modified, with the focus shifting away from physician-mandated prescriptions and proscriptions and toward assisting the patients in finding the "it works for me" approach (McCord & Brandenberg, 1995).

COGNITIVISM

Learning theories based on cognitivism are designed to allow the learner to organize and integrate what is perceived into an overall pattern or gestalt. This type of learning cannot be observed directly as it involves a change in the individual's ability to respond (Woolfolk & Nicolich, 1980). The learner is viewed as an active participant in a process that involves seeking out information, problem solving, and drawing from past experience to gain understanding. Cognitive learning may be viewed as either inductive or deductive. Inductive learning involves using specifics to discover general concepts. Deductive learning involves moving from a general understanding of concepts to understanding specifics. Regardless of the type of learning that is occurring, the educator must (a) understand the learner's level of understanding, and (b) develop carefully sequenced learning experiences that build on previous knowledge. Hilgard and Bower (1966) describe six principles emphasized in cognitive theory:

1. The perceptual features of the problem given the learner are important conditions of learning—figure-ground relations, directional signs, sequence, organic interrelatedness. Hence, a learning problem should be so structured and presented that the essential features are open to the inspection of the learner.

2. The organization of knowledge should be an essential concern of the teacher or educational planner so that the direction from simple to complex is not from arbitrary, meaningless parts to meaningful wholes, but instead from simplified wholes to more complete wholes.

3. Learning is culturally relative, and both the wider culture and the subculture to which a learner belongs may affect a learner's ability to learn.

4. Cognitive feedback confirms correct knowledge and corrects faulty learning. The learner tries something and then accepts or rejects what he or she does on the basis of its consequences.

5. Goal setting by the learner is important as motivation for learning, and successes and failures

determine how a learner sets future goals.

6. Divergent thinking, which leads to inventive problem solving or the creation of novel and valued products, is to be nurtured along with convergent thinking, which leads logically to correct answers.

To illustrate how occupational therapy practitioners educate their clients, consider the challenge of teaching total hip precautions to older adults who have undergone hip replacements. If an educational session on the structure and function of the hip joint is linked to the problem that brought the client to the hospital (such as osteoarthritis) and to activities of daily living rather than to unrelated examples, the patient will perceive the anatomy and physiology, the discussed condition, and the effect on the patient as a whole. The occupational therapy practitioner leading that session would give special attention to how the information is presented to foster learning. Outlines might be used to help the patient identify relevant information. The occupational therapy practitioner could also ask the patient to paraphrase information presented to make sure that the patient is successfully distinguishing critical details.

BEHAVIORISM

A behavioral approach to teaching concentrates on eliminating faulty behaviors and acquiring new, more adaptive ones (Chiodo, Rosenstein, & Clark, 1986). According to Milholland and Forisha (1972), the behaviorist orientation considers a person to be a passive organism governed by stimuli supplied by the external environment. Individuals can be manipulated; that is, their behavior can be controlled by manipulating environmental stimuli. Learning is evidenced by changes in behavior that are both observable and measurable. Specific behaviors are expected to increase when paired with positive reinforcers and decrease when paired with negative reinforcers (Brown, 1961; Geis et al., 1965; Whaley & Malott, 1971). Positive reinforcers, to be effective, must be both desirable and realistically available (Chiodo et al., 1986). From a behavioral standpoint, complex behavior is shaped through the process of successive approximation, in which each action that leads to a more complicated behavior is reinforced. Whether immediate or delayed, the reward serves to motivate and reinforce the actions or behavior itself, not the goal of the behavior, since the goal may be long term and not readily observable to be patient (Chiodo et al., 1986). Reinforcement can be given on a fixed or variable basis. On the one hand, feedback after every trial does not seem to affect learning and retention of information (Winstein & Schmidt, 1990). On the other hand, feedback at random intervals may assist with processing relevant information and developing error-detection abilities (Poole, 1995).

The occupational therapy practitioner's role in behavioral practice is to shape behavior by controlling environmental conditions. This learning concept is much different from the approach used in cognitive and humanistic therapies in which cognitive and motivational influences on learning and behavior are recognized.

Given that behavioral approaches stem from a limited view of the human organism, to be compatible with the nature of occupational therapy practice, the use of behavioral strategies, such as positive reinforcement and successive approximation, is appropriate only after time is spent exploring the following:

1. A patient's level of awareness

2. His or her concern about the issue at hand

3. His or her understanding of the benefits of behavior change.

When the client and occupational therapy practitioner agree on a course of action, behavioral strategies such as positive reinforcement and successive approximation can be used to promote behavior change.

For example, if a patient decides that learning T'ai Chi is important to improve balance, flexibility, and conditioning, the patient could decide to reward himself or herself for each step made toward accomplishing that goal. Such steps might include exploring community resources, purchasing a tape, or attending a class. The "rewards" could be items that further support the patient in exercising (new sneakers), or they may be unrelated to the goal (a special lunch with friends).

SELF-EFFICACY THEORY

Self-efficacy concerns one's judgment of personal ability to execute specific behaviors that can control events (Bandura, 1986). Self-efficacy is behavior-specific and future oriented. That is, it pertains to an individual's ability to use particular cognitive or behavioral skills in a specific situation at some point in the future. Self-efficacy is a cognitive process. According to Bandura (1989), individuals who have a high sense of self-efficacy visualize success scenarios that provide positive guides for performance, and they cognitively rehearse good solutions to potential problems. Those who judge themselves as inefficacious are more inclined to visualize failure scenarios and to dwell on how things will go wrong. Such inefficacious thinking weakens motivation and undermines performance. Numerous studies have shown that cognitive simulations in which individuals visualize themselves executing activities skillfully enhance subsequent performance. (Bandura,

1986; Corbin, 1972; Feltz & Landers, 1983, Kazdin, 1978). Improvement in self-efficacy is therefore associated with positive changes in behavior and health status (Bandura, 1986; O'Leary 1985; Strecher et al., 1986; Lorig et al., 1989).

Occupational therapy practitioners working with older adults may find self-efficacy theory useful given that older adults (a) may be subject to stereotyping that can undermine their confidence in their ability to maintain and improve their quality of life, and (b) often experience major life changes in rapid succession. These changes, such as disability, retirement, relocation, and loss of friends or spouses, place demands on interpersonal skills as new relationships often need to be developed in order to maintain personal well being (Bandura, 1989). Perceived social inefficacy increases the vulnerability of older people to stress and depression, both directly and indirectly, by impeding development of social supports that serve to buffer against life stressors. (Holahan & Holahan, 1987a, 1987b).

Gonzalez et al. (1990) identified four empirically verified ways to enhance self-efficacy: skills mastery, modeling, reinterpretation of signs and symptoms, and persuasion.

Mastering of Skills

Skills mastery is probably the most powerful way to enhance self-efficacy. Because skills mastery is generally achieved by first breaking skills into small, manageable tasks, activity analysis is highly relevant to social learning theory. Acquisition and mastery of skills are further facilitated by identifying goals, sequencing subtasks, and practicing the skill in simulated and, later, natural environments.

Modeling

Modeling can be achieved through mutual patient aid, health education media (books, videos, pamphlets), and support groups. Creation of patient networks, in fact, has been shown to improve the likelihood that a target group or individual will adopt a new behavior. To be effective, models should appear to be realistic figures for self-comparison.

Reinterpretation of Signs and Symptoms

What people believe about their disease or how they interpret symptoms can affect their ability to deal with it (Bandura, 1982). For example, individuals with early Chronic Obstructive Pulmonary Disease may interpret shortness of breath as a normal result of physical exertion, and an indicator of personal, physical inefficacy, instead of using it as a cue to use a compensatory technique such as pursed-lip breathing. Reinterpreting such mislabeled symptoms may therefore improve an individual's sense of self-efficacy and foster adaptive behaviors.

Persuasion

Persuasion can help people believe it is possible for them to develop the skills needed to meet a given situational demand (Bandura, 1982). Using feedback from peers in small groups and developing short-term, realistic goals are two ways health educators can incorporate persuasion into practice.

ANDRAGOGY

Malcolm Knowles's theory of adult learning and motivation is known as andragogy. The andragogical model, which differs from pedagogy, the learning model for children, incorporates principles from various other theories and assumptions about adult learners.

Specifically, andragogy is based on the following assumptions about adults (Knowles, 1984):

1. **The need to know:** Adults need to know why they need to learn.

2. **The learner's self-concept:** Adults believe they are responsible for their own decisions, for their own lives. Because adult learners see themselves as capable of self-direction, they will resist learning experiences in which this capability is not acknowledged.

3. **The role of the learner's experience:** Adults bring both more and a different quality of experience to learning situations than youths do. Because of this broad range of experience, adult education emphasizes individualization of teaching and learning experience. In addition, the collective experiences of a group of adult learners can be used as resources for learning.

4. **Readiness to learn:** Adults come ready to learn those things they need to know and are able to do so to cope effectively with their real-life situations.

5. **Orientation to learning:** Adults are life centered (or task centered or problem centered) in their orientation to learning. Adults are motivated to devote energy to learning something to the extent that they perceive that it will help them perform tasks or deal with problems that they confront in their life situations.

6. **Motivation:** While adults are responsive to some external motivations (better jobs, promotions, or higher salaries), the most potent motivations are internal pressures (desire for job satisfaction, self-esteem, or quality of life).

By contrasting andragogy and pedagogy, the unique characteristics of andragogy and the model's relevance to health education become evident. Table 16–1 provides this comparison.

As a process model, andragogy is concerned with providing procedures and resources for helping learners acquire information and skills. These procedures are outlined as follows (Knowles, 1984):

1. Establishing a climate conducive to learning that is characterized by physical comfort, mutual trust and respect, mutual helpfulness, freedom of expression, and acceptance of differences

2. Creating a mechanism for mutual planning

3. Diagnosing the needs for learning

4. Formulating program objectives that will meet those needs

5. Designing a pattern of learning experiences

6. Conducting the learning experiences with suitable techniques and materials

7. Evaluating the learning outcomes and rediagnosing learning needs.

Knowles strongly advocated the use of contract learning to reconcile the needs and expectations of an organization, profession, or society and the individual's internal needs and interests (Knowles, 1984). An example of a typical learning contract is depicted in figure 16–1.

Occupational therapy practitioners working with older adults can use principles of adult learning in a number of ways. Consider the task of training a group of older adults about rheumatoid arthritis and joint protection techniques. The group can decide if, how, and when topics related to the subject should be covered. In an adult learning environment, the experience of the group members would be as important (if not more important) than the occupational therapist's knowledge.

Table 16–1. A Comparison of the Assumptions and Designs of Pedagogy and Andragogy

Assumptions			Design Elements		
	Pedagogy	Andragogy		Pedagogy	Andragogy
Self-concept	Dependency	Increasing self-directedness	**Climate**	Authority-oriented Formal Competitive	Mutuality Respectful Collaborative Informal
Experience	Of little worth	Learners are a rich resource for learning	**Planning**	By teacher	Mechanism for mutual planning
Readiness	Biological development social pressure	Developmental tasks of social roles	**Diagnosis of need**	By teacher	Mutual self-diagnosis
Time perspective	Postponed application	Immediacy of application	**Formulation of objectives**	By teacher	Mutual negotiation
Orientation to learning	Subject centered	Problem centered	**Design**	Logic of the subject matter Content units	Sequenced in terms of readiness Problem units
			Activities	Transmittal techniques	Experiential techniques (inquiry)
			Evaluation	By teacher	Mutual rediagnosis of needs Mutual measurement of program

Source: *The Adult Learner: A Neglected Species,* by Malcolm Knowles, copyright 1990 by Gulf Publishing Company, Houston, TX. Reprinted with permission. All rights reserved.

Figure 16–1. A typical learning contract form.

Learning Contract for:			
Name _____			
Activity _____			
Learning Objectives	Learning Resources and Strategies	Evidence of Accomplishment of Objectives	Criteria and Means for Validating Evidence

Influences on Learning and Behavior Change

Green et al. (1980) describe predisposing, enabling, and reinforcing factors as follows (see table 16–2):

- Predisposing factors are factors antecedent to behavior that provide the rationale or motivation for the behavior. Included are knowledge, attitudes, beliefs and values.

- Enabling factors are factors antecedent to the behavior that allow a motivation or aspiration to be realized. Included are personal skills and resources as well as community resources.

- Reinforcing factors are factor subsequent to behavior that provide the continuing reward, incentive, or punishment for a behavior and contribute to its persistence or extinction. Included are social as well as physical benefits, and tangible as well as imagined or vicarious rewards. Use of the classification by Green et al., of enabling, reinforcing, and predisposing influences on health behavior will now be explored.

PREDISPOSING FACTORS

Knowledge

"Knowledge is a necessary, but not sufficient, factor in changing health behavior" (Green et al., 1980). Sensorimotor and cognitive changes associated with aging, which could limit learning abilities, are presented in chapter 4.

The Diffusion of Innovation Model describes a process of disseminating (or diffusing) information about *new* products or ideas by transferring information from the resource to the user. It also describes how different communication patterns influence decisions

Table 16–2. Three Categories of Factors Contributing to Health Behavior

Predisposing Factors:
Knowledge
Beliefs
Values
(Selected demographic variables)

Enabling Factors:
Availability of health resources
Accessibility of health resources
Community or government priority and commitment to health
Health-related skills

Reinforcing Factors:
Family
Peers
Teachers
Employer
Health providers

Source: From *Health Education Planning,* by Green et al. Copyright 1980 by Mayfield Publishing Company. Reprinted with permission.

regarding whether to adopt and maintain a new, innovative behavior. According to the model's developer, E. R. Rogers (1983), diffusion is the process by which an innovation is communicated through certain channels over time among members of a social system.

The diffusion model suggests that the adaptation of a new health-related behavior is less a function of individual assessment of the scientific merit of adaptation, and more a function of who in one's environment adopts the innovation. According to Rogers (1983), "people depend mainly upon a subjective evaluation of an innovation that is conveyed to them from individuals like themselves who have previously adopted the innovation."

The heart of the diffusion process, then, lies in the modeling and imitation of near peers who serve as social

models. Rogers (1983) emphasizes that more-effective communication occurs when two individuals are homophilous. The personal, social, and language differences between health care professionals, who are the sources for information, and clients, the information recipients, can be barriers to effective communication.

According to Rogers (1983), mass-media channels are more effective in creating *knowledge* of innovations, whereas interpersonal channels, optimally between near peers, are more effective in forming and changing *attitudes* toward a new idea and in influencing the decision to adopt or reject a new idea or behavior.

The Diffusion of Innovation Model supports the use of individual or group role models in treatment. Obviously, communication between near peers is not always possible. Consequently,

Table 16-2. Health Belief Model Components That Provoke Health Behavior

Component	Definition	Example
Perceived susceptibility	Subjective probability of becoming ill	High risk
Perceived severity	Subjective evaluations of the negative consequences of illness	Mastectomy, death
Perceived benefits	Beliefs about efficacy and feasibility of health behavior	Healthy diet, exercise
Perceived barriers	Negative aspects of health behavior	Cost
Self-efficacy	Belief in one's ability to perform behavior that obtains good outcomes	Confidence about competence in self-care

Source: Data from Rosenstock (1990) and Bandura (1977a, 1977b); compiled by Padilla and Bulcavage (1991).

occupational therapy practitioners must be diligent in using language and presentation styles that are most comparable to a client's learning preferences.

Beliefs

Beliefs are influenced by personal experiences, culture, and society. The Health Belief Model (Hochbaum, 1958; Rosenstock, 1966) suggests that the adaptation of health-related behaviors is a function of an individual's perception of the severity of the health problem, personal susceptibility to the problem, efficacy of the behavior to be adopted, and barriers to adaptation. Components of the Health Belief Model are shown in table 16–3.

The Health Belief Model reminds us that when information suggesting the need for a behavior change is presented to a client, that individual is weighing the costs and benefits of the suggestion. Changing behavior requires

decision making. The decision-making process involves consideration of several factors including (but not limited to) financial variables, social implications, and personal preferences. For example, an older adult woman who is deciding whether or not to use a walker may consider herself to be at high risk for a fall, which could result in a serious injury (hip fractures). However, she may believe that using the walker could actually increase her fall risk because she is not confident of her ability to use the walker properly. The client may be concerned that if she uses the walker, she will be perceived as being "disabled" or dependent on others. The client might know that using the walker will make her family happy, but the perceived benefit would not be enough to motivate her to use the walker consistently, given the presence of the barriers described.

Exploring a client's beliefs during that decision-making process enables the client and occupational therapy practitioner to work together to identify health and self-care practices that are compatible with the patient's lifestyle and culture. By including self-efficacy as a factor that influences health behavior, the Health Belief Model emphasizes that the client is the agent for change. Although the Diffusion of Innovations Model suggests that the heart of the diffusion process is in the modeling of peers, the Health Belief Model suggests a kind of individual level of analysis of costs and benefits (Peterson & Howland, 1995). Interestingly, research suggests that interventions that combine variables from the two models are more effective than interventions that incorporate a single perspective (Peterson & Howland, 1995).

Values

Whether explicitly stated or implicitly suggested by decisions and actions, patients' values influence their interactions with health care practitioners. For example, an older adult client who highly values autonomy, free will, and self-sufficiency may have difficulty accepting the role of "patient" if he or she associates that role with dependence and vulnerability. Treatment can be enhanced by

- Recognizing values held by clients
- Developing treatment plans that do not conflict with clients' values.

Attitudes

According to Green et al. (1980), "an attitude is a rather constant feeling that is directed toward an object (be it a person, an action, or an idea); and inherent in the structure of an attitude is evaluation, a good-bad dimension." As predisposing factors, attitudes also influence the degree to which a patient is motivated to make a behavior change.

ENABLING FACTORS

Without necessary skills or resources, even a highly motivated client may fail to take recommended actions to manage his or her illness. By evaluating performance components, occupational therapy practitioners typically have a good appreciation for the actual skill level of a client and can consider those enabling factors when developing treatment plans. However, inadequate financing, transportation, physical space, or equipment may hinder a client's ability to apply skills learned in therapy (such as work simplification or joint protection), despite a desire to do so. Consideration of resources is important throughout the treatment process, but it is critical prior to a client's discharge into the community. Occupational therapy practitioners must ask clients or family members about resources available, or not available, to them in their home and community.

Occupational therapy practitioners can help ensure that a client will be supported in his or her home environment by telling clients and their families about available, community-based services. Health education is an ongoing process, as a client's physical, social, and emotional needs will change over time. Therefore, informal communications between occupational therapy practitioners and their clients after discharge can help facilitate a client's ability to access new community services as needs arise.

REINFORCING FACTORS

Health education is an ongoing process during which a client encounters numerous decision points. A fundamental principle of human behavior is that rewarded behavior tends to be repeated. Positive reinforcing factors, such as decreased pain, improved self-care abilities, or increased enjoyment from socialization, can positively influence a client's decision to stay with a given treatment program. Other powerful forms of reinforcement include social supports.

Social support is a significant predictor of successful adaptation to disability. One means of increasing social support is to involve the patient's immediate and extended family (Belgrave, 1991). Turner and Alston (1994) describe the following predictors that serve as a foundation for their model of the family's role in psychosocial adaptation:

- Individuals develop in a systemic context as opposed to an isolated environment. The family system provides the most salient social milieu. Moreover, the family will be affected by the member with a disability and will be active participants in the adjustment to the disability.

- All individuals and families display some measure of competence, and any effective intervention will involve acknowledging and using those competencies.

- Ethnicity and culture strongly influence family process. As a result, family rules and family patterns, along with family context, must be considered when providing therapy to an individual who is disabled.

- Time plays a significant role in the adjustment process. The effects of a disability are both dynamic and developmental. The impact of the disability is neither nonstatic nor isolated but operates reciprocally and reverberates over time.

Several authors have asserted that psychosocial adaptation to disability is influenced by race and culture (Atkins, 1986; Alston & Turner, 1994; Wright, 1988). Therefore, in addition to the general assumptions listed above, occupational therapy practitioners must consider how a family's race and culture will impact the rehabilitation process. For example, kinship bonds, role flexibility, strong religious orientation, and strong work and education ethics have been identified as characteristics common to black families (Hill, 1971; Hines & Boyd-Franklin, 1952). These strengths can be incorporated into the therapeutic process to facilitate an African-American individual's psychosocial adaptation to physical disability (Turner & Alston, 1994). Narrative interviewing can be used by occupational therapy practitioners to begin to understand influences on behavior that include both the social and cultural contexts in which a client lives.

Program Planning for Health Education

The first step in changing behavior is to identify its causes. If the causes of patient behavior can be understood, health professionals can intervene with the most appropriate combination of patient education, training, resource development, support, and rewards to influence the factors that predispose, enable, or reinforce the behavior (Bartlett, 1983). An intervention linked to diagnosed problems among these factors has the greatest chance of success (Bruhn, 1983). Assessment of older adults is described in detail in chapter 11 of this manual. Health education is a dynamic process that includes assessment and reassessment. As the PRECEDE model reminds us, a variety of factors interact and change over time to influence health behavior of the older adult.

Developing Learning Objectives

The process of developing learning objectives is a mutual effort between the occupational therapist and the client. Findings from the assessment process will guide the occupational therapist and the client in selecting and prioritizing learning objectives. Learning is commonly categorized into three domains. These domains of learning were identified by Bloom and include *cognitive* behaviors, or behaviors that relate to knowledge and information; *affective behaviors,* which relate to values and attitudes; and *psychomotor behaviors,* which relate to the ability to perform tasks or skills (Bloom, 1956).

Psychomotor goals are given the most attention in practice. This is because, in occupational therapy, documentation of evaluation results must include long-term functional goals that reflect the changes to occur by the end of an intervention (AOTA, 1995). These functional changes, as psychomotor behaviors, are observable and measurable. Although occupational therapy practitioners are required to write goals that reflect changes in behavior or skills, the affective and cognitive aspects of learning that predispose or motivate clients to make positive changes in health behavior should not be minimized.

PRINCIPLES OF BEHAVIOR CHANGE AND HEALTH EDUCATION

General Considerations

Green and Frankish (1994) describe several principles of behavior change and health education that help occupational therapists design education programs. These principles, although described by Green and Frankish in the context of an asthma-prevention program, are relevant to any health education program. The following principles reflect the common elements from the theories of learning and behavior change that were described earlier in this chapter. (Green & Frankish, 1994, pp. 219S–222S):

- **Principle of hierarchy:** States that there is a natural order in the sequence of factors influencing behavior.

- **Principle of cumulative learning:** States that experiences must be planned in a sequence that takes into account the patient's prior learning experiences and the concurrent incidental learning experiences or opportunities to which patients may be exposed.

- **Principle of participation:** States that changes in behavior will be greater if patients have identified their own needs for change and have actively selected the methods or approaches that they believe will enable them to change.

- **Principle of situational specificity:** States that there is nothing inherently superior or inferior about any method of intervention or patient education, but that the effectiveness and efficiency of any program will depend on the circumstances and the characteristics of the patient or the change agent, i.e., physician, nurse educator.

- **Principle of multiple methods:** States that comprehensive behavior change programs should employ different methods or components in consideration of the interaction of person-specific and situation-specific factors.

- **Principle of individualization:** Individualization or tailoring of patient education interventions applies the principles of participation, situational specificity, and cumulative learning in producing interventions that are both patient- and situation-relevant.

- **Principle of relevance:** States that the more relevant the contents and methods used are to the patient's circumstances and interests, the more likely the learning and behavior process is to be successful.

- **Principle of feedback:** States that provision of feedback allows the patient to adapt both the learning process and the resultant behavioral responses to his or her own situation and pace.

- **Principle of reinforcement:** States that behavior that is rewarded tends to be repeated.

- **Principle of facilitation:** Involves the degree to which an intervention provides the means for patients to take action or reduces the barriers to action.

SPECIAL CONSIDERATION FOR OLDER ADULTS

Effective communication is essential to all health education efforts. Special consideration must be given to the physical and psychological needs of older adults during all communications, whether written or verbal. These considerations are clearly outlined in chapter 11.

Educational Strategies

An overview of strategies for teaching in the cognitive, affective, and psychomotor domains is presented here. Strategies for teaching cognitive and affective skills are presented first, as they underlie behavioral skills.

COGNITIVE SKILL DEVELOPMENT

Concept learning and decision making are two important skills encompassed in the cognitive domain. With respect to teaching concepts, individual instruction of older adults as opposed to group lecture is preferred for several reasons. First, presentation of general concepts is often the first step in an educational process. In the first phases of treatment, establishment of rapport between the health professional and client is critical. Clients who perceive health professionals as helpful and genuinely concerned about their well being are more likely to return for future teaching. Second, a clear understanding of basic concepts, such as joint protection or energy conservation, is the basis for future teaching. Occupational therapy practitioners must be assured that a basic understanding of information relevant to future teaching has occurred. Third, individual instruction allows the occupational therapy practitioner to better attend to the special learning needs of the older adult learner (i.e., consideration of sensory changes). Fourth, although understanding of concepts can be enhanced by pointing out relevant characteristics of the concept and by using examples, the subject presented will often be brand new to the client. Individual instruction provided in a supportive, relaxing climate will invite older adult learners to ask questions as needed.

Cognitive skill development occurs along a hierarchical continuum that is made up of six major domains: knowledge, comprehension, application, analysis, synthesis, and evaluation (Bloom, 1956). Once the occupational therapist is assured that clients are familiar with basic concepts, group activities can be used to improve the level of understanding on a particular subject.

Audiovisual aids, such as slide-tape programs or video cassettes, are helpful in supplementing and reinforcing the concepts presented via individual or group instruction. Occupational therapy practitioners must make themselves available to clients for questioning during or after an audiovisual presentation. Likewise, printed materials are useful resources. However, special attention must be given to the reading level and print size of the material.

Problem solving is a process beginning with identification of a problem and proceeding through gathering data, general solutions, and evaluating the solutions chosen (Reilly & Oermann, 1992). Written assignments, such as keeping a diary to monitor problem situations and problem-solving skills, however, may be foreign to older adults who have not had prior experience with such activities. Computer-assisted instruction may encounter similar difficulties. Simulations and role-play activities are alternatives for promoting problem-solving skills. Group exercises often provide valuable opportunities for peer feedback.

AFFECTIVE SKILL DEVELOPMENT

Clients open to exploring their own values, beliefs, and attitudes will gain a better appreciation of how these affective, predisposing factors influence decision making and behaviors. Research shows that optimal performance requires not only the necessary skills but also adaptive self-conceptions (Bandura, 1989). Those who have lower confidence and those who believe they have little control over outcomes show poorer performance (Barry, West, & Dennehey, 1989; Hertzog, Dixon, & Hulsch, 1990; Lachman, Steinberg, & Trotter, 1987). Whether they are accurate or not, negative self-conceptions can have

far-reaching effects. Negative self-conceptions include being dependent on others, avoiding physical exercise, remaining isolated and homebound, seeking unneeded medical attention, being over-reliant on medications, and experiencing anxiety and decreased motivation to engage in activities (Bandura, 1989; Lachman, 1991). Because many older persons hold maladaptive views about their activities and potential for improvement, the success of an intervention depends on promoting adaptive beliefs in conjunction with teaching specific skills. Negative self-conceptions in older adults can be changed using cognitive restructuring techniques (Lachman et al., 1992; Rodin, 1983).

Cognitive restructuring interventions are designed to educate individuals about their self-conceptions and promote more realistic and adaptive views. Cognitive restructuring was heavily used in an intervention developed by the Roybal Center for Applied Gerontology, located at the New England Research Institute in Watertown, Massachusetts. (The Roybal Center was under a grant from the National Institutes on Aging of the National Institutes of Health.) The Roybal Center developed the intervention with the goal of changing attitudes and self-conceptions to reduce fear of falling. In that intervention, the cognitive restructuring component consisted of three elements:

1. **Education about adaptive and maladaptive conceptions:** Education about adaptive and maladaptive conceptions can take place through discussion (group or individual) or through videotapes in which contrasting coping styles are modeled. When educating older adults about adaptive and maladaptive conceptions, discussing the implications of mal-

adaptive conceptions on quality of life may be helpful.

2. **Promotion of adaptive conceptions:** This is best accomplished through group discussion in which examples of data illustrating the credibility of adaptive perspectives are presented. Faulty assumptions and erroneous beliefs that underlie concerns must be considered in a supportive atmosphere. In addition, older adult learners can generate personal examples demonstrating the advantages of taking control and increasing confidence in many areas of their lives.

3. **Self-instructional training to implement adaptive conceptions:** Older adults can learn to identify their own cognitions related to adaptive or maladaptive views. Therapists can help clients recognize "strategy-relevant" versus "strategy-interfering" thoughts during conversations occurring in treatment. Older adults may be asked to write down negative thoughts in a log and try to formulate positive statements to counter the fears.

A growing body of evidence suggests that peer relationships are a rich potential source of support in old age. (Blau, 1973; Arling, 1976; Wood & Robertson, 1978; Johnson, 1983). Supportive groups provide a safe place where older adults can share and compare beliefs and attitudes that can significantly impact on their quality of life.

PSYCHOMOTOR SKILL DEVELOPMENT

Activities that are primarily movement and that emphasize overt physical response bear the label *psychomotor* (Singer, 1975). The performance of transfers, self-care activities, and biomechanically based treatment techniques, such as scar massage or active range-of-motion exercises, are all examples of psychomotor skills that may be learned in therapy. Occupational therapy practitioners teaching these skills are concerned not only with the outcome of the motor skills but also the *process* that eventually leads to the designed outcome. Optimally, skill in psychomotor performance progresses from imitation to naturalization, in which a task is accomplished with a high degree of coordination and speed and the sequence of actions is automatic. Skills identified as being priorities in treatment can be taught as either discrete behaviors (individually distinctive behaviors that stand alone) or chained behaviors (a routine or skill involving a sequence of discrete behaviors) (Snell, 1994). Naylor and Briggs (1961) suggest that practice of discrete behaviors, *part practice*, is more effective in skills that are highly complex and have low organization (few individual components in the task.) *Whole practice* is more effective and highly organized, with increased component interaction. Singer (1975) poses questions to be answered in relation to the complexity criteria of a skill:

1. How difficult does the learner perceive the task to be?

2. How many things does the learner have to think about or remember from previous related experiences?

3. To what extent is it possible to forget the task over time? Does the skill pose a challenge for the learner to remember it?

Some psychomotor skills may be approached from a problem-solving methodology. Clients able to explore alternative methods to achieve psychomotor goals should be encouraged to do so as long as the alternative process does not compromise safety or undermine future learning. Regardless of how a skill is taught, the goal of the learning experience is for the client to gain insight into the total process by understanding how steps are related and integrated. Motor-skill learning requires practice, optimally under natural conditions, to generalize learning. Practice typically follows a demonstration of the desired skill. Demonstration can be provided by other clients who have learned the targeted skill, by models on videotapes, or by therapists. Use of peer models allows clients to appraise their capabilities through social comparison with their age mates. By maintaining or improving their relative standing among age mates, older adults can preserve their sense of self-efficacy in the face of changing capabilities (Frey & Ruble, 1989).

Evaluation

Throughout this chapter, thought has been given to developing effective health education programs. The quality or effectiveness of a given intervention can be assessed at four different levels:

- Formative evaluation
- Process evaluation
- Impact evaluation
- Outcome evaluation.

The evaluation methods used will depend upon the level of evaluation called for in a given situation.

A *formative evaluation* provides information used during the beginning stages of a program. Such an evaluation is not concerned with outcomes, but rather the development, design, and improvement of an intervention. An increasingly popular component of the formative evaluation is the *focus-group interview,* which is a qualitative approach to learning about the feelings, ideas and perceptions of population subgroups (Walker & Howland, 1992). Information gleaned from focus-group interviews can stimulate new ideas for treatment plans that address the specific needs of a particular client population.

Process evaluations are used after an intervention has been developed and involve documenting the actual implementation of a program. Formative evaluation assesses whether specific elements such as facilities, staff space, or services are being provided or are established according to the given program plan (Windsor, Baranowski, Clark, & Cutter, 1984). Process evaluations describe what was done for a patient or group of patients and how well it was done. Data from process evaluations can be used to justify fiscal expenditures to insurers and health care managers and to establish provider competency. Most continuous quality improvement (CQI) programs involve some type of process evaluation. Monitoring program use, analyzing participant surveys, pretesting materials developed for a particular program, and observing clients involved in educational experiences are all examples of process evaluation methods.

The third level of evaluation is *impact evaluation.* Impact evaluations assess intermediate variables in a causal chain. Take for example the following logic:

Knowledge → Attitudes → Behavior Change → Reduction of Incidence of a Problem

This model says that knowledge leads to changes in attitudes, that changes in attitudes lead to changes in behavior, and that changes in behavior lead to a reduction in the problems of interest. Impact evaluation measures changes in knowledge, attitudes, and behaviors (Howland, 1993).

To determine whether observed cognitive, attitudinal, or behavioral changes can be attributed to a specific program or intervention, more sophisticated research methods must be used. These methods will be discussed in the context of outcome evaluation.

Outcome evaluation assesses changes or improvement in morbidity, mortality, or other health-status indicator for a specified group of people (Windsor et al., 1984). Attributing an observed impact or outcome to a specific intervention implies a causal relationship between the dependent variable (outcome, behavior, attitude or condition), and the independent variable (the specific program implemented). Alternative explanations for an observed, significant impact have to be ruled out (Cook & Campbell, 1983). A randomized, controlled trial is the most effective research design for comparing alternative programs, educational or otherwise. Random assignment and subsequent establishment of the comparability of two groups is the best way to ensure that the groups to be compared will be as similar as possible in every respect, so that differences observed during the trial can be attributed to the interventions themselves, rather than to pre-existing differences between members of the group. Impact and outcome evaluation research is typically not a part of the evaluation of independent hospital programs due to their complexity. However, an understanding of the hierarchy of research design will enable occupational therapy practitioners to interpret observations with more accuracy.

Summary

Health education involves the use of a variety of teaching strategies to facilitate voluntary behavior changes that are conducive to health. In the first component of this chapter, five theories of learning, from which health education principles are drawn, were described. The PRECEDE model was presented in the second component of this chapter as a framework for examining factors that influence behavior change. As described by the PRECEDE model, predisposing factors affecting learner readiness and motivation, and enabling factors in the form of skills, are important intrinsic influences on health behavior. External influences on behavior include resource availability and reinforcing factors. Reinforcing factors include not only the perceived benefits of a given program but also the social supports. Occupational therapy practitioners must elicit a client's story to identify and understand the predisposing, enabling, and reinforcing factors operating. Failure to do so can result in miscommunications and unrealistic treatment planning. In addition, patients who perceive that their needs are not understood or appreciated may be less likely to use services offered by health care providers in the future.

The third component of this chapter described the steps involved in program planning for health education. Health education has been presented as encompassing cognitive, affective, and psychomotor learning. Teaching strategies designed to foster development of cognitive, affective, and psychomotor skills were discussed with the recognition that the educational techniques used vary depending on the goal of the learning experience. Finally, this chapter discussed ways in which health education programs can be evaluated to help occupational therapy practitioners monitor the quality and effectiveness of the health education interventions they use in practice.

Activities

1. Consider your own education in occupational therapy. Name two cognitive, two affective, and two psychomotor skills that you have learned during your studies.
2. Review Case Study 1. Describe the following:
   - One strategy used by Ms. Jon that used principles from humanism
   - One strategy that used principles from cognitivism
   - One strategy that used principles from behaviorism.
3. Review Case Study 2. Describe the following:
   - One strategy used by Mr. T or Ms. V that used principles from self-efficacy theory
   - One strategy that used principles from adult learning theory.

Review Questions

1. Why are health education principles compatible with principles that guide occupational therapy practice?
2. Identify and describe the basic tenets of five learning theories that have contributed to the development of the PRECEDE model of health education.
3. Compare the assumptions and designs of pedagogy and andragogy.
4. Describe predisposing, enabling, and reinforcing factors that contribute to behavior change in older adults.
5. Describe and contrast the cognitive, affective, and psychomotor domains of learning.
6. Describe and contrast formative evaluation, process evaluation, impact evaluation, and outcome evaluation.

Case Studies ══

CASE STUDY 1

Mrs. W is an 81-year-old woman who sustained a right Colle's fracture after a fall at home. One month after the injury, Mrs. W was diagnosed with reflex sympathetic dystrophy (RSD) and referred to occupational therapy. Mrs. W's occupational therapy practitioner, Ms. Jon, began the first treatment session by asking about Mrs. W's experiences over the past month. Ms. Jon listened carefully to Mrs. W and began to understand how Mrs. W's injury and subsequent diagnosis of RSD had left her feeling frustrated, saddened and "unlike herself." Ms. Jon learned that Mrs. W had given up her role as volunteer in a community hospital and was feeling ineffective in her roles as wife, grandmother, and artist. Ms. Jon commented to Mrs. W that her injury appeared to represent a loss of independence that Mrs. W had been fighting for in the face of the osteoarthritis that affected her knees and limited her standing tolerance. Mrs. W verified this observation and began to explore further the impact the wrist fracture had had on her and her family. She realized that since the fall her social outlets had been limited as had her ability to cook and take care of herself. Mrs. W stated that she did not want to risk further injury by walking with crowds of people in a mall or reaching for pots and pans in the kitchen. Further, Mrs. W described how she had become more dependent on her husband, daughter, and grandchildren. Mrs. W realized that she also expected her physician and occupational therapist, as "experts" to "fix" her right hand. Mrs. W was surprised to acknowledge this shift in her thinking since she thought of herself as typically self-reliant with a strong work ethic. Mrs. W subsequently began to acknowledge that she had the most responsibility for her rehabilitation, but her family and health care team could be valuable resources for her.

As Ms. Jon listened, she became more and more aware of how Mrs. W's family was an important source of support to her. Ms. Jon wondered why Mrs. W's family had not been coming with her into the clinic during therapy, since at least one of Mrs. W's family members typically drove her to the hospital where the clinic was located. When asked about this, it was clear that Mrs. W's family thought that the presence of family members would be a distraction during therapy. Because Mrs. W was eager to have her family sit in, an invitation to be a part of occupational therapy was extended to the family. From that point, at least one family member accompanied her to therapy. Mrs. W's family became invaluable to the rehabilitation process, since they provided ideas to help Mrs. W manage her daily tasks. Ms. Jon was sure to express her gratitude for the family's contributions. Ms. Jon was also impressed at how the family adapted to support Mrs. W and still got the family's work done. For example, Mrs. W's grandchildren took on new responsibilities for laundry and cooking, although Mrs. W was encouraged to help as she was able.

Over the course of the first month in therapy, Ms. Jon provided Mrs. W and her family with information about RSD and treatment options available. Charts and texts were used to show how RSD develops and why specific interventions are recommended. Ms. Jon encouraged Mrs. W and her family to gather information on RSD and gave them suggestions regarding how to access that information. Pros and cons of different treatment approaches were discussed. Ms. Jon, who believed that learning occurs deductively, presented general information on subjects she felt were critical to therapy, such as stellate ganglion blocks and problems associated with disuse of an extremity. She added to Mrs. W's knowledge base over subsequent sessions by using nontechnical language to describe what she considered to be subordinate content. This subordinate content included information on basic anatomy and the circulatory system. Specific skills such as active exercise programs and retrograde massage were practiced in the clinic and at home where the family set time aside to help Mrs. W as needed. Mrs. W was also encouraged to teach other clients the skills she had learned as opportunities arose. Throughout treatment, Ms. Jon was careful to listen to how the time and effort spent toward rehabilitation were affecting Mrs. W and her household. During their conversations, Mrs. W was encouraged to reflect on her own personal strengths, such as concern for others and a sense of humor, that had enabled her to overcome previous difficulties in her life. Mrs. W recognized that her own self-determination would be an essential element to her recovery, which was taking longer than she had expected.

Armed with information from her occupational therapy practitioner and physician, Mrs. W began a series of stellate ganglion block injections. Mrs. W and Ms. Jon jointly developed a home program that consisted of a progression of at-home activities that could be carried out after the injections. Ms. Jon developed a chart upon which Mrs. W could document the daily completion of her home program. Mrs. W treated herself to the purchase of new canvases and paints (which she used to exercise her right hand) as a reward for each of the weeks in which she completed the designated tasks. Mrs. W became dedicated to her rehabilitation program. Her accomplishments, seen as a work in progress, became a source of encouragement for other outpatients in the clinic.

CASE STUDY 2

The treatment strategies described in this case study were drawn from an intervention offered through the Edward R. Roybal Center for Research in Applied Gerontology, located at the New England Research Institute in Watertown, Massachusetts.

Mrs. M is an 81-year-old woman with a history of osteoarthritis, who has been receiving occupational therapy as an outpatient since she was diagnosed with reflex sympathetic dystrophy (RSD) 5 months ago. The RSD developed after Mrs. M sustained a Colle's fracture during a fall. Mrs. M lives with her very supportive family. She values her roles as wife, mother, grandmother, and artist. In the course of treatment, Mrs. M's therapist, Mr. T, recognized that Mrs. M's fear of falling was limiting her willingness to socialize and resume her previous household responsibilities. This concern about falling was assessed by Mr. T after direct and indirect questioning and through observation. For example, Mr. T asked Mrs. M directly if there were things she would like to do but did not do because she was afraid of falling. Although Mrs. M denied she was "afraid" of falling, she did indicate that she felt she was being "sensible" in avoiding activities like walking on sidewalks when possible. Mr. T inquired about Mrs. M's level of confidence in performing daily activities, ranging from getting up from a chair to climbing stairs and getting into and out of the bathtub. Mrs. M reported that she was dressing and bathing herself but stated that she often asked her granddaughter to stand by when she was getting into the bathtub "just in case."

Mr. T's concern about Mrs. M's apparent fear of falling was supported by Ms. V, the COTA working in the clinic. Ms. V observed Mrs. M's hesitancy toward walking in hospital corridors and noted that getting to and from the clinic was an effort for Mrs. M, both physically and mentally, despite the assistance of family members.

To address this fear of falling, Mrs. M, Mr. T, and Ms. V took the following steps:

1. Mr. T informed other members of Mrs. M's health care team of Mrs. M's concerns and encouraged the team members to raise the issue of falls with her in a context that was relevant to their disciplines. Mr. T encouraged the team to approach the issue as a "concern" or "worry" about falls instead of as a "fear" of falling since the word "fear" might not accurately represent Mrs. M's feelings.

2. Mr. T initiated conversations about falls with Mrs. M, since she had difficulty bringing up the subject. During those conversations, Mr. T was careful to listen to the beliefs that were driving her concerns. For example, Mrs. M believed that falls were an "inevitable" consequence of old age. Mr. T gently pointed out that the view that falls were not preventable was not supported by his own clinical experience or research. In subsequent conversations, Mr. T praised Mrs. M when she made statements that reflected that she felt she had control over her health and the quality of her life.

3. Ms. V discussed specific fall-prevention strategies, addressing environmental and behavioral risk factors with Mrs. M and her family. Ms. V, Mrs. M, and Mrs. M's family decided on five potential environmental hazards that would be addressed first. Mrs. M and her family then worked out step-by-step plans to remove potential fall hazards at home and later reviewed the plans with Ms. V during treatment.

4. Mrs. M and her family were given several suggestions regarding how to access exercise programs appropriate for older adults in their community. Concerns raised by Mrs. M and her family regarding exercising were addressed by Mr. T and Ms. V initially and later by Mrs. M's physician, who ultimately gave approval for Mrs. M to participate in a pool exercise program offered locally.

5. Ms. V organized group activities that involved Mrs. M and other patients who expressed a concern about falling. For example, surveys of the hospital for environmental hazards were conducted by the outpatient group. Feedback from these surveys and suggestions for improvement were given to hospital management. Such exercises gave Mrs. M and the other group members the opportunity to use their problem-solving skills and reinforced the importance of assertiveness in fall prevention.

Together, these activities demystified fall prevention for Mrs. M and encouraged her to develop strategies that would work best for her and her family. The feedback Mrs. M received from the health care team, her family, and peers led to her having increased confidence in her own problem-solving skills and her ability to be more active. The relationships that Mrs. M established with other outpatients became particularly important sources of reinforcement.

References

Abraham, C., & Sheeran, P. (1994). Modeling and modifying young heterosexuals' HIV-preventive behavior: A review of theories, findings and educational implications. *Patient Education and Counseling, 23,* 173–186.

Alston, R. J., & Magadi, S. P. (1992). The interaction between disability status and the African-American experience: Implications for rehabilitation counseling. *Journal of Applied Rehabilitation Counseling, 23,* 10–14.

Alston, R. J., & Turner, W. L. (1994). A family strength model of adjustment to disability for African-American clients. *Journal of Counseling Development, 72,* 378–383.

American Occupational Therapy Association. (1995). *Elements of clinical documentation.* Prepared for the AOTA Commission on Practice by L. K. Thomson & M. Foto. Baltimore: AOTA.

Anderson, R. M. (1986). The personal meaning of having diabetes: Implications for patient behavior and education or kicking the bucket theory. *Diabetic Medicine, 3,* 85–89.

Arling, G. (1976). The elderly widow: Her family and friends. *Journal of Marriage and Family, 38,* 737.

Atkins, B. J. (1986). Innovative approaches and research in addressing the needs of nonwhite disabled persons. In S. Walker, F. Z. Belgrave, A. M. Banner, & R. W. Nicholls (Eds.), *Equal to the challenge: Perspective, problems, and strategies in rehabilitation of the Non-White Disabled.* Proceedings from the National Conference of the Howard University Model to Improve Rehabilitation Services to Minority Populations with Handicapping Conditions. Syracuse, NY: ERIC Clearinghouse on Information Resources. ERIC Document Reproduction Services No. ED 276 198.

Bandura, A. (1977a). *A social learning theory.* Englewood Cliffs, NJ: Prentice-Hall.

Bandura, A. (1977b). Self-efficacy: Toward a unifying theory of behavior change. *Psych Rev., 84,* 191–215.

Bandura, A. (1982). Self-efficacy mechanism in human agency. *Am Psychol, 37,* 122–147.

Bandura, A. (1986). *Social foundations of thought and action: A social cognitive theory.* Englewood Cliffs, NJ: Prentice-Hall.

Bandura, A. (1986b). Self-efficacy mechanism in physiological activation and health-promoting behavior. In J. Madden IV., S. Mathysse, & J. Barchas (Eds.), *Adaptations, learning and affect.* New York: Raven.

Bandura, A. (1989). Regulation of cognitive processes through perceived self-efficacy. *Developmental Psychology, 25,* 729–735.

Barry, J. M., West, R. L., & Dennehey, D. M. (1989). Reliability and validity of the memory self-efficacy questionnaire. *Developmental Psychology, 25,* 701–713.

Bartlett, E. (1983). Educational self-help approaches in childhood asthma. *Journal Allergy Clin Immunol. 72,* 545–555.

Belgrave, F. Z. (1991). Psychosocial predictors of adjustment to disability in African-Americans. *Journal of Rehabilitation, 57,* 37–40.

Blau, Z. (1973). *Old age in a changing society.* New York: New Viewpoints.

Bloom, B. S. (Ed.). (1956). *Taxonomy of educational objectives: Handbook I, cognition domain.* New York: D. McKay.

Bonder, B. R., (1994). Growing old in the United States. In B. R. Bonder & M. B. Wagner (Eds.), *Functional performance in older adults* (p. 12). Philadelphia: F. A. Davis.

Brown, J. S. (1961). *The motivation of behavior.* New York: McGraw-Hill.

Bruhn, J. (1983). The applications of theory in childhood asthma self-help programs. *J Allergy Clin Immunol., 72,* 561–578.

Chiodo, G. T., Rosenstein D. I., & Clark, J. H. (1986). Counseling principles for more effective patient education. *Community Dent Oral Epidemio., 14,* 190–192.

Cook, T. D., & Campbell, D. T. (1983). The design and conduct of quasi-experiments and true experiments in field settings. In M. D. Dannette (Ed.), *Handbook of industrial and organizational psychology.* New York: John Wiley & Sons.

Corbin, C. (1972). Mental practice. In W. Morgan (Ed.), *Ergogenic aids and muscular performance* (pp. 93–118). New York: Academic Press.

Feltz, D. L., and Landers, D. M. (1983). Effects of mental practice on motor skill learning and performance: A meta-analysis. *Journal of Sport Psychology, 5,* 25–57.

Ferrell, B. R., Ferrell, B. A., Abril, C., & Tran, K. (1994). Pain management for elderly patients with cancer at home. *Cancer, 74*(7 Suppl), 2139–2146.

Geis, G. L., Stebbins, W. C., & Lundin, R. W. (1965). *Reflex and operant conditioning.* New York: Appleton, Century, Crofts.

Gonzalez, V. M., Goeppinger, J., & Lorig, K. (1990). Four psychosocial theories and their application. *Arthritis Care and Research, 3,* 132–143.

Green, L. W., Kreuter, M. W., Deeds, S. G., & Partridge, K. B. (1980). *Health education planning: A diagnostic approach.* Mountain View, CA: Mayfield.

Green, L. W., and Frankish, C. J. (1994). Theories and principles of health education applied to asthma. *Chest, 106,* 219S–222S.

Hertzog, C., Dixon, R. A., & Hulsch, D. F. (1990). Relationships between metamemory, memory predictions and memory task performance in adults. *Psychology and Aging, 5,* 215–227.

Hilgard, E. R., & Bower, G. H. (1966). *Theories and learning.* New York: Appleton, Century, Crofts.

Hill, R. B. (1972). *The strengths of black families.* New York: Emerson Hall.

Hines, P. M., Boyd-Franklin, N. (1982) Black families. In M. McGoldrick, J. Pearce, & J. Giordano (Eds.), *Ethnicity and family therapy* (pp. 84–107). New York: Guilford.

Hochbaum, G. M. (1958). *Public participation in medical screening programs: A social psychological study.* Public Health Service Publication No. 572. Washington, DC: U.S. Government Printing Office.

Holahan, C. K., & Holahan, C. J. (1987a). Life stress, hassles, and self-efficacy in aging: A replication and extension. *Journal of Applied Social Psychology, 17,* 574–592.

Holahan, C. K., & Holahan, C. J. (1987b). Self-efficacy, social support, and depression in aging: A longitudinal analysis. *Journal of Gerontology, 42,* 65–68.

Howland, J. (1993). Process evaluation. Lecture presented at Boston University School of Public Health, Boston.

Johnson, C. (1983). Dyadic family relations and social support. *Gerontologist, 23*, 377.

Jourard, S. M. (1961) *Healthy personality.* New York: McGraw-Hill.

Kazdin, A. E. (1978). Covert modeling-therapeutic application of imagined rehearsal. In J. L. Singer & K. S. Pope (Eds.), *The power of human imagination: New methods in psychotherapy.* Emotions, personality, and psychotherapy (pp. 225–278). New York: Plenum.

Knowles, M. (1984). *The adult learner: A neglected species.* Houston, TX: Gulf Publishing.

Lachman, M. E. (1991). Perceived control over memory and aging developmental and intervention perspectives. *Journal of Social Issues, 47*, 159–175.

Lachman, M. E., Steinberg, E. S., & Trotter, S. D. (1987). The effects of control beliefs and attributes on memory self assessments and performance. *Psychology and Aging, 2*, 266–271.

Lachman, M. E., Weaver, S. L., Bandura, M., Elliot, E., & Lwekowicz, C. (1992). Improving memory control beliefs through cognitive restructuring and self-generated strategies. *Journal of Gerontology: Psychological Sciences, 47*, 293–299.

Lorig, K., Seleznick, M., Lubeck, D., Ung, E., Chastain, R., & Holman, H. R. (1989). The beneficial outcomes of arthritis self-management course are inadequately explained by behavior change. *Arthritis Rheum, 32*, 91–95.

McCord, E. C., & Brandenburg C. (1995). Beliefs and attitudes of persons with diabetes. *Family Medicine, 27*, 267–271.

McKenna, G. (1995). Learning theories made easy: Humanism. *Nursing Standard, 9*, 29–31.

Milhollan, F., & Forisha, B. (1972). *From Skinner to Rogers.* Lincoln, NE: Professional Publications.

Naylor, J., & Briggs, G. (1961). *Long-term retention of learned skills: A review of the literature.* Academy of Educational Development Technical Report, U.S. Department of Commerce, No. 61, 390.

O'Leary, A. (1985). Self-efficacy and health behavior. *Res. Ther., 23*, 437–451.

Office of Cancer Communications, National Cancer Institute. *Making health communications work, a planners guide.* (NIH Publication No. 89–1493). Bethesda, MD: National Institutes of Health.

Padilla, G. V., & Bulcavage, L. M. (1991). Theories used in patient/health education. *Seminars in Oncology Nursing, 7*, 87–96.

Peterson, E. W., & Howland, J. (1995). Predicting radon testing among university employees. *Journal of the Air and Water Management Association.* (In press).

Poole, J. L. (1995). Learning. In C. A. Trombly (Ed.), *Occupational therapy for physical dysfunction* (pp. 265–276). Baltimore, MD: Williams & Wilkins.

Reilly, D. E., & Oermann M. H. (1992). *Clinical teaching in nursing education.* New York: National League for Nursing.

Rodin, J. (1983). Behavioral medicine: Beneficial effect of self-control training in aging. *International Review of Applied Psychology, 132*, 153–181.

Rogers, C. R. (1983). *Freedom to learn for the 80s.* Ohio: Merrill.

Rogers, E. R. (1983). *Diffusion of innovations.* NY: Macmillan Publishing.

Rosenstock, I. M. (1966). Why people use health services. *Milbank Q, 44*, 94–124.

Rosenstock, I. M. (1990). The health belief model: Explaining health behavior through expectancies. In K. Glanz, F. M. Lewis & B. K. Rimer (Eds.), *Health behavior and health education: Theory, research and practice* (pp. 39–62). San Francisco: Jossey-Bass.

Singer, R. (Ed.). (1975). *Motor learning and human performance*. New York: Macmillan Publishing.

Snell, M. E. (1994). Principles for teaching self-care skills. In C. Christiansen (Ed.), *Ways of living: Self-care strategies for special needs* (pp. 77–100). Rockville, MD: American Occupational Therapy Association.

Strecher, V. J., McEvoy-DeVellis, B., Becker, M. H., & Rosenstock, I. M. (1986). The role of self-efficacy in achieving health behavior change. *Health Education Quarterly, 13,* 73–91.

Turner, W. L., & Alston, R. J. (1994). The role of the family in psychosocial adaptation to physical disabilities for African-Americans. *Journal of the National Medical Association, 86,* 915–921.

Walker, J. E., & Howland, J. (1992). Exploring dimensions of the fear of falling: Use of the focus group interview. *American Occupational Therapy Association Gerontology Special Interest Section Newsletter, 15,* 1–3.

Whaley, D. L., & Malott, R. W. (1971). *Elementary principles of behavior.* New York: Appleton, Century, Crofts.

Windsor, R. A., Baranowski, T., Clark, N., & Cutter, G. (1984). *Evaluation of health promotion and education programs.* Mountain View, CA: Mayfield Publishing.

Winstein, C. J., & Schmidt, R. A. (1990). Reduced frequency of knowledge of results enhances motor skill learning. *Journal of Experimental Psychology, 16,* 677–691.

Wood, V., & Robertson, J. (1978). Friendship and kinship interaction: Differential effect on the morale of the elderly. *Journal of Marriage and Family, 40,* 367.

Woolfolk, A. E., & Nicolich, L. M. (1980). *Educational psychology for teachers.* Englewood Cliffs, NJ: Prentice-Hall.

Wright, T. J. (1988). Enhancing the professional preparation of rehabilitation counselors for improved services to ethnic minorities with disabilities. *Journal of Applied Rehabilitation Counseling, 19,* 4–9.

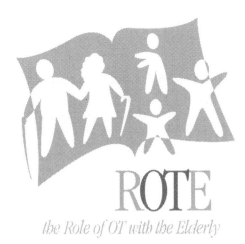

ROTE

the Role of OT with the Elderly

Client- and Family-Practitioner Relationships: Collaboration as an Effective Approach to Treatment

Deborah Walens, MHPE, OTR/L, FAOTA
Laurie Rockwell-Dylla, MS, OTR/L

Abstract

Traditional health care often takes for granted the important role clients[1] and families play in the process of rehabilitation and recovery. If our emerging system of care, with increased reliance on technology and managed care, is to be more cost-efficient, we have the

> … potential to inhibit the development of the relationships that practitioners need to form with clients in the context of their communities and with other practitioners in order to provide comprehensive, integrated care (Tresolini & the Pew-Fetzer Task Force, 1994, p. 16).

This chapter presents a model for practice that recognizes the importance of the relationship between the client, family, and practitioner in the day-to-day rehabilitation and recovery process—whether in the hospital, a long-term care facility, or at home. The authors propose a model of caring for the elderly that is client- and family-centered using a collaborative approach between service providers and service receivers. An essential component of the collaborative process is understanding and appreciating the client's and family's perspective and valuing their input in making decisions with respect to care options.

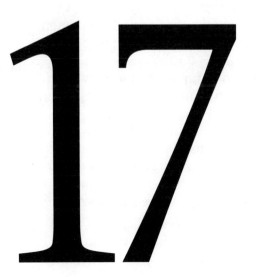

A review of literature on caregiving, the humanization of the caring process, and the process of collaboration will be presented. Actual stories of older adults and their families will be used to assist the reader in a synthesis of occupational therapy's roles in working with the elderly. This chapter illustrates the experiences, daily dilemmas, and adaptive strategies used by the elderly and their caregivers, as well as a deeper understanding of the knowledge, skills and attitudes necessary to engage in a collaborative relationship with the elderly and their families.

Magnitude of Caregiving

As a group, the elderly are more likely than younger people to suffer from multiple, chronic, and often disabling conditions that leave them physically and socially dependent (Stoto, Behrens, & Rosemont, 1990, p. 40). Over the next 15 years, the United States will see a rapid increase in the number of persons older than 65 that will lead to a shift in the burden of health care from an acute to a chronic disease process (Shugars, O'Neil, & Bader, 1991, p. 6).

A key question practitioners will need to answer is "What can be done to support and enable families to continue providing care in the home?" (Stone, 1991, p. 47). At any given time, more than 13 million spouses and adult children of disabled elderly persons, or one in 11 full-time workers, face making decisions about the long-term care of an older adult family member. According to Stone, under one-third of the 13 million provide help with activities of daily living to disabled spouses or parents living at home, and another three million relatives, friends, or neighbors are active caregivers. Still others provide informal care to elders in nursing homes.

The National Family Caregivers Association (NFCA) estimated that 18 million family caregivers provide services valued at $190 billion a year, compared with $22 billion worth of services being provided by professional caregivers in the home (Mintz, 1995, p. 7). Home care is estimated to be one of the fastest growing parts of the health care industry—the number of persons older than age 65 is projected to increase from one out of five to one out of four by the year 2020. These demographics represent challenges not only to older adults and their families, but also to health care providers and policy makers. The economic realities of providing health care require a reexamination of the traditional medical model of practice as health care providers engage in caring for older adults with their families and communities.

Caregiver Needs

Managed care and cutbacks in professional caregiving in the hospital and home have resulted in family members providing more direct hands-on medical care in addition to custodial care and social support for their aging and disabled spouses and parents. According to Baginski, "Most people can care for family members over the short term; it is the months and years of caregiving that can take a tremendous toll" (1995, p. 30). Since caregiving is rarely a role family members anticipate or prepare for, they need education and support as they assume this role. For quality caring to take place, families need to have information, resources, and support to sustain them in their caregiving. When asked to identify their needs, caregivers listed the following as most significant:

- Information on diagnosis and prognosis of an illness, information on community resources (eligibility and cost), information on nutrition and delivery of therapeutic meals, and information on where to get legal advice

- Assistance with managing housekeeping, cooking, house maintenance and yard work
- Help with feelings of resentment and guilt, as well as with loneliness, isolation, and depression of the older adult being cared for, and help with caregiver stress due to lack of visitors and personal contact
- Respite care for weekends or vacations
- Spiritual comfort and the promise that someone else cares and supports their caregiving as worthwhile (Baginski, 1995, p. 31).

At first glance, the above list seems out of the realm of what professional caregivers are prepared to provide; however, on closer examination, caregivers can do much to ease the burden. By educating and offering support, professionals strengthen the family's ability to provide effective care and maintain elderly family members in least-restrictive environments. As professionals become more cognizant and responsive to the needs of older adults and their caregivers, the outcomes of professional caregiving will be more satisfying for all involved.

LEO AND TILLIE'S STORY

The following story represents the dilemma faced by millions of spouses and adult children of older adults—coping with the long-term care needs of the elderly and making arrangements to prevent radical reorganization of their households. This story is presented to illustrate the adaptive strategies used by the elderly and their families to cope with changing needs and the role the occupational therapist can

assume to deal with changes in occupational performance.

Leo, 83, a retired paint manufacturer, has adjusted successfully to the disabling effects of arthritis resulting in three hip replacement surgeries, a lumbar laminectomy, and a cerebrovascular accident. However, his wife, Tillie, 84, described how the cancer preying on Leo's body resulted in a critical turning point in *both* of their lives:

> Cancer started gnawing at him and he got so weak and started falling. He tripped on a cane, once, and broke that, if you can believe breaking a quad cane! He would fall going up stairs, he would fall off the toilet, he would fall in the hall, he was falling off the kitchen chair onto the floor.

Life at home became a series of daily crises and struggles to cope with increasing vulnerability to perceived obstacles in their home. One of the biggest barriers was climbing the stairs to the second floor. Once taken for granted, the task now became a treacherous activity as Leo weakened from cancer. Rather than be constrained by his home environment, Leo and Tillie began to employ a series of strategies to adapt to the situation. A supportive family system provided the physical assistance Leo required. Tillie described,

> Our son and grandson would come over every night to help him. They came over, two of them, every night, and one would take the foot and lift it up and my son would take his arm.

The arrangement of physically assisting Leo worked for a while, but finally Tillie and Leo realized they would have to find another method. When discussing the dilemma with the home-health occupational therapist, she recommended they purchase an electric chairlift. The chairlift proved to be invaluable, as it allowed Leo the freedom to be either upstairs or downstairs and not confined to one area. Leo and Tillie felt "it paid for itself a thousand times" and considered it as a "godsend." They successfully met this and other challenges that arose, until 2 years later when Leo suffered a second right cerebrovascular incident. According to Tillie, the second stroke was worse. This time his bladder was affected, his left arm became weaker, and, if he tried to get up, he would fall over. Compounding the effects of the stroke was the presence of a cancerous tumor on the bowel; the removal of the tumor weakened Leo more.

While in the hospital, Leo received only limited amounts of physical therapy. Despite his efforts during physical therapy, the physiatrist and neurologist felt he was not an appropriate rehab candidate. Tillie was advised to put Leo in a nursing home, as it was determined he would be too much for her to handle. Tillie would not hear of it, and Leo wanted very much to go home. This lack of understanding of the "patient's" and family's goals on the part of the medical team reflects the divergence (Kaufman, 1988) that often occurs between the patient's and family's perspectives and the medical team's perspective. Leo and Tillie made the decision to return to the comfort and familiarity of home. In part because of the medical team's lack of understanding their goal, Leo and Tillie soon realized they were faced with unanticipated challenges. In the preceding 2 years, they had accommodated to Leo's changing abilities, but a second stroke necessitated more intensive caregiving.

Leo's loss of bowel and bladder control and need for help with self-care and transfers required nursing and occupational therapy home-health services. Tillie arranged to have a full-time home-health aide to assist her so Leo would not be a burden to the family. The increasing presence of medical equipment—chairlift, wheelchair, electric hospital bed, commode, bath seat, and grab bars—transformed their home into a mini-hospital. Even a space in the master bedroom was designated as the "therapy corner." Not only was Leo's and Tillie's space altered, but also their daily routine and habits were drastically affected. In order to meet all of Leo's needs, Tillie orchestrated his care into a stringent daily plan, which she carried out with the assistance of Pearl, the home-health aide.

A typical day for Leo and Tillie is as follows:

7:00 a.m.—Tillie administers Leo's pills; he falls back to sleep.

9:00 a.m.—Tillie assists with hygiene activities; they have breakfast, with Tillie providing cues to slow down. After breakfast Tillie monitors Leo's breathing exercises.

9:30 a.m.—Pearl arrives to take over the self-care tasks; initially, Pearl spends time with Tillie and Leo, hearing a report of their night.

10:00 a.m.—Pearl transfers Leo to the commode.

10:20 a.m.—Pearl shaves and sponge bathes Leo in bed.

11:00 a.m.—Pearl puts splints on Leo's left arm and leg; Leo naps for 45 minutes.

11:45 a.m.—Pearl carries out the daily exercise program with Leo: range-of-motion exercises, bridging exercises, and standing and reaching exercises.

12:15 p.m.—Pearl gets Leo dressed.

12:45 p.m.—Pearl transfers Leo to the wheelchair on the second floor and moves him to the chairlift. Leo rides the chairlift downstairs, where Pearl transfers him into a second wheelchair.

1:00 p.m.—Leo has his lunch in the den, feeding himself with his right hand, with cues from Pearl and Tillie to slow down.

2:00 p.m.—Pearl takes Leo in his wheelchair to the park. At the park, he and Pearl sit under a shade tree, and Leo talks with friends who congregate there.

3:30 p.m.—Pearl and Leo return from the park.

3:45 p.m.—Pearl brings Leo upstairs via the chairlift, reversing the process used earlier. Upstairs, Pearl transfers Leo into bed, does range-of-motion exercises, and changes his catheter.

4:30 p.m.—Pearl puts the splints back on, and Leo wears them while he naps. Pearl leaves for the day.

5:30 p.m.—Tillie takes the splints off and sets Leo up for dinner.

6:00 p.m.—Tillie brings dinner upstairs, warms it in a microwave, and they eat dinner together.

7:00 p.m.—Tillie and Leo watch television together.

8:00 p.m.—Leo falls asleep.

Tillie explained how such a routine has ensured that Leo's needs are met and his dignity maintained.

> Yeah, we really do have a down-pat routine. And if we get slightly off it, it just seems to upset him. Get one thing turned around, especially the bowel pattern, if he's not on the commode, or if Pearl doesn't get to him right after breakfast, it's just a worry to him all day. He's so fastidious about his personal cleanliness and stuff.

Tillie found that, without the structure of a daily routine, Leo became confused. The occupational therapist validated this observation and acknowledged the ritualization of caregiving tasks and their importance to Tillie. A structured daily routine enabled her to manage both Leo's care and other aspects of the household in an efficient manner. While this routine served a useful function, all spontaneity was relinquished. As Leo stated, "I've lost a lot of adventure," and Tillie commented that their "social life is nil." The daily pattern of their life was replaced by a regimented routine and a redefinition of Leo's and Tillie's roles.

Tillie assumed her former role as a nurse, caring for Leo by administering medication, checking to be sure he did his breathing exercises, and making sure his bowel and bladder were regulated. Additionally, Leo's household duties were relegated by Tillie, and she was faced with many unfamiliar tasks.

> Well, see, I have to manage everything now. Pay the bills and all that. A lot of things he can help with. I never did get things ready for the taxes and all that. Boy, did I have to learn fast!

As Leo relinquished a number of his roles, Tillie helped him maintain a sense of dignity and connectedness by doing "identity work" (Corbin & Strauss, 1990, p. 64). Tillie involved him in household decisions by asking his advice on what information to give their accountant and having him monitor their stocks. Tillie combined "identity work" along with activities to enhance his quality of life and remain "connected" to significant aspects of his life experiences. Activities that were used in maintaining his identity included continuing to give him the "business section" of the *Tribune* with his breakfast, watching *Jeopardy* in the den to keep his mind sharp, relaxing in the sunny Florida room, and continuing to hold family gatherings in the dining room and living room as before.

Other members of the family, while not directly involved in Leo's daily needs, played a vital role in maintaining Leo's identity. Leo's son visited frequently, and they would discuss the family business and topics of interest, like sports. At other times, Leo would involve himself in making a project for someone in the family. Leo's home-health occupational therapy practitioner understood Leo's love of working with colors in decorating his home, as his career had been that of a paint manufacturer. Therefore, she engaged Leo in craft projects that involved bright colors, allowing that part of his identity to still be expressed. Leo made candy dishes, paperweights, and candlestick holders, and gave them as gifts to family and friends. His occupational therapy practitioner helped him "to do" for others, which was very important and gave him pleasure. As Leo said, "I get a big kick out of doing things for others."

Leo's life was also enriched by making opportunities for him to get outside as often as possible, so he didn't feel confined. Tillie helped Leo keep "socially connected" by making sure Leo routinely had visits with neighbors and took him out for car rides to favorite places.

Both Leo and Tillie were comfortable with the adaptations they made to prevent placing Leo in a nursing home. They attribute their success in preventing institutionalization to much trial and error over the years, involvement from family members, and having the support of caring home-health professionals.

The chronic and complex nature of Leo's condition, Leo's and Tillie's desire to keep Leo at home, and the increasing demands for caregiving, raise multiple issues involving how professional caregivers support older adults and their families who assume the primary task of caring for persons with limited functional abilities. Tillie's life now revolved around, "getting things done, taking care of Leo's health and well-

being, and taking care of her own health and well-being." These three themes are consistent with Hasselkus's (1989, pp. 650–652) findings on the dilemmas of family caregivers: How can professional caregivers assist and support spouses and families who care for older adults at home?

Reframing Caregiving: Meaning Versus Task

Suzanne Mintz, cofounder of NFCA, states that the "one overriding complaint (of caregivers), is that no one understands what they are going through" (Mintz, 1995, p. 8). Professionals often do not take the time to find out what the family knows about the care receiver or to understand the feelings associated with the responsibilities of caregiving. The family's contributions often go unnoticed and have been labeled the invisible work of the caregiver.

The process of caregiving is much more complex than the performance of or assistance with personal tasks (bathing, grooming, or toileting), instrumental tasks (transporting, preparing meals, doing laundry, cleaning, or giving financial assistance), and skilled care (injections, wound care, or catheter care). Families are often thrust into the role with little or no forethought or may assume the role of caregiving over time, until it gradually becomes all consuming. As family caregivers provide the emotional link between the professional caregivers and the identified client, professional caregivers need to appreciate that families provide "a service one cannot pay another to provide" (Mintz, 1995, p. 8).

In an attempt to understand better the caregiver's perspective, professionals should examine not only the tasks that caregivers engage in but also the *mean-*

ing behind these tasks. Bowers (1987) discusses caregiving by defining its purpose. This framework gives meaning not only to the explicit behaviors on the part of the caregiver but also the mental activities that are part of the invisible work of the caregiver. Five categories of caregiving identified by Bowers included anticipatory, preventive, supervisory, instrumental, and protective care. These categories describe not the task itself but the purpose or meaning behind the behavior:

- **Anticipatory caregiving:** Caring behavior and decisions that anticipate the possible needs of the older adult. An example would be deciding to move closer to a parent in anticipation of needs down the road.

- **Preventive caregiving:** Activities engaged in to prevent illness, injury, complications, and physical and mental deterioration. An example would be active monitoring or supervising of an older adult's daily routine. This also could include altering the physical environment for increased safety, regular questioning about symptoms, or monitoring medications.

- **Supervisory caregiving:** Situations in which the caregiver is engaged in active and direct involvement with the older adult. Activities include arranging for, checking up on, making sure, setting up, and checking out services that are needed by the older adult. This may be done with or without the older adult's awareness.

- **Instrumental caregiving:** Caregiving that includes doing for, assisting with, providing for, and giving care. Activities include hands-on caregiving for the purpose of maintaining an older adult's physical integrity and health status.

- **Protective caregiving:** This type of caregiving is experienced as the most difficult and important type of care provided. Often these activities are done by the caregiver to prevent threats to the older adult's self-image or physical well-being. This type of protective caring is very prevalent when spouses and children are attempting to maintain the older adult's identity and self-worth (Bowers, 1987, p. 25).

Because of the critical role spouses and families undertake, professional caregivers need to include them as active members of the health care team and offer them opportunities to share their perspectives, as well as help them be effective caregivers.

Home Care Experience

In his book *Mosaic of Care: Frail Elderly and Their Families in the Real World*, Gubrium (1991) recognizes that

> … the home is becoming an important component of the health care system. The high costs of institutionalization combined with the growing population of frail elderly, the availability of transportable care apparatus, and the development of a home care industry bring the household into a realistic focus as a care setting (Gubrium, 1991, p. 49).

Gubrium emphasizes that very little is understood about the interpersonal dynamics and the practical activities that are being carried out in the home setting. Gubrium feels there are a number of important questions that need to be answered, such as

> What is the meaning of familial responsibility to those concerned? How do families learn what they are, and are not, responsible for in caring for frail elderly at home? How do those involved evaluate, in their own terms, the quality of home care?

How much caregiving is enough? What kind of care is sufficient? What does it mean to care in the first place? How do interpersonal ties of the family shape members' sense of responsibility? (Gubrium, 1991, p. 50).

Gubrium refers to the original three caregiving factors:

1. The frail elderly family member's level of impairment

2. The family caregiver's felt burden or stress

3. The likelihood of institutionalization, as the basis of the "care equation" that grew out of research being done in home care of persons with Alzheimer's disease (Gubrium, 1991, p. 50).

In regard to this care equation, Gubrium stated:

> In the original reasoning, as the care receiver's impairment worsens, it presents an increasing burden of care to the caregiver, which, in turn, affects the caregiver's tolerance, eventually requiring the care receiver's institutionalization. Overall, the model is framed negatively; one bad thing leads to another (p. 51).

With the caregiver literature developing primarily in the care of persons with Alzheimer's disease over the past 10 years, "There is no notion that families might define care in both the short and long run as an ordinary domestic matter" (Gubrium, 1991, p. 51).

Gubrium acknowledges that the original care equation has been embellished to include a number of intervening variables like social support, the caregiver's precrisis attitude toward the suitability of nursing home care, and the personal well-being of the caregiver. With these added dimensions, "what emerged is a greater awareness of the need to consider the *meaning* of the care equation's factors to those

concerned" (Gubrium, 1991, p. 52). Gubrium regards the ideas of burden, stress, strain, and caregiver tolerance as a negative and linear view and that the focus should be on the care *experience* (1991, p. 53).

Gubrium believes that

> ... the native experiences of caregiving are more realistically captured when a linear, service-oriented framework is set aside and replaced by a view toward caregiving's complex and dynamic relationships."

That is an understanding "grounded in the real world of the actual, lived experience or interpretive practices of those concerned."

Humanizing Health Care

A common dilemma faced by professional caregivers is that the needs of the elderly and their caregivers often seem overwhelming and clearly would take a larger investment of time and money than is often available and feasible. A side effect of using technology and business principles to streamline medical care is a system lacking a sense of caring, unless professionals consciously safeguard against dehumanized care. The best and possibly the easiest way to humanize care is to humanize the relationship between professional caregivers and the client (Studt, 1975, p. 220).

The moral conflicts associated with dehumanized care confront health professionals daily. Professional caregivers need to reflect on and assess their own behaviors and values for what constitutes humanized caring, as well as dehumanized care. Howard (1975, p. 66) summarizes dehumanizing behavior in the following way:

> ... Depersonalized people are viewed as inanimate, unfeeling objects or machines to be manipulated, experi-

mented upon, fragmented into problems, and treated with detachment. In more extreme cases they are isolated, alienated, stripped of dignity, and given few if any opportunities to escape from the static, sterile, degrading environments in which they are enmeshed. Their care is often substandard in accord with society's perception of their lesser worth (p. 66).

Unfortunately, older adults are particularly vulnerable to dehumanized care due to their decreased physical, mental, social, and economic abilities. Professional caregivers are in a unique position to establish and perpetuate the ways in which the caring process is engaged. Central to the health professional's education is learning to form caring relationships.

> Practitioners need to develop as reflective learners who understand the client as a person, recognize and deal with multiple contributors to health and illness, and understand the nature of healing relationships (Tresolini & Pew-Fetzer Task Force, 1994, p. 39).

Howard identifies eight factors that constitute humanized care in the health professions. The following ways of viewing the client and the family help to define the values inherent in creating humanized care (As a practitioner, to what extent do you hold the following beliefs about the people you care for?):

- Human beings have *inherent worth* regardless of their ethnicity, sexual orientation, religious beliefs, social or economic status (Howard, 1975). The diversity of our society requires that practitioners understand differences in how various cultures approach health care and make decisions with respect to its use.

- People (older adults) are *unique* and *irreplaceable* and need to be treated as individuals with different needs, hopes, and dreams. By noting the individual differences of clients, providers can avoid making health care uniform with the expectation that everyone fits the same framework (Howard, 1975). (This is particularly challenging in a cost conscious environment.)

- People have very *complex lives* that embrace many behavioral milieus. At any one time, a person's experience is influenced by both the past and the present, depending on which is more salient. When health care professionals are concerned only with that part of the individual that is relevant to being a client, they run the risk of fragmenting and viewing the person as a condition or diagnosis (Howard, 1975). In doing so, practitioners fail to understand the meaning of illness in an individual's life.

- "Human relations are predicated on *freedom of choice*" (Howard, 1975). When a person becomes a client, practitioners assume the person is willing to have considerable dependence on others for self-care. Practitioners need to keep in mind that all people have considerable control over their destinies even when denied essential freedoms.

- A humanized relationship relies on *basic* respect and a *sense of equality* (Howard, 1975). Even though the client-practitioner relationship assumes that the practitioner has a degree of expertise, the practitioner needs to acknowledge that the client has the unique expertise of knowing himself or herself better than anyone else. The client's unique perspective of his or her illness is critical to therapeutic caring.

- *Shared decision making* and responsibility logically follow in a humanistic relationship where individuals regard each other as having inherent worth, uniqueness, wholeness of self, freedom of action, and equality. The emerging frame of reference accepts that "all older adults have a right and perhaps a duty to participate as much as possible in decisions about their care" (Howard, 1975).

- In a humanized relationship, the practitioner has the *ability to empathize* with and care about a client. By being able to see the world from the client's vantage point, the practitioner can more readily understand the client's needs and respond appropriately.

- In person-to-person interaction, where human beings are valued, caring can take place. Affective neutrality, although considered by some as a characteristic of professionalism, is in essence depersonalizing. When a health practitioner is able to replace affective neutrality with *positive affect*, he or she is able to develop an emotional commitment that shows sincerity and concern (Howard, 1975).

When clients (and families) share responsibility for their care, at least three assumptions are implicit: they have behavioral options with respect to their illness, the quality and quantity of their lives are at stake, and they deserve significant control over choices of possible regimens and lifestyles (Howard, 1975, p. 81).

When clients and families share in the decision making to the extent that they are competent, they need to be informed and educated about diagnosis, prognosis, available interventions, risks, and cost of available therapies. Practitioners who involve their clients and family caregivers in understanding what is going on and what can be expected from professional caregiving create alternatives so clients and families can make informed decisions.

Competent Caring

The challenge of caring in a climate that is focused on efficiency and measurable results is to preserve and enhance caring. With increased dependency on technology and objectivism, occupational therapy risks alienation from the very roots of its history. Yerxa reminds us

Our practice in the future should be evaluated not only on the basis of measurable scientific outcomes, but also by what it contributes to individual human dignity, a sense of mastery, and self-respect (1980, p. 534).

It seems logical that client-practitioner partnerships would be a "win-win" situation. When practitioners view clients and families as having strengths and abilities, clients and families are empowered to pursue needs, hopes, and dreams. The "caring is not the taking-care-of the person, but helping the person learn to take care of himself or herself" (Gilfoyle, 1980, p. 519).

What is competent caring? Peloquin (1989) discusses the client-practitioner relationship as a blending of both competence and caring. The client's vision of the practitioner is embodied in the relationship that develops in the process of providing occupational therapy. Benner and Wrubel (1989) discuss caring in the following way:

Because caring sets up what matters to a person, it also sets up what counts as stressful, and what options are available for coping. Caring creates possibility. This is the first way in which caring is primary. It determines both what will be stressful and what will count as coping. Caring (having things matter) puts the person in a place of risk and vulnerability. Relationships, things, events, and projects do not show up as stressful unless they matter. If the person does not care, an event cannot be stressful. But the nature of caring is such that it also sets up what coping options are available and acceptable to the person.

As practitioners shift their paradigm for caring to a collaborative model, professionals will need to acknowledge and value their personal capacity to be self-reflective. With a commitment of providing services that reflect an understanding of the elderly client and his or her family, and a sensitivity to the individual's expressed needs, practitioners need to maintain their ability to continue to care. Active reflection on one's self and work will be essential for self-awareness and self-growth. A valuing of self-awareness is essential to valuing other individuals and the basis for understanding the life experiences of the persons being cared for. Without self-knowledge our own emotional responses can become barriers to helping others. Self-care is essential as practitioners become a resource for older adults in need (Tresolini & Pew-Fetzer Task Force, 1994).

Collaborative Versus Expert Model

Historically and currently, the use of expert models dominates the medical profession and reflects a professional's viewing her- or himself as having total expertise and control over decision making (Cunningham & Davis, 1985, p. 12). Practitioners socialized in an expert model of hands-on treatment position themselves to control evaluation, treatment, and decision making. Often the client and family feel as if the intervention is being done to them, and they are rendered submissive in the process.

The common belief that clients and their families are passive in the process of receiving health care is changing

both in the hospital and the home. One of the changes occurring in the relationship between the client, family, and practitioner is that the relationship itself is recognized as providing a source of satisfaction and positive outcome for all involved. (Tresolini & Pew-Fetzer Task Force, 1994). A practitioner's blending of scientific knowledge and understanding of the client's experience of illness is being realized as essential to expert practice (Benner & Wrubel, 1989; Harvath, Archbold, Stewart, Gadow, Kirschling, Miller, Hagan, Brody, & Schook, 1995; Tresolini & Pew-Fetzer Task Force, 1994).

Changing to Collaboration

Many professionals have worked in environments where they provided the care, made the decisions, and controlled the flow of information to the client, family, and other professionals. Because of prior learning and socialization, changing to a collaborative model is much more challenging than developing new skills.

> Collaboration is defined as an approach to therapeutic relationships that incorporates flexibility to address each consumer's specific needs, lifestyle, and personal values. The purpose of collaboration is to involve the client actively in identifying the problems he or she considers to be most pressing and develop plans for achieving relevant outcomes (Corcoran, 1993, p. 22).

Collaboration is an ongoing process and is characterized by the professional's use of the following skills and strategies (Johnson, McGonigel, & Kaufmann, 1989; Bazyk & Trombino, 1990):

- Active listening
- Honest, clear, and jargon-free communication
- Mutual respect for knowledge and skills

- Two-way sharing of information
- Recognition and support of individual and family values, customs, and beliefs
- Understanding and empathy
- Shared evaluation, planning, and decision making
- Accessibility and responsiveness
- Absence of judgment and labeling.

The cornerstone of collaboration is effective communication. To establish an effective partnership, professionals not only need to change attitudes but also must develop new skills and practice them.

One aspect that is essential to effective collaboration is the ability to elicit the client and caregiver's stories to understand individual and family needs and to develop a plan that is relevant and meaningful. Practitioners should understand the client's and family's view of illness, how the illness is experienced, the meaning it has in the person's life, and what goals and needs the client and family have. Ultimately, this understanding will lead to more effective treatment (Kaufman, 1988). Because the rehabilitation and recovery process is often long and is dramatically influenced by demographic, psychological, sociocultural, and medical variables, it affects all dimensions of the older adult's and family's life (Kaufman, 1988).

Practitioners' relationships are central to integrating caring, healing, and community. When clients and families take more active roles in shaping the health care services they use, they are able to adapt and function in the face of change. When practitioners pay attention to the whole person, older adults and their families are offered wider options for caring that provide the moral, ethical, and spiritual basis for support and self-care (Tresolini &

Pew-Fetzer Task Force, 1994). Effective caring demands that practitioners approach the client-practitioner relationship using models of practice that actively engage the client and family in assessment, planning, and intervention processes. Collaboration is an effective way to achieve this outcome. When engaging in a collaborative model, the client and family have ultimate control over decisions about their care and are seen as having knowledge and expertise that are critical to the outcome of the situation (Cunningham & Davis, 1985).

For the most part, the family, not the professional, is the constant in an elderly person's life. This necessitates collaboration with the client and family at all points on the continuum of care (Shelton, Jeppson, & Johnson, 1992). The professional acts as a consultant and guide to the client and family while providing direct service when necessary. (When you think of the word *collaboration,* what comes to mind for you? How would you describe the collaborative process? When reflecting on your current practice, how many of the following principles are consistent with the ways in which you interact with the elderly and their families?)

Principles of Client-Family and Practitioner Relationships

When engaged in a collaborative process, the practitioner needs to do the following:

- Promote a relationship in which client, family members, and practitioners work together to ensure the best services for the client and the family.
- Recognize and respect the knowledge, skills, and experience that the

client and family bring to the relationship.

- Acknowledge that the development of trust is an integral part of a collaborative relationship.

- Facilitate open communication so that the client and family feel free to express themselves.

- Create an atmosphere in which the cultural traditions, values, and diversity of the client and his or her family are acknowledged and honored.

- Recognize that negotiation is essential in a collaborative relationship.

- Bring to the relationship the mutual commitment to meet the needs of the client and his or her caregivers (Bishop, Woll, & Arango, 1993).

The Collaboration Process

Collaboration can be compared to team building (Bishop et al., 1993). When a team is effective, the whole team shares in the responsibilities of defining what, how, when, and by whom. The client, family, and practitioners form a partnership with the purpose of facilitating the best functioning of the older adult. This requires a shift in thinking from a model in which practitioners assume control to a model where the client and family are recognized and valued for their knowledge, skills, and expertise. The client and family have two kinds of expertise: "They know more than anyone else [about] how their illness affects their functioning and they do the basic work of getting well" (Studt, 1975, p. 218). Therefore, the client and family make a critical contribution to the development and success of a good health care plan.

For collaborative relationships to work, trust and mutual respect must develop between the client, family, and practitioner. Trust develops over time and is facilitated by open communication and a willingness to discuss issues openly and honestly.

A collaborative relationship is a trusting relationship where expectations, hopes, and sometimes dreams are shared. Trust does not require agreement on all issues, nor does it require perfect solutions. When disagreements occur, it is easier to resolve them within the context of a trusting relationship (Bishop et al., 1993, p. 23).

Practitioners have a special responsibility in developing trust (Bishop et al., 1993) with the elderly and their families. As the elderly and their families are often dependent on the services being provided, they may not easily risk placing themselves in a vulnerable position. Practitioners need to understand that when the elderly or their families have placed their trust in them, the families assume that the practitioner will be sensitive to their needs and will be honest in sharing information.

Open, honest, and timely communication are central to all collaborative relationships.

Collaborative relationships are characterized by dialogue—an ongoing effort by all persons to discuss the issues and concerns at hand, to exchange information, provide feedback, share reactions and ideas, and create solutions (Bishop et al., 1993, p. 26).

As a dialogue develops between the older adult, family, and practitioner, the practitioner should recognize that listening is just as important as sharing ideas and giving information in a clear and open way.

All relationships occur in a context that is shaped by individual cultural traditions, values, and beliefs. One of the greatest challenges practitioners face is understanding and respecting the unique beliefs, values, and customs (Bishop et al., 1993) of older adults and their families.

In order to develop sensitivity to the diverse background of individuals and their families five elements are necessary: an awareness and acceptance of differences, an awareness of the influence of the professional's culture on how he or she thinks and acts, an understanding of the dynamics of difference in the helping process, knowledge of the family's culture, and the ability to adapt practice skills to fit the family's cultural context (Bishop et al., 1993, p. 29).

The ability to negotiate is essential in a collaborative relationship. "Negotiation is the process of laying on the table different options, priorities, and preferences of all team members" (Bishop et al., 1993, p. 32). In doing so the client, family, and practitioner can discuss and determine the best plan. Throughout the process, the practitioner must be ready to engage in simple negotiations, such as appointment times, or more complex issues, such as whether the older adult is going to become independent in dressing or allow his or her spouse to assume the responsibility. Decisions need to be understood in the context of the older adult's needs and wishes and those of the family. Given an older adult's desire for more meaningful activities, the practitioner may work with the client and spouse to direct limited energy to the pursuit of a leisure interest instead of focusing on self-care that the spouse is willing to take more responsibility for.

Last, older adults live in communities where there are varying levels of commitment to the elderly. Understanding the resources of a community and the types of services offered to support families can be an essential resource. Communities often provide services that can decrease the burden experienced by older adults and their families. Community programs (such as meals on wheels, senior day care centers, transportation for the disabled, lending closets for adaptive equipment, respite services, and grocery and pharmacy delivery services) and programs (such as the "baby brigade" or adopt-a-grandparent) provide opportunities for older adults to meet relational needs and improve their quality of life.

To ensure that older adults and their families receive the best service possible, practitioners need to build and nurture working relationships with older adults and their families. Practitioners need to be cognizant that this shift in philosophy of creating partnerships with older adults and their families leads to shared responsibility and satisfaction in the outcome.

The Samanski Family: "A House with a Kitchen and Five Bedrooms"

The following story depicts a collaborative relationship between a home-health occupational therapy practitioner, an older adult couple, and their two daughters. The story highlights the collaborative process used to gain an understanding of the issues and concerns faced by the family and to develop a meaningful and relevant treatment plan that met the needs of the clients and caregivers. The names Samanski, Joan, Anne, Deborah, and Art are pseudonyms.

The occupational therapy practitioner, Vickie, began working with the family after receiving a referral for Mrs. Samanski, a 79-year-old woman diagnosed with myxedema (a thyroid condition that causes an extreme amount of edema). During the initial phone contact, Vickie learned that Mrs. Samanski lived with her husband, Art, and her two daughters, Deborah and Anne. Deborah and Anne helped take care of their mother. The Samanskis lived in a middle-class section of the northwest side of Chicago in a two-story house.

Deborah answered the door. On entering the home, Vickie paid close attention to the possessions displayed in the home to give her insight into Mrs. Samanski as a person. Vickie also noted potential physical barriers, such as the staircase leading to the second floor. She wondered how Mrs. Samanski managed going up and down.

As Vickie walked through the home, she was struck by the presence of a queen-size bed all made up with a comforter and embroidered pillows in the living room. She found Mrs. Samanski in this room. Mrs. Samanski was a frail-looking woman sitting in a high-backed recliner. To gain understanding of the family's situation, Vickie began interviewing Anne and Deborah, who provided most of the information, as Mrs. Samanski was very fatigued.

GAINING UNDERSTANDING

The first questions determined the family's life before Mrs. Samanski's hospitalization and what led to the referral for home health. Vickie also asked them to share what their life was like at present, including the challenges they encountered and the strategies they had devised. Using an ethnographic interview, Vickie elicited Mrs. Samanski's story. (Refer to table 17–1 for details on ethnographic interviewing.)

Mrs. Samanski had a history of congestive heart failure, emphysema and asthma. As a result of the myxedema, she experienced shortness of breath when exerting herself. She was able to care for herself, do the cooking and cleaning, and enjoyed crocheting and visiting with friends. She had difficulty, however, in climbing the thirteen steps to reach her bedroom. She began spending more time on the first floor and even began to sleep on the first floor in the recliner.

Her daughters convinced her to move her bed into the living room where she could relax and be more comfortable. Altering a public space into more of a private space was the first adaptation they made to accommodate Mrs. Samanski's changing needs. At this time, Mrs. Samanski was still able to care for herself, her husband, and her home.

A few years later, Deborah's and Anne's caregiver "careers" began when Mrs. Samanski experienced increasing difficulty breathing and fluid retention to the point her legs were swollen to four times their normal size. For the first time, Mrs. Samanski found it difficult to care for herself and the home that she had managed for 60-plus years. She was hospitalized with a resurgence of her thyroid condition. When stabilized, her physician strongly recommended inpatient rehabilitation, but Mrs. Samanski was adamant about returning home. So, in collaboration with her physician, Mrs. Samanski and her family agreed that she would return home with home nursing, occupational therapy, and physical therapy.

At home, Deborah and Anne assisted Mrs. Samanski with bathing, dressing, and hygiene; administered her medications; and managed her nursing and therapy regime. Her daughters monitored her medical status and informed her nurse and doctor of significant changes. In addition to caring for Mrs. Samanski, they took over management of the household, including grocery shopping, cooking, cleaning, and upkeep of the family home. Their only saving grace was that their father, in his mid-80s, was in good health and able to care for himself, do the household bookkeeping and gardening, and was content puttering in the house and garage. Since Deborah and Anne were each spending increasing amounts of time away from their homes, they decided to move back in with their parents.

During the interview, Vickie decided she would need to address Mrs. Samanski's decreased functioning, and Deborah's and Anne's caregiver needs. The interview defined a current "typical day," but Vickie also wanted to understand more about their lives prior to becoming caregivers. What were they most concerned about, and what would help them in their caregiver role? Anne, the eldest, was divorced and had lived near her parents in an apartment. Deborah was single and had lived in a condominium before she moved back home. She was trying to balance caregiving with a career as a freelance artist.

They wanted Mrs. Samanski to be independent—walking to the kitchen to get a drink, getting in and out of bed, and going to the toilet. They hoped she could be left alone for short periods of time while they took care of other responsibilities. Another major concern was Mrs. Samanski's ability to manage in an emergency situation.

Vickie tried to engage Mrs. Samanski in conversation to better understand her goals. She explained that she did not like to think about the future, because the future holds more sickness, more loss of friends, and more loss of independence. She did, however, express a desire to do some of the things she did before, like cooking and crocheting. Vickie took this opportunity to see some of her personal possessions as another window into her world.

Everyone agreed on a plan that included two sessions a week in which Mrs. Samanski would work on activities to increase strength, learn ways to simplify self-care and homemaking activities to conserve energy, learn to maneuver safely around the house, master strategies for dealing with emergency situations, and reengage in familiar activities. The occupational therapist's role was to guide the process and consult with Anne and Deborah so Mrs. Samanski would see herself as an active family member and not a prisoner of her living room. Then Vickie addressed Anne and Deborah's caregiver needs by promoting Mrs. Samanski's overall quality of life and helping the daughters access community resources that would help them adjust to their roles as caregivers.

Part of the negotiation process during treatment planning involved scheduling visits for afternoon or early evenings, as they had always been a "late rising family." They also requested that the occupational therapy practitioner and the physical therapist coordinate their schedules so that sessions were on alternate days, so Mrs. Samanski could derive optimal benefit from each session.

PROVIDING MEANINGFUL TREATMENT

Vickie learned more about Mrs. Samanski as they talked during the exercise sessions about activities she enjoyed. Vickie drew upon Mrs. Samanski's interest in cooking by asking her to share favorite recipes and helpful cooking tips. Since cooking had been a major part of her life, and her daughters wanted Mrs. Samanski to do more for herself, many sessions focused on activities in the kitchen. The sessions began first with the "simple" tasks like getting a drink, progressing to pouring coffee, retrieving items from the refrigerator, sitting at the table to peel vegetables and "supervising" Anne and Deborah during meal preparation. When Mrs. Samanski was strong enough to cook a favorite dish, they learned that preparing a whole meal was too taxing, and the role of "kitchen supervisor" was more in keeping with her physical capabilities.

Since crocheting was an activity Mrs. Samanski loved to do, Vickie asked Deborah to get the materials Mrs. Samanski would need to work on a small project. With encouragement, Mrs. Samanski crocheted a little each day and made a pot holder similar to the ones she had crocheted years ago.

For nearly a year, Mrs. Samanski's world had been limited to the living room. While she was able to go the kitchen, she preferred to stay in the security of the recliner which had become a cocoon for her. So each session involved reacquainting Mrs. Samanski with the rooms of her house until she became less fearful of moving about the first floor and the back porch. Mrs. Samanski also eventually climbed the steps to the second floor and ventured outside. One therapy session was devoted to helping Mrs. Samanski maneuver safely outside for a trip to the corner mailbox and around the block in a wheelchair. This therapeutic "trip" provided her with the opportunity to reacquaint herself with her neighbors and see the outside world. Her daughters were astonished to see she could safely venture out and enjoy the trip. In another session, an emergency was simulated so Mrs. Samanski could practice summoning help and exiting her home safely and quickly. The "fire drill" offered peace of mind to Deborah and Anne.

Vickie helped fulfill Deborah's and Anne's other needs by listening to their frustrations in dealing with both the physical and emotional aspects of caring for their mother. In each session,

Vickie encouraged them to express their concerns and frustration and reminded them of the importance of taking care of themselves and addressing their own physical, social, and emotional needs. With her help they found information on a support group (Children of Aging Parents), read articles on coping and caring for aging parents, and found that being listened to and having their experiences and concerns acknowledged was most beneficial. They valued observing Mrs. Samanski's increased activities and used Vickie as a model for developing ways to engage and modify activities to use with their mother.

Just as Mrs. Samanski progressed to the point where she had reached her goals and where Deborah and Anne were getting situated in their roles and routines as caregivers, another incident occurred that forced them to reorganize their lives and household once again.

MR. SAMANSKI'S STORY

Mr. Samanski suddenly became critically ill. The focus now shifted from caring for Mrs. Samanski to dealing with Mr. Samanski's life-or-death situation. Mr. Samanski had no prior medical conditions, but at 87 he experienced a rupture of his esophagus, a condition referred to as Boorhave Syndrome, which generally results in immediate death. Mr. Samanski was rushed to the hospital, where he had emergency surgery. Deborah sat vigil in the intensive care unit until he stabilized. During this time, Anne took over household chores and primary caregiving responsibility for Mrs. Samanski. Mrs. Samanski's status had improved with home therapy but started to decline because of the emotional impact of Mr. Samanski's hospitalization. Literally speaking, Deborah's and

Anne's caregiving responsibilities had increased exponentially overnight.

Mr. Samanski improved after two months of rehabilitation and was able to return home with home health care. Since Vickie was familiar with the family, she was specifically requested to work with Mr. Samanski. Vickie needed to understand how this most recent incident impacted their lives. Once again, she used an ethnographic interview to understand Mr. Samanski's illness experience and the challenges now facing Deborah and Anne.

CARING FOR MR. AND MRS. SAMANSKI

After two years of caring for their mother, Deborah and Anne were adept in managing "home care" for their father. They monitored his pulse, blood pressure, daily nutritional intake and output, and provided wound care where a J-tube had been inserted. Additionally they assisted him with self-care activities, participated in the therapy program, tried to keep up his spirits, and took over the household tasks for which he had been responsible.

When Vickie entered the Samanski home, it had undergone another transformation. This time, the dining room, which served as Mr. Samanski's bedroom, had been equipped with an electric hospital bed and tray. While Mrs. Samanski was content to be in the living room, Mr. Samanski had a very special regard for his bedroom upstairs and wanted to resume sleeping and spending time upstairs. He described his bedroom as a "wall of dreams" where he would reminisce while looking at pictures and memorabilia on the walls. He often dreamed about a particular event represented in the pictures when he napped and found this very relaxing and pleasurable. Mr. Samanski expressed how much he loved puttering in the basement, garage, and garden. Now, the stairs were an obstacle for getting to these places.

MR. SAMANSKI'S TREATMENT PLAN

Because Deborah and Anne knew the importance of Mr. Samanski's activities, they had set up a table in the corner of the dining room that served as his office. They hung photographs, postcards, and get well cards on the wall replicating the "wall of dreams" upstairs. A chair was put by the window so he could view his garden, and Vickie suggested woodworking projects and indoor gardening in his new space. These activities were important to Mr. Samanski, as they reflected his interests and restored those aspects of his identity that were important to him. These activities were a divergence from the custodial, instrumental, and medical aspects of caring for their parents. By engaging in activities that focused on the relational aspects of care, both parents and daughters were able to re-engage in activities that were a valued part of the family tradition.

Mr. Samanski progressed to the point where he could maneuver safely but required guidance climbing steps to spend time in his "real" bedroom. He resumed some of his self-care and spent time recreating his bedroom on the first floor, working on household bookkeeping and indoor gardening, and talking with his daughters. He attributed his adjustment to a somewhat normal way of life to the care provided by his daughters and the therapy that helped him get back into a routine.

The onset of Mrs. Samanski's and then Mr. Samanski's illnesses directly impacted roles, routines, and relationships for everyone in the family, as well as the physical and symbolic environment of their home. Their home became a space they jokingly referred to as a "house with a kitchen and five bedrooms."

The Clinical Reasoning Process

The occupational therapist drew upon the model of human occupation as a frame of reference guiding her clinical reasoning. An important part of her reasoning process involved a phenomenological perspective in which the clients' illness and family's caregiving experiences were a focal point. Key to this perspective was viewing the clients and family as "experts" and "teachers." Vickie viewed herself as the "learner."

Hasselkus (1990, p. 10) advocates using "ethnographic interviewing to elicit an understanding of the interviewee's point of view. Its aim is to gain insight into the subjective perspective of the person being interviewed." While Hasselkus used ethnographic interviewing with family caregivers, ethnographic interviewing also can be used successfully with the older adult client to understand his or her values, beliefs, and experiences. With an understanding of the client and the family caregiver's perspectives, a therapeutic plan can be developed that consists of treatment goals and outcomes that are mutually satisfying to all.

Table 17–1 provides general guidelines for using ethnographic interview-

Table 17–1. Ethnographic Interviewing

- The client and caregiver are viewed as experts and an understanding of their knowledge, views, beliefs, values, and customs is critical to develop a meaningful and relevant plan. The therapist is considered a facilitator in this process and a learner.

- The occupational therapy practitioner should avoid assuming an authoritative role during the interview by giving advice or telling the interviewee what to do.

- The interview is semistructured with a focus on learning more about the person's occupational history. The therapist should develop four to six global questions to guide the interview. The Occupational Performance History Interview (Kielhofner, Henry, & Walens, 1989) can be used as a reference.

- A helpful technique when interviewing is to incorporate terms used by the client or caregiver. This will require active listening on the part of the interviewer and clarification of terms to be sure the interviewee's point of view is understood.

- The occupational therapy practitioner should express interest in what the interviewee is saying. Verbal and nonverbal communication must be congruent.

- The occupational therapy practitioner should be honest with the interviewee by asking for clarification when something is not understood. This is an opportunity to better understand the interviewee.

- The interview should be asymmetrical, with the interviewee doing most of the talking.

- When learning to interview, the therapist should practice with an older adult who is willing to be a mentor, obtaining permission to audiotape the interview. When the interview is completed, the therapist should then analyze the audiotape and critique his or her ability to follow the above suggestions.

Table 17–2. The Client's Interview

The open-ended questions used during the ethnographic interview included:

1. What was your hospital and therapy experience like?
2. What was your typical day prior to hospitalization?
3. How did you spend your time prior to your hospitalization? With whom did you spend time? Where did you spend your time in your home? Where in the community did your spend time? What routines did you have? What roles did you have?
4. What is a typical day currently? Note what changes have occurred in your roles, routine, and environment.
5. In the present living situation, who are you residing with, what responsibilities do they have, what challenges or barriers do you face, and what strategies or adaptations have you found to be helpful?
6. What is of most concern to you?
7. How do you envision yourself in a month? What do you hope to accomplish with therapy?

Table 17-3. The Caregiver's Interview

The open-ended questions asked during the ethnographic interview included:

1. What was your typical day prior to assuming a "caregiver" role?
2. What is your typical day now? Note what changes have occurred in your roles, routine, and environment.
3. What is your present living situation? What responsibilities do you have? What challenges do you encounter? What strategies have you used?
4. What are you most concerned about?
5. What do you feel would help you most in your role as caregiver?
6. What do you hope therapy will accomplish?

ing. For more detailed information, the reader is referred to Hasselkus (1990) and Spradley (1979).

In the case study at the end of this chapter, the home-health therapist used ethnographic interviewing to gain understanding of each member of the family. Tables 17–2 and 17–3 provide a general outline of the questions used by the therapist to elicit the older adult client's and caregiver's perspectives. These are typical questions asked by an occupational therapist in an interview, but what makes the ethnographic interview different is the therapist's approach to understanding the experience of the client and caregiver. The prior discussion on ethnographic interviewing clarified the role and process used by the interviewer, which are critical to a productive interview.

ENVIRONMENTAL ASSESSMENT

Understanding physical and symbolic aspects of the home environment was an important part of understanding the Samanski family. Typically, the physical aspects of the client's environment are the focus, such as the number of steps, width of doorways, or the height of the bathtub. This information is important for ensuring the older adult's safe functioning in his or her home. However, the symbolic aspects of the environment reveal insight into the older adult's and family members' values and interests, which are critical in developing a meaningful treatment plan. In the Samanski's situation, to better understand both the physical and symbolic environments, the occupational therapist used an observation and interview guide that included:

1. Observing possessions such as photographs, knick-knacks, and mementos and asking about them during the interview

2. Understanding what events transpire in various rooms

3. Understanding the "surveillance zone" from the rooms in which clients spend most of their time

4. Noting rooms that older adults would like to access but that are "closed off" because of stairs or other barriers

5. Determining whether there are "special places" clients would like to escape to, like a workshop or hobby area, and if this "special place" could be recreated somewhere else in the home

6. Asking if clients get outside and have the opportunity to stay connected to their community.

For more resources on understanding the meaning of the home and assessing the physical and symbolic features of home environments, refer to

- Rowles, G. D. (1991). Beyond performance: Being in place as a component of occupational therapy. *American Journal of Occupational Therapy, 45*(3), 265–271.

- Rowles, G. D. (1983). Place and personal identity in old age: Observations from Appalachia. *Journal of Environmental Psychology, 3,* 299–313.

- Rowles, G. D. (1981). The surveillance zone as meaningful space for the aged. *Gerontologist, 21,* 304–311.

- Rubinstein, R. L. (1989). The home environment of older people: A description of the psycho-social processes linking person to place. *Journal of Gerontology, 44,* S45–S53.

- Rockwell-Dylla, L. (1992). Older adults, meaning of environment: Hospital and home. Unpublished master's thesis: Chicago: University of Illinois at Chicago.

Activities

Gaining Skills in Ethnographic Interviewing

This activity allows the interviewer to understand the older adult client and the family caregiver's needs, concerns, and experiences better. Each student will need to identify an older adult and a caregiver who are willing to be "mentors" for this exercise. For best results choose mentors who are verbal and willing to share their experiences. Ideally, the older adult mentor and caregiver should be a pair.

Before beginning the process, get permission from each to audiotape the interviews. Elicit the older adult's and caregiver's stories separately by using ethnographic interviews. These interviews should provide insight into the older adult's illness experience and the caregiver's experience. A minimum of two interview opportunities with each mentor is recommended.

Structure the interview with the questions Kaufman (1988) suggests to understand the client's and family's view of illness, how the illness is experienced, the meaning it has in the person's life, and what goals and needs the client and family have. After completing the interviews, listen to the audiotape and compare the two sets of interviews for themes that are similar and different. What assumptions were made about the older adult and the caregiver before meeting them? What was learned through the mentoring experience? How does the older adult frame the illness experience? How does the caregiver frame the illness experience? How have the older adult and the caregiver adapted to decreased abilities? What has been lost? What has replaced prior routines and roles?

The final part of this exercise is to have the student write a paper which synthesizes the above questions. This discussion on paper can also be the focus of a small group discussion with students sharing their interview experiences.

Consulting with Caregivers

This activity gives the reader an opportunity to develop skills in identifying and implementing services that assist and support family members to do the following:

- Take care of the care receiver
- Take care of themselves
- Get things done (Hasselkus, 1988).

Use Bower's five categories of caregiving to identify an approach (information, resources, support, strategies) an occupational therapist could use to address each of the caregiving areas.

- Anticipatory caregiving
- Preventive caregiving
- Supervisory caregiving
- Instrumental caregiving
- Protective caregiving.

Review Questions

1. List the most commonly expressed needs of caregivers.
2. Identify and give examples of the five categories of caregiving identified by Bowers.
3. Explain why is it important to consider the *meaning* of the client's and caregiver's experiences in planning treatment.
4. List and discuss the eight factors identified by Howard that constitute humanized care in the health professions.
5. Identify and discuss the skills that an occupational therapy practitioner needs to effectively collaborate with older adult clients and family members.
6. List and discuss the principles involved in client and family-practitioner collaboration.
7. List and discuss the general guidelines for ethnographic interviewing.
8. Identify assessment tools that can be used to understand the life story of an older adult client and caregiver.

Case Studies

CASE STUDY 1

The following is a case story designed for the occupational therapy student.

Katherine is a 60-year-old woman who last year suffered a left hemisphere CVA. At that time, she lived alone in a three-room apartment in a continuing care community complex. She received home-health occupational therapy and physical therapy and progressed to the point at which she was able to complete her self-care, cooking, and light-cleaning tasks independently, despite limited use of her right hand. She enjoyed cooking Italian food and visiting with friends she had made in the apartment building. She looked forward to her visits with her nieces, who are her only form of family support.

Recently, she suffered a fall, severely injuring herself, and was hospitalized for a month. She is now unable to return to her own apartment because of her inability to care for herself; she needs moderate assistance for ambulation, transferring, and completing self-care activities. Because of her decline in functioning, she had to relinquish her apartment and now resides on the second floor of the nursing home that comprises one of the levels of care in the continuing care community. Her physician has ordered OT and PT services.

As the OT on this case, identify what process you would use to gain understanding of Katherine's current situation. Identify the questions that would comprise your interview guide, and other assessment tools you would use to gain further understanding of Katherine's world. Discuss what goals and potential treatment activities you would suggest to Katherine, given the significant change in her functioning and place of residence.

CASE STUDY 2

The following is a case designed for the OT practitioner.

Walter is an 87-year-old man with a history of early stage Alzheimer's, a recent, mild left hemisphere CVA, and a history of two TIAs that occurred within the past month. Prior to the CVA and TIAs, he was able to drive and lived alone in a bungalow in a Chicago suburb. Due to further cognitive impairment, his doctors advised him to stop driving and recommended to his daughter that he not be left alone. His daughter Debbie has placed him in an adult day care program 2 days a week near her home, which is a 30-minute drive from Walter's own home.

Walter is able to ambulate independently and completes most of his self-care; however, he is unsteady at times. Walter says that he "doesn't have any problems," but according to Debbie, Walter has difficulty using his right hand for writing, cutting meat, tying, and zipping. She also feels he is unable to live alone and would like him to move in with her and her husband. Her father wishes to remain in his own home and community where he has resided for the past 40 years. Debbie would like her father to be able to use his right hand better and to be involved in activities to keep him occupied when at her house. She is trying to manage her own family, business, and home responsibilities, as well as take care of her father's needs.

As the OT practitioner referred to this case, consider what assessments and interventions you would use with Walter and Debbie. What questions would you ask Walter to understand his needs and goals better? What questions would you ask Debbie to understand her concerns with respect to Walter and her goals better?

Appendix.
Resources

INTERVIEW TOOLS

1. Kielhofner, G., Henry, A., & Walens, D. (1989). *A user's guide to the Occupational Performance History Interview*. Rockville, MD: American Occupational Therapy Association.

The Occupational Performance History Interview (OPHI) is a semi-structured interview tool providing a framework for gathering information about a client's life story. The interview is guided by a set of recommended questions that reflect a specific frame of reference and cover five content areas relevant to occupational performance: (a) organization of daily living routines; (b) life roles; (c) interests, values, and goals; (d) perceptions of ability and responsibility; and (e) environmental influences. The interview uses a five-point rating scale to determine the person's level of adaptation, and the interviewer writes a "Life History Narrative" describing the person's pattern of adaptation with respect to the five content areas. For specific information refer to the OPHI manual.

2. Baron, K., & Curtin, C. (1990). *A manual for use with the Self-Assessment of Occupational Functioning*. Unpublished manuscript, Department of Occupational Therapy, University of Illinois at Chicago.

The Self-Assessment of Occupational Functioning (SAOF) was designed to assist in collaborative treatment planning between the occupational therapy practitioner and the client. The SAOF consists of a series of self-statements corresponding to the model of human occupation and results in a profile of strengths and weaknesses from the client's point of view. For specific information, refer to the SAOF manual, which is available from the University of Illinois at Chicago.

3. Spradley, J. P. (1979). *The ethnographic interview*. Fort Worth, TX: Harcourt Brace Jovanovich College Publishers.

Hasselkus, B. R. (1990). Ethnographic interviewing: A tool for practice with family caregivers for the elderly. *Occupational Therapy Practice, 2*(1), 9–16.

Spradley and Hasselkus provide excellent resources for learning ethnographic interviewing. Hasselkus' article should be reviewed prior to giving an ethnographic interview.

4. For more information on interview tools, refer to

Kielhofner, G., Mallinson, T., & de las Heras, C. G. (1995). Methods of data gathering. In G. Kielhofner (Ed.), *A model of human occupation: Theory and application*. Baltimore: Williams & Wilkins.

CAREGIVER ASSESSMENT TOOLS

5. Lalonde, B. (1988). *Quality assurance manual of the home care association of Washington*. Edmonds, WA: Home Care Association of Washington.

The Caregiver Strain Scale was developed by the Home Care Association of Washington for eliciting information on the perceived subjective and objective stress experienced by family caregivers. This tool can be obtained from The Home Care Association of Washington, P.O. Box C-2016, Edmonds, WA 98020. Telephone: (206) 775-8120. For information on applying this tool in practice, refer to

Brittingham, K., & Dempster, M. (1990). Occupational therapists in home health care: Ensuring positive outcomes through collaboration. *OT Practice, 2*, 32–44.

References

Baginski, Y. (1995). Supporting family caregivers: It makes good business sense, too. *Caring Magazine, 14*(4), 30–34.

Baron, K., & Curtin, C. (1990). *A manual for use with the Self-Assessment of Occupational Functioning*. Unpublished manuscript, Department of Occupational Therapy, University of Illinois at Chicago.

Bazyk, S., & Trombino, B. (1990). Occupational therapy practice: Practice dilemmas. In P. M. Dougherty & M. V. Ramski (Eds.), *OT Practice, 2*(1), 84–89.

Benner, P., & Wrubel, J. (1989). *The primacy of caring: Stress and coping in health and illness*. Menlo Park, CA: Addison-Wesley.

Bishop, K. K., Woll, & Arango, P. (1993). *Family/professional collaboration for children with special health needs and their families*. Burlington, VT: Department of School Work, University of Vermont.

Bowers, B. J. (1987). Intergenerational caregiving: Adult caregivers and their aging parents. *Advances in Nursing Science, 9*(2), 20–31.

Corbin, J. M., & Strauss, A. (1990). Making arrangements. In J. F. Gubrium & A. Sankar (Eds.), *The Home care experience: Ethnography and policy*. Newbury Park: Sage.

Corcoran, M. A. (1993). Collaboration: An ethical approach to effective therapeutic relationships. *Topics in Geriatric Rehabilitation, 9*(1), pp. 21–29.

Cunningham, C., & Davis, H. (1985). *Working with parents: Frameworks for collaboration*. Philadelphia: Open University Press.

Gilfoyle, E. M. (1980). Caring: A philosophy for practice. *American Journal of Occupational Therapy, 34*(8), 517–521.

Gubrium, J. F. (1991). *The mosaic of care: Frail elderly and their families in the real world*. New York: Springer Publishing.

Harvath, T. A., Archbold, P. G., Stewart, B. J., Gadow, S., Kirschling, J. M., Miller, L., Hagan, J., Brody, K., & Schook, J. (1995). Establishing partnerships with family caregivers: Local and cosmopolitan knowledge. *Caring Magazine, 15*(4), 22–29.

Hasselkus, B. R. (1990). Ethnographic interviewing: A tool for practice with family caregivers for the elderly. *OT Practice, 2*(1), 9–16.

Hasselkus, B. R. (1988). Meaning in family caregiving: Perspectives on caregiver/professional relationships. *Gerontologist, 28*(5), 686–691.

Hasselkus, B. R. (1989). The meaning of daily activity in family caregiving for the elderly. *American Journal of Occupational Therapy, 43*(10), 649–656.

Howard, J. (1975). Humanization and dehumanization of health care. In J. Howard & A. Strauss (Eds.), *Humanizing Health Care*. New York: John Wiley & Sons.

Johnson, B. H., McGonigel, M. J., & Kaufmann, R. K. (Eds.). (1989). *Guidelines and recommended practices for the individualized family service plan*. Washington, DC: National Early Childhood Technical Assistance System, U.S. Department of Education.

Kaufman, S. R. (1988). Stroke rehabilitation and the negotiation of identity. In S. Reiharz & G. D. Rowles (Eds.), *Qualitative gerontology*. New York: Springer.

Kielhofner, G., Mallinson, T., & de las Heras, C. G. (1995). Methods of data gathering. In G. Kielhofner (Ed.), *A model of human occupation: Theory and application*. Baltimore: Williams & Wilkins.

Kielhofner, G., Henry, A., & Walens, D. (1989). *A user's guide to the occupational performance history interview.* Rockville, MD: American Occupational Therapy Association.

Lalonde, B. (1988). *Quality assurance manual of the home care association of Washington.* Edmonds, WA: Home Care Association of Washington.

Mintz, S. (1995). Family caregivers. *Caring Magazine, 14*(4), 7–10.

Rockwell-Dylla, L. (1992). *Older adults' meaning of environment: Hospital and home.* Unpublished master's thesis, University of Illinois at Chicago.

Rowles, G. D. (1983). Place and personal identity in old age: Observations from Appalachia. *Journal of Environmental Psychology, 3,* 299–313.

Rowles, G. D. (1981). The surveillance zone as meaningful space for the aged. *Gerontologist, 21,* 304–311.

Rowles, G. D. (1991). Beyond performance: Being in place as a component of occupational therapy. *American Journal of Occupational Therapy, 45*(3), 265–271.

Rubinstein, R. L. (1989). The home environment of older people: A description of the psychosocial processes linking person to place. *Journal of Gerontology, 44,* S45–S53.

Shelton, T. L., Jeppson, E. S., & Johnson, B. H. (1992). *Family-centered care for children with special health care needs.* Bethesda, MD: Association for the Care of Children's Health.

Shugars, D. A., O'Neil, E. H., & Bader, J. D. (Eds.). (1991). *Healthy America: Practitioners for 2005, an agenda for action for U.S. health professional schools.* Durham, NC: The Pew Health Professions Commission.

Spradley, J. P. (1979). *The ethnographic interview.* Fort Worth, TX: Harcourt Brace Jovanovich College Publishers.

Stone, R. (1991). Familial obligation: Issues for the 1990s. *Generations, 5*(Summer/Fall), 47–50.

Stoto, M. A., Behrens, R., & Rosemont, C. (1990). *Health people 2000: Citizens chart the course.* Washington, DC: National Academy Press.

Studt, E. (1975). Altering role relationships. In J. Howard & A. Strauss (Eds.), *Humanizing Health Care.* New York: John Wiley & Sons.

Tresolini, C. P., & the Pew-Fetzer Task Force. (1994). *Health Professions Education and Relationship-Centered Care.* San Francisco: Pew Health Professions Commission.

Yerxa, E. J. (1980). Occupational therapy's role in creating a future climate of caring. *American Journal of Occupational Therapy, 34*(8), 529–534.

Endnotes

1. Throughout this chapter the word *client* is used instead of *patient* to refer to older adults receiving services at any point on the continuum of care. Implicit in the word client is an understanding and expectation that the client, family, and practitioners actively collaborate in defining care options that best suit individual needs. This change in paradigm requires that practitioners reframe their thinking and behavior from a medieval or expert model of practice to a collaborative model in which client, family, and practitioners become partners in the caring process.

2. Note: This activity could be easily used as a professional development activity by a study group for therapists wanting to learn ethnographic interviewing.

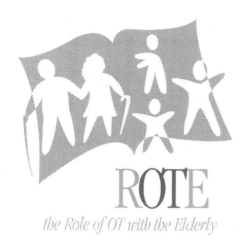

ROTE

the Role of OT with the Elderly

Keeping Current with Laws and Public Policy Issues That Influence Practice

Jeffrey L. Crabtree, MS, OTR/L, FAOTA

Abstract

This chapter teaches the basics of how to keep up with the information and policies that influence your practice. It offers a how-to approach to keeping current with the latest legal information and public mandates specifically related to occupational therapy services for older adults.

This chapter is divided into three sections. The first includes the generic categories of statutory law, written by the U.S. Congress, and administrative law, or rules and regulations, written by federal agencies. This section explains general sources and processes by which these laws are enacted. The second section focuses on specific programs, such as Medicare and the Older Americans Act. The third section discusses public policy issues, such as managed care. Each section provides the "first line" of resources for advances and changes in specific topics in the law, regulations, specific programs, and public policy issues.

The same resource organization may be noted several times. This practice should help the reader by placing the resource close to the topic discussed. The addresses and telephone numbers of resource organizations are in the alphabetical index of Resource Organizations at the end of this chapter.

The resources in this chapter are limited. If an exhaustive search of a law, a federal program, or a public mandate is necessary, additional resources will be required.

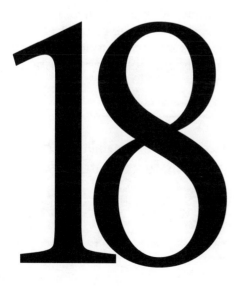

Section 1. Keeping Current with Legislation

Federal Legislation

Proposed legislation may be originated by a number of sources, from the President to a private citizen. Proposals are most often introduced as bills and numbered separately for the Senate and House in the order of their introduction during that congressional session. Other congressional actions similar to bills include joint resolutions, concurrent resolutions, and simple resolutions.

Once a bill is introduced, it is given a title and legislative number, and notice of its introduction is printed in the *Congressional Record*. The bill will go through a complex legislative process, the explanation of which is beyond the scope of this chapter. After its introduction and committee assignment, the proposed bill is sent to the U.S. Government Printing Office (GPO) for printing and made available to the public from the document rooms of both houses of Congress.

For example, Senate Bill S. 933 and its companion, H.R. 2273, were introduced in the Senate by Senator Harkin and in the House of Representatives by Representative Coelho on May 9, 1989

(see table 18–1). The purpose of these bills, according to their authors, was to establish a prohibition of discrimination on the basis of disability.

Upon either presidential approval or a congressional override of the president's veto, a bill becomes law. Its first official version is published in pamphlet form known as slip law. Copies of slip laws are available in all depository libraries or from Congress. S. 933 and H.R. 2273, once signed by

Table 18–2

Americans with Disabilities Act Cited as Public Law:
Americans with Disabilities Act of 1990,
Public Law P. L. 101–336
Congress #/ \Law #

the president, became The Americans with Disabilities Act of 1990 and Public Law 101–336 on July 26, 1990 (see table 18–2).

At the end of each session of Congress, the U.S. Government Printing Office publishes the *U.S. Statutes at Large*. This publication arranges laws in chronological order by date enacted. Each volume includes a subject index and tables that refer the reader to previous laws affected. Public Law 101–336, July 26, 1990, was published

Table 18–1

Americans with Disabilities Act in Bill Form
S. 933
H.R. 2273
Congressional Body/ \Bill #

Table 18–3

Americans with Disabilities Act as Cited in the *U.S. Statutes at Large*
Statute volume #\
Public Law P. L. 101–336   104 Stat. 327
Congress #/   \Law #   \page #

in volume 104, page 327, of the *U.S. Statutes at Large* (see table 18–3).

A law is formally referred to as an act. Title XVIII of the Social Security Act (P.L. 74–271), which established Health Insurance for the Aged or Disabled, or Medicare, is one example. Frequently, a law is also known by its popular name, by its sponsors, or by a later law amending the original legislation. For example, the Social Security Act is often referred to as the Social Security Amendments of 1965 (P.L. 89–97). Laws are also known by their public law number. One such law, P.L. 94–142, The Education for All Handicapped Children Act of 1975, is known to many occupational therapists as the law that mandates occupational therapy services to school-aged children with disabilities. The hyphenated number of a public law refers to the Congress in which the law was enacted and the chronological number of the law—in that order. Therefore, P.L. 94–142 was enacted during the 94th Congress (1975–76) and was the 142nd law passed in that Congress.

As though the names and numbers of laws are not confusing enough, laws are periodically codified and renumbered according to the Code of Laws of the United States. Table 18–4 indicates how the ADA is cited in the *United States Code (USC)*. As the chairman of the Committee on the Revision of the Laws of the House of Representatives explained when Congress first decided to institute a Code of Laws in 1926, the USC "is the official restatement in convenient form of the general and permanent laws of the United States" (USCA, 1983, p. xi). There are 50 titles of *United States Code*. Those of particular interest to occupational therapists who work with older adults are Title 29, which includes the ADA, and Title 42, which includes the Social Security Amendments of 1965 and the Older Americans Act of 1965.

Most laws and regulations contain large amounts of information not specifically related to occupational therapy services. Much of the information about reimbursement or about service eligibility, for example, is embedded in the verbiage of the law or regulations. Some sources have indexes that will help pinpoint the information, but others do not. In any case, while the search for needed information is seldom easy, the rewards are often worth the effort.

Information on the status of a bill can be found using the following resources:

1. Free copies of bills, committee reports, conference reports, and public laws are available through either the House or Senate Document Room, U.S. Capitol, Washington, D.C. Probably the easiest way to get copies of these is to call or write the local office of a U.S. representative or senator. Typically, a staff person will be able to send a copy of the bill or slip law requested. These offices are listed in the "U.S. Government" section of the telephone book, or the American Occupational Therapy Association (AOTA) can help.

2. Public and academic libraries, especially those with a government documents section, will have copies of slip laws and a variety of refer-

Table 18-4

Americans with Disabilities Act in U.S. Code as Law
42 USC §§12101-12213
Title #/ \Sections #

ence materials helpful in finding information about bills and laws.

The following list contains selected government sources of information about bills or public laws. Unless otherwise noted, these sources can be obtained from the U.S. Government Printing Office, Superintendent of Documents:

1. *The Congressional Record* provides daily coverage of House and Senate proceedings. *The Congressional Record* includes an index for each congressional session. The index includes a chronological history of Senate and House bills and resolutions. It is available on microfiche.

2. The *Monthly Catalog of U.S. Government Publications* offers a listing of the committee hearings, reports, and other information not published in *The Congressional Record.*

3. *Digest of Public General Bills and Resolutions,* published by the Library of Congress, Washington, DC, provides descriptions of daily legislative proceedings.

4. At the end of each session of Congress, the U.S. Government Printing Office publishes *U.S. Statutes at Large.* This publication arranges laws in chronological order by date enacted. Each volume includes a subject index and tables that refer the reader to any previous laws that may be affected by the current legislation.

Numerous commercial publications are helpful in gaining information about bills and public laws:

1. The *Congressional Information Service Index* (*CIS Index*) is a monthly service that includes catalogs, abstracts, and indexes of congressional publications issued during the previous month. Included in this service is the CIS/Microfiche Library containing bills organized by congressional numbers, and a *CIS/Annual* that includes abstracts of congressional publications and legislative history for all public laws enacted during the year. These are published by the Congressional Information Service, Inc.

2. The *Congressional Index,* published by Commerce Clearing House, a for-profit publisher, contains references to a wide variety of sources, including bills, committee hearings, and voting records of members of Congress.

3. The *CQ Weekly Report* and *Congressional Quarterly Almanac* are published by Congressional Quarterly. The *CQ Weekly Report* provides complete coverage of weekly legislative activity with quarterly indexes. The *Congressional Quarterly Almanac* furnishes a condensation of the *CQ Weekly Report's* coverage with commentary and summaries. For subscription information, contact Congressional Quarterly, Customer Services.

Special interest and trade groups can be an excellent source of information about bills and their status in Congress:

1. The American Occupational Therapy Association (AOTA) is one example of a special interest group that keeps current information about federal and state legislation of importance to occupational therapists. AOTA publishes information on federal legislative and regulatory developments regularly in *OT Week,* in *OT Practice,* and in the *AOTActionLine,* a bulletin published by the association's Government Relations Department. Additional resources, such as testimony and position papers, are available from the GRD.

2. The League of Women Voters is an example of a special interest group that focuses on issues of interest to the general public. The League often studies and reports on specific issues as well. The League of Women Voters of the United States has state and local chapters, which are listed in the telephone book.

3. American Association of Retired Persons (AARP) is a special interest group for older adults. They publish a number of resources useful to occupational therapists, and they track legislation they consider to be important to older Americans.

4. Families U.S.A. has grassroots lobbyists throughout each state. It publishes *Update* and a number of other publications containing information about federal legislation and federal agency actions important to older adults and their families.

5. National Citizens' Coalition for Nursing Home Reform (NCCNHR) is an advocacy group for residents of nursing homes, nursing home operators, and others who want to improve the care of people living in nursing homes. NCCNHR publishes a newsletter and a number of other publications related to nursing home laws and regulations.

6. American Federation of Home Health Agencies (AFHHA) represents interests of freestanding, hospital-based, and chain Medicare-certified home-health care agencies (HHA) in legislative and regulatory processes. Its publications include the *Insider* newsletter.

7. American Health Care Association (AHCA) is a national federation of associations representing more than 10,000 nonprofit and for-profit long-term-care (nursing home) providers. The AHCA publishes the *Provider* monthly.

8. American Hospital Association (AHA) represents more than 5,000 hospitals and has a number of personal membership groups. AHA publishes *Hospitals & Health Networks* and offers a number of educational activities, including national conferences.

9. National Association for Home Care (NAHC) is an association for providers of home-health and hospice-care services. The NAHC offers networking opportunities through its annual conference and regional meetings. This organization's publications include *Caring Magazine* and *Homecare News*.

10. Visiting Nurse Associations of America (VNAA) is an organization of more than 450 nonprofit community-based Visiting Nurse Associations that provide a wide range of services, including occupational therapy to older adults in their homes.

The following are sources of laws published in codified form:

1. Every 6 years a new edition of the *United States Code (USC)* is published. These editions cumulate, codify by topic, and incorporate by title the public laws appearing in *U.S. Statutes at Large*. The *USC* can be purchased from the Superintendent of Documents, U.S. Government Printing Office.

2. *United States Code Annotated (USCA)* is published by West Publishing Company. It is updated periodically and is organized according to the official code of laws of the United States. It includes annotations from federal and state courts.

State Legislation

Each state implements federal law differently; and, of course, each state generates its own laws. Despite this diversity, all states have elements in common: to become law, bills are written and passed in state legislatures and signed by the governor, and each state codifies those laws.

There are three generic sources of information about state laws related to occupational therapy services for older adults:

1. The American Occupational Therapy Association (AOTA), Government Relations Department, provides its members with local contacts and information about laws that pertain to individual states. In addition, the AOTA offers a number of publications on topics related to occupational therapy services to older adults.

2. State professional organizations have resources and information about specific state laws and will be able to put you in contact with individuals who are knowledgeable about issues specific to a state. In addition, trade associations, such as the American Federation of Home Health Agencies (AFHHA), the American Health Care Association (AHCA), the American Hospital Association (AHA), National Association for Home Care (NAHC), and the Visiting Nurse Associations of America (VNAA), have resources and information about specific state laws.

3. Some public and many academic libraries will have state government publications indexes as well as copies of state bills, statutory laws, administrative laws, and rules and regulations.

Federal Rules and Regulations

Administrative law consists of the rules and regulations issued by federal agencies, bureaus, commissions, and other units of the executive branch of the federal government. While statutory laws identify and prescribe legal directives, regulations and rules specify implementation of those laws. For example, the Health Care Financing Administration (HCFA) of the Department of Human and Health Services (DHHS) writes rules, regulations, and manuals that specify how Title XVIII of the Social Security Amendments of 1965, or Medicare, will be implemented. In this case, HCFA writes regulations that establish criteria for eligibility, delivery, and payment of federal health programs and services.

Once a government agency writes a draft of the regulations, they are published in the *Federal Register* as proposed rules for public response (see table 18–5). After a period of public review and after the agency has finalized the rules, they are published as Final Rules (regulations) in the *Federal Register* and are legally binding (see table 18–6). Annually, the final rules are codified by topic and added to the *Code of Federal Regulations (CFR)* (see table 18–7). The *CFR* and *U.S. Code* often share common title numbers. For example, Title 42, Public Health, of the *U.S. Code* and of the *CFR* includes law and regulations, respectively, dealing with Medicare. In the case of Medicare and Medicaid, the HCFA also publishes Medicare manuals that further explain the policies and procedures related to implementing Medicare services.

Table 18–5:

Americans with Disabilities Act in *Federal Register* as a Proposed Rule:

56 FR 8578 (February 28, 1991)
volume #/   \page #

Table 18–6

Americans with Disabilities Act in *Federal Register* as a Final Rule

56 FR 35544 (July 26, 1991)
volume #/   \page #

Table 18–7

Americans with Disabilities Act in *Code of Federal Regulations* as a Regulation:

36 CFR §1150
Title #/   \Section #

Information about the status of rules and regulations and how to find the actual wording of the rule or regulation can be found using the following government resources:

1. *The Federal Register (FR)* is a daily publication of the Office of Federal Register, National Archives and Records Service.

2. The U.S. Department of Commerce, National Technical Information Service (NTIS) publishes a comprehensive catalog of its holdings. Of the many useful publications available through NTIS, the HCFA Medicare manuals may be of the greatest value. These include the *Medicare: Coverage Issues Manual* (HCFA Pub. No. 6); *Outpatient Physical Therapy Provider Manual* (HCFA Pub. No. 9), which includes Occupational Therapy Services; and *Medicare: Skilled Nursing Facility Manual* (HCFA Pub. No. 12), to name only a few. These manuals,

along with HCFA laws and regulations, are also available on CD-ROM.

The following selected commercial publications are useful resources for researching rules and regulations:

1. *Health Administration: Laws, Regulations and Guidelines.* (Kander & May, 1977) offers commentary, explanation, and interpretive guidelines written by administrative agencies. The publication is updated at least quarterly.

2. *CCH Medicare and Medicaid Guide*, in four volumes, is published biweekly by Commerce Clearing House. This publication contains an overview of the programs and topical indexes (Vol. I); audits, usage, and quality review (Vol. II); federal Medicare requirements and state Medicaid requirements (Vol. III); and Medicare regulations, amendments, and a cumulative index (Vol. IV).

3. *Nursing Home Regulations: Survey, Certification and Enforcement Manual* is published by the Thompson Publishing Group. This is an annual subscription service that includes the basic manual containing the HCFA regulations pertinent to nursing homes and long-term care administration, monthly updates of changes in the regulations, and a monthly newsletter that, according to the publisher, offers accurate and timely information that will keep the subscriber "one step ahead" of frequent changes to the regulations.

4. *St. Anthony's Color-Coded Medicare Coverage Manual* is published by St. Anthony Publishing, Inc.

5. The Center for Medicare Advocacy, Inc., provides legal advice, self-help materials, and representation to the elderly and disabled of Connecticut who are unfairly denied Medicare coverage. While this free service is

offered exclusively to Connecticut residents, their self-help materials are very useful and apply to all Americans. The Center for Medicare Advocacy publishes a quarterly newsletter, *Center News*.

The primary government source of codified regulations is the *Code of Federal Regulations*. It is published by the Office of Federal Register, National Archives and Records Service, General Services Administration, Washington, D.C., and can be purchased from the Superintendent of Documents, U.S. Government Printing Office.

State Regulations

The states vary in how they implement federal laws; and, of course, each state has laws, rules, and regulations that are unique to that state. Despite this diversity, each state's implementation shares one element. Once a bill becomes law, some department or agency of the state government must write rules and regulations that explain how that law is to be implemented. Three generic sources of information about state rules and regulations relate to occupational therapy services for older adults.

1. The American Occupational Therapy Association (AOTA), Government Relations Department provides its members with local contacts and information about regulations that pertain to individual states. In addition, the AOTA offers a number of publications on topics of occupational therapy services to older adults.

2. State professional organizations have resources and information about specific state regulations and are able to make reference to individuals who are knowledgeable about specific issues. In addition, trade associations, such as the American Federation of Home Health Agencies (AFHHA), the American Health Care Association (AHCA), the American Hospital Association (AHA), National Association for Home Care (NAHC), and the Visiting Nurse Associations of America (VNAA) have resources and information about specific state rules and regulations.

3. Some public and many academic libraries have state government publications indexes and other resources for learning about state rules and regulations.

Section 2. Keeping Current with Government Programs

The Americans with Disabilities Act (ADA)

ADA provides a clear and comprehensive national mandate to end discrimination against individuals with disabilities and to bring persons with disabilities into the economic and social mainstream. In addition, the ADA is meant to provide enforceable standards addressing discrimination against individuals with disabilities. This law extends civil rights protections in employment, public accommodations, services provided by state and local governments, public and private transportation, and telecommunication relay services.

Primary resources for the text of the ADA (P.L. 101–336) and regulations can be found in the *United States Code* and the *Code of Federal Regulations,* respectively. Section I lists other resources, such as the *Congressional Information Service Index,* that are helpful in gaining information about ADA.

Various public and private institutions have useful information about specific portions of the ADA:

1. The American Occupational Therapy Association (AOTA) provides its members with the names of local occupational therapy experts and information about the ADA that pertains to individual states.

2. National Council on Disability is an independent federal agency working with the President and Congress to increase the inclusion, independence, and empowerment of all Americans with disabilities. The Council recently issued two reports, one titled *The Americans with Disabilities Act: Ensuring Equal Access to the American Dream,* and the other titled *Voices of Freedom: America Speaks Out on the ADA.* These reports offer information about the implementation, effectiveness, and impact of the ADA.

3. U.S. Architectural and Transportation Barriers Compliance Board (Access Board) disseminates information about building and transportation barriers related to the ADA.

4. U.S. Department of Justice, Civil Rights Division, Office on the Americans with Disabilities Act, disseminates information about public accommodation related to the ADA.

5. The Equal Employment Opportunity Commission, Office of Legal Counsel, is in charge of explaining and enforcing ADA's employment provisions.

6. The President's Committee on Employment of People with Disabilities offers brochures, fact sheets, and other general information on ADA.

7. Council of State Administrators of Vocational Rehabilitation refers inquiries to local vocational rehabilitation agencies.

8. State Governors' Committee on Employment of People with Disabilities offers brochures, fact sheets and other general information on ADA.

9. Trade and professional associations, such as the Aging Design Research Program of the AIA/ACSA Council on Architectural Research, the Human Factors and Ergonomics

Society, and the Interdisciplinary Society for the Advancement of Rehabilitative and Assistive Technology (RESNA), will have information about portions of the ADA.

Medicare

In very simple terms, Medicare is a federal health insurance program for people 65 or older, certain people with disabilities under 65, and people of any age who have permanent kidney failure. This program provides reimbursement for basic services, including occupational therapy in many circumstances, but it does not cover all medical expenses. There are two parts of Medicare: hospital insurance, often referred to as "Part A," and medical insurance, often referred to as "Part B." The hospital insurance is financed through part of the payroll tax that also pays for Social Security, and the medical insurance is financed in part by monthly premiums paid by enrollees.

Primary resources for the text of the Medicare law and regulations can be found in the *United States Code* and the *Code of Federal Regulations*, respectively. In addition, Section I lists other resources, such as the *Congressional Information Service Index*, the National Technical Information Service, and the American Occupational Therapy Association, as important sources of information about Medicare.

Medicaid

Medicaid, called MediCal in California, is a state-run program designed primarily to help those with low income and few or no resources. While the federal government helps pay for Medicaid, states have flexibility on eligibility standards and coverage of services.

Principal resources for the text of the Medicaid law and regulations can be found in the *United States Code* and the *Code of Federal Regulations*, respectively. Section I also lists publications such as the *Congressional Index* and the *Congressional Information Service Index* that contain useful information about Medicaid. In addition, the American Occupational Therapy Association, the National Association for Home Care, and the Visiting Nurses Associations of America mentioned in Section I also offer useful information about Medicaid.

Older Americans Act

The Older Americans Act of 1965 (OAA) is the creator of the Aging Network—a nationwide system of federal, state, and local agencies dedicated to providing support, nutrition, and other social services to older individuals. At the federal level, the Administration on Aging (AOA), within the Department of Health and Human Services, administers the majority of the OAA programs. The AOA oversees a network of state and area agencies on aging, which maintain responsibility for funding, coordinating, and managing the broad array of services, programs, and other initiatives for the elderly that are authorized by the OAA. Except for access services, in-home services, and legal assistance (priority areas specified in the act), OAA services are designed and funded in response to the needs of the elderly in individual communities.

Under the OAA structure, state agencies on aging receive federal funds for implementation of AOA-approved state plans on aging. Area agencies on aging (AAAs) then develop and fund services based on state-approved area plans on aging. AAAs deliver social services to the elderly population within their jurisdictions primarily through subgrants and contracts with local service providers.

The Older Americans Act, like many acts, requires Congressional reauthorization. Consequently, a number of Congressional reports of hearings and workshops, as well as government publications, are available. An example is a report of a workshop conducted by the Senate Special Committee on Aging. (Special Committee on Aging, U.S. Senate. [1991.] *Older Americans Act: 25 Years of Achievement: Findings and Policy Recommendations of the 1990 Workshops*. Washington, DC: U.S. Government Printing Office.)

See the Index of Resource Organizations for a list of the U.S. Administration on Aging Regional Offices. State and local agencies on aging should be listed in the blue pages of the telephone book.

Section 3.
Keeping Current with Public Policy Issues

Professional Education

Health care personnel shortages, especially in rural areas of the country, and personnel costs are among the compelling reasons for revamping professional education. Within the last few years, a number of states and organizations have undertaken studies and other activities to resolve these shortages and to reverse the rising cost of health care. One of the ideas generated from these efforts includes cross-training professionals to perform common tasks where there may be an overlap in certain patient-care settings between occupational therapy and other professions. An example might be to train nurses to make splints and train occupational therapists to give medications.

Information about this and other professional education issues and policies can be found using the following resources:

1. The American Occupational Therapy Association provides its members with information about a wide range of topics related to professional education. This effort includes continuing professional education by offering workshops across the country and presenting a major annual conference, with several days of institutes, courses, and other educational opportunities. The AOTA also keeps its members informed of policy trends in professional education and offers a number of publications on topics concerning occupational therapy services to older adults. Also, professional associations like the American Society on Aging (ASA), the Gerontological Society of America (GSA), and the Association for Gerontology in Higher Education (AGHE) offer support for professional education in the area of aging and provide direct educational experience to professionals.

2. Various government and private organizations have studied the personnel needs of the growing population of older adults. The National Institute on Aging (NIA), one of the National Institutes of Health, conducts and supports biomedical and behavioral research to increase the knowledge of the aging process and associated physical, psychological, and social factors resulting from advanced age. The NIA publishes a number of reports on the research it supports and on other issues. One such report is *Personnel for Health Needs of the Elderly Through the Year 2020*. (NIH Pub. No. 87–2950) Washington, DC: Department of Health and Human Services, 1987.

3. The Pew Health Professions Commission, as stated in a recent report, "was inspired by the belief that the education and training of health professionals is out of step with the evolving health needs of the American people" (Shugars, O'Neil, & Bader, 1991). Despite the controversial nature of the commission's recommendations, they are being taken seriously by education leaders and public policy makers.

Disease Prevention and Health Promotion

The Public Health Service's report, *Healthy People 2000: National Health Promotion and Disease Prevention Objectives* (1990) outlines the United States's disease prevention and health promotion agenda. As the report's introduction states, "This report frames the elements of that agenda from the perspective of the potential to prevent unnecessary disease and disability and to achieve a better quality of life for all Americans." Within the wide scope of this mandate, a number of prevention and health promotion goals related to older adults exist. These goals include reducing hip fractures and increasing the proportion of people with chronic and disabling conditions who receive information about community and self-help resources.

Information about disease prevention and health promotion issues and policies can be found using the following national resources and published reports:

1. Public Health Service. (1990). *Healthy people 2000: National health promotion and disease prevention objectives.* (DSHS Pub. No. [PHS] 91–50212). Washington, DC: U.S. Government Printing Office.

2. Public Health Service. (1993). *Healthy people 2000 review: National health promotion and disease prevention objectives. Midcourse revisions.* (DSHS Pub. No. [PHS] 91–1232–1). Washington, DC: U.S. Government Printing Office.

3. National Center for Health Statistics. (1983). *Health, United States, 1983.* (DHHS Pub. No. [PHS] 84–1232). Public Health Service. Washington, DC: U.S. Government Printing Office.

4. National Center for Health Statistics, Public Health Service, Centers for Disease Control and Prevention, U.S. Department of Health and Human Services, among its many functions, collects, maintains, analyzes, and disseminates national data on health status and health services. One such publication is as follows:

    Van Nostrand, F., Furner, S. E., Suzman, R. (1993). (Eds.). Health data on older Americans: United States, 1992. *Vital Health Statistics 3*(27).

5. U.S. Senate Special Committee on Aging, the American Association of Retired Persons, the Federal Council on the Aging, and the U.S. Administration on Aging. (1991). *Aging America: Trends and projections.* (DHHS Pub. No. [FCoA] 91–28001). Washington, DC: U.S. Department of Health and Human Services.

Each state varies in how it implements national mandates. There are three generic sources of information about state disease prevention and health promotion related to occupational therapy services to older adults:

1. The American Occupational Therapy Association (AOTA) Government Relations Department provides its members with local contacts and information about health promotion efforts that pertains to individual states. In addition, the AOTA offers a number of publications on topics of occupational therapy services to older adults.

2. State professional organizations have resources and information about state-level disease prevention and health-promotion efforts. Also, trade associations, such as the American Federation of Home Health Agencies (AFHHA), and the Visiting Nurse Associations of America (VNAA), have state-level affiliates that have useful resources for information about state-level disease prevention and health promotion mandates.

3. Most public and academic libraries will have information about state government and private efforts to prevent disease and promote health.

Managed Care and Health Care Reform

Managed care is a difficult term to define. It seems to mean very different things to different people. In simplistic terms, the phrase is used to describe a broad range of delivery systems meant to control quality and use of services, as well as control clinical cost and operational expense. Health care reform, on the other hand, probably conjures similar images for most people in the health care field: Rising health care costs, overuse of technology and other services, cost shifting, excess capacity, uneven distribution of health care professionals, and many other problems.

Within the political context of managed care and health care reform, the Government Relations Department of the AOTA actively lobbies for needed changes in bills and existing laws and regulations. Many recent proposed bills included in the rubric of managed care or health care reform have serious implications for the population occupational therapists typically serve, as well as for occupational therapy practitioners themselves. One is the establishment of protections for patient rights, such as access to occupational therapy in Medicare and Medicaid managed care plans. "AOTA is seeking antidiscrimination or nonexclusion language prohibiting health plans from arbitrarily eliminating entire classes of health professionals from their networks based solely on the license or certification they hold and ensuring that health plans have sufficient number, mix, and distribution of health care professionals to meet consumer needs" (*OT Week*, October 5, 1995).

AOTA provides its members information about a wide range of topics related to managed care, from addresses and phone numbers of HCFA Regional Offices and state insurance commissioners, to specific information about recent decisions and long-term trends in managed care and health care reform. In addition, the AOTA offers a number of publications on topics concerning occupational therapy services to older adults.

Information about managed care and other health care reform issues and policies can be found using other resources, including books and article review subscription services, that help track trends in managed care:

1. Faulkner & Gray's Healthcare Information Center offers a twice-monthly publication entitled *Medical outcomes and guidelines alert*. This publication, according to its publishers, offers news and analysis on developments and issues from business, payers, insurers, and providers related to medical outcomes and practice guidelines.

2. *Inside Health Care Reform* is a monthly publication that includes news and analysis of administration proposals, bills in Congress, and positions of the American Hospital Association, the American Medical Association, and other leading organizations in the field of health care. This is published by Atlantic Information Services, Inc.

3. O'Leary, M. R., et al. (1994). *Lexikon: Dictionary of health care terms, organizations, and acronyms for the era of reform*. Oakbrook Terrace, IL: Joint Commission on Accreditation of Healthcare Organizations.

4. Weiner, & de Lissovy, (1993). Raising a tower of Babel—A taxonomy of managed care & health insurance plans. *The Journal of Health Politics, Policy, and Law, 18*(1), 75–103. This article includes a comprehensive glossary of terms, reviews past and current trends in

the market for nontraditional health benefit plans, and proposes a system of classification that will aid in understanding how managed care plans differ from conventional health insurance.

5. Fazen, M. F. (1994). *Managed Care Desk Reference: The Complete Guide to Terminology and Resources*. Dallas: HCS Publications. This useful book contains a comprehensive glossary and information about government and private resources important to understanding managed care.

6. Trade associations, such as American Hospital Association (AHA), National Association for Home Care (NAHC), and the Visiting Nurse Associations of America (VNAA), have state-level affiliates that are useful resources for information about managed care and health reform mandates.

Standards of Care and Quality of Care

American taxpayers and beneficiaries of federally mandated programs, such as Medicare, have a stake in getting the best quality of service possible given the existing resources. The means of securing quality of services includes government regulations, organizational accreditation, professional standards of practice, and institutional internal quality improvement programs, to name a few. Federal laws, such as the Social Security Act, often mandate particular standards of care for nursing homes and other Medicare providers, and government regulations spell out how those standards are to be met. In addition, professional organizations such as the AOTA publish position papers, guidelines, and practice standards for their members.

A few recent examples of articles published by the AOTA are cited here:

1. American Occupational Therapy Association. (1995). Statement: Psychosocial concerns within occupational therapy practice. *American Journal of Occupational Therapy, 49*(10), 1011–1013.

2. American Occupational Therapy Association. (1995). Elements of clinical documentation (Revision). *American Journal of Occupational Therapy, 49*(10), 1032–1035.

3. American Occupational Therapy Association. (1994). Uniform terminology (3rd edition). *American Journal of Occupational Therapy, 48*(11), 1047–1054.

4. American Occupational Therapy Association. (1994). Statement: Occupational therapy services for persons with Alzheimer's disease and other dementias. *American Journal of Occupational Therapy, 48*(11), 1029–1031.

5. American Occupational Therapy Association. (1994). Statement of occupational therapy referral. *American Journal of Occupational Therapy, 48*(11), 1034.

6. American Occupational Therapy Association. (1994). Position paper: Occupational therapy and long-term services and supports. *American Journal of Occupational Therapy, 48*(11), 1035–1036.

7. American Occupational Therapy Association. (1994). Occupational therapy code of ethics. *American Journal of Occupational Therapy, 48*(11), 1037–1038.

8. American Occupational Therapy Association. (1994). Standards of practice for occupational therapy. *American Journal of Occupational Therapy, 48*(11), 1039–1043.

9. American Occupational Therapy Association. (1994). Guide for supervision of occupational therapy personnel. *American Journal of*

Occupational Therapy, 48(11), 1045–1046.

10. American Occupational Therapy Association. (1993). Position paper: Occupational therapy and the Americans with Disabilities Act (ADA). *American Journal of Occupational Therapy, 47*(12), 1083–1084.

11. American Occupational Therapy Association. (1993). Core values and attitudes of occupational therapy practice. *American Journal of Occupational Therapy, 47*(12), 1085–1086.

Many institutions that provide services to older adults are accredited by The Joint Commission on Accreditation of Healthcare Organizations (JCAHO). JCAHO was established in 1951 as a private, not-for-profit organization whose mission is to improve the quality of health care provided to the public. JCAHO accredits ambulatory care, home care, hospital long-term care, and mental health institutions. JCAHO offers a number of services in addition to accreditation of health care organizations. These include standards setting, evaluation, education, consultation, and publication of information pertinent to current standards of care and quality of care. One such publication is *A Guide to Establishing Programs for Assessing Outcomes in Clinical Settings.*

In terms of national governmental oversight, the Health Care Financing Administration (HCFA), which administers the Medicare program nationally, typically contracts with state agencies to monitor how Medicare providers meet Medicare standards of care. In addition, ombudsman offices mandated by the Older Americans Act respond to complaints about care received from Medicare providers.

Three generic sources of information about state-level efforts to establish and monitor standards of health care for older adults will be useful:

1. The American Occupational Therapy Association (AOTA) has a cadre of Quality Assurance Consultants. In addition, the AOTA offers a number of publications on topics concerning occupational therapy services to older adults.

2. State professional organizations have resources and information about specific state efforts and can make references to individuals who are knowledgeable about specific issues. Also, trade associations such as the American Health Care Association (AHCA), the American Hospital Association (AHA), and the Visiting Nurse Associations of America (VNAA), have state-level affiliates with useful resources for information about state-level professional standards and quality-of-care mandates.

3. Some public and many academic libraries have information about state agency contracts with HCFA to monitor Medicare providers' performance, in addition to local government efforts to establish standards and quality of care.

General Information Resources

1. The American Occupational Therapy Association (AOTA) provides its members with information and services relating to virtually all of the topics and issues contained in this chapter. The AOTA offers a number of publications on topics concerning occupational therapy services to older adults.

2. World Health Organization. (1980). *International Classification of Impairments, Disabilities, and Handicaps.* Geneva: World Health Organization.

3. *Healthcare Leadership Review*, according to COR Healthcare Resources, the publishers, sifts through more than 150 health care journals, newsletters, and magazines to pull out the most innovative ideas, significant trends, and developing issues and publishes these in readable summaries.

4. *HeadsUp*, a subscription service of Individual, Inc., provides customized reports by allowing subscribers to choose up to 10 specific topics within six health care categories. The categories include general health care (e.g., health economics, Medicare, and Medicaid), medical delivery services (e.g. home-health services, long-term care, and national managed care companies), and clinical areas and pharmaceuticals (e.g., central nervous system disorders, gerontology, and muscular and neuromuscular diseases).

5. National Archive of Computerized Data on Aging (NACDA) is a project of the Interuniversity Consortium for Political and Social Research. This organization concentrates on domestic and international issues on aging and health issues. It provides data on these issues through media such as magnetic tape, diskettes, and electronic network file transfers. In addition, NACDA publishes a bulletin and catalogue of its collections and offers seminars.

6. The Agency for Health Care Policy and Research (AHCPR) is a new organization within the Public Health Service (PHS) and may be eliminated in the wake of health care reform. The agency's primary goals are to promote effective, appropriate, high-quality health care, increase access to care, and improve the way health services are organized, delivered, and financed.

These goals are realized through a number of AHCPR offices and centers (e.g., the Center for Medical Effectiveness Research and the Office of Health Technology Assessment). These components of AHCPR award grants for a wide range of activities including examination of managed care and assessment of the quality of the process, outcomes of coordinated care, and health care of the aged and disabled, including long-term care. For more information contact: Information and Publications Division, Agency for Health Care Policy and Research, Executive Office Center, 2101 East Jefferson Street, Suite 501, Rockville MD 20852, (800)358–9295, (301)594–2283 (Fax).

7. Thomas, R. K., Pol, L. G., & Sehnert, W. F. (1994). *Health Care Book of Lists*. GR Press, Inc. This book contains 338 tables of data and other information about a range of topics from health status and mortality to demographics and data on medical and health education.

8. Nolan, J. R., & Nolan-Haley, J. M. (1990). *Black's Law Dictionary*. St. Paul, MN: West Publishing.

A number of professional organizations, including AOTA, exist to support service, education, and research in the area of aging. Among these are the American Society on Aging (ASA) and the Gerontological Society of America (GSA):

1. The ASA offers forums, networks, and affiliate groups, such as the Mental Health and Aging and the Aging, Disability, and Rehabilitation Networks, within ASA for those interested in specific areas of aging. The ASA holds an annual conference and multiple seminars throughout the country for professionals and the public. It also pub-

lishes newsletters of the specialty networks and *Generations*, an in-depth quarterly journal that deals with one issue at a time.

2. GSA is composed of professionals representing a variety of disciplines. It holds an annual conference and other meetings throughout the year. It publishes a newsletter and three bimonthly journals: *The Gerontologist; The Journal of Gerontology Series A: Biological Sciences and Medical Sciences; and The Journal of Gerontology Series B: Psychological Sciences and Social Sciences.*

In addition to professional organizations, many centers and institutes exist, often associated with universities that, while not dedicated specifically to aging, provide resources about ethics and aging. These include but are not limited to the following three:

1. The Hastings Center is a nonprofit, nonpartisan organization that carries out educational and research programs on ethical issues in medicine, the life sciences, and the professions. The Hastings Center publishes the bimonthly journal entitled *Hastings Center Report.*

2. Kennedy Institute of Ethics, which operates the National Reference Center for Bioethics Literature, Georgetown University, Washington, D.C.

3. The Center for Biomedical Ethics, University of Minnesota, publishes a newsletter and a number of "Reading Packets" and special reports on subjects of interest to those working with older adults.

Each component of the health care industry has its trade association. The following is a list of many trade associations of interest to occupational therapists working with older adults.

Virtually all of these organizations have state-level affiliates that are useful resources for information about government programs and public mandates:

1. American Federation of Home Health Agencies (AFHHA). This group represents interests of free-standing, hospital-based, and chain Medicare-certified home health care agencies (HHA) in legislative and regulatory processes. Its publications include the *Insider* newsletter.

2. American Health Care Association (AHCA) is a national federation of associations representing over 10,000 nonprofit and for-profit long-term-care (nursing home) providers. The AHCA publishes the *Provider* monthly.

3. American Hospital Association (AHA) represents more than 5,000 hospitals and has a number of personal membership groups. AHA publishes *Hospitals* and *Health Networks* and offers a number of educational activities including national conferences.

4. National Association for Home Care (NAHC) is an association for providers of home health and hospice care services. The NAHC offers networking opportunities through its annual conference and regional meetings. This organization's publications include *Caring Magazine* and *Homecare News.*

5. Visiting Nurse Associations of America (VNAA) is an organization of more than 450 nonprofit, community-based Visiting Nurse Associations that provide a wide range of services, including occupational therapy to older adults in their homes.

Appendix A.

RESOURCE ORGANIZATIONS

Agency for Health Care Policy and
    Research (AHCPR)
Publications Clearing House
P.O. Box 8547
Silver Spring, MD 20907–8547
(800) 358-9295
(301) 594-2280 (Fax)

Aging Design Research Program
AIA/ACSA Council on Architectural
    Research
1735 New York Avenue, NW
Washington, DC 20006
(202) 626-7300

American Association of Retired
    Persons
601 E Street, NW
Washington, DC 20049
(202) 434-2277

American Federation of Home Health
    Agencies (AFHHA)
1320 Fenwick Lane, Suite 100
Silver Spring, MD 20910
(301) 588-1454
(301) 588-4732 (Fax)

American Health Care Association
    (AHCA)
1201 L Street, NW
Washington, DC 20005-4014
(202) 842-4444
(202) 842-3860

American Hospital Association (AHA)
One N. Franklin
Chicago, IL 60606
(312) 442-3000
(312) 442-4796 (Fax)

American Occupational Therapy
    Association (AOTA)
4720 Montgomery Lane
P.O. Box 31220
Bethesda, MD 20824-1220
(301) 652-2682 (Nonmembership
    number)
(800) 729-2682 (Membership
    service line)
(800) 377-8555 (TDD)

American Psychiatric Association
1400 K Street, NW
Washington, DC 20005
(202) 682-6000
(202) 682-6114

American Society on Aging (ASA)
833 Market Street, Suite 511
San Francisco, CA 94103-1824
(415) 974-9600
(415) 974-0300 (Fax)

Association for Gerontology in Higher
    Education (AGHE)
1001 Connecticut Avenue, NW,
    Suite 410
Washington, DC 20036-5504
(202) 429-9277

Atlantic Information Services, Inc.
1100 17th Street, NW, Suite 300
Washington, DC 20036
(202) 775-9008
(202) 331-9542

Center for Biomedical Ethics
University of Minnesota
UMHC Box 33
Harvard Street at East River Road
Minneapolis, MN 55455
(612) 625-4917

Center for Medicare Advocacy
P.O. Box 350
Willimantic, CT 06266
(203) 456-7790

Commerce Clearing House (CCH)
4025 W. Peterson Avenue
Chicago, IL 60646
(312) 866-6000
(312) 866-3895

Congressional Information Service, Inc.
    (CIS)
4520 East-West Highway
Bethesda, MD 20814
(301) 654-1550
(301) 654-4033 (Fax)

Congressional Quarterly (CQ)
    Customer Services
1414 22nd Street, NW
Washington, DC 20037
(800) 854-9043

COR Healthcare Resources
P.O. Box 40959
Santa Barbara, CA 93140-0959
(805) 564-2177
(805) 564-2146 (Fax)

Council of State Administrators of
Vocational Rehabilitation
P.O. Box 3776
Washington, DC 20007
(202) 638-4634

Equal Employment Opportunity
Commission
Office of Legal Counsel
1801 L Street, NW
Washington, DC 20507
(800) 872-3362
(202) 663-4691
(202) 663-7026 (TDD)

Faulkner & Gray's Healthcare
Information Center
P.O. Box 27758
Washington, DC 20077-1343

Families U.S.A.
1334 G Street, NW
Washington, DC 20005
(202) 737-6340

Gerontological Society of America
(GSA)
1275 K Street, NW, Suite 350
Washington, DC 20005-4006
(202) 842-1275

Governor's Committee on
Employment of People with
Disabilities
Hastings Center
255 Elm Road
Briarcliff Manor, NY 10510
(914) 762-8500

Human Factors and Ergonomics
Society
P.O. Box 1369
Santa Monica, CA 90406
(310) 394-1811
(310) 394-2410

Individual, Inc.
8 New England Executive Park
Burlington, MA 01803
(800) 414-1000

Interdisciplinary Society for the
Advancement of Rehabilitative
and Assistive Technology (RESNA)
1700 N. Moore Street, Suite 1540
Arlington, VA 22209
(703) 524-6686
(703) 524-6630 (Fax)

Joint Commission on Accreditation of
Healthcare Organizations (JCAHO)
One Renaissance Boulevard
Oakbrook Terrace, IL 60181
(708) 916-5800

Kennedy Institute of Ethics
National Reference Center for
Bioethics Literature
Georgetown University
Washington, DC 20057
(202) 687-3885

League of Women Voters of the
United States
1730 M Street, NW
Washington, DC 20036

Medicode (formerly Med-Index
Publications)
5225 Wiley Post Way, Suite 500
Salt Lake City, UT 84116-2889
(800) 999-4600

National Archive of Computerized
Data on Aging (NACDA)
Inter-University Consortium for
Political and Social Research
P.O. Box 1248
Ann Arbor, MI 48106
(313) 764-8392

National Association for Home Care
(NAHC)
519 C Street, NE
Washington, DC 20002-5809
(202) 547-7424
(202) 547-3540 (Fax)

National Center for Health Statistics
Centers for Disease Control and
Prevention
Public Health Service
U.S. Department of Health and
Human Services
6525 Belcrest Road
Hyattsville, MD 20782
(301) 436-8500

National Citizens' Coalition for
  Nursing Home Reform (NCCNHR)
  1224 M Street, NW, Suite 301
  Washington, DC 20005
  (202) 393-2018

National Council on Disability
  1331 F Street, NW, Suite 1050
  Washington, DC 20004-1107
  (202) 272-2004
  (202) 272-2074 (TTD)
  (202) 272-2022 (Fax)

National Council on the Aged, Inc.
  (NCOA)
  600 Maryland Avenue, SW
  West Wing 100
  Washington, DC 20024

National Health Council, Inc.
  350 5th Avenue, Suite 1118
  New York, NY 10118
  (212) 268-8900

National Technical Information Service
  (NTIS)
  5285 Port Royal Road
  Springfield, VA 22161
  (703) 487-4630
  (703) 321-8547 (Fax)

Office of Federal Register
  National Archives and Records
  Service
  General Services Administration
  Washington, DC

Pew Health Professions Commission
  UCSF Center for Health
  Professions
  1388 Sutter Street, Suite 805
  San Francisco, CA 94109
  (415) 476-8181
  (415) 476-4113

President's Committee on Employment
  of People with Disabilities
  1331 F Street, NW, Room 636
  Washington, DC 20004
  (202) 372-6200
  (202) 372-6219 (Fax)

St. Anthony Publishing, Inc.
  P.O. Box 96561
  Washington, DC 20090
  (800) 632-0123

U.S. Architectural and Transportation
  Barriers Compliance Board,
  Office of General Counsel
  (Access Board)
  1331 F Street, NW, Suite 1000
  Washington, DC 20004-1111
  (800) 872-2253 (voice or TDD)
  (202) 653-7834

U.S. Department of Justice
  Civil Rights Division
  Office on the Americans with
  Disabilities Act
  P.O. Box 66118
  Washington , DC 20035-6118
  (202) 514-0301
  (202) 514-0381 (TDD)

U.S. Government Printing Office
  P.O. Box 371954
  Pittsburgh, PA 15250-7954
  (202) 512-2250
  (202) 512-1800 (Fax)

Visiting Nurse Associations of America
  (VNAA)
  3801 E. Florida Avenue, Suite 206
  Denver, CO 80210
  (303) 753-0218
  (303) 753-0258 (Fax)

West Publishing Company
  P.O. Box 64779
  St. Paul, MN 55164-0779
  (612) 228-2500

Appendix B

U.S. ADMINISTRATION ON AGING REGIONAL OFFICES

Region I
(Rhode Island, Vermont,
Connecticut, Maine,
Massachusetts, and New
Hampshire)
Administration on Aging
John F. Kennedy Building,
Room 2075
Boston, MA 02203
(617) 565-1158

Region II
(New York, New Jersey, Puerto Rico,
and Virgin Islands)
Administration on Aging
26 Federal Plaza, Room 38–102
New York, NY 10278
(212) 264-2978 or 2977

Region III
(District of Columbia, Maryland,
Virginia, Delaware, Pennsylvania,
and West Virginia)
Administration on Aging
P.O. Box 13716—Stop 23
Philadelphia, PA 19101
(215) 596-6891 or 6900

Region IV
(Alabama, Florida, Mississippi,
South Carolina, Tennessee, North
Carolina, Kentucky, and Georgia)
Administration on Aging
101 Marietta Towers, Suite 903
Atlanta, GA 30323
(404) 331-5900

Region V
(Illinois, Indiana, Michigan,
Minnesota, Ohio, and Wisconsin)
Administration on Aging
105 West Adams Street, 20th Floor
Chicago, IL 60603
(312) 353-3141

Region VI
(Arkansas, Louisiana, Oklahoma,
New Mexico, and Texas)
Administration on Aging
1200 Main Tower Building,
Room 1000
Dallas, TX 75201
(214) 767-2972

Region VII
(Iowa, Kansas, Missouri, and
Nebraska)
Administration on Aging
601 East 12th Street, Room 384
Kansas City, MO 64106
(816) 426-2955

Region VIII
(Colorado, Montana, Utah,
Wyoming, North Dakota, and
South Dakota)
Administration on Aging
1961 Stout Street, Room 308
Federal Office Building
Denver, CO 80294
(303) 844-2951

Region IX
(California, Nevada, Arizona,
Hawaii, Guam, Northern Mariana
Islands, and American Samoa)
Administration on Aging
50 United Nations Plaza, Room 480
San Francisco, CA 94102
(415) 556-6003

Region X
(Alaska, Idaho, Oregon, and
Washington)
Administration on Aging
Blanchard Plaza, RX-33, Room 1202
2201 Sixth Avenue
Seattle, WA 98121
(206) 553-5341

References

Adams, P. F., & Marano, M. A. (1995). Current estimates from the National Health Interview Survey, 1994. *Vital and Health Statistics, (10)*, 193.

Egan, M. (1992). HMO contracts: Partnerships for the future. *OT Week, (6)*40, 14–15.

Fazen, M. F. (1994). *Managed care desk reference: The complete guide to terminology and resources.* Dallas: HCS.

Feinleib, M. (Ed.). Proceedings of the 1991 International Symposium on Data on Aging. *Vital Statistics (5)*7.

Fulton, J. P., Katz, S., Jack, S. S., & Hendershot, G. E. (1989). Physical functioning of the aged: United States, 1984. *Vital Statistics (10)*167.

Kander, M. L., & May, K. (Eds.). (1977). *Health administration: Laws, regulations, and guidelines.* Owings Mills, MD: National Health Publishing Limited Partnership.

Kearney, D. S. (1992). *The new ADA: Compliance and costs.* Kingston, MA: R. S. Means Company.

National Center for Health Statistics. (1983). *Health, United States, 1983.* (DHHS Pub. No. [PHS] 84-1232.) Public Health Service, Washington, DC: U.S. Government Printing Office.

O'Leary, J. R., et al. (1994). *Lexikon: Dictionary of health care terms, organizations, and acronyms for the era of reform,* Oakbrook Terrace, IL: Joint Commission on Accreditation of Healthcare Organizations.

O'Neil, E. H., Shugars, D. A., & Bader, J. D. (Eds.). (1993). *Health professions education for the future: Schools in service to the nation.* San Francisco: Pew Health Professions Commission.

Pew Health Professions Commission. (1995). Critical challenges: Revitalizing the health professions for the twenty-first century. San Francisco: UCSF Center for the Health Professions.

Public Health Service. (1990). *Healthy people 2000: National health promotion and disease prevention objectives.* (DSHS Pub. No. [PHS] 91-50212). Washington, DC: U.S. Government Printing Office.

Public Health Service. (1993). *Healthy people 2000 review. National health promotion and disease prevention objectives. Midcourse revisions.* (DSHS Pub. No. [PHS] 91-1232-1). Washington, DC: U.S. Government Printing Office.

Robinson, J. S. (1993). *Tapping the government grapevine: The user-friendly guide to U.S. government information sources* (2nd ed.). Phoenix: Oryx.

Roper, F. W., & Boorkman, J. A. (1984). *Introduction to reference sources in the health sciences.* Chicago: Medical Library Association.

Sears, J. L., & Moody, M. K. (1994). *Using government information sources: Print and electronic* (2nd ed.). Phoenix: Oryx.

Shugars, D. A., O'Neil, E. H., & Bader, J. D. (1991). *Healthy Americans: Practitioners for 2005, an agenda for action for U.S. health professional schools.* Durham, NC: Pew Health Professions Commission.

Thomas, R. K., Pol, L. G., & Sehnert, W. F. (1994). *Health care book of lists.* GR Press.

U.S. Senate Special Committee on Aging, American Association of Retired Persons, Federal Council on Aging, and Administration on Aging. (1991). *Aging America: Trends and projections.* (DHHS Pub. No. [FCoA] 91-28001.) Washington, DC: U.S. Department of Health and Human Services.

Van Nostrand, J. F., Furner, S. E., & Suzman, R. (Eds.). (1993). *Health data on older Americans: United States, 1992. Vital Health Statistics* 3(27).

Wickliffe, J., & Sowada, E. (1992). *The Federal Register: What it is and how to use it.* Washington, DC: Office of the Federal Register, National Archives and Records Administration.

World Health Organization. (1980). Geneva: World Health Organization.

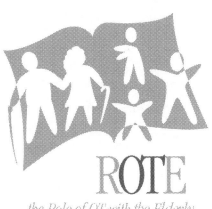

Index

the Role of OT with the Elderly

Index

Note: Page numbers in bold type indicate tables and figures, while page numbers in italic type indicate photographs.

Americans With Disabilities Act. *See also* Federal government
  environmental considerations and, 391, 398
  nonhuman environment tools of practice and, 128
  provisions, 29, 149–150
  reasonable accommodation and, 708–709, 711
  resources, 863, 869–870
  work and, 707–709

AMPS. *See* Assessment of Motor and Process Skills

Analysis and synthesis as tools of practice, 126–127, 730

Analytic frames of reference, 114, 115

Andragogy, 810–812, **812**

Angina pectoris, description, 184

An Annotated Index of Occupational Therapy Evaluation Tools, 522

Anticipation, as adaptive strategy, 60

Anticipatory caregiving, 839

Anxiety, as problem of the elderly, 610–611

AoA. *See* U.S. Administration on Aging

A-ONE. *See* Arnadottir OT-ADL Neurobehavioral Evaluation

AOTF. *See* American Occupational Therapy Foundation

Apartments, environmental considerations, 384

ARDs. *See* Alzheimer's related disorders

Area agencies on aging, resources, 870–871

Arm movement, environmental considerations, 393

Arnadottir OT-ADL Neurobehavioral Evaluation, 528, 531

Arteriosclerosis, description, 183

Arthritis
  depression and, 223
  joint changes in older adults and, 180
  joint replacement, 56
  occupational therapy needs, 26
  pain response testing and, 553–554
  sexual function and, 682
  sleep disturbances and, 243

Arthritis Foundation (OH), 431

Arts and crafts groups, 783

Asian culture, view of aging, 271–272

Assessment of Motor and Process Skills

cross-cultural application of, 521
description, 31
  inpatient rehabilitation evaluation process and, 352

Assessment of the Elderly, 522

Assessments, 31–32. *See also* Evaluation considerations; Outcome measures; *specific assessments by name; specific areas of practice, e.g., Community-based practice; specific performance area, context, or component by name*
  adult day care OT role and, 462–463
  considerations for assessing older adults
    auditory acuity, 518–519
    cognitive function and sensory loss, 519–520
    cultural considerations, 520–521
    factors in, 515–518
    tactile discrimination and motor performance, 519
    visual acuity, 518
  defining the levels of function addressed by, 510–513
  for falls, 656–658
  health education and, 817, 819
  purposes of, 508
  resources, 522, 857
  review questions, 532
  specific examples
    disability level of function/dysfunction, 526–528
    functional level of function/dysfunction, 528
    impairment level of function/dysfunction, 529–530
    pathophysiology level of function/dysfunction, 530–531
    societal limitation level of function/dysfunction, 522–526
  top-down and bottom-up approaches to, 513–514, 548
  types of, 508–510

Assistance codes, 582, 583, 584, 586, 588

Assisted living
  environmental considerations, 386–387
  future needs for, 21
  isolation and, 264

Assistive devices. *See also* Assistive equipment; Durable medical equipment
  activities of daily living and, 636
  funding for equipment, 698–699
  general concepts, 636
  home management and, 717
  leisure activities and, 731

bones, 178–179
joints, 179–180
muscles, 180–182
sensory changes
hearing, 175–177
somatosensory system, 177–178
taste and smell, 177
vestibular system or balance, 178
vision, 172–175

Biological models of aging as inevitable decline, 17

Biological programming theory of maturation, 48

Biomechanical model of practice, description, 111–112

Biophysical theories of maturation, 47–48
biological aging conclusions, 48

Bires, Jeannie, 432

Board member role for occupational therapists, 472

Bobath techniques, 32, 113

Bone changes in older adults, 178–179

Botkin, S.P., physiological analyses of older people, 17

Bottom-up approach to assessments, 513–514, 548

Box and Block Test, 557

Brief Cognitive Rating Scale, 106

"Broadening the Construct of Independence," 441

Brokos, Pat, 432

BRS. *See* Behavioural Rating Scale

Building codes, designed housing, 385

Butler, Robert, biomedical research advances prediction, 20–21

Canadian-American Conference, on economic factors in OT service delivery, 420

Canadian Occupational Performance Measure, 527

Canadian Occupational Performance Measure, inpatient rehabilitation evaluation process and, 350

CANAM Conference. *See* Canadian-American Conference

Cancer, sexual function and, 682

Canes, description, 640

CAPE. *See* Clifton Assessment Procedures for the Elderly

Cardiac arrest, description, 184

Cardiovascular disease
cognition and, 204
coronary artery disease, 184–185
definition, 184
sexual function and, 682

Cardiovascular system
cardiovascular disease and, 184–186
heart
functional changes, 182–183
structural changes, 182
vascular system
arteriosclerosis and, 183
hypertension and, 183–184

Caregiver education, 86, 635. *See also* Adult education; Education; Health education; Patient and family education
about dementia, 579
about falls, 658
adult day care programs, 458–459, 468–470
collaborative model of care and, 833–857
community-based practices, 419, 429
home health agencies, 375
inpatient rehabilitation units, 354
Medicare teaching requirements and, 372
skilled nursing facilities, 365
subacute care evaluation and, 333
transition to home from hospital or rehabilitation program and, 695–696

Caregiver Options for Practical Experiences
background, 597–598, 602
case studies, 603–607
findings, 601–602
format of groups, 600
method, 599–600
objectives, 600–601
results, 601
subjects, 599
theoretical foundation, 598–599

Caregiver perspectives on occupational therapy. *See* Evaluation considerations; Outcome measures

Caregivers. *See also* Caregiver education
adult day care and, 455
assessment tools and, 525
community-based practices and, 422
COPE group, 597–607
definition, 346

AOTA documents reflecting issues in, 440–441
barriers to
  assumptions about the aging process, 435–437
  health model-social services model differences, 437–438
  isolation of practitioners, 439–440
  language barrier, 438–439
case studies, 443–447
consultation levels
  case-centered consultation, 428
  educational consultation, 428
  program or administrative consultation, 428
consultation models
  clinical or treatment model, 428–429
  collegial or professional model, 429
  educational model, 429
depression treatment and, **619, 620, 621, 622**
exercises, 449–450
impact of change on
  activity limitations and, 418
  aging as a global phenomenon and, 420–421
  awareness of successful aging strategies and, 419–420
  caregiver education and, 419
  demographic shifts and, 417–418
  health care systems and, 417
  need to expand OT services in, 421
network of community aging services
  AoA and, 423–425
  elder housing opportunities and, 426–427
  key players in, 422
  OAA and, 422–423, 424
  practitioner use of, 425–426
  types of services in, 425
scope of activities in, 427–428
strategies for, 429–430
survey of community-based OT practitioners, 430–435
Community colleges, adult education programs, 83–84
Community facility services
  collaborative model of care and, 846
  community-based practices and, 425
Community reintegration. *See also* Discharge planning
  advanced functional goals outcome level and, 320
  resources for elders, **89–91**

Comorbidity of depression and physical illness, 611, 613
Compensation. *See also specific performance areas by name*
  as adaptive strategy, 60, 559–562
  cues for memory, 201
Compensatory learning. *See* Patient and family education
Competence-environmental press model of practice, 598
Competent caring, 842–843
Comprehensive outpatient rehabilitation facilities, growth of, 318
Compression of Morbidity theory of disability, 239
Computers
  assistive equipment location via, 403–404
  cyberspace for seniors, **265**
  information superhighway use by older adults, 21
Con games, 720–721
Concept learning, 819
Conceptual models of practice
  biomechanical model, 111–112
  cognitive disabilities model, 112
  cognitive-perceptual model, 112
  components, 110–111
  group work model, 112–113
  model of human occupation, 113
  motor control model, 113
  sensory integration model, 113–114
  spatiotemporal adaptation, 114
  types of, 110
Confidentiality, 152–153
Conflict group model, 780
Conflict in groups. *See* Group models and theories
Conflicts of interest, 155
Congestive heart failure, description, 185
Congregate housing. *See* Senior and congregate housing
Congressional Record, 862
Conservator process, 718–719, 720
Constructive team approach, 788
Consultant role for occupational therapists, 28, 140–141
  adult day care and, 466–467

community-based practices and, 417–450

rehabilitation health care systems and, 311–312, 315–316, 325

skilled nursing facilities and, 362

team approach and, 793

Consultation, definition, 427–428

Consumer-driven services, evolution of, 310

A Consumer's Guide to Home Adaptation, 351

Consumers' perspectives on assistive equipment, 402–403

Continuing care retirement communities description, 82

environmental considerations, 385

transition to home after hospitalization or rehabilitation program and, 690–692

Continuing education programs, 711–712

Continuity, as adaptive strategy, 59–60

Continuity of care

rehabilitation health care systems case study, 324

Continuum of care, transition to home after hospitalization or rehabilitation program and, 690–692, 696

Contract agencies, subacute programs and, 331

Contract learning, 811, **813**

Control

as buffer against stress, 214–215

relation to health, 214

Cooking groups, 783

Coordination training, 564. *See also* Exercise; Sensorimotor performance component

COPD. *See* Chronic obstructive pulmonary disease

COPE. *See* Caregiver Options for Practical Experiences

Coping strategies. *See also* Stress

age-related changes, 212–213

definition, 212

emotion-focused, 212–213

functions of coping, 212

widowed persons and, 251–252

COPM. *See* Canadian Occupational Performance Measure

Corcoran, Mary, 434

CORFs. *See* Comprehensive outpatient rehabilitation facilities

Coronary artery disease, description, 184–185

Cost issues. *See* Economic factors; Reimbursement for occupational therapy services

COTAs. *See* Certified occupational therapy assistants

Cowdry, E.V., 17

CPT. *See* Cognitive Performance Test

Criterion-based tests, 551–552. *See also* specific tests by name

Cross-cultural considerations. *See* Cultural considerations; Cultural environment; Cultural sensitivity; Racial and ethnic factors

Cross-linkage theory of maturation, 48

Crystallized intelligence, 203, 205

CTSIB. *See* Clinical Test for Sensory Interaction in Balance

Cultural considerations. *See also* Cultural environment; Cultural sensitivity; Racial and ethnic factors

in adult day care, 473, 477

American cultural characteristics, 795–797

assessments and, 520–521

collaborative model of care and, 845–846

cross-cultural view of aging, **799**

health education and, 817

in home health agencies, 366, 370

inpatient rehabilitation evaluation process and, 352

in OT service delivery, 345–346

in primary care service delivery, 335, 337

team approach to occupational therapy and, 795–799

Cultural environment. *See also* Cultural considerations; Racial and ethnic factors

aging and culture, 271–273

case studies, 275–276

euphemisms for older adults, 271

role loss and, 273–274

transition to home and, 692–693

work and productive activities and, 706

Cultural sensitivity. *See also* Cultural considerations; Racial and ethnic factors

family intervention and, 31
patient and family education and, 37
role of grandparents in Hispanic families, 31
Cumulative learning behavior change principle, 818
CVAs. *See* Cerebrovascular accidents
Cybernetic-growth group model, 780
Cyberspace for seniors, **265**
Cyclic life course, 21

Daily life tasks. *See* Activities of daily living; Daily living activities; Evaluation considerations; Occupational performance; Outcome measures; Performance problems; *specific performance area, context, or component by name*
Daily living activities. *See also* Activities of daily living; *specific performance area, context, or component by name*
activities, 255
case studies, 256–257
discretionary activities, 231, 232–233
goals of occupational therapy, 230
impairment, disability, and task ability, 254–255
leisure activities, 241–242
obligatory activities, 230, 231–232
occupational therapy implications, 234, 242–243
performance areas, 234–235
productive activities and activities of daily living, 235–240
roles of older adults, 243–253
time allocation factors, 233–234
time use and, 230–231
work-related productive activities, 240
Dark adaptation
changes in older adults, 174, 175
environmental considerations, 395
Databases. *See* Computers; *specific databases by name*
Date of onset of medical condition, 539
DCRSP. *See* Dementia Care and Respite Services Program
Decision-making skills, health education and, 815–816, 819
Declaration of Objectives for Older Americans, community-based practice and, 422
Deductive learning, 808

Defense mechanisms, 212
Deily, Joyce, 430–431
Delirium, dementia and, 222
The Delta Society, 562
Dementia. *See also* Alzheimer's disease; Cognitive integration/cognitive performance component
assessment tools, 524–525
caregiver stress and, 88, 222
cerebrovascular accidents and, 185, 186
classification of, 221
clinical characteristics
behavioral impairment, 576–578
cognitive impairment, 574–575
functional impairment, 575–576
cognitive disabilities model of practice and, 112
COPE group, 597–607
day care and respite care, 32, 457
delirium and, 222
dementia syndrome of depression, 223–224
description, 221, 573–574
environment as compensation method, 32
environmental considerations, 389–391, 399–400
factors specific to rehabilitation for, 578–579
home safety issues, 701
leisure activities and, 733–734
memory difficulties and, 201, 202
rehabilitative efforts, 222
reversible causes of, 221–222
sexual function and, 681–682
transition to home from hospital or rehabilitation program and, 696
Dementia Care and Respite Services Program, adult day care, 457
Dementia units, 389–391
Democratic groups, 777
Demographics of the aging population
age-based public policies, 20
changing family patterns, 20
community-based practices and, 417–418, 420–421
costs of caregiving and, 834
economic status, 17
family settings, 16
growth in number of older Americans, 15–16
long-lasting bonds and, 19–20

inpatient rehabilitation evaluation process and, 352–353
legislative influences, 391
OT service objectives and, 344
for the Samanski family, 846–853
single-family dwellings or apartments, 384

Epidemiological Catchment Area Program, 610

Episodic memory, 574–575

Epstein, Cynthia, 419

Equilibrium group model, 780

Erikson, Erik, personality theory of maturation, 49

ERISA. *See* Employees Retirement Income Security Act

Estrogen replacement therapy, sexual function and, 191

Ethical considerations. *See also Code of Ethics*
in adult day care, 474, 477
allocation of resources, 144, 157–158
complexity of treatment and, 144
confidentiality, 152–153
conflicts of interest, 155
differentiating unethical from illegal, 152
documentation responsibilities, 152–153
federal, state, and local laws and regulations, 148–152
funding of OT services, 376
Hippocratic Oath and, 146–147
historical background, 145–146
licensure, 148
in OT service delivery, 345
overcharge reports by GAO, 154
patient referrals, 155
personal autonomy, 714–715
personal biases, 156–157
in primary care service delivery, 335
rationing of services, 144
reimbursement for OT services, 366
team approach to occupational therapy and, 798–799
unethical activities example, 152
values and ethics in gerontic practice, 145–147

Ethnic factors. *See* Cultural considerations; Cultural environment; Cultural sensitivity; Racial and ethnic factors

Ethnogeriatrics, definition, 272

Ethnographic interviewing, 847, 850, **851**, 851–852, **852**, 854

Ethnographic perspective
emic approach, 694
informant identification, 694
interpreting information, 694–695
self-reflection, 694

Euphemisms
for death and dying, 744
for older adults, 271

Euthanasia, 744–745

Evaluation considerations. *See also* Assessments; Interventions; Outcome measures; Outcome-oriented rehabilitation; *specific areas of practice, e.g.,* Community-based practice; *specific performance area, context, or component by name*
acute care evaluation, 331–333
clinical OT role and, 313
framework for OT services and, 345
health education programs, 822–823
home health agencies, 369–373
inpatient rehabilitation units, 349–355
skilled nursing facilities, 362–365
subacute care evaluation, 333–334
treatment planning and, 540

Evaluative assessments, 509

Exercise. *See also* Sensorimotor performance component
aging process and, 56
cognition and, 204
exercise groups, 783
heart function and, 183
memory and, 204
motor skills testing and, 552
muscle strength changes and, 181
osteoporosis and, 179
reaction time improvement and, 202
wellness and, 58

EXIT euthanasia organization, 745

Expert models of care, collaborative models comparison, 843

Exploratory actions cognitive level, 582–583

External case management, 791. *See also* Case management

External continuity, as adaptive strategy, 59–60

Eyes. *See* Vision changes in older adults

Facilitation behavior change principle, 819

Fair Housing Act Amendments
    adaptations to homes and, 717
    environmental considerations and, 391

Fairfax County Health Department (VA), 434–435

Falls
    assessment for, 554, 656–658
    case study, 661
    cognitive-behavior therapy for prevention of, 658–659
    demographics of, 653
    environmental considerations, 398–399
    extrinsic factors, 654
    home assessment checklist for fall hazards, 657, 664–666, 715
    increased risk for in older adults, 178
    intrinsic factors, 653–654
    occupational therapy intervention, 658–659
    posture and, 637
    prevention model, 654, 655
    review questions, 660
    role of occupational therapy in prevention, 655–659
    studies on, 655
    toileting and, 646

Falls Efficacy Scale, 656

Falls Interview Schedule, 656, 662–663

"Falls Safety Self Study Packet," 655

Familiarity and meaning, as environmental consideration, 401

Families. *See also* Cultural considerations; Patient and family education
    as caregivers, 20, 31, 64
    depression treatment and, 619, **622**
    health education and, 817
    hospice programs and, 750, 753
    leisure activities and, 731
    long-lasting bonds with, 19–20
    social support from, 213

Family intervention. *See also* Patient and family education
    necessity of involving the family in treatment, 31, 37, 64

FAST. *See* Functional Assessment and Safety Tool

Fecal incontinence, toileting and, 647

Federal government. *See also* Health care reform; Public policy issues; *specific programs and legislative acts by name*

ADA as legislative process example
    in bill form, **862**
    cited as public law, **862**
    as cited in the *U.S. Statutes at Large*, **862**
    in *Code of Federal Regulations* as a regulation, **867**
    in *Federal Register* as a final rule, **867**
    in *Federal Register* as a proposed rule, **866**
    in *United States Code* as a law, **863**
    government program resources, 869–871
    legislation resources, 862–865
    rules and regulations resources, 866–868

Federal Register, 866, **867**

Fee-for-service plans. *See* Insurers

Feedback. *See also* Positive reinforcement
    feedback behavior change principle, 819
    to remediate motor skills, 564–565

Feeling-oriented discussion groups, 783

FHAA. *See* Fair Housing Act Amendments

Fieldwork education, 140

55 ALIVE/MATURE DRIVING driver refresher course, 672

Figure-ground discrimination, environmental considerations, 396

Filipino elders, 272

FIM. *See* Functional Independence Measure

FIS. *See* Falls Interview Schedule

Floor and ground treatments, *398*, 398–399

Fluid intelligence, 203

Focus-group interviews, health education programs and, 822

Follow-up in the home, discharge planning and, 335

Food consistency. *See also* Eating
    nutrition and, 642
    swallowing and, 643–644

Food management. *See also* Eating
    assistance with, 645

Food Stamps, elderly persons and, 149

For-profit organization funding of community-based practices, 424–425. *See also* *specific organizations by name*

Formative evaluations, health education programs and, 822

Foster Grandparent Program, 248

Foto, Mary, on adult day care services, 476

Fractures
from falls, 653
osteoporosis and, 179

Frames of reference
acquisitional, 114, 115–116
analytic, 114, 115
behaviors and physical signs, 114
developmental, 114, 115
function-dysfunction continua, 114
postulates regarding change, 114
theoretical base, 114

Framington longitudinal study, 56

Fraud, risk factors for seniors, 720–721

Free radical theory of maturation, 48

Freestanding outpatient rehabilitation centers. *See also* Inpatient rehabilitation
growth of, 318

Friendly Visitor program, 86

Friendship in older adults
loss of long-lasting friends, 252
quality of, 252

Function
definitions, 165–166
as focus of gerontology, 36, 57–58
hierarchy of function/dysfunction, **511**, 511–513

Functional Activities Questionnaire, 715

Functional Assessment and Safety Tool, 523, 524

Functional goals. *See also* Evaluation considerations; Interventions; Outcome-oriented rehabilitation, outcome levels; Treatment planning; *specific performance area, context, or component by name*
health education and, 818–819
home health agencies, 372–373
inpatient rehabilitation units, 353–355
OT service objectives, 343–344
skilled nursing facilities, 364–365

Functional impairment. *See* Impairment

Functional independence, definitions of, 104–107

Functional Independence Measure
disability assessments, 526
inpatient rehabilitation evaluation process and, 351, 356

Functional limitation level of function/dysfunction
assessment examples, 528
definition, 511, 512

Functional limitations. *See specific performance area, context, or component by name*

Funding issues. *See* Economic factors; Reimbursement for occupational therapy services

GCNS. *See* Gerontologic clinical nurse specialists

Geller, Paulette, 457

Gender factors
Alzheimer's disease, 188
discretionary activities, 232–233
family caregivers, 16, 601–602
instrumental activities of daily living, 238
joint changes in older adults, 179–180
life expectancy, 15–16
maturation research, 51
money handling, 286
obligatory activities, 231
osteoporosis, 178–179
sexual function, 191, 680–681
time allocation, 233
work-related activity performance, 240

Gene theory of maturation, 48

General Accounting Office, overcharge reports, 154

Generic names taxonomy, 404

Geriatric Education Center (WA), 432–433

Geriatric inpatient rehabilitation. *See* Inpatient rehabilitation

Geriatric nurse practitioners, description, 79–80

Geriatric physical therapists, description, 81–82

Geriatric researchers. *See also* specific researchers by name
description, 82

Geriatric social workers, description, 81

Geriatricians, description, 78–79

Geriatrics
definition, 25
need for occupational therapists with training in, 318

Gerontic, definition, 25–26

Gerontic occupational therapists. *See also* Occupational therapists
definition, 26
description, 81

Gerontic occupational therapy. *See also*
Clinical occupational therapy;
Occupational therapy
clinical role and, 311–312
function and activity focus
advocating occupational therapy,
38–39, 57–58
patient and family education and,
37–38
future trends, 35, 40
historical perspective
assessments, 31–32
early years, 26–27
environmental and sociolegal
changes, 28–30
family intervention, 30–31
increasing knowledge of aging
changes, 30
rehabilitation movement, 27
managed health care and, 35–36
program development
Gerontology Special Interest Section,
33–35, 40
treatment modalities, 32–33
recognition of as special area of practice,
26
therapist education, 39–40

Gerontic rehabilitation. *See* Medical rehabilitation

Gerontologic clinical nurse specialists,
description, 80–81

Gerontological Society of America, founding of, 18

Gerontology
activities, 22
biological models of aging as inevitable
decline, 17
chronological age and, 57
definition, 17, 25, 56–57
demographics of the aging population,
15–17
developing interest in older adults,
17–19
education programs, 19
federal government legislation, 18–19
first major studies, 17
founding of Gerontological Society of
America, 18, 57
function and, 57–58
future directions, 20–21
longitudinal studies, 18
need for occupational therapists with
training in, 318

psychology aging and, 57
review questions, 22
social aging and, 57
social gerontology subfield, 57
social trends, 19–20
U.S. national policy for older adults,
17–18

Gerontology Special Interest Section,
establishment of, 33

Gitlin, Laura, 434

Glare
environmental considerations, 394–395
vision changes and, 173

Glaucoma, description, 174

Global Deterioration Scale for Assessment
of Primary Degenerative Dementia, 106
early dementia stage, 584
late confusional predementia stage, 583
late dementia stage, 588
middle dementia stage, 586, 587

Global outcome, description, 319

GNPs. *See* Geriatric nurse practitioners

Goal-directed activity cognitive level,
583–584

Goals. *See* Functional goals

Government funding. *See* Economic factors; Federal government; Reimbursement for occupational therapy services; State governments; *specific agencies, programs, and organizations by name*

Government programs. *See* Federal government; *specific programs by name*

Government regulation. *See* Federal government; State governments; *specific agencies, programs, and legislative acts by name*

GPO. *See* U.S. Government Printing Office

Grab bars, *392*

Grandparent role of older adults
distant figure style, 250
formal style, 249
fun-seeking style, 249, 250
meaning of, 249
patterns of grandparenting, 249–250
repository of wisdom style, 249–250
surrogate style, 249

"Granny dumping," 281–282

Grasping and pinching, 393, 557

Great American Smokeouts, 59

Grief. *See* Bereavement

Grooming. *See* Hygiene and grooming

Group approach to occupational therapy. *See* Team approach to occupational therapy

Group dynamics model of practice, 598

Group education. *See also* Adult education; Education; Health education
benefits, 133–134
settings, 132–133

Group models and theories
communication in groups, 782
conflict in groups, 782
contemporary groups in OT practice, 783–784
developmental stages of groups, 781
education groups with older adults, 783, 784–785, 802
emotional patterns of groups, 781
formation of small groups, 781
importance of studying groups, 776
leadership style impacts on groups, 777–778
models of group treatment, 782–783
primary groups, 780–781
roles within groups, 778–779
small group definition, 776–777
small group models, 779–780

Group work model of practice, description, 112–113

Group work with depressed persons, 618–620

Growth groups, 783

GSA. *See* Gerontological Society of America

Guardianship process, 718–719, 720

Guide for Supervision of Occupational Therapy Personnel, 788–789

Guide to Classification of Occupational Therapy Personnel, 154–155

Gustation. *See* Taste and smell changes in older adults

Gustatory sensation testing, 555

Hall, G. Stanley, 17

The Handicapped Driver's Mobility Guide, 672

Handicaps. *See also* Disabilities
ICIDH concept of, 166

Handrails, *388*

Havighurst, Robert, 18

Havighurst, Robert, personality theory of maturation, 49, 50

HCFA. *See* U.S. Health Care Financing Administration

Health Belief Model of learning, 806, **815**, 815–816

Health care reform. *See also* Federal government; Public policy issues; State governments
adult day care and, 461
rehabilitation service trends and, 376–377
resources, 874–875

Health care systems. *See also* specific types of rehabilitation facility by name
activities, 92
belief systems about health and aging
gerontology, 56–58
medical model, 55–56
wellness and prevention, 58–60
community-based practices and, 417
humanizing, 840–842
rehabilitation health care systems, 307–325
service systems for older adults
acute care, 61–63, **70–71**
adult day care, 74–75
community reentry after medical treatment, 86–91
definition of terms, 61–78
geriatric specialists, 78–82
home health care, 72–74
hospice programs, 75–78, **76**
long-term-care facilities, 67, 69–72, **70–71**
medical/social models of delivery, 60–61
outpatient rehabilitation, 65–66
rehabilitation settings, 63–65
subacute care, 66–67, **68**
wellness and prevention, 82–86

Health education. *See also* Adult education; Caregiver education; Education; Patient and family education
activities, 824
case studies, 825–827
educational strategies
affective skills development, 818, 820–821
cognitive skills development, 818, 819–820
psychomotor skills development, 818, 821–822

inpatient rehabilitation units and, 354–355

review questions, 532, 543

skilled nursing facilities and, 364–365

treatment planning and treatment approaches, 538–542

Interviews of clients and caregivers

activities of daily living and, 634

ethnographic interviewing, 847, 850, **851**, 851–852, **852**, 854

health education programs and, 822

in home health agencies, 370–371

in inpatient rehabilitation units, 350–351

resources, 857

in skilled nursing facilities, 364

Intradisciplinary interagency case management, 792. *See also* Case management

Intradisciplinary intraagency case management, 791. *See also* Case management

Intrapsychic groups, 782, 783

Ischemic heart disease. *See* Coronary artery disease

Isolation

of occupational therapists

in community-based practices, 439–440

in home health care, 368–369

of older adults

physical environment and, 264–266

social environment and, 283

J CAHO. *See* Joint Commission on Accreditation of Healthcare Organizations

Joint changes in older adults, 179–180. *See also* Musculoskeletal system changes in older adults

Joint Commission on Accreditation of Healthcare Organizations

home health care definition, 72

standards of care, 329, 876

subacute care definition, 67

subacute care guidelines, 66

Journal of Gerontology, founding of, 18

K ansas City Studies of Adult Life, 18

Kevorkian, Dr. Jack, 745

Kiernat, Jean, 433–434

Kinesthetic changes in older adults. *See* Sensory changes in older adults

Kitchen safety, 701

Kitchen Task Assessment, 528

Knowledge, as influence on health behavior, 813–815

Kohlman Evaluation of Living Skills, 106, 111

KTA. *See* Kitchen Task Assessment

Language. *See also* Cultural considerations; Semantic memory

as barrier in OT service delivery, 438–439, 530

Large-print books, 266

Late confusional predementia stage, 583

Late dementia stage, 588

Later adult developmental tasks, clinical OT role and, 314–315

Latino culture. *See* Hispanic and Latino cultures

Leadership styles, impact on small groups, 777–778

Learned helplessness

sense of control and, 214

treatment planning and, 539–540

Learning. *See also* Cognition; Education; Memory

learning contracts, 811, **813**

learning theories and health education, 806–813

limitations on, 635

memory and, 199, 200

normal aging and, 30

principles for older persons

clinical OT role and, 315

health education, 805–827

treatment planning and, 541–542

sleep disturbances and, 243

LEC. *See* Life Experiences Checklist

Lee, Valerie, 431

Legal issues. *See also* Documentation of occupational therapy services; Reimbursement for occupational therapy services; specific legislative acts by name

adult day care, 474, 477

helping another person to die, 744–745

specialized housing, 426

Legibility, as environmental consideration, 401

Legislative issues. *See also* Health care reform; *specific legislative acts by name*

multiskilled caregivers and, 38–39
occupational therapy and, 35–36
rehabilitation settings and, 63
resources, 874–875
subacute care and, 66
treatment planning and, 540–541

"Manipulative help rejecters," 614

Manual actions cognitive level, 584–586

Manual dexterity. *See* Psychomotor skills; Sensorimotor performance component

Manual muscle test, 557

Manual wheelchairs, description, 640

Marriage. *See also* Sexual function
length of, 19–20
retirement and, 710–711

Maryland Easter Seal Society for Disabled Children and Adults, 432

Maslow, Abraham, pyramid of needs theory of maturation, 49–50

Maturation of the older adult. *See also* Later adult developmental tasks
assessment considerations and, 515–521
biophysical theories, 47–48
definition, 47
development as a lifelong process, 47, 57
gender and culture issues, 51
personality theories, 48–50
social theories, 50–51

Maximum cognitive assistance code, 586–587

MBPC. *See* Memory and Behavior Problem Checklist

McDonald's, hiring of older workers, 709

MDS. *See* Minimum Data Set

Meal preparation, 645

Meals on Wheels program, 64, 716

Meals on Wheels (VA), 430–431

MEAMS. *See* Middlesex Elderly Assessment of Mental State

Meaning. *See* Familiarity and meaning

Mechanical presbycusis, description, 176–177

Medic Alert, 700

Medicaid. *See also* Medicare
adult day care and, 455, 460, 475, 477
description, 149
fraud and abuse provisions, 153–154
funding for assistive devices, 699

inpatient rehabilitation unit reimbursement, 358
long-term-care coverage, 330
resources, 866, 870

Medical day care. *See* Adult day care

Medical model. *See also specific types of care facility by name*
benefits of, 61
community-based practices comparison, 418, 437–438, 442
description, 30
disease cure and prevention, 56, 691
as framework for occupational therapy, 345
pathology and reductionism, 55–56
service delivery
acute care, 61–63, **70–71**
adult day care, 74–75, 456
definition, 61
general themes, 60
geriatric specialists, 78–82
home health care, 72–74
hospice programs, 75–78, **76**
long-term care, 67, 69–72, **70–71**
outpatient rehabilitation, 65–66
rehabilitation settings, 63–65
subacute care, 66–67, **68**

Medical rehabilitation. *See also* Rehabilitation health care systems; Rehabilitation services; *specific areas of service, e.g.,* Primary care services
description, 316–317
older adult needs for, 318–319
outcome levels, 319–320
outcome-oriented rehabilitation, 319
therapeutic focus on, 317–318

Medical schools, geriatrics training, 79

Medicare. *See also* Medicaid
adult day care and, 455, 460–461, 475
assistance codes, 582, 583, 584, 586, 588
description, 149
eligibility, 57
fraud and abuse provisions, 153–154
functional-based evaluation and treatment guidelines, 332
funding for assistive devices, 699
home health agency reimbursement, 368, 369–370, 374, 375
home health care and, 73
hospice programs, 77, 746
implementation of, 28
inpatient rehabilitation unit reimbursement, 358–359

dexterity testing, 557
function testing, 556–557
performance assessment, 519

Motorized scooters, description, 640

MrFIT. *See* Multiple Risk Factor
Intervention Trials

Multi-infarct dementias. *See* Vascular
dementias

Multidisciplinary teams, definition, 787

Multiple medical diagnoses
rehabilitation health care systems case
study, 324
treatment planning and, 538–539

Multiple methods behavior change principle, 818

Multiple Risk Factor Intervention Trials, 58

Muscle changes in older adults
muscle diseases, 181–182
muscle-wasting and decline in strength,
180–181

Musculoskeletal system changes in older
adults. *See also* Assessments
assessment considerations, 519,
556–557
bones, 178–179
joints, 179–180
muscles, 180–182
treatment considerations, 562–565

Myocardial infarction
depression and, 223
description, 184–185

National Cancer Institute, health education and, 806

National Center for Health Statistics,
Health Interview Survey, 16, 235, 403

National Center for Medical Rehabilitation
Research, hierarchy of function/dysfunction, **511**, 511–513

National Center on Elder Abuse, fraud
reports, 720

National Council on Aging. *See also*
National Institute on Adult Daycare
volunteers and, 248

National Executive Service Corps, volunteers and, 248

National Family Caregivers Association, on
costs of caregiving, 834

National Health Interview Survey
assistive equipment and environmental
modification costs, 403

self-assessment of health, 16
Supplement on Aging
disability statistics, 235

National Hospice Organization, 746

National Institute of Mental Health,
Epidemiological Catchment Area
Program, 610

National Institute on Adult Daycare
adult day care definition, 74
adult day care standards and guidelines,
455, 459, 461, 462–463, 477
on day care terminology, 454
on goals of adult day care, 459
support of adult day services movement
by, 477

National Institute on Aging
establishment, 19
longitudinal studies, 18
research funding from, 434

National Institute on Alcohol Abuse and
Alcoholism, estimates of alcohol abuse
in older adults, 225

National Institutes of Health. *See also specific components by name*
Baltimore Longitudinal Studies of aging,
18

National Long-Term Care Demonstration,
691

National Medical Expenditure Survey, on
activity limitations, 418

Native Americans
community-based practices and, 423
views of aging, 272

NCMRR. *See* National Center for Medical
Rehabilitation Research

Neglect, 279, **280–281**

Negotiation skills, collaborative model of
care and, 846

Nervous system
central nervous system, 186–187
peripheral nervous system, 187–189

Neugarten, Bernice, diverse patterns of
adaptation to aging conclusion, 18

Neural presbycusis, description, 176

Neurological disorders. *See* Cognitive integration/cognitive performance component; *specific disorders by name*

Neuromusculoskeletal functions testing,
556–557

Neuropsychologists, inpatient rehabilitation role, 348

Prostate enlargement, sexual function and, 191

Provider-driven services, evolution of, 310

Psychiatric conditions. *See* Psychosocial/ psychological performance component; *specific conditions by name*

Psychological aging, 57

Psychological Assessment of the Elderly, 522

Psychomotor skills. *See also* Assessments; Sensorimotor performance component

assessment, 519

development, 818, 821–822

Psychosocial issues. *See also* Psychosocial/ psychological performance component; *specific disorders and conditions by name*

health education and, 817

home health agencies, 372–373

Psychosocial/psychological performance component

anxiety in older adults, 610–611

case studies, 623–626

clinical presentations of depression in the elderly

assessments, 615

depressive pseudodementia, 613

personality disorders, 613–615

somatization, 613

comorbidity of depression and physical illness, 611, 613

criteria for depression and dysthymia, 611, **612**

depression in older adults, 610

description, 121

review questions, 627

role of OT practitioners in, 610, 619–620

schizophrenia in older adults, 611

treatment planning and group work

activities of daily living, 618, **619**

families and, 619, **622**

leisure activities, 618–619, **620**

work and productive activities, 619, **621**

treatment planning and individual work, 615–618

Psychotic symptoms, 577–578

Public aging network. *See specific components of, e.g.,* U.S. Administration on Aging

Public libraries, adult education programs, 84

Public policy issues. *See also* Federal government; State governments; *specific issues*

disease prevention and health promotion resources, 872–873

general information resources, 876–878

managed care and health care reform resources, 874–875

policy issue assessments, 510

professional education resources, 872

resource organizations, 879–881

standards of care and quality of care resources, 875–876

Purposeful activity, 103, 126

Quality assurance assessments, 509–510

Quality of care. *See also* Omnibus Budget Reconciliation Act; Standards of care

criteria for evaluating, 345–346

resources, 875–876

Quality of life, 36

activities of daily living and, 235

hospice programs and, 746–747, 748, 749–750, 752

transition to home from hospital or rehabilitation program and, 691

Quasi-mechanical group model, 779

Racial and ethnic factors. *See also* Cultural considerations; Cultural environment; Cultural sensitivity

demographics of older population, 16

difficulties with activities of daily living, 16

health education and, 817

home health care, 73

hospice programs, 75

maturation research, 51

nutrition, 642

patients in rehabilitation settings, 63–64

views of aging, 271–273

wellness, 59

RAI. *See* Resident Assessment Instrument

Ramps, ADA recommendations for, 398

Range of motion, 556–557

Rapid-eye-movement sleep, 243

Razors, safe handling of, 645

RBI. *See* Role Adaptation Bereavement Inventory

Reaction time

age-related changes, 202

driving and, 670

Reality orientation
reality-oriented discussion groups, 783
as therapy, 32

Recordings for the Blind and Dyslexic, 266

Recordkeeping. *See* Documentation of
occupational therapy services

Recreation. *See* Leisure activities

Recreational therapists, skilled nursing
facility role, 362

Reductionism, 55–56

Referral source role for occupational therapists, 155, 425, 472

Rehabilitation health care systems. *See also*
Rehabilitation services; *specific types of
services, e.g.,* Primary care services
case study, 322–324
client-centered delivery of services,
310–311
clinical OT role, 313–315
complexity of gerontic practice,
308–309
consultant OT role, 315–316
gerontic OT role, 311–312, 325
medical rehabilitation as a major focus
in, 316–319
multidimensional health care problems,
309
outcome-oriented rehabilitation,
319–320
trends in, 376–377
well-being of older adults and, 307–308,
309

Rehabilitation model, 27, 30, 32

Rehabilitation services. *See also* Medical
rehabilitation; Rehabilitation health care
systems; *specific areas of service, e.g.,*
Primary care services; *specific types of
rehabilitation facility by name*
challenges facing OT practitioners,
344–346
home health agencies, 366–375, 375
inpatient rehabilitation, 347–360
objectives of, 343–344
review questions, 378
skilled nursing facilities, 360–366
treatment planning and, 540–541
trends in, 376–377

Rehabilitation settings. *See also* Outpatient
rehabilitation; *specific settings by name*
advantages and disadvantages, 65
elder patients and, 63–64

length of stay, 63
nonhuman environment tools of practice and, 128
objective of, 63
occupational therapists and, 64–65
team approach to care, 63, 64

Rehabilitation teams. *See specific types of
rehabilitation facility by name*

Reimbursement assessments, 510

Reimbursement for occupational therapy
services. *See also* Documentation of
occupational therapy services;
Economic factors; *specific sources of payment, e.g.,* Medicare
adult day care, 460–461, 475–476, 477
community-based practices, 423–425,
437–438
home health agencies, 368, 369–370
inpatient rehabilitation units, 358–360
skilled nursing facilities, 362, 365–366

Reinforcement behavior change principle,
819

Reinforcing influences on health behavior,
809, 816–817, 819

Reinterpretation of signs and symptoms,
enhancing self-efficacy via, 810

Relationships between service providers
and receivers. *See* Collaborative model
of care

Relevance behavior change principle, 819

RELIABLE SOURCE, 404

Religious affiliation
health and, 253
hospice programs and, 750–751
wellness and, 85–86

Reminiscences
clinical OT role and, 314
consultant OT role and, 316
as therapy, 32

Researcher role for occupational therapists,
470–471

Resident, definition, 360

Resident Assessment Instrument, skilled
nursing facility services and, 363

Resident Assessment Protocol, 149

Residential integration. *See* Home or residential integration

Respect, collaborative model of care and,
845

Respiratory system, age-related changes,
189–191

Respite care
dementia and, 32
discharge planning and, 88

Respite Report: Special Issue, on adult day care services, 475–476

Restorative model of adult day care, 456

Retired homemaker role of older adults, 253

Retired Senior Volunteer Program, 248

Retired Senior Volunteer Services, 711

Retirement. *See also* Worker-retiree role
adjustment phases, 246
average age for, 19
company policies and, 245
early retirement, 709
education during, 711–712
extended period of, 19
forced retirement at age 65, 26
health status and, 710
marital relationship and, 710–711
market opportunities for work, 245
original purpose of, 17, 19
planning for, 710, 717–718
psychosocial aspects, 710–711
as reward for work, 709
satisfaction factors, 246
transition to, 710
volunteer work and, 711
work substitutes, 711

Retirement Research Foundation, 420

Riley, Matilda and John, 20

Rising. *See* Sitting and rising

Ritualistic team approach, 788

Rivermead Perceptual Assessment Battery, 518, 530

Rocking behavior, environmental considerations, 400

Rogers, Joan, support for Gerontology Special Interest Section, 33

Role Adaptation Bereavement Inventory, 523

Role Checklist, 522, 523

Role loss. *See also* Roles of older adults
adaptation to, 273–274
hospice programs and, 748

Role of Occupational Therapy with the Elderly
curriculum, 34
development of, 33
expert panel review, 35
surveys, 34–35

Roles of groups. *See* Group models and theories

Roles of occupational therapy practitioners. *See specific types of practitioner and rehabilitation facility by name*

Roles of older adults. *See also* Role loss
caregiver, 250–251
cross-cultural view of aging, **799**
friend, 252
grandparent, 248–250
leisure participant, 246–247
occupational therapy implications, 253–254
religious participant, 253
retired homemaker, 253
role definition, 243
volunteer, 247–248
widowed person, 251–252
worker-retiree, 244–246

ROM. *See* Range of motion

Routine Task Inventory, 589

Roybal Center for Applied Gerontology, cognitive restructuring techniques, 820–821

RPAB. *See* Rivermead Perceptual Assessment Battery

RTI. *See* Routine Task Inventory

Rural areas, isolation and, 264

"Safe and Sound Through the Senior Years" (WA), 432–433

SAFER. *See* Safety Assessment of Function in the Environment for Rehabilitation

Safety. *See also* Driving; Environmental considerations; Falls; Home evaluations
assessment considerations, 524
cognitive levels of rehabilitation and, 583, 584–588
home management and, 715–716
preparation for emergencies, 699–701

Safety Assessment of Function in the Environment for Rehabilitation, 523, 524, 715–716

The Samanski family, 846–853

Saunders, Dame Cicely, hospice movement and, 745

Scams, 720–721

Scheduling of home visits, 369

Schizophrenia, 611

SCORE. *See* Service Corps of Retired Executives

outpatient rehabilitation, 65–66
rehabilitation settings, 63–65
subacute care, 66–67, **68**
wellness and prevention
adult education, 83–84
community services, 82–83
religious affiliations, 85–86
retirement planning, employee assistance programs, and volunteer work, 85
self-help/support groups, 84–85
Sexual function. *See also* Marriage
age-related changes, 191, 680–681
biopsychosocial approach to therapy, 680
conceptual framework, 679–680
cultural stereotypes, 679, 681
demographic factors, 681
myths about, **284**, 285
physical conditions and, 682
PLISSIT Model and, 683, 686–687
primary, secondary, and tertiary care options, 682–683
psychological conditions and, 681–682
research findings, 683
review questions, 685
social environment and, 283–285, **284**
sociocultural attitudes and, 681
studies of, 679
uniform terminology definition, 679
Seymour, Karen, 433
Shared responsibility for care. *See* Collaborative model of care
Shock, Nathan, 18
Short-term memory. *See* Primary memory
Shoshanna, Shamberg, 434
Shull, Pat, 460–461
Single-family dwellings. *See also specific types of housing by name*
environmental considerations, 384
Sitting and rising
environmental considerations, 393
sitting to standing transfers, 639, 641
Situational specificity behavior change principle, 818
Skilled intervention requirements, home health agencies, 374–375
Skilled nursing facilities. *See also* Long-term-care facilities
bathing and, 647–648
discharge planning, 365
documentation of services, 365

growth of, 318
OT evaluation process
achieving goals through intervention, 364–365
guidelines for, 362–363
identifying problems by observing, 364
interviewing for information, 364
setting goals through collaboration, 364
outcome measures, 365
rehabilitation process overview, 360–361
reimbursement for services, 365–366
roles of rehabilitation professionals, 361–362
Skills mastery, enhancing self-efficacy via, 810
Sleep, 243
"small changes, BIG DIFFERENCES," 424
Small groups. *See* Group models and theories; *specific type of group by name*
Smell changes in older adults. *See* Taste and smell changes in older adults
Smell Identification Test, 556
Smoking cessation programs, 58–59
SNFs. *See* Skilled nursing facilities
Social aging, 57
Social environment. *See also* Social support
abandonment and, 281–282
abuse and, 279, **280–281**, 281
activities, 287
bereavement and, 282–283
case studies, 288–290
economic insecurity, 285–286
isolation and loneliness, 283
neglect and, 279, **280–281**
sexual intimacy and expression, 283–285
slow or rapid changes in, 278
transition to home and, 692
Social gerontology, 57, 58
Social/Health Maintenance Organization, 691
Social model of adult day care, 456
Social Security
earnings limitation, 57
eligibility for, 245
Social Security Act, 17–18
amendments, 19, 455, 863
keeping current with legislation, 863, 875

Social Service programs, adult day care and, 455

Social services model. *See* Consultant role for occupational therapists

Social support. *See also* Social environment adaptation and, 213
definition, 213
health education and, 817

Social system groups, 782, 783

Social theories of maturation
activity level, 50
disengagement, 50
identity continuity, 50–51

Social workers. *See also* Case management discharge planning role, 334–335
geriatric social worker description, 81
inpatient rehabilitation role, 347, 355–356, 360
skilled nursing facility role, 361

Socialization, as environmental consideration, 401

Societal limitation level of function/dysfunction
assessment examples, 522–526
definition, 511, 512

Societal perspective on occupational therapy. *See* Evaluation considerations; Outcome measures

Sociology of groups. *See* Group models and theories; Team approach to occupational therapy

Somatization, 613

Somatosensory system changes in older adults, 177–178

SOTOF. *See* Structured Observational Test of Function

Source Book of Geriatric Assessment, 522

South Carolina Long-Term Demonstration Project, 691

Spatiotemporal adaptation model of practice, 114

Special care units, environmental considerations, 389–391

Special-purpose adult day care, 457

Specialized adult day care, 457

Specialized housing. *See also specific types of housing by name*
community-based practices and, 426–427

Speech and language pathologists
home health agency role, 368, 369–370
inpatient rehabilitation role, 348
skilled nursing facility role, 361

Spinal spondylosis, description, 180

SPLAT assessment for falls, 657

Splints, 562

SSI. *See* Supplemental Security Income

Stability, environmental considerations, *392,* 392–393

Stair climbing, 639

Stand-by/supervision cognitive assistance code, 582–583

Standards and Guidelines for Adult Daycare, 459, 462–463

Standards for Adult Daycare, 455

Standards of care. *See also* Quality of care
for adult day care, 455, 459, 461, 462–463, 477
JCAHO and, 329, 876
resources, 875–876

Stanford Geriatric Education Center, 272–273

State governments. *See also* Health care reform; Public policy issues; *specific agencies, programs, and legislative acts by name*
government program resources, 870
legislation resources, 865–866
resource organizations, 879–881
rules and regulations resources, 868

State University of New York at Buffalo, OT student survey, 34–35

Stereognosis testing, 553

Stereotypes and stigma
labels, 263
negative and positive, 271
physical environment and, 263, 266–267
sexual function, 679, 681
treatment planning and, 540

Stigma. *See* Stereotypes and stigma

Storytelling. *See* Life histories; Life stories; Reminiscences

Strengthening programs, 562–563. *See also* Exercise

Stress
caregivers and, 31, 88, 222, 250, 578, 579, 713
patients in long-term-care facilities, 69
sense of control and, 214–215

Stroke. *See* Cerebrovascular accidents

Structural-functional group model, 780

Structured Observational Test of Function, 521, 527–528

Subacute care. *See also* Acute care; Inpatient rehabilitation; *specific types of rehabilitation facility by name*
  acute care comparison, 329–330, 330–331
  advantages and disadvantages, 67
  definition of, 67
  levels for, **68**
  managed care and, 66
  medical rehabilitation as a focus in, 318
  patient needs, 66
  primary care services case study, 339–340
  subacute care evaluation, 333–334

Successive approximation, health education and, 809

Suicide
  depression and, 224–225
  hospice programs and, 744
  indirect or passive, 224
  physician-assisted suicide, 745
  prevalence, 224
  widowed persons and, 251

Sun City Community Health Education and Resource Center (AZ), 433–434

Sundown Syndrome, environmental considerations, 390

Supervision
  administrator OT role and, 467–468
  COTA-OTR partnerships and, 788–789
  educator OT role and, 469–470

Supervisory caregiving, 839

Supplemental Security Income
  description, 149
  provisions, 19

Swallowing
  assistance with, 643–644
  food consistency and, 643–644

Tactile and touch changes in older adults. *See also* Assessments; Sensorimotor performance component
  assessment considerations, 519, 552–553
  environmental considerations, 398

Tactile discrimination assessment, 519, 552–553

Task groups, 783

Task lighting, *394*

Task-oriented approach to assessments. *See specific performance area, context, or component by name*

Task performance. *See* Activities of daily living; *specific performance area, context, or component by name*

Taste and smell changes in older adults, 177. *See also* Assessments
  assessment considerations, 555–556
  environmental considerations, 397
  treatment considerations, 562

Teaching materials, 34. *See also* Health education

Teaching models, 34. *See also* Health education

Team approach to occupational therapy. *See also specific types of care facility by name*
  advantages of, 786–787
  case management and, 789–793
  case study, 800–801
  collaborative model of care, 833–857
  consultancy and, 793
  COTA-OTR partnership, 788–789
  cross-cultural considerations, 795–799
  cross-cultural view of aging, **799**
  ethical considerations, 798–799
  group models and theories, 776–785, 802
  interdisciplinary team definition, 786, 787–788
  multidisciplinary team definition, 787

Tech Act. *See* Technology-Related Assistance to Individuals with Disabilities Act

Technology. *See* Assistive devices; Assistive equipment; Assistive listening devices; Computers

Technology-Related Assistance to Individuals with Disabilities Act, 401, 424

Telephone assistance programs, 697

Telephone reassurance programs, 699–700

Terminal drop hypothesis, 204

Terminal illness. *See* Hospice programs

Theft, 720–721

Theories of groups. *See* Group models and theories

Therapeutic recreation specialists, inpatient rehabilitation role, 348

Uniform terminology for occupational therapy, 118–119, 123–124, 126, 166–167

The Uniform Terminology for Occupational Therapy, 118, 166–167, **167**, 440–441, 679

United States Code, 863, **863**, 866

Universal design, 263, 269, 402

University of Chicago
gerontology education program, 19
Kansas City Studies of Adult Life, 18

University of Michigan, gerontology education program, 19

University of Washington, Center for Health Promotion in Older Adults, 58

Upward gaze, environmental considerations, 396

U.S. Administration on Aging
community-based practice and, 423–425
establishment of, 18
regional offices, 882
resources, 870

U.S. Bureau of Labor Statistics, occupational therapy projection, 35

U.S. Civil Aeromedical Institute, work performance of older adults, 244

U.S. Code. *See* United States Code

U.S. Congress. *See also* U.S. House of Representatives
community-based practices funding and, 423
federal legislative process, 862–863
keeping current with government programs, 871

U.S. Department of Health and Human Services. *See also* U.S. Administration on Aging
National Medical Expenditure Survey, 418

U.S. Department of Housing and Urban Development, housing complaints, 717

U.S. Department of Labor, work performance of older adults, 244

U.S. Government Printing Office, 862, 864

U.S. Health Care Financing Administration
federal rules and regulations, 866
Long-Term-Care Survey, 418, 419
overcharges for occupational therapy, 158

U.S. House of Representatives. *See also* U.S. Congress
conference on health care professionals caring for elderly patients, 79

U.S. Small Business Administration, support for Service Corps of Retires Executives, 248

U.S. Statutes at Large, **862**, 862–863

Utility assistance programs, 697

VA. *See* Veterans' Administration

Values. *See also* Cultural considerations
health education and, 816

Vascular dementias, 186, 573

Vascular system
arteriosclerosis and, 183
hypertension and, 183–184

Vestibular function testing, 554

Vestibular retraining, 560

Vestibular system changes in older adults, 178. *See also* Assessments
environmental considerations, 398–399

Veterans' Administration
adult day care and, 460, 475
elderly persons and, 149

Vision changes in older adults. *See also* Assessments
assessment considerations, 518, 554–555
cataracts, 173
cornea, 173–174
driving and, 670
environmental considerations, 394–396
exterior structures, 175
isolation and, 266, 283
lens, 172–173
physiological changes, 30
retina, 174–175
sclera, 174
treatment considerations, 560–561
vitreous humor, 174

Visiting Nurses Association, 64

VISTA. *See* Volunteers in Service to America Program

Visual acuity assessments, 518

Visual perception testing, 554–555

Visual perceptual retraining, 560–561

Vital capacity of lungs, 189–190, 637

Volunteer work
ADA reasonable accommodation provisions and, 711
barriers to volunteering, 247